Atherosclerotic and Cardiometabolic Disease: From Molecular Basis to Therapeutic Advances

Atherosclerotic and Cardiometabolic Disease: From Molecular Basis to Therapeutic Advances

Editors

Eva Kassi
Harpal S. Randeva
Ioannis Kyrou

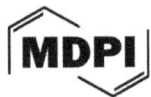

Basel • Beijing • Wuhan • Barcelona • Belgrade • Novi Sad • Cluj • Manchester

Editors
Eva Kassi
Department of Biochemistry
Medical School of Athens
National and Kapodistrian
University of Athens
Athens
Greece

Harpal S. Randeva
Warwick Medical School
University of Warwick
Coventry
United Kingdom

Ioannis Kyrou
Laboratory of Dietetics and
Quality of Life, Department
of Food Science and Human
Nutrition, School of Food and
Nutritional Sciences,
Agricultural University of
Athens
Athens
Greece

Editorial Office
MDPI
St. Alban-Anlage 66
4052 Basel, Switzerland

This is a reprint of articles from the Special Issue published online in the open access journal *International Journal of Molecular Sciences* (ISSN 1422-0067) (available at: www.mdpi.com/journal/ijms/special_issues/atherosclerotic_cardiometabolic).

For citation purposes, cite each article independently as indicated on the article page online and as indicated below:

Lastname, A.A.; Lastname, B.B. Article Title. *Journal Name* **Year**, *Volume Number*, Page Range.

ISBN 978-3-0365-8603-8 (Hbk)
ISBN 978-3-0365-8602-1 (PDF)
doi.org/10.3390/books978-3-0365-8602-1

© 2023 by the authors. Articles in this book are Open Access and distributed under the Creative Commons Attribution (CC BY) license. The book as a whole is distributed by MDPI under the terms and conditions of the Creative Commons Attribution-NonCommercial-NoDerivs (CC BY-NC-ND) license.

Contents

About the Editors . . . . **vii**

Preface . . . . **ix**

Eva Kassi, Ioannis Kyrou and Harpal S. Randeva
Atherosclerotic and Cardio-Metabolic Diseases: From Molecular Basis to Therapeutic Advances
Reprinted from: *Int. J. Mol. Sci.* **2023**, 24, 9737, doi:10.3390/ijms24119737 1

Heyu Meng, Jianjun Ruan, Zhaohan Yan, Yanqiu Chen, Jinsha Liu and Xiangdong Li et al.
New Progress in Early Diagnosis of Atherosclerosis
Reprinted from: *Int. J. Mol. Sci.* **2022**, 23, 8939, doi:10.3390/ijms23168939 7

Michal Kowara and Agnieszka Cudnoch-Jedrzejewska
Different Approaches in Therapy Aiming to Stabilize an Unstable Atherosclerotic Plaque
Reprinted from: *Int. J. Mol. Sci.* **2021**, 22, 4354, doi:10.3390/ijms22094354 21

Narjes Nasiri-Ansari, Eliana Spilioti, Ioannis Kyrou, Vassiliki Kalotychou, Antonios Chatzigeorgiou and Despina Sanoudou et al.
Estrogen Receptor Subtypes Elicit a Distinct Gene Expression Profile of Endothelial-Derived Factors Implicated in Atherosclerotic Plaque Vulnerability
Reprinted from: *Int. J. Mol. Sci.* **2022**, 23, 10960, doi:10.3390/ijms231810960 39

Yin-Chia Chen, Jiunn-Jye Sheu, John Y. Chiang, Pei-Lin Shao, Shun-Cheng Wu and Pei-Hsun Sung et al.
Circulatory Rejuvenated EPCs Derived from PAOD Patients Treated by CD34$^+$ Cells and Hyperbaric Oxygen Therapy Salvaged the Nude Mouse Limb against Critical Ischemia
Reprinted from: *Int. J. Mol. Sci.* **2020**, 21, 7887, doi:10.3390/ijms21217887 62

Stathis Dimitropoulos, Vasiliki Chara Mystakidi, Evangelos Oikonomou, Gerasimos Siasos, Vasiliki Tsigkou and Dimitris Athanasiou et al.
Association of Soluble Suppression of Tumorigenesis-2 (ST2) with Endothelial Function in Patients with Ischemic Heart Failure
Reprinted from: *Int. J. Mol. Sci.* **2020**, 21, 9385, doi:10.3390/ijms21249385 80

Alida Taberner-Cortés, Ángela Vinué, Andrea Herrero-Cervera, María Aguilar-Ballester, José Tomás Real and Deborah Jane Burks et al.
Dapagliflozin Does Not Modulate Atherosclerosis in Mice with Insulin Resistance
Reprinted from: *Int. J. Mol. Sci.* **2020**, 21, 9216, doi:10.3390/ijms21239216 91

Marios Sagris, Emmanouil P. Vardas, Panagiotis Theofilis, Alexios S. Antonopoulos, Evangelos Oikonomou and Dimitris Tousoulis
Atrial Fibrillation: Pathogenesis, Predisposing Factors, and Genetics
Reprinted from: *Int. J. Mol. Sci.* **2021**, 23, 6, doi:10.3390/ijms23010006 109

María Aguilar-Ballester, Gema Hurtado-Genovés, Alida Taberner-Cortés, Andrea Herrero-Cervera, Sergio Martínez-Hervás and Herminia González-Navarro
Therapies for the Treatment of Cardiovascular Disease Associated with Type 2 Diabetes and Dyslipidemia
Reprinted from: *Int. J. Mol. Sci.* **2021**, 22, 660, doi:10.3390/ijms22020660 126

Yoshimi Kishimoto, Kazuo Kondo and Yukihiko Momiyama
The Protective Role of Sestrin2 in Atherosclerotic and Cardiac Diseases
Reprinted from: *Int. J. Mol. Sci.* **2021**, 22, 1200, doi:10.3390/ijms22031200 153

Glória Conceição, Diana Martins, Isabel M. Miranda, Adelino F. Leite-Moreira, Rui Vitorino and Inês Falcão-Pires
Unraveling the Role of Epicardial Adipose Tissue in Coronary Artery Disease: Partners in Crime?
Reprinted from: *Int. J. Mol. Sci.* **2020**, *21*, 8866, doi:10.3390/ijms21228866 . . . . **165**

Gavin H. C. Richards, Kathryn L. Hong, Michael Y. Henein, Colm Hanratty and Usama Boles
Coronary Artery Ectasia: Review of the Non-Atherosclerotic Molecular and Pathophysiologic Concepts
Reprinted from: *Int. J. Mol. Sci.* **2022**, *23*, 5195, doi:10.3390/ijms23095195 . . . . **183**

Christina-Maria Flessa, Narjes Nasiri-Ansari, Ioannis Kyrou, Bianca M. Leca, Maria Lianou and Antonios Chatzigeorgiou et al.
Genetic and Diet-Induced Animal Models for Non-Alcoholic Fatty Liver Disease (NAFLD) Research
Reprinted from: *Int. J. Mol. Sci.* **2022**, *23*, 15791, doi:10.3390/ijms232415791 . . . . **194**

Theodoros Androutsakos, Narjes Nasiri-Ansari, Athanasios-Dimitrios Bakasis, Ioannis Kyrou, Efstathios Efstathopoulos and Harpal S. Randeva et al.
SGLT-2 Inhibitors in NAFLD: Expanding Their Role beyond Diabetes and Cardioprotection
Reprinted from: *Int. J. Mol. Sci.* **2022**, *23*, 3107, doi:10.3390/ijms23063107 . . . . **228**

Narjes Nasiri-Ansari, Chrysa Nikolopoulou, Katerina Papoutsi, Ioannis Kyrou, Christos S. Mantzoros and Georgios Kyriakopoulos et al.
Empagliflozin Attenuates Non-Alcoholic Fatty Liver Disease (NAFLD) in High Fat Diet Fed ApoE$^{(-/-)}$ Mice by Activating Autophagy and Reducing ER Stress and Apoptosis
Reprinted from: *Int. J. Mol. Sci.* **2021**, *22*, 818, doi:10.3390/ijms22020818 . . . . **260**

About the Editors

Eva Kassi

Dr. Eva Kassi graduated with distinction from the Medical School of Aristotle University of Thessaloniki in 1991. She then completed her internal medicine training and residency in endocrinology, diabetes and metabolism in the Department of Endocrinology, Diabetes and Metabolic Diseases at "G.Gennimatas" General Hospital of Athens, and she became a certified endocrinologist (2001). She was a research fellow in the Department of Endocrinology and Metabolic Diseases at the University of Leiden, the Netherlands (2000). She received her PhD in Biochemistry in 2004. Since 2021, she is a Professor of Endocrinology and Biochemistry, Unit of Endocrinology, Diabetes Mellitus and Metabolic Diseases, 1st Department of Propaedeutic and Internal Medicine, LAIKO Hospital, National and Kapodistrian University of Athens, Greece. She is a Representative of LAIKO General Hospital of Athens in the European Reference Network on rare endocrine conditions (Endo-ERN).

She is an author or a co-author of more than 150 peer-reviewed publications published in international scientific journals with 6390 citations, and an h-index of 34. Her current research interests focus on 1) atherosclerosis and atherosclerosis-related diseases, metabolic syndrome, and NAFLD, and 2) rare diseases of calcium and phosphate disorders.

She serves as an Associate Editor for *Hormones-International Journal of Endocrinology* and *Metabolism* and as a member of the Editorial Board for *Molecular and Cellular Endocrinology* and *Journal of Geriatric Cardiology*. She also serves as a regular peer reviewer for more than 35 international journals, including the *Journal of the American College of Cardiology* and *Diabetologia*. She has given more than 100 invited talks in national and international congresses.

Harpal S. Randeva

Prof. Harpal S. Randeva graduated in Medicine from the University of Dundee, and is a clinical academic at Warwick Medical School, University of Warwick, as well as a Consultant in Endocrinology, Diabetes and Metabolism at University Hospital Coventry & Warwickshire (UHCW), NHS Trust. Prof. Randeva is the Head of Endocrinology, Diabetes and Metabolism at the Warwickshire Institute for the Study of Diabetes, Endocrinology and Metabolism (WISDEM) and the Director of R&D at UHCW. Prof. Randeva is also a Fellow of the Academy of Translational Medicine, the Royal College of Physicians, and the Royal Society of Medicine and Association of Physicians of England and Ireland. He has been involved in biomedical research since his medical training years in Oxford and London, with a primary interest in PCOS, diabetes, obesity, NAFLD and other dysmetabolic states. Currently, he is leading a multidisciplinary research team at UHCW and University of Warwick, with significant experiences in clinical trials and translational research. Prof. Randeva has published more than 250 papers in leading peer-reviewed journals (H-index: 75; >18000 citations), and presents regularly as an invited speaker at both national and international scientific meetings.

Ioannis Kyrou

Dr. Ioannis Kyrou has a Medical Diploma (Athens Medical School, Greece), a PhD in Medicine (Warwick Medical School, UK), and a Master of Education (Aston University, UK). Dr. Kyrou is an Ass. Prof. of Metabolic Medicine and Nutrition, and a GMC registered endocrinologist with over 15 years of clinical and translational research experience in the field of cardio-metabolic diseases, endocrinology, nutrition, aging, and public health, having led multiple research studies in these subjects. His current research focuses on obesity/diabetes, metabolism, nutrition, physical activity/exercise, PCOS, NAFLD, and cardiovascular and mental health, with a particular interest in women's health and older populations. To date, his overall research output has resulted in important publications in high-impact, peer-reviewed, biomedical journals (>110 papers in PubMed; >6800 citations; h-index: 41), as well as in numerous announcements in national and international biomedical congresses. In addition, Dr. Kyrou has authored more than 25 chapters in biomedical textbooks. Finally, Dr. Kyrou is also a Fellow of the UK Higher Education Academy (Advance HE) and a member of multiple scientific/medical societies.

Preface

In recent years, important progress has been made in the field of molecular biology concerning atherogenesis. However, there are still gaps in current knowledge regarding its underlying pathogenesis. Moreover, various diseases, such as non-alcoholic fatty liver disease/steatohepatitis, diabetes mellitus, arterial hypertension, dyslipidemia, and metabolic syndrome, are tightly connected with atherosclerosis, sharing, at least in part, common molecular pathogenetic mechanisms.

Although cardiovascular diseases (CVDs) still remain the leading cause of death globally, lifestyle modification interventions, as well as pharmacological therapies (e.g., anti-hypertensive, lipid-lowering drugs) and advances in cardiovascular surgery, have led to a reduction in CVD mortality.

This reprint of a Special Issue aims to provide new data and discuss recent advances in the field of atherosclerosis and atherosclerosis-related diseases. An improved understanding of the common pathophysiological processes that result in cardio-metabolic diseases will help in the identification of effective prevention strategies and the development of innovative therapeutic targets which can be introduced in routine clinical practice. This reprint can meet the interests of professionals across a wide range of specialties, including endocrinologists, cardiologists, gastroenterologists, molecular biologists, and basic clinical and translational researchers with a particular focus on the field of cardiovascular endocrinology.

Professor Eva Kassi, Professor Harpal S. Randeva, and Ass. Professor Ioannis Kyrou edit this Special Issue and acknowledge all authors for the contributed articles.

Eva Kassi, Harpal S. Randeva, and Ioannis Kyrou
Editors

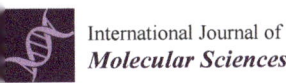

Editorial

Atherosclerotic and Cardio-Metabolic Diseases: From Molecular Basis to Therapeutic Advances

Eva Kassi [1,2,*], Ioannis Kyrou [3,4,5,6,7] and Harpal S. Randeva [3,4,*]

1. Department of Biological Chemistry, Medical School, National and Kapodistrian University of Athens, 11527 Athens, Greece
2. Endocrine Unit, 1ST Department of Propaedeutic Internal Medicine, Laiko Hospital, National and Kapodistrian University of Athens, 11527 Athens, Greece
3. Warwick Medical School, University of Warwick, Coventry CV4 7AL, UK; kyrouj@gmail.com
4. Warwickshire Institute for the Study of Diabetes, Endocrinology and Metabolism (WISDEM), University Hospitals Coventry and Warwickshire NHS Trust, Coventry CV2 2DX, UK
5. Research Institute for Health & Wellbeing, Coventry University, Coventry CV1 5FB, UK
6. Aston Medical School, College of Health and Life Sciences, Aston University, Birmingham B4 7ET, UK
7. Laboratory of Dietetics and Quality of Life, Department of Food Science and Human Nutrition, School of Food and Nutritional Sciences, Agricultural University of Athens, 11855 Athens, Greece
* Correspondence: ekassi@med.uoa.gr (E.K.); harpal.randeva@uhcw.nhs.uk (H.S.R.)

Cardiovascular diseases (CVDs) still remain the major cause of death worldwide; however, CVD-related mortality has been reduced due to lifestyle modification interventions, as well as novel pharmacological therapies and advances in cardiovascular surgery. Notably, a spectrum of diseases which are closely connected with atherosclerosis, such as non-alcoholic fatty liver disease (NAFLD), dyslipidaemia, arterial hypertension, and metabolic syndrome, appear to share common molecular pathogenetic mechanisms. In the present Special Issue, we focus on this spectrum of atherosclerosis-related cardio-metabolic diseases, aiming to offer a better understanding of their common molecular backgrounds, which can further help in designing prognostic/diagnostic tools and developing novel therapeutic tools.

In their review, Meng et al. describe and discuss the latest methods in the early diagnosis of coronary atherosclerosis via imaging, the evaluation of gene and protein markers, and trace elements [1]. Among imaging techniques, computed tomography coronary angiography (CCTA) can replace invasive coronary angiography (ICA) in individuals with suspected acute coronary syndrome (ACS) who have a low or medium pre-test risk of coronary artery disease (CAD). Furthermore, multiple studies have reported numerous miRNAs that are expressed in ACS and stable CAD, with miR-1, miR-133, miR-208a, and miR-499 considered to be ACS biomarkers. However, the authors noted that the use of such miRNAs in clinical practice needs additional work to address any current methodological, technical, or analytical shortcomings.

In the review by Kowara and Cudnoch-Jedrzejewska, different approaches directed at the specific molecular pathways involved in atherosclerotic plaque vulnerability and destabilisation are presented [2]. Metabolic approaches target lowering LDL particles and increasing HDL, whilst cell survival approaches aim at promoting cell survival mechanisms, such as efferocytosis and autophagy in VSMC and macrophages, as well as the M2 anti-inflammatory phenotype polarisation of macrophages. Furthermore, anti-inflammatory approaches focus on a reduction in T cell infiltration and migration as well as cytotoxic T cell activity, while antioxidant approaches are directed towards the neutralisation of reactive oxygen species. Finally, targeting intra-plaque neovascularisation via the inhibition of VEGF receptors and extracellular matrix (ECM) fragmentation is considered to be plaque-stabilising. As the authors discuss, microRNAs emerge as a potential therapeutic option, as they can control all stages of atherosclerotic plaque progression via regulating

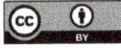

the corresponding mRNAs. Thus, applying agomirs of stabilising miRNAs or antagomirs of destabilising miRNAs could be promising in the prevention of plaque vulnerability.

Interestingly, according to the "timing hypothesis", HRT appears to be safe and even protective in younger postmenopausal women who are asymptomatic for CVD and within 10 years of menopause onset [3]. This means that, once atherosclerotic plaque has been formed, oestrogen may be potentially harmful. The favourable effects of oestrogen in the early stages of the atheromatosis process (endothelium activation/dysregulation) have been widely investigated; however, data on the role of oestrogen in the factors involved in the later stages of the atherogenesis process which lead to plaque vulnerability/rupture are insufficient.

Nasiri-Ansari et al. aimed to investigate the effects of oestradiol (E_2) on the expression of the molecules implicated in atherosclerotic plaque vulnerability, resembling a low-grade inflammatory state that occurs in atherosclerosis, using an established endothelial in vitro system [4]. They also tried to clarify whether these effects are mediated by ERα, ERβ, or GPR-30 receptors. Their research findings showed that in the absence of low-grade inflammation, an overexpression of ERα can initiate the atherosclerosis process via increasing the expression of MCP-1 and MMP-2 activity. Moreover, under low-grade inflammation, E_2 can promote the destabilisation of atherosclerotic plaque via increasing the expression of MCP-1 and MMP-9, as well as the activity of MMP-2 in human arterial endothelial cells (HAECs), an effect mediated via GPR-30. Accordingly, the authors conclude that the balance of the expression of the various ER subtypes may play an important role in the paradoxical characterisation of oestrogen as being both beneficial and harmful, since E_2 induces different effects in either the early stages of atheromatosis or atheromatous plaque instability via different ERs. Further studies will identify the exact role of each ER subtype in the atherosclerosis inflammatory process, which could potentially lead to the development of specific ER agonists/antagonists with an improved benefit/risk ratio.

Research on novel heart failure (HF) biomarkers is currently being strongly promoted, particularly using a multi-marker rather than a single-biomarker approach. Among such biomarkers is the soluble suppression of tumorigenesis-2 (sST2), which acts as a decoy receptor for IL-33. Indeed, sST2 has been shown to be associated with endothelial dysfunction, acute decompensated heart failure, myocardial fibrosis, and adverse remodelling.

Dimitropoulos et al., in their research article, examined the association between arterial wall properties and sST2 levels in patients with HF of ischemic aetiology [5]. Their findings show that sST2 levels were associated with the HF status and functional capacity of the patients as assessed using the NYHA classification, although the levels of sST2 were not associated with left ventricular ejection fraction (LVEF). No association between sST2 and pulse wave velocity (PWV, a marker of arterial stiffness) was found; however, an inverse association between sST2 levels and FMD was observed, underscoring the interplay between endothelial dysfunction and HF pathophysiologic mechanisms. Although the authors note that a conclusion about a causal connection between sST2 and endothelial dysfunction in patients with HF of ischemic aetiology cannot be supported by this study, their findings add additional information on endothelial dysfunction occurring in those with decompensated heart failure underlined by myocardial remodelling/fibrosis. Further studies are needed before suggesting sST2 with prognostic significance in clinical practice.

Chen et al. investigated whether treatment with endothelial progenitor cells (EPCs) derived from patients with peripheral arterial occlusive disease (PAOD) would protect limbs against critical limb ischemia (CLI) in adult male nude mice [6]. Notably, they found that only rejuvenated EPCs (the EPCs received combined $CD34^+$ cell and hyperbaric oxygen treatment) could restore blood flow and salvage CLI in this mouse model. Although the underlying mechanisms may differ between mice and humans and the exact mechanistic basis of xenogeneic EPC therapy still needs to be fully elucidated, the rejuvenated EPC therapy may serve as an innovative therapy for CLI/severe PAOD patients.

SGLT2 inhibitors (SGLT2is) have been approved for use as anti-diabetic medication due to their favourable effects on reducing hyperglycaemia and metabolism via increasing glucosuria and natriuresis. Additional effects of SGLT2is have been recognised, such as weight loss due to urinary loss of calories, improved renal function and blood pressure, and direct actions in the myocardium. Moreover, SGLT2i treatment has been shown to improve insulin β cell function and insulin sensitivity in patients with type 2 diabetes mellitus (T2DM). In the research article by Taberner-Cortés et al., the possible benefit of dapagliflozin (a selective SGLT2i) in atherosclerosis was investigated using an $ApoE^{-/-}Irs2^{+/-}$ mouse model. Under atherogenic dietary conditions, it exhibited insulin resistance and accelerated atherosclerosis, but not hypertension or hyperglycaemia [7]. According to their results, dapagliflozin reduced glucose-stimulated insulin secretion from islets and insulin-signalling in adipose tissue, without altering glucose levels. Moreover, in contrast with other studies showing that SGLT2is can attenuate the atherosclerosis process, the authors found that treatment with dapagliflozin did not affect the atherosclerosis lesion size and plaque stability, nor the circulating inflammatory markers [8,9]. Further research will elucidate whether or not the beneficial effects of SGLT2is on the atherosclerosis process are exerted only in the presence of insulin resistance and hypercholesterolemic conditions.

A comprehensive review by Sagris et al. summarised the existing data on the predisposing factors of atrial fibrillation (AF), including dietary habits, sedentary lifestyle, and potential genetic factors which regulate pathogenic mechanisms, such as fibrosis, oxidative stress, and inflammatory processes [10]. The latter includes mutations/polymorphisms in potassium and sodium channel genes, as well as mutations in the gap junctional protein. The authors emphasised that lifestyle modifications including alcohol reduction and Mediterranean diet combined with extra virgin olive oil, weight loss, and cardio-metabolic risk factor management are fundamental in AF prevention. Moreover, medications, such as anti-inflammatory agents, angiotensin-converting enzyme inhibitors, angiotensin receptor blockers, aldosterone antagonists, and the novel SGLT2i, have revealed beneficial effects on AF inducibility.

Aguilar-Ballester et al., in their review, present and discuss new pharmacological treatments which, in addition to their anti-diabetic and lipid-lowering effects, appear to also have direct beneficial effects on CVD [11]. As such, incretin-based therapies, SGLT2is, and proprotein convertase subtilisin kexin 9 inactivating therapies (PCSK9is) can act directly on the cells implicated in the atherosclerosis process (endothelial, VMCs, immune cells), as well as on cardiomyocytes. Within this work, the authors summarised experimental studies and randomised control trials (RCTs) which provide strong evidence for the potential effects of these new treatments on the cardiovascular system, beyond metabolic control.

Sestrin2 is an antioxidant protein that was originally identified as hypoxia-induced gene 95 (Hi95). It is expressed and secreted mainly by macrophages, T lymphocytes, endothelial cells, cardiac fibroblasts, and cardiomyocytes [12]. Kishimoto et al. analysed the protective role of sestrin2 against the progression of atherosclerotic and cardiac diseases [13]. From a pathophysiological point of view, sestrin2 appears to be upregulated as a response to stress stimuli (i.e., oxidative, ER, and genotoxic stress) and activates two signalling pathways—Kelch-like ECH-associated protein 1 (Keap1)/Nrf2 and AMPK/mTORC1— which leads to decreased ROS accumulation, apoptosis and inflammation, and increased autophagy. Clinical studies have shown that the plasma levels of sestrin2 were positively correlated with the severity of both CAD and carotid atherosclerosis, possibly reflecting a compensatory response to increased oxidative stress. However, further studies are needed to elucidate the exact role of sestrin2 and its potential therapeutic use in atherosclerotic diseases.

A growing body of evidence suggests that adipose tissue anatomic specificity is pivotal to the pathophysiology of various cardio-metabolic diseases [14]. Specifically, epicardial adipose tissue (EAT) has emerged as a very interesting fat depot, which surrounds the coronary arteries and appears to have specific metabolic properties. Of note, several studies have identified EAT as being an independent predictor of CAD. The review by Conceição et al. published in this Special Issue provides an overview of the potential effects of dysfunctional EAT on CAD pathophysiology [15]. Using integrative bioinformatics analysis, they identified 46 up- or downregulated proteins which are mainly implicated in inflammatory processes to modulate the local environment and the formation and progression of coronary atherogenesis. Future studies will assess whether targeting the paracrine and endocrine communication between EAT and coronary arteries (e.g., via molecules with anti-inflammatory properties) could be considered as a promising therapeutic approach for those with CAD.

Coronary artery ectasia (CAE) is a relatively common coronary angiographic finding which is associated with atherosclerosis in 50% of cases [16]. In their review article, Richards et al. presented the proposed mechanisms underlying vascular remodelling in the pathogenesis of CAE [17]. Although CAE and CAD share common pathogenetic pathways, such as oxidative stress, vascular endothelial dysfunction, lipid dysregulation, and altered extracellular matrix regulation, there are significant differences in the cytokine milieu and metabolite profile in CAE compared to CAD, which strongly implies that there is a distinct pathogenesis of CAE that potentially requires a different therapeutic approach.

NAFLD refers to a spectrum ranging from benign liver steatosis to non-alcoholic steatohepatitis (NASH), liver fibrosis, and eventually cirrhosis and hepatocellular carcinoma. Over recent decades, NAFLD has evolved as a major health problem. Notably, considering its underlying pathogenesis, which involves mechanisms such as ER stress, apoptosis, and autophagy, as well as the spectrum of NAFLD-associated cardio-metabolic disorders, the term metabolic (dysfunction)-associated fatty liver disease (MAFLD) has been proposed [18–20].

Flessa et al. presented the most common mouse models used in NAFLD research [21]. Notably, several such models are being used, involving dietary interventions (e.g., the MCD, AMLN, GAN, and fast-food-like diets), genetic manipulations (e.g., *Prostaglandin E2*-deficient mice and the APOE2ki, *ApoE$^{-/-}$*, *Krt18$^{-/-}$*, *Mat1a$^{-/-}$*, and NEMO^{LPC-KO} mice), the administration of chemical substances (e.g., carbon tetrachloride, CCl$_4$; streptozotocin), and/or a combination of these to replicate either the entire NAFLD spectrum or a particular disease stage (e.g., NASH). Given that there is no ideal animal model for the NAFLD spectrum yet, the specific research hypothesis/objectives of each study will drive the selection of the most suitable model in order to investigate the NAFLD-related pathophysiologic mechanisms and/or treatments.

SGLT2is have been investigated as a potential treatment for NAFLD. The exact molecular mechanisms mediating these effects have not been fully elucidated. In their narrative review, Androutsakos et al. provided an overview of the current evidence on the mechanisms underlying the pathogenesis of NAFLD and the potential impact of SGLT2is on NAFLD development and progression, summarising data from in vitro, animal, and human studies [22]. Relevant data indicate that a reduction in hyperglycaemia, improvement in systematic insulin resistance, increased caloric loss, and decreased body weight mostly due to glycosuria contribute to the alleviation of NAFLD. Apart from this, SGLT2is exert a hepato-protective effect by decreasing hepatic inflammation and hepatic de novo lipogenesis and increasing hepatic beta-oxidation. An augmented number of clinical studies have highlighted the favourable effects of SGLT2is on NAFLD in patients with T2DM, estimated using non-invasive biomarkers, imaging techniques, or even liver biopsy, while data on non-diabetic patients remain limited. Interestingly, the authors noted that different effects between members of the SGLT2i class have been observed, suggesting that there are features specific to these individual drugs regarding the underlying mechanism(s) of action and their corresponding effects on NAFLD. Future mechanistic studies would expand our understanding of the specific mechanisms underlying the pathogenesis of NAFLD and the potential favourable actions of SGLT2is for NAFLD treatment.

Nasiri-Ansari et al., in their research article published in this Special Issue, investigated the impact of empagliflozin (a selective SGLT2i) in NAFLD using high fat diet (HFD)-fed ApoE$^{(-/-)}$ mice [23]. Empagliflozin led to reduced fasting glucose, as expected, but also decreased the NAFLD activity score. The latter was accompanied by a decreased expression of lipogenic enzymes (*Fasn*, *Screbp-1c*, and *Pck-1*) and inflammatory molecules (*Mcp-1* and *F4/80*). Focusing on the underlying mechanisms, the authors demonstrated for the first time that empagliflozin treatment for five weeks attenuates NAFLD progression in ApoE$^{(-/-)}$ mice by promoting autophagy, reducing ER stress, and inhibiting hepatic apoptosis. The authors point out that further research is required in order to delineate the possible dose- and duration-dependent differential effects of empagliflozin on NAFLD development and progression.

The original articles and reviews published in this Special Issue aim to provide new data and discuss the recent advances in the field of atherosclerosis and atherosclerosis-related diseases. An improved understanding of the common pathophysiological processes that result in cardio-metabolic diseases will help in the identification of effective prevention strategies and the development of innovative therapeutic targets which can be introduced in routine clinical practice.

Author Contributions: Conceptualisation, E.K. and I.K.; writing—original draft preparation, E.K.; writing—review and editing, E.K., I.K. and H.S.R. All authors have read and agreed to the published version of the manuscript.

Conflicts of Interest: The authors declare no conflict of interest.

References

1. Meng, H.; Ruan, J.; Yan, Z.; Chen, Y.; Liu, J.; Li, X.; Meng, F. New Progress in Early Diagnosis of Atherosclerosis. *Int. J. Mol. Sci.* **2022**, *23*, 8939. [CrossRef]
2. Kowara, M.; Cudnoch-Jedrzejewska, A. Different Approaches in Therapy Aiming to Stabilize an Unstable Atherosclerotic Plaque. *Int. J. Mol. Sci.* **2021**, *22*, 4354. [CrossRef] [PubMed]
3. Kassi, E.; Spilioti, E.; Nasiri-Ansari, N.; Adamopoulos, C.; Moutsatsou, P.; Papapanagiotou, A.; Siasos, G.; Tousoulis, D.; Papavassiliou, A.G. Vascular Inflammation and Atherosclerosis: The Role of Estrogen Receptors. *Curr. Med. Chem.* **2015**, *22*, 2651–2665. [CrossRef]
4. Nasiri-Ansari, N.; Spilioti, E.; Kyrou, I.; Kalotychou, V.; Chatzigeorgiou, A.; Sanoudou, D.; Dahlman-Wright, K.; Randeva, H.S.; Papavassiliou, A.G.; Moutsatsou, P.; et al. Estrogen Receptor Subtypes Elicit a Distinct Gene Expression Profile of Endothelial-Derived Factors Implicated in Atherosclerotic Plaque Vulnerability. *Int. J. Mol. Sci.* **2022**, *23*, 960. [CrossRef] [PubMed]
5. Dimitropoulos, S.; Mystakidi, V.C.; Oikonomou, E.; Siasos, G.; Tsigkou, V.; Athanasiou, D.; Gouliopoulos, N.; Bletsa, E.; Kalampogias, A.; Charalambous, G.; et al. Association of Soluble Suppression of Tumorigenesis-2 (ST2) with Endothelial Function in Patients with Ischemic Heart Failure. *Int. J. Mol. Sci.* **2020**, *21*, 9385. [CrossRef] [PubMed]
6. Chen, Y.C.; Sheu, J.J.; Chiang, J.Y.; Shao, P.L.; Wu, S.C.; Sung, P.H.; Li, Y.C.; Chen, Y.L.; Huang, T.H.; Chen, K.H.; et al. Circulatory Rejuvenated EPCs Derived from PAOD Patients Treated by CD34(+) Cells and Hyperbaric Oxygen Therapy Salvaged the Nude Mouse Limb against Critical Ischemia. *Int. J. Mol. Sci.* **2020**, *21*, 7887. [CrossRef]
7. Taberner-Cortes, A.; Vinue, A.; Herrero-Cervera, A.; Aguilar-Ballester, M.; Real, J.T.; Burks, D.J.; Martinez-Hervas, S.; Gonzalez-Navarro, H. Dapagliflozin Does Not Modulate Atherosclerosis in Mice with Insulin Resistance. *Int. J. Mol. Sci.* **2020**, *21*, 9216. [CrossRef]
8. Dimitriadis, G.K.; Nasiri-Ansari, N.; Agrogiannis, G.; Kostakis, I.D.; Randeva, M.S.; Nikiteas, N.; Patel, V.H.; Kaltsas, G.; Papavassiliou, A.G.; Randeva, H.S.; et al. Empagliflozin improves primary haemodynamic parameters and attenuates the development of atherosclerosis in high fat diet fed APOE knockout mice. *Mol. Cell. Endocrinol.* **2019**, *494*, 110487. [CrossRef]
9. Nasiri-Ansari, N.; Dimitriadis, G.K.; Agrogiannis, G.; Perrea, D.; Kostakis, I.D.; Kaltsas, G.; Papavassiliou, A.G.; Randeva, H.S.; Kassi, E. Canagliflozin attenuates the progression of atherosclerosis and inflammation process in APOE knockout mice. *Cardiovasc. Diabetol.* **2018**, *17*, 106. [CrossRef]
10. Sagris, M.; Vardas, E.P.; Theofilis, P.; Antonopoulos, A.S.; Oikonomou, E.; Tousoulis, D. Atrial Fibrillation: Pathogenesis, Predisposing Factors, and Genetics. *Int. J. Mol. Sci.* **2021**, *23*, 6. [CrossRef]
11. Aguilar-Ballester, M.; Hurtado-Genoves, G.; Taberner-Cortes, A.; Herrero-Cervera, A.; Martinez-Hervas, S.; Gonzalez-Navarro, H. Therapies for the Treatment of Cardiovascular Disease Associated with Type 2 Diabetes and Dyslipidemia. *Int. J. Mol. Sci.* **2021**, *22*, 660. [CrossRef] [PubMed]
12. Sun, W.; Wang, Y.; Zheng, Y.; Quan, N. The Emerging Role of Sestrin2 in Cell Metabolism, and Cardiovascular and Age-Related Diseases. *Aging Dis.* **2020**, *11*, 154–163. [CrossRef]
13. Kishimoto, Y.; Kondo, K.; Momiyama, Y. The Protective Role of Sestrin2 in Atherosclerotic and Cardiac Diseases. *Int. J. Mol. Sci.* **2021**, *22*, 1200. [CrossRef] [PubMed]
14. Matloch, Z.; Cinkajzlova, A.; Mraz, M.; Haluzik, M. The Role of Inflammation in Epicardial Adipose Tissue in Heart Diseases. *Curr. Pharm. Des.* **2018**, *24*, 297–309. [CrossRef]
15. Conceicao, G.; Martins, D.; Miranda, M.I.; Leite-Moreira, A.F.; Vitorino, R.; Falcao-Pires, I. Unraveling the Role of Epicardial Adipose Tissue in Coronary Artery Disease: Partners in Crime? *Int. J. Mol. Sci.* **2020**, *21*, 8866. [CrossRef] [PubMed]

16. Eitan, A.; Roguin, A. Coronary artery ectasia: New insights into pathophysiology, diagnosis, and treatment. *Coron. Artery Dis.* **2016**, *27*, 420–428. [CrossRef]
17. Richards, G.H.C.; Hong, K.L.; Henein, M.Y.; Hanratty, C.; Boles, U. Coronary Artery Ectasia: Review of the Non-Atherosclerotic Molecular and Pathophysiologic Concepts. *Int. J. Mol. Sci.* **2022**, *23*, 5195. [CrossRef]
18. Nasiri-Ansari, N.; Androutsakos, T.; Flessa, C.M.; Kyrou, I.; Siasos, G.; Randeva, H.S.; Kassi, E.; Papavassiliou, A.G. Endothelial Cell Dysfunction and Nonalcoholic Fatty Liver Disease (NAFLD): A Concise Review. *Cells* **2022**, *11*, 2511. [CrossRef]
19. Flessa, C.M.; Kyrou, I.; Nasiri-Ansari, N.; Kaltsas, G.; Kassi, E.; Randeva, H.S. Endoplasmic reticulum stress in nonalcoholic (metabolic associated) fatty liver disease (NAFLD/MAFLD). *J. Cell Biochem.* **2022**, *123*, 1585–1606. [CrossRef]
20. Flessa, C.M.; Kyrou, I.; Nasiri-Ansari, N.; Kaltsas, G.; Papavassiliou, A.G.; Kassi, E.; Randeva, H.S. Endoplasmic Reticulum Stress and Autophagy in the Pathogenesis of Non-alcoholic Fatty Liver Disease (NAFLD): Current Evidence and Perspectives. *Curr. Obes. Rep.* **2021**, *10*, 134–161. [CrossRef]
21. Flessa, C.M.; Nasiri-Ansari, N.; Kyrou, I.; Leca, B.M.; Lianou, M.; Chatzigeorgiou, A.; Kaltsas, G.; Kassi, E.; Randeva, H.S. Genetic and Diet-Induced Animal Models for Non-Alcoholic Fatty Liver Disease (NAFLD) Research. *Int. J. Mol. Sci.* **2022**, *23*, 15791. [CrossRef] [PubMed]
22. Androutsakos, T.; Nasiri-Ansari, N.; Bakasis, A.D.; Kyrou, I.; Efstathopoulos, E.; Randeva, H.S.; Kassi, E. SGLT-2 Inhibitors in NAFLD: Expanding Their Role beyond Diabetes and Cardioprotection. *Int. J. Mol. Sci.* **2022**, *23*, 3107. [CrossRef] [PubMed]
23. Nasiri-Ansari, N.; Nikolopoulou, C.; Papoutsi, K.; Kyrou, I.; Mantzoros, C.S.; Kyriakopoulos, G.; Chatzigeorgiou, A.; Kalotychou, V.; Randeva, M.S.; Chatha, K.; et al. Empagliflozin Attenuates Non-Alcoholic Fatty Liver Disease (NAFLD) in High Fat Diet Fed ApoE((−/−)) Mice by Activating Autophagy and Reducing ER Stress and Apoptosis. *Int. J. Mol. Sci.* **2021**, *22*, 818. [CrossRef] [PubMed]

Disclaimer/Publisher's Note: The statements, opinions and data contained in all publications are solely those of the individual author(s) and contributor(s) and not of MDPI and/or the editor(s). MDPI and/or the editor(s) disclaim responsibility for any injury to people or property resulting from any ideas, methods, instructions or products referred to in the content.

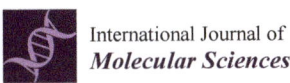

Review

New Progress in Early Diagnosis of Atherosclerosis

Heyu Meng [1,2,3,†], Jianjun Ruan [1,2,3,†], Zhaohan Yan [1,2,3], Yanqiu Chen [1,2,3], Jinsha Liu [1,2,3], Xiangdong Li [1,2,3] and Fanbo Meng [1,2,3,*]

1. Jilin Provincial Precision Medicine Key Laboratory for Cardiovascular Genetic Diagnosis, Jilin Provincial Cardiovascular Research Institute, Jilin University, Changchun 130033, China
2. Jilin Provincial Engineering Laboratory for Endothelial Function and Genetic Diagnosis of Cardiovascular Disease, Jilin Provincial Cardiovascular Research Institute, Jilin University, Changchun 130033, China
3. Jilin Provincial Molecular Biology Research Center for Precision Medicine of Major Cardiovascular Disease, Jilin Provincial Cardiovascular Research Institute, Jilin University, Changchun 130033, China
* Correspondence: mengfb@jlu.edu.cn; Tel.: +86-15948346855
† These authors contributed equally to this work.

Abstract: Coronary atherosclerosis is a potentially chronic circulatory condition that endangers human health. The biological cause underpinning cardiovascular disease is coronary atherosclerosis, and acute cardiovascular events can develop due to thrombosis, platelet aggregation, and unstable atherosclerotic plaque rupture. Coronary atherosclerosis is progressive, and three specific changes appear, with fat spots and stripes, atherosclerosis and thin-walled fiber atherosclerosis, and then complex changes in arteries. The progression and severity of cardiovascular disease are correlated with various levels of calcium accumulation in the coronary artery. The therapy and diagnosis of coronary atherosclerosis benefit from the initial assessment of the size and degree of calcification. This article will discuss the new progress in the early diagnosis of coronary atherosclerosis in terms of three aspects: imaging, gene and protein markers, and trace elements. This study intends to present the latest methods for diagnosing patients with early atherosclerosis through a literature review.

Keywords: coronary atherosclerosis; computed tomography coronary angiography; genes; protein; trace element

1. Introduction

Coronary atherosclerosis is a life-threatening chronic cardiovascular condition. Coronary atherosclerosis is one of the leading causes of death among the aged. The localized deposition of fat in the arteries, along with the development of smooth muscle cells and a fibrous matrix, is the primary issue with atherosclerosis. Over time, this encourages the formation of atherosclerotic plaques [1]. The biological root of cardiovascular disease is atherosclerosis, and thrombosis, platelet aggregation, and unstable atherosclerotic plaque rupture will result in arterial stenosis or occlusion, resulting in acute cardiovascular illness [2,3]. Because inflammation plays a major part in all stages of coronary atherosclerosis's progression, it is commonly regarded as a chronic inflammatory disease. Inflammation is the common cause of the physiological and pathological alterations that occur throughout the onset and progression of coronary atherosclerosis. Years of extensive research have revealed that coronary atherosclerosis has a complicated etiology, with lipid buildup and chronic inflammation in the artery wall being the crucial attributes [4].

Typically, atherosclerosis of the coronary arteries is linked with alterations in lipid metabolism and hypercholesterolemia [5]. Increased low-density lipoprotein (LDL) levels are known cardiovascular disease risk factors [6]. However, the pathophysiology of the disease appears to be more complex than alterations in lipid metabolism, involving numerous variables, with inflammation being the most significant [7]. Local endothelial dysfunction, which may be induced by blood flow instability near an artery's bend or bifurcation, is the pathological cause of the development of atherosclerosis. The activation of vascular endothelial cells in response to mechanical stress results in the recruitment of circulating immune cells. An atherosclerotic plaque is developed by circulating monocytes adhering to and infiltrating into the affected area of the artery wall, differentiating into macrophages, aggressively taking up lipids through phagocytosis, and producing a significant number of foam cells [8].

Fat spots and stripes, atherosclerosis, thin-walled fiber atherosclerosis, and eventually complicated arteries are the three types of particular changes that develop in sequence as atherosclerosis progresses [9,10]. According to the disease's course, the American College of Cardiology divides them into six groups [11,12]. The Type I and Type II early phases can be identified by lipid patches. Yellow patches and a few foam cell accumulations can be seen in the artery's intima. Lipid droplets and smooth muscle cells that T lymphocytes have penetrated are present in the intima. Preplaque, or Type III, is characterized by more extracellular lipid droplets generating lipid nuclei between the layers of smooth muscle cells in the intima and mesomembrane without forming a lipid pool. The stage of atherosclerotic plaque production is Type IV. Since the lipids are more concentrated, the lipid pool has already formed. The artery wall is distorted, and the intimal structure is obliterated. The development of thin-walled fibro-atheroma is a hallmark of Type V. It is the lesion of atherosclerosis that is most recognizable. Lumen stenosis develops when white plaque enters the artery lumen. A proliferative fibrous cap encircles the lipid pool, and the intima of the plaque surface is obliterated. Type VI is referred to as a complicated atherosclerotic lesion, which is a serious lesion. It is distinguished by bleeding, necrosis, ulceration, calcification, and fibrous plaque wall thrombosis.

Calcification is a key cause of coronary atherosclerosis [13] and a good marker to forecast future heart problems. Heart disease worsens and spreads at different rates depending on how much calcium builds up in the body [14]. Coronary atherosclerosis is treated and has a favorable prognosis when the amount and extent of calcification are determined early [15]. The purpose of the present study is to discuss the new progress in the early diagnosis of coronary atherosclerosis in terms of three aspects: imaging, gene and protein markers, and trace elements (see Figure 1 for details).

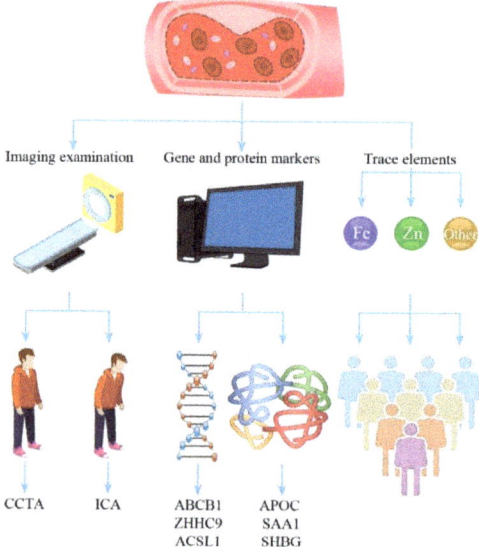

Figure 1. Flow chart of the three examination modes of coronary atherosclerosis. From left to right are imaging examination, gene and protein marker examination, and trace element examination.

2. Imaging Examination

High-spatial-temporal-resolution invasive coronary angiography (ICA) is the gold standard for examining coronary lumens [16–18]. Over the last three decades, computed tomography coronary angiography (CCTA) has evolved into an effective and inexpensive imaging tool for assessing coronary artery disease (CAD). Because normal CTCA images have a strong negative predictive value, they can effectively eliminate substantial CAD, minimizing the requirements for additional imaging tests and lowering ICA use in patients with low and intermediate CAD risk [19–22]. Because of its cost-effectiveness and clinical efficacy, the National Institutes of Health guidelines in 2016 advised that CCTA be used as a first-line survey in all suspected stable CAD patients [23]. The Society of Cardiovascular Computed Tomography's steering committee developed acceptable standards for using CCTA to guide doctors [24].

CCTA is widely used to identify (a) patients with indicative coronary heart disease who have a low or moderate pre-test probability of coronary heart disease and (b) patients with a low or moderate pre-test probability of coronary heart disease who have newly diagnosed heart failure and no known ischemic heart disease, as well as (c) in the evaluation of cardiac health before surgery in patients thought to have a low or moderate risk of coronary heart disease. The risk factors for atherosclerosis include smoking, older age, diabetes, high cholesterol, and hypertension. As mentioned earlier, these are the fundamental elements, and a person with these risk factors will undoubtedly have a higher probability of developing coronary heart disease. These risks serve as the foundation to determine which patients should undergo CCTA when determining whether their risks are high or low. Several studies have demonstrated that CCTA provides patients with suspected or established CAD with good prognostic and therapeutic potential. With a sensitivity of 0.90 and a specificity of 0.92, CCTA revealed high diagnostic accuracy for coronary plaques compared to intravascular ultrasound (IVUS) as a reference standard, per a meta-analysis [25].

CCTA can substitute ICA in individuals with suspected acute coronary syndrome (ACS) who have a low or medium pre-test risk of CAD. When analyzing over 3000 low-risk patients with suspected ACS, four randomized controlled trials compared CCTA to the standard of therapy [26–29]. These trials confirmed what was already known about the negative predictive value of CCTA. They showed again and again that it is safe to send CCTA-negative patients home from the emergency room with a very low rate of major cardiovascular adverse events (MACE) (<1%). This reduces the time required to leave the hospital and the length of stay, saving money and allowing processes to run more smoothly. However, for patients likely to have CAD before the test, ICA should be the first imaging test because CCTA has a low negative predictive value in this group [30].

Using conventional retrospective cardiac gating approaches, the cumulative mean radiation dosage, and CCTA in adult patients varied from 6 to 20 mSv in the past (equivalent to 300–1000 chest radiographs). Incorporating prospective cardiac gating into CCTA can minimize radiation exposure by around 70% [31]. With the introduction of new generations of CT scanners, the radiation dose, contrast dose, and patient turnover time of CCTA have all lowered dramatically, while image quality has also increased. The number of layers on the multi-slice spiral CT (MSCT) scanner has been increased from 64 to 128, 256, 320, and 640. This allows for the precise measurement of the degree of coronary artery stenosis and the composition of the coronary atherosclerotic plaque. The CT coronary artery calcium score and CCTA radiation dose can now be reduced further (equal to <50 chest radiographs), and sub-millimeter accuracy can be reached with the latest 640-slice CT scanner or third-generation DSCT scanner [32].

Additionally, the contrast load can be decreased from an average of 80 mL to 35 mL by using these faster scanners, lowering the risk of contrast nephropathy [33,34]. Further technological advances have resulted in faster CT scanners, ranging from 640-layer dynamic-volume CT scanners to spectral CT and third-generation DSCT. The X-ray tube is the primary focus of DSCT advancement. The transition from static to rotating X-ray tubes, with improvements in its properties, such as a larger heat capacity and cooling speed, enhances the CT scanner's efficiency and allows for a higher rack speed [35]. Using a DSCT scanner with two X-ray tubes increases the efficiency of obtaining entire data sets. Each X-ray tube must be rotated 90°, reducing the picture radiation exposure and acquisition time. The third-generation DSCT scanner can greatly boost the tube power at low potential, significantly lowering radiation exposure [35].

Accurate cross-sectional vascular information can be obtained using intravascular ultrasonography (IVUS) imaging. According to the most recent research, clinicians may accurately assess pathophysiological changes in blood vessels, illness development, and the impact of therapeutic interventions using IVUS data collected at two different times [36]. As an early indicator of arterial injury, the endothelium with osmotic dysfunction is thought to be the main factor in atherosclerosis. Tools and other methods based on magnetic resonance imaging (MRI) enable us to understand the role of endothelial permeability in cardiovascular disease and the risks in vivo [37]. The most widely used radioactive tracer in vascular research and a different marker of plaque inflammation is 18-F-fluorodeoxyglucose (18-F-FDG). Increasingly, 18-F-FDG and other PET (positron emission tomography) tracers are employed to provide imaging endpoints for cardiovascular intervention trials. Using biological processes, PET imaging can characterize the high-risk traits of susceptible atherosclerotic plaques. Inflammation, microcalcification, hypoxia, and neovascularization can all be tracked using current radioactive tracers in susceptible plaques. Developing novel PET radioactive tracers, imaging techniques, and hybrid scanners may improve the effectiveness and accuracy of characterizing high-risk plaques [38]. Plaque features are identified through a novel atherosclerosis identification approach. Plaque detection frequently uses multi-mode/hybrid imaging systems and near-infrared fluorescence imaging. In both clinical and experimental settings, Indocyanine Green (ICG) targets human plaques with endothelial anomalies and offers fresh insights into its targeting mechanism [39].

3. Gene and Protein Markers

3.1. Gene Level

MicroRNA (miRNA), which plays an important role in regulating pathophysiological processes such as cell adhesion, proliferation, lipid uptake, efflux, and the production of inflammatory mediators, offers a new molecular understanding for investigating their effects on these pathways in coronary atherosclerosis and helps to pinpoint potential therapeutic approaches. MiRNA's potential as a diagnostic, prognostic, or therapy response biomarker for cardiovascular disease has been particularly increased by the realization that miRNA may be detected outside of cells, even in circulating blood [40]. Figure 2 illustrates the connection between genes and proteins.

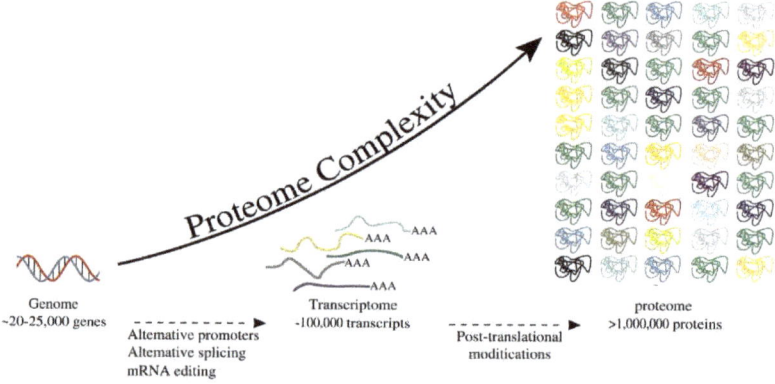

Figure 2. The entire process from gene to protein.

Cholesterol homeostasis is essential to the physiology of the cell. Variations in cellular or systemic cholesterol concentrations are linked to metabolic disorders. In circulation, cholesterol is transported by lipoproteins, which maintain cholesterol homeostasis by transferring (such as low-density lipoprotein (LDL)) and removing (such as high-density lipoprotein (HDL)) cholesterol from cells and tissues. High-level low-density lipoprotein cholesterol (LDLC) and/or low-level high-density lipoprotein cholesterol (HDLC) imbalances that encourage cell cholesterol buildup can induce coronary atherosclerosis. Recent discoveries of genes that regulate the abundance and function of low-density lipoprotein (LDL) and high-density lipoprotein (HDL) have significantly increased our knowledge of the regulatory circuits that regulate plasma lipoprotein levels [4,5,11].

MiRNA regulates lipoprotein metabolism and associated diseases such as metabolic syndrome, obesity, and atherosclerosis [41]. miR-33 regulates macrophage activation and mitochondrial metabolism. Furthermore, recent research has indicated that miR-33 controls vascular homeostasis and cardiac responsiveness to pressure stress. Aside from miR-33 and miR-122, single-nucleotide polymorphisms near the miRNA gene were linked to abnormal levels of human circulation lipids. Some of these miRNAs, such as miR-148a and miR-128-1, target proteins involved in cellular cholesterol metabolisms, such as the low-density lipoprotein receptor (LDLR) and the ATP binding cassette A1 (ABCA1) [42].

MiR-122 is a microRNA implicated in the metabolism of lipoproteins, and its expression is substantially enriched in the liver [43]. MiR-122 is a critical regulator of cholesterol and fatty acid production and hence a crucial regulator of lipoprotein homeostasis, as shown by tests in mice and non-human primates, where its function was inhibited [43,44]. It should be noted that miR-122 acts on specific genes in hepatocytes, rather than participating in all lipid metabolism pathways [45]. MiR-223 and miR-27b, on the other hand, as major post-transcriptional regulatory centers, regulate the gene network of cholesterol and lipoprotein metabolism [46,47]. MiR-223 suppresses the hmgs1, sc4mol, and srb1 genes involved in HDL absorption and cholesterol production, resulting in higher levels of HDL-C and total cholesterol in the liver and plasma in miR-223 mice [46].

Coronary atherosclerosis can easily occur on the artery wall due to ongoing hyperlipidemia and fluctuating shear stress. Endothelial cells experience several molecular and cellular conformational changes in response to biomechanical and biochemical stimuli, aiding coronary atherosclerosis development. For instance, leukocyte migration to the arterial wall, which may be one of the primary indicators connected to new plaques, is aided by the early elevation of the expression of adhesion molecules such as vascular adhesion molecule (VCAM)-1, intracellular adhesion molecule (ICAM)-1, and E-selectin [48]. Some miRNAs can directly target the 3′-UTR of these molecules as a result of miR-17-3p (targeting ICAM-1) and miR-31 (targeting E-selectin), which are connected to coronary atherosclerosis [49]. These molecules induce an increase in macrophages in the process of atherosclerosis [50–52]. It is unclear how these two miRNAs function in experimental coronary atherosclerosis. In addition to these molecules that promote adhesion, several other pro-inflammatory and pro-thrombotic factors are also activated by nuclear factor (NF)-κB signaling, which is a significant route. Two cytokine-reactive miRNAs, miR-181b and miR-146a, control NF-κ. Different components of the B signal have a protective effect on coronary atherosclerosis [53].

Elevated plasma levels of miR-146a-5p and miR-21-5p have been established in studies as general biomarkers of ACS circulation [54]. According to Amanpreet et al., the most prevalent miRNAs in CAD (miR-1, miR-133a, miR-208a, and miR-499) are significantly expressed in the heart and have an important role in cardiac physiology [55]. Even though studies found that numerous miRNAs are expressed in ACS, and stable CAD, miR-1, miR-133, miR-208a, and miR-499 are typically considered ACS biomarkers [41], these biomarkers, particularly miR-499, whose concentration gradient level is associated with myocardial damage, are most likely to diagnose ACS and stable CAD [55,56].

Ariana et al.'s study demonstrates that miR-132 is both required and sufficient to cause the formation of pathogenic cardiomyocytes, a hallmark of unfavorable cardiac remodeling.

As a result, miR-132 can be employed as a therapeutic target for heart failure (HF). At the same time, anti-miR-132 therapy demonstrated good pharmacokinetics, safety, tolerability, a dose-dependent PK/PD relationship, and high clinical promise [39,57]. Several pathologic cellular effects and molecular signaling pathways relevant to atherosclerosis are continuously regulated and fine-tuned by miRNA [40]. The progression and balance of atherosclerotic plaques are regressed due to changes in these pathways—for instance, ventricular hypertrophy (miR-208 and miR-133), fibrosis (miR-21 and miR-29), and ventricular arrhythmias (miR-1, miR-328, and miR-133) [58]. Table 1 describes the miRNAs mentioned above.

Table 1. Description of miRNAs.

Name	miR-122 miR-223 miR-27 miR-33 miR-128 miR-148a	miR-17 miR-31	miR-181 miR-146	miR-146 miR-21 miR-1 miR-133a miR-208a miR-499	miR-132	miR-1 miR-133 miR-328	miR-21 miR-29	miR-208 miR-133
Role	Lipid metabolism	Inflammatory	Proliferation and differentiation	ACS	Heart failure	Arrhythmias	Fibrosis	Ventricular hypertrophy

There are potential drawbacks of using miRNA to identify atherosclerosis, including differences in the reliability of different screening methods [59]. The challenge of isolating miRNA using conventional RNA reagents necessitates the optimization of miRNA isolation from complex materials. Detection methods vary as well, with Qubit and microRNA assays offering the lowest variation (%CV 5.47, SEM ± 0.07), followed by Nano Drops (%CV 7.01, SEM ± 0.92) and the Agilent Biological Analyzer (%CV 59.21, SEM ± 1.31) [59]. The long-term clinical use of miRNAs necessitates additional work to address current methodological, technical, or analytical shortcomings. Standard operating protocols, coordinated miRNA isolation, and quantification techniques are necessary to increase repeatability among different investigations [60].

The advancement of genome-wide analysis, particularly microarray analysis, is critical in identifying clinical indicators of coronary atherosclerosis [61,62]. Whole-blood gene expression profiles can reveal illness status dynamics and suggest putative disease causes [63]. Many prevalent illnesses, such as AMI [64–67] and various forms of atherosclerosis [68], have distinct gene expression profiles. Differential gene expression in peripheral blood cells can provide more information on disease dynamics and better forecast the likelihood of cardiovascular events than currently employed approaches [63]. Changes in gene expression in peripheral blood cells have high sensitivity and specificity for diagnosing coronary heart disease (CAD) [69]. The expression level of the adior2 gene, for example, is linked to the advancement of coronary atherosclerosis [70]. Meng et al. revealed that numb ABCB1, ACSL1, ZHHC9, and other genes have important roles in the pathogenesis of atherosclerosis [71–74]. Furthermore, a study from the University of Washington discovered that the SVEP1 gene causes atherosclerosis in the absence of cholesterol [75].

3.2. Protein Levels

Protein is the stage following the gene level and the product of gene translation. Coronary atherosclerosis develops due to a complex combination of environmental and hereditary variables. According to recent research, smoking and stress can quickly lead to cardiovascular disease [76,77]. While genetic variables are uncontrollable, adjustments in certain environmental effects, such as lifestyle and smoking behaviors, may alleviate cardiovascular symptoms [78,79]. It is important to note that genetic factors account for 50% of the risk of atherosclerosis. As a result, early patient diagnosis using reliable genetic indicators of atherosclerosis can result in prompt and precise therapy choices. Therefore, finding new molecular markers is crucial in coronary heart disease for early detection, prompt warning, early intervention, and improved prognosis [80,81]. APOC3 and APOC4 have been confirmed to be involved in the process of atherosclerosis [82–84]. Meng et al. found that different proteins were present in different types of coronary atherosclerosis and that different protein markers identified different phases of atherosclerosis. Six genes (*ALB, SHBG, APOC, APOC3, APOC4,* and *SAA4*) were found to be responsible for its regulation [68].

4. Trace Elements
4.1. Zinc Ion

The rise in patients with coronary heart disease in the United States, Europe, and China is related to diet-associated raised blood cholesterol and blood glucose levels, as well as poor lifestyle habits such as smoking and genetic factors [85]. Smoking, blood sugar, lipids, and hypertension are the four main risk factors for coronary heart disease. These four independent risk variables were found to be primary predictors of coronary atherosclerosis [86–88]. Simultaneously, an intriguing relationship has surfaced. The prevalence of coronary heart disease in underdeveloped nations is positively connected with the human development index.

In contrast, it is inversely correlated with the human development index in developed countries ($\rho = 0.47$ and 0.34, accordingly). Furthermore, the incidence of coronary heart disease has increased in emerging nations over the last few decades, while it has decreased ($p = 0.021$ and 0.002) in developed countries [89–92]. This is due to dietary imbalances and differences in the serum concentrations of several trace elements [93].

As a result, it is worthwhile to investigate the differences in trace element concentrations in the human body and their associations with coronary heart disease. An analysis reveals that coronary heart disease and other diseases are associated with trace elements in the body [94–96]. Zinc ion helps to control many cellular metabolic processes, such as how proteins, lipids, and carbohydrates are broken down and used by the body [97,98]. Zinc is a crucial component of over seventy enzymes, including superoxide dismutase and glutathione peroxidase. As a cofactor of copper-zinc superoxide dismutase (Cu, Zn SOD), zinc can influence CD. Research has demonstrated that zinc supplementation can lower the activity of copper-zinc superoxide dismutase due to an antagonistic relationship between excessive zinc consumption and copper absorption [99]. Zinc also has anti-inflammatory and antioxidant effects [94]. An increased zinc concentration enhances cell antioxidant capability and ensures the maintenance of appropriate endothelium function. Due to zinc's involvement in enzymes, humoral mediators, and mitosis, the immune system relies on zinc to function. Zinc deficiency is associated with sensitivity to oxidative stress, IL-1 and tumor necrosis factor expression, and endothelial cell death [94]. These factors are all involved in atherosclerosis progression. A decline in zinc ion concentration is associated with coronary heart disease in non-smoking older patients and women, particularly post-menopausal women. Patients with coronary artery disease benefit from taking zinc ions in the appropriate amounts [100].

4.2. Iron Ion

Iron is required for numerous physiological activities. Iron-containing proteins and enzymes serve as an essential part of cellular metabolism. These enzymes and proteins are essential for cell proliferation, cell death, DNA synthesis, DNA repair, and mitochondrial function [101–103]. Iron is the principal component of hemoglobin, which is needed to produce red blood cells and transfer oxygen. Iron is also potentially harmful in high concentrations due to its tendency to produce reactive oxygen species (ROS) and damage biomolecules via Fenton reaction-generated hydroxyl radicals [104]. It is also a significant component in determining bacterial toxicity [92].

Iron consumption or outflow irregularities can result in disease. Iron was originally implicated in coronary atherosclerosis development [104,105]. Low-density lipoprotein oxidation can be accelerated by free iron [106]. LDL receptors on macrophages then absorb

LDL, causing foam cells to be recruited. Foam cell infiltration and necrotic core enlargement are crucial steps in coronary atherosclerosis development [107]. In atherosclerotic plaques, many macrophage subtypes have been identified [108]. Macrophages have a significant role in the progression of coronary atherosclerosis. Lipid absorption, which can cause the production of inflammatory cytokines and the formation of foam cells, is the principal cause of M1 macrophage activation in plaques [109]. M1 macrophages are considered to induce coronary atherosclerosis by paracrine stimulating SMC migration and proliferation from the middle membrane to the intima.

Hydrolyzing collagen fibers in the fiber cap, MMP-1, MMP-3, and MMP-9 produced by M1 cells might cause plaque instability [110]. In addition, Th2 cytokines (such as IL-4, IL-10, and IL-13) activate M2 macrophages to create anti-inflammatory cytokines. The inflammatory response is assumed to be balanced by M2 macrophages, which also support tissue repair and inflammation remission. The M1/M2 model offers a condensed structure for comprehending macrophage behavior in a damaged environment. While M2 macrophages can export and metabolize iron, M1 macrophages have high ferritin content and are superior in terms of iron accumulation. Coronary atherosclerosis may result from the variation in the iron turnover rate between M1 and M2 macrophages. The relationship between the peripheral blood iron concentration and coronary atherosclerosis was validated by a cross-sectional study involving more than 4000 individuals. Loss of peripheral blood iron ions can be used as a biomarker for coronary atherosclerosis prognosis [64].

4.3. Other Trace Elements

Trace elements significantly influence cardiovascular disease by directly or indirectly altering the circulatory process [111–113]. Blood metal levels and childhood and adolescent obesity have been demonstrated to correlate positively, according to research by Fan et al. [114]. It was discovered that obesity was associated with an increase in superoxide dismutase (SOD) levels and total circulation copper concentrations. Metal ions influence the expression of leptin in adipocytes by regulating the release of free fatty acids and glucose uptake, highlighting that obesity is a significant coronary heart disease risk factor [114,115]. As per Kalita et al., variations in trace elements can improve insulin resistance in people with type 2 diabetes [116]. Numerous diabetes-related enzymes utilize magnesium and manganese as cofactors. Their insufficiency raises the risk of metabolic syndrome, impairs glucose metabolism, and may lead to atherosclerosis [116,117]. The serum selenium level was substantially linked with all-cause mortality in both men and women, particularly women with coronary heart disease, according to Li et al. [118]. Consequently, alterations in trace element concentrations in the body are regarded as the most important factor in the development of some diseases and in transitioning from health to illness.

This article has certain limitations. The study only discusses imaging, genes and proteins, and trace elements related to atherosclerosis, but other facets of the disease should also be examined. The key to the early detection of atherosclerosis is the combination of more cutting-edge diagnostic procedures and various examination techniques.

5. Conclusions

It is viable to assess coronary atherosclerosis risk using genes and trace elements. In patients with definite symptoms of coronary heart disease, it is reasonable to perform noninvasive investigations such as CCTA. One of the therapy methods for coronary artery disease is the detection of trace elements, which is important for prognosis.

Author Contributions: Manuscript preparation, H.M., F.M. and J.R.; review, Y.C. and Z.Y.; editing, X.L. and J.L. All authors have read and agreed to the published version of the manuscript.

Funding: This research received no external funding.

Institutional Review Board Statement: Not applicable.

Informed Consent Statement: Not applicable.

Data Availability Statement: Not applicable.

Conflicts of Interest: The authors declare no conflict of interest.

Abbreviation

LDL	Low-density lipoprotein
ICA	Invasive coronary angiography
CCTA	Computed tomography coronary angiography
CAD	Coronary artery disease
ACS	Acute coronary syndrome
MACE	Major cardiovascular adverse events
MSCT	Multi-slice spiral CT
DSCT	Dual-source computed tomography
IVUS	Intravascular ultrasound
MRI	Magnetic resonance imaging
18-F-FDG	18 -F-fluorodeoxyglucose
PET	Positron emission tomograph
NIR	Near-infrared imaging
ICG	Indocyanine green
miRNA	MicroRNA
CV	Coefficient of variation
ABCA1	ATP binding cassette A1
HDL	High-density lipoprotein
LDLC	Low-density lipoprotein cholesterol
HDLC	High-density lipoprotein cholesterol
VCAM	Vascular adhesion molecule
ICAM	Intracellular adhesion molecule
NF	Nuclear factor
ACS	Acute coronary syndrome
HF	Heart failure
PK/PD	Pharmacokinetics/pharmacodynamics
AMI	Acute myocardial infarction
ROS	Reactive oxygen species
SOD	Superoxide dismutase

References

1. Ross, R. Atherosclerosis—An inflammatory disease. *N. Engl. J. Med.* **1999**, *340*, 115–126. [CrossRef] [PubMed]
2. Kanter, J.E.; Kramer, F.; Barnhart, S.; Averill, M.M.; Vivekanandan-Giri, A.; Vickery, T.; Li, L.O.; Becker, L.; Yuan, W.; Chait, A.; et al. Diabetes promotes an inflammatory macrophage phenotype and Atherosclerosis through acyl-CoA synthetase 1. *Proc. Natl. Acad. Sci. USA* **2012**, *109*, E715–E724. [CrossRef]
3. Li, J.J.; Chen, J.L. Inflammation may be a bridge connecting hypertension and Atherosclerosis. *Med. Hypotheses* **2005**, *64*, 925–929. [CrossRef]
4. Falk, E. Pathogenesis of Atherosclerosis. *J. Am. Coll. Cardiol.* **2006**, *47* (Suppl. 8), C7–C12. [CrossRef] [PubMed]
5. Miname, M.H.; Santos, R.D. Reducing cardiovascular risk in patients with familial hypercholesterolemia: Risk prediction and lipid management. *Prog. Cardiovasc. Dis.* **2019**, *62*, 414–422. [CrossRef] [PubMed]
6. Summerhill, V.I.; Grechko, A.V.; Yet, S.F.; Sobenin, I.A.; Orekhov, A.N. The atherogenic role of circulating modified lipids in Atherosclerosis. *Int. J. Mol. Sci.* **2019**, *20*, 3561. [CrossRef] [PubMed]
7. Taleb, S. Inflammation in Atherosclerosis. *Arch. Cardiovasc. Dis.* **2016**, *109*, 708–715. [CrossRef]
8. Cheng, F.; Torzewski, M.; Degreif, A.; Rossmann, H.; Canisius, A.; Lackner, K.J. Impact of glutathione peroxidase-1 deficiency on macrophage foam cell formation and proliferation: Implications for atherogenesis. *PLoS ONE* **2013**, *8*, e72063. [CrossRef]
9. Falk, E.; Nakano, M.; Bentzon, J.F.; Finn, A.V.; Virmani, R. Update on acute coronary syndromes: The pathologists' view. *Eur. Heart J.* **2013**, *34*, 719–728. [CrossRef]
10. Rognoni, A.; Cavallino, C.; Veia, A.; Bacchini, S.; Rosso, R.; Facchini, M.; Secco, G.G.; Lupi, A.; Nardi, F.; Rametta, F.; et al. Pathophysiology of atherosclerotic plaque development. *Cardiovasc. Hematol. Agents Med. Chem.* **2015**, *13*, 10–13. [CrossRef]
11. Stary, H.C.; Chandler, A.B.; Glagov, S.; Guyton, J.R.; Insull, W., Jr.; Rosenfeld, M.E.; Schaffer, S.A.; Schwartz, C.J.; Wagner, W.D.; Wissler, R.W. A definition of Atherosclerosis's initial, fatty streak, and intermediate lesions. A report from the Committee on Vascular Lesions of the Council on Arteriosclerosis, American Heart Association. *Circulation* **1994**, *89*, 2462–2478. [CrossRef] [PubMed]

12. Virmani, R.; Kolodgie, F.D.; Burke, A.P.; Farb, A.; Schwartz, S.M. Lessons from sudden coronary death: A comprehensive morphological classification scheme for atherosclerotic lesions. *Arterioscler. Thromb. Vasc. Biol.* **2000**, *20*, 1262–1275. [CrossRef] [PubMed]
13. Yahagi, K.; Kolodgie, F.D.; Lutter, C.; Mori, H.; Romero, M.E.; Finn, A.V.; Virmani, R. Pathology of human coronary and carotid artery atherosclerosis and vascular calcification in Diabetes mellitus. *Arterioscler. Thromb. Vasc. Biol.* **2017**, *37*, 191–204. [CrossRef] [PubMed]
14. Wang, X.; Matsumura, M.; Mintz, G.S.; Lee, T.; Zhang, W.; Cao, Y.; Fujino, A.; Lin, Y.; Usui, E.; Kanaji, Y.; et al. In vivo calcium detection by comparing optical coherence tomography, intravascular ultrasound, and angiography. *JACC Cardiovasc. Imaging* **2017**, *10*, 869–879. [CrossRef] [PubMed]
15. Miller, J.M.; Rochitte, C.E.; Dewey, M.; Arbab-Zadeh, A.; Niinuma, H.; Gottlieb, I.; Paul, N.; Clouse, M.E.; Shapiro, E.P.; Hoe, J.; et al. Diagnostic performance of coronary angiography by 64-row CT. *N. Engl. J. Med.* **2008**, *359*, 2324–2336. [CrossRef] [PubMed]
16. Assante, R.; Klain, M.; Acampa, W. Use coronary artery calcium scanning as a triage for invasive coronary angiography. *J. Nucl. Cardiol.* **2019**, *26*, 613–615. [CrossRef] [PubMed]
17. Morris, P.D.; Gunn, J.P. Computing Fractional Flow Reserve From Invasive Coronary Angiography: Getting Closer. *Circ. Cardiovasc. Interv.* **2017**, *10*, e005806. [CrossRef]
18. Minhas, A.; Dewey, M.; Vavere, A.L.; Tanami, Y.; Ostovaneh, M.R.; Laule, M.; Rochitte, C.E.; Niinuma, H.; Kofoed, K.F.; Geleijns, J.; et al. Patient Preferences for Coronary CT Angiography with Stress Perfusion, SPECT, or Invasive Coronary Angiography. *Radiology* **2019**, *291*, 340–348. [CrossRef]
19. National Research Council. *Health Risks from Exposure to Low Levels of Ionizing Radiation: BEIR VII Phase 2*; The National Academies Press: Washington, DC, USA, 2006.
20. Collet, J.P.; Thiele, H.; Barbato, E.; Barthelemy, O.; Bauersachs, J.; Bhatt, D.L.; Dendale, P.; Dorobantu, M.; Edvardsen, T.; Folliguet, T.; et al. 2020 ESC Guidelines for the management of acute coronary syndromes in patients presenting without persistent ST-segment elevation. *Eur. Heart J.* **2020**, *42*, 1289–1367. [CrossRef]
21. Collet, C.; Onuma, Y.; Andreini, D.; Sonck, J.; Pompilio, G.; Mushtaq, S.; La Meir, M.; Miyazaki, Y.; de Mey, J.; Gaemperli, O.; et al. Coronary computed tomography angiography for heart team decision-making in multivessel coronary artery disease. *Eur. Heart J.* **2018**, *39*, 3689–3698. [CrossRef]
22. Mushtaq, S.; Andreini, D.; Pontone, G.; Bertella, E.; Bartorelli, A.L.; Conte, E.; Baggiano, A.; Annoni, A.; Formenti, A.; Trabattoni, D.; et al. Prognostic value of coronary CTA in coronary bypass patients: A long-term follow-up study. *JACC Cardiovasc. Imaging* **2014**, *7*, 580–589. [CrossRef] [PubMed]
23. National Institute for Health and Clinical Excellence. *Chest Pain of Recent Onset: Assessment and Diagnosis of Recent Onset Chest Pain or Discomfort of Suspected Cardiac Origin*; Royal College of Physicians: London, UK, 2010.
24. Taylor, A.J.; Cerqueira, M.; Hodgson, J.M.; Mark, D.; Min, J.; O'Gara, P.; Rubin, G.D.; American College of Cardiology Foundation Appropriate Use Criteria Task Force; Society of Cardiovascular Computed Tomography; American College of Radiology; et al. ACCF/SCCT/ACR/AHA/ASE/ASNC/NASCI/SCAI/SCMR 2010 appropriate use criteria for cardiac computed tomography. A report of the American College of Cardiology Foundation Appropriate Use Criteria Task Force, the Society of Cardiovascular Computed Tomography, the American College of Radiology, the American Heart Association, the American Society of Echocardiography, the American Society of Nuclear Cardiology, the North American Society for Cardiovascular Imaging, the Society for Cardiovascular Angiography and Interventions, and the Society for Cardiovascular Magnetic Resonance. *J. Cardiovasc. Comput. Tomogr.* **2010**, *4*, 407. [PubMed]
25. Voros, S.; Rinehart, S.; Qian, Z.; Joshi, P.; Vazquez, G.; Fischer, C.; Belur, P.; Hulten, E.; Villines, T.C. Coronary atherosclerosis imaging by coronary CT angiography: Current status, correlation with intravascular interrogation and meta-analysis. *JACC Cardiovasc. Imaging* **2011**, *4*, 537–548. [CrossRef] [PubMed]
26. Goldstein, J.A.; Chinnaiyan, K.M.; Abidov, A. CT-STAT Investigators The CT-STAT (Coronary Computed Tomographic Angiography for Systematic Triage of Acute Chest Pain Patients to Treatment) trial. *J. Am. Coll. Cardiol.* **2011**, *58*, 1414–1422. [CrossRef]
27. Litt, H.I.; Gatsonis, C.; Snyder, B.; Singh, H.; Miller, C.D.; Entrikin, D.W.; Leaming, J.M.; Gavin, L.J.; Pacella, C.B.; Hollander, J.E. CT angiography for safe discharge of patients with possible acute coronary syndromes. *N. Engl. J. Med.* **2012**, *366*, 1393–1403. [CrossRef]
28. Hoffmann, U.; Truong, Q.A.; Schoenfeld, D.A. ROM ICAT-II Investigators Coronary CT angiography versus standard evaluation in acute chest pain. *N. Engl. J. Med.* **2012**, *367*, 299–308. [CrossRef]
29. Hamilton-Craig, C.; Fifoot, A.; Hansen, M.; Pincus, M.; Chan, J.; Walters, D.L.; Branch, K.R. Diagnostic performance and cost of CT angiography versus stress ECG—A randomized prospective study of suspected acute coronary syndrome chest pain in the emergency department (CT-COMPARE). *Int. J. Cardiol.* **2014**, *177*, 867–873. [CrossRef]
30. Arbab-Zadeh, A.; Miller, J.M.; Rochitte, C.E.; Dewey, M.; Niinuma, H.; Gottlieb, I.; Paul, N.; Clouse, M.E.; Shapiro, E.P.; Hoe, J.; et al. Diagnostic accuracy of computed tomography coronary angiography according to pre-test probability of coronary artery disease and severity of coronary arterial calcification. The CORE-64 (coronary artery evaluation using 64-row multidetector computed tomography angiography) International Multicenter Study. *J. Am. Coll. Cardiol.* **2012**, *59*, 379–387.
31. Kuchynka, P.; Lambert, L.; Černý, V.; Marek, J.; Ambrož, D.; Danek, B.A.; Linhart, A. Coronary CT angiography. *Cor Vasa* **2015**, *57*, e425–e432. [CrossRef]

32. Halliburton, S.S.; Abbara, S.; Chen, M.Y.; Gentry, R.; Mahesh, M.; Raff, G.L.; Shaw, L.J.; Hausleiter, J.; Society of Cardiovascular Computed Tomography. SCCT guidelines on radiation dose and dose-optimization strategies in cardiovascular CT. *J. Cardiovasc. Comput. Tomogr.* **2011**, *5*, 198–224. [CrossRef]
33. Zhang, F.; Yang, L.; Song, X.; Li, Y.N.; Jiang, Y.; Zhang, X.H.; Ju, H.Y.; Wu, J.; Chang, R.P. Feasibility study of low tube voltage (80 kVp) coronary CT angiography combined with contrast medium reduction using iterative model reconstruction (IMR) on standard BMI patients. *Br. J. Radiol.* **2016**, *89*, 20150766. [CrossRef] [PubMed]
34. Raju, R.; Thompson, A.G.; Lee, K.; Precious, B.; Yang, T.H.; Berger, A.; Taylor, C.; Heilbron, B.; Nguyen, G.; Earls, J.; et al. Reduced iodine load with CT coronary angiography using dual-energy imaging: A prospective randomized trial compared with standard coronary CT angiography. *J. Cardiovasc. Comput. Tomogr.* **2014**, *8*, 282–288. [CrossRef] [PubMed]
35. Ulzheimer, S.; Flohr, T. Multislice CT: Current Technology and Future Developments. In *Medical Radiology*; Springer: Berlin/Heidelberg, Germany, 2009; pp. 3–23.
36. Tsiknakis, N.; Spanakis, C.; Tsompou, P.; Karanasiou, G.; Karanasiou, G.; Sakellarios, A.; Rigas, G.; Kyriakidis, S.; Papafaklis, M.; Nikopoulos, S.; et al. IVUS Longitudinal and Axial Registration for Atherosclerosis Progression Evaluation. *Diagnostics* **2021**, *11*, 1513. [CrossRef] [PubMed]
37. Lavin, B.; Andia, M.E.; Saha, P.; Botnar, R.M.; Phinikaridou, A. Quantitative MRI of Endothelial Permeability and (Dys)function in Atherosclerosis. *J. Vis. Exp.* **2021**, *178*, e62724. [CrossRef] [PubMed]
38. Sriranjan, R.S.; Tarkin, J.M.; Evans, N.R.; Le, E.P.V.; Chowdhury, M.M.; Rudd, J.H.F. Atherosclerosis imaging using PET: Insights and applications. *Br. J. Pharmacol.* **2021**, *178*, 2186–2203. [CrossRef]
39. Verjans, J.W.; Osborn, E.A.; Ughi, G.J.; Calfon Press, M.A.; Hamidi, E.; Antoniadis, A.P.; Papafaklis, M.I.; Conrad, M.F.; Libby, P.; Stone, P.H.; et al. Targeted Near-Infrared Fluorescence Imaging of Atherosclerosis: Clinical and Intracoronary Evaluation of Indocyanine Green. *JACC Cardiovasc. Imaging* **2016**, *9*, 1087–1095. [CrossRef]
40. Feinberg, M.W.; Moore, K.J. MicroRNA Regulation of Atherosclerosis. *Circ. Res.* **2016**, *118*, 703–720. [CrossRef]
41. Seronde, M.F.; Vausort, M.; Gayat, E.; Goretti, E.; Ng, L.L.; Squire, I.B.; Vodovar, N.; Sadoune, M.; Samuel, J.-L.; Thum, T.; et al. Circulating microRNAs and Outcome in Patients with Acute Heart Failure. *PLoS ONE* **2015**, *10*, e0142237. [CrossRef]
42. Aryal, B.; Singh, A.K.; Rotllan, N.; Price, N.; Fernández-Hernando, C. MicroRNAs and lipid metabolism. *Curr. Opin. Lipidol.* **2017**, *28*, 273–280. [CrossRef]
43. Esau, C.; Davis, S.; Murray, S.F.; Yu, X.X.; Pandey, S.K.; Pear, M.; Watts, L.; Booten, S.L.; Graham, M.; McKay, R.; et al. miR-122 regulation of lipid metabolism revealed by in vivo antisense targeting. *Cell Metab.* **2006**, *3*, 87–98. [CrossRef]
44. Elmen, J.; Lindow, M.; Schutz, S.; Lawrence, M.; Petri, A.; Obad, S.; Lindholm, M.; Hedtjarn, M.; Hansen, H.F.; Berger, U.; et al. LNA-mediated microRNA silencing in non-human primates. *Nature* **2008**, *452*, 896–899. [CrossRef] [PubMed]
45. Elmen, J.; Lindow, M.; Silahtaroglu, A.; Bak, M.; Christensen, M.; Lind-Thomsen, A.; Hedtjarn, M.; Hansen, J.B.; Hansen, H.F.; Straarup, E.M.; et al. Antagonism of microRNA-122 in mice by systemically administered LNA-antimiR leads to up-regulation of a large set of predicted target mRNAs in the liver. *Nucleic Acids Res.* **2008**, *36*, 1153–1162. [CrossRef] [PubMed]
46. Vickers, K.C.; Landstreet, S.R.; Levin, M.G.; Shoucri, B.M.; Toth, C.L.; Taylor, R.C.; Palmisano, B.T.; Tabet, F.; Cui, H.L.; Rye, K.A.; et al. MicroRNA-223 coordinates cholesterol homeostasis. *Proc. Natl. Acad. Sci. USA* **2014**, *111*, 14518–14523. [CrossRef]
47. Vickers, K.C.; Shoucri, B.M.; Levin, M.G.; Wu, H.; Pearson, D.S.; Osei-Hwedieh, D.; Collins, F.S.; Remaley, A.T.; Sethupathy, P. MicroRNA-27b is a regulatory hub in lipid metabolism and is altered in dyslipidemia. *Hepatology* **2013**, *57*, 533–542. [CrossRef] [PubMed]
48. Libby, P.; Ridker, P.M.; Hansson, G.K. Progress and challenges in translating the biology of Atherosclerosis. *Nature* **2011**, *473*, 317–325. [CrossRef]
49. Suarez, Y.; Wang, C.; Manes, T.D.; Pober, J.S. Cutting edge: TNF-induced microRNAs regulate TNF-induced expression of E-selectin and intercellular adhesion molecule-1 on human endothelial cells: Feedback control of inflammation. *J. Immunol.* **2010**, *184*, 21–25. [CrossRef]
50. Shi, Z.G.; Sun, Y.; Wang, K.S.; Jia, J.D.; Yang, J.; Li, Y.N. Effects of miR-26a/miR-146a/miR-31 on airway inflammation of asthma mice and asthma children. *Eur. Rev. Med. Pharmacol. Sci.* **2019**, *23*, 5432–5440.
51. Zhou, F.; Liu, P.; Lv, H.; Gao, Z.; Chang, W.; Xu, Y. miR-31 attenuates murine allergic rhinitis by suppressing interleukin-13-induced nasal epithelial inflammatory responses. *Mol. Med. Rep.* **2021**, *23*, 42. [CrossRef]
52. An, J.H.; Chen, Z.Y.; Ma, Q.L.; Wang, H.J.; Zhang, J.Q.; Shi, F.W. LncRNA SNHG16 promoted proliferation and inflammatory response of macrophages through miR-17-5p/NF-κB signaling pathway in patients with Atherosclerosis. *Eur. Rev. Med. Pharmacol. Sci.* **2019**, *23*, 8665–8677.
53. Sun, X.; Belkin, N.; Feinberg, M.W. Endothelial microRNAs and Atherosclerosis. *Curr. Atheroscler. Rep.* **2013**, *15*, 372. [CrossRef]
54. Zhelankin, A.; Stonogina, D.; Vasiliev, S.; Babalyan, K.; Sharova, E.; Doludin, Y.; Shchekochikhin, D.; Generozov, E.; Akselrod, A. Circulating Extracellular miRNA Analysis in Patients with Stable CAD and Acute Coronary Syndromes. *Biomolecules* **2021**, *11*, 962. [CrossRef] [PubMed]
55. Kaur, A.; Mackin, S.T.; Schlosser, K.; Wong, F.L.; Elharram, M.; Delles, C.; Stewart, D.J.; Dayan, N.; Landry, T.; Pilote, L. Systematic review of microRNA biomarkers in acute coronary syndrome and stable coronary artery disease. *Cardiovasc. Res.* **2020**, *116*, 1113–1124. [CrossRef] [PubMed]
56. Viereck, J.; Thum, T. Circulating Noncoding RNAs as Biomarkers of Cardiovascular Disease and Injury. *Circ. Res.* **2017**, *120*, 381–399. [CrossRef] [PubMed]

57. Foinquinos, A.; Batkai, S.; Genschel, C.; Viereck, J.; Rump, S.; Gyöngyösi, M.; Traxler, D.; Riesenhuber, M.; Spannbauer, A.; Lukovic, D.; et al. Preclinical development of a miR-132 inhibitor for heart failure treatment. *Nat. Commun.* **2020**, *11*, 633. [CrossRef] [PubMed]
58. Melman, Y.F.; Shah, R.; Das, S. MicroRNAs in heart failure: Is the picture becoming less miRky? *Circ. Heart Fail.* **2014**, *7*, 203–214. [CrossRef]
59. Wright, K.; de Silva, K.; Purdie, A.C.; Plain, K.M. Comparison of methods for miRNA isolation and quantification from ovine plasma. *Sci. Rep.* **2020**, *10*, 825. [CrossRef] [PubMed]
60. de Gonzalo-Calvo, D.; Pérez-Boza, J.; Curado, J.; Devaux, Y.; EU-CardioRNA COST Action CA17129. Challenges of microRNA-based biomarkers in clinical application for cardiovascular diseases. *Clin. Transl. Med.* **2022**, *12*, e585. [CrossRef]
61. McPherson, R. Chromosome 9p21 and coronary artery disease. *N. Engl. J. Med.* **2010**, *362*, 1736–1737. [CrossRef]
62. Ardissino, D.; Berzuini, C.; Merlini, P.A.; Mannucci, P.M.; Surti, A.; Burtt, N.; Voight, B.; Tubaro, M.; Peyvandi, F.; Spreafico, M.; et al. Influence of 9p21.3 genetic variants on clinical and angiographic outcomes in early-onset myocardial infarction. *J. Am. Coll. Cardiol.* **2011**, *58*, 426–434. [CrossRef]
63. Aziz, H.; Zaas, A.; Ginsburg, G.S. Peripheral blood gene expression profiling for cardiovascular disease assessment. *Genom. Med.* **2007**, *1*, 105–112. [CrossRef]
64. Meng, H.; Wang, Y.; Ruan, J.; Chen, Y.; Wang, X.; Zhou, F.; Meng, F. Decreased iron ion concentrations in the peripheral blood correlate with coronary Atherosclerosis. *Nutrients* **2022**, *14*, 319. [CrossRef] [PubMed]
65. Meng, H.; Wang, X.; Ruan, J.; Chen, W.; Meng, F.; Yang, P. High expression levels of the SOCS3 gene are associated with acute myocardial infarction. *Genet. Test. Mol. Biomark.* **2020**, *24*, 443–450. [CrossRef] [PubMed]
66. Ruan, J.; Meng, H.; Wang, X.; Chen, W.; Tian, X.; Meng, F. Low expression of FFAR2 in peripheral white blood cells may Be a genetic marker for early diagnosis of acute myocardial infarction. *Cardiol. Res. Pract.* **2020**, *2020*, 3108124. [CrossRef]
67. Tan, B.; Liu, L.; Yang, Y.; Liu, Q.; Yang, L.; Meng, F. Low CPNE3 expression is associated with risk of acute myocardial infarction: A feasible genetic marker of acute myocardial infarction in patients with stable coronary artery disease. *Cardiol. J.* **2019**, *26*, 186–193. [CrossRef] [PubMed]
68. Meng, H.; Ruan, J.; Chen, Y.; Yan, Z.; Shi, K.; Li, X.; Yang, P.; Meng, F. Investigation of specific proteins related to different types of coronary atherosclerosis. *Front. Cardiovasc. Med.* **2021**, *8*, 758035. [CrossRef]
69. Elashoff, M.R.; Wingrove, J.A.; Beineke, P.; Daniels, S.E.; Tingley, W.G.; Rosenberg, S.; Voros, S.; Kraus, W.E.; Ginsburg, G.S.; Schwartz, R.S.; et al. Development of a blood-based gene expression algorithm for assessing obstructive coronary artery disease in non-diabetic patients. *BMC Med. Genom.* **2011**, *4*, 26. [CrossRef]
70. Ikonomidis, I.; Kadoglou, N.; Tsiotra, P.C.; Kollias, A.; Palios, I.; Fountoulaki, K.; Halvatsiotis, I.; Maratou, E.; Dimitriadis, G.; Kremastinos, D.T.; et al. Arterial stiffness is associated with increased monocyte expression of adiponectin receptor mRNA and protein in patients with coronary artery disease. *Am. J. Hypertens.* **2012**, *25*, 746–755. [CrossRef]
71. Meng, H.; Li, L.; Ruan, J.; Chen, Y.; Yan, Z.; Liu, J.; Li, X.; Mao, C.; Yang, P. Association of Low Expression of NUMB in Peripheral Blood with Acute Myocardial Infarction. *Cardiol. Res. Pract.* **2022**, *2022*, 7981637. [CrossRef]
72. Ruan, J.; Meng, H.; Chen, Y.; Yan, Z.; Li, X.; Meng, F. Expression of ATP-binding cassette subfamily B member 1 gene in peripheral blood patients with acute myocardial infarction. *Bioengineered* **2022**, *13*, 11095–11105. [CrossRef]
73. Li, T.; Li, X.; Meng, H.; Chen, L.; Meng, F. ACSL1 affects Triglyceride Levels through the PPARγ Pathway. *Int. J. Med. Sci.* **2020**, *17*, 720–727. [CrossRef]
74. Li, L.; Meng, H.; Wang, X.; Ruan, J.; Tian, X.; Meng, F. Low ZCCHC9 Gene Expression in Peripheral Blood May Be an Acute Myocardial Infarction Genetic Molecular Marker in Patients with Stable Coronary Atherosclerotic Disease. *Int. J. Med. Sci.* **2022**, *15*, 1795–1804. [CrossRef] [PubMed]
75. Jung, I.H.; Elenbaas, J.S.; Alisio, A.; Santana, K.; Young, E.P.; Kang, C.J.; Kachroo, P.; Lavine, K.J.; Razani, B.; Mecham, R.P.; et al. SVEP1 is a human coronary artery disease locus that promotes Atherosclerosis. *Sci. Transl. Med.* **2021**, *13*, eabe0357. [CrossRef] [PubMed]
76. Wirtz, P.H.; von Känel, R. Psychological stress, inflammation, and coronary heart disease. *Curr. Cardiol. Rep.* **2017**, *19*, 111. [CrossRef] [PubMed]
77. Jokinen, E. Obesity and cardiovascular disease. *Minerva Pediatr.* **2015**, *67*, 25–32.
78. Khot, U.N.; Khot, M.B.; Bajzer, C.T.; Sapp, S.K.; Ohman, E.M.; Brener, S.J.; Ellis, S.G.; Lincoff, A.M.; Topol, E.J. Prevalence of conventional risk factors in patients with coronary heart disease. *JAMA* **2003**, *290*, 898–904. [CrossRef]
79. Jayashree, S.; Arindam, M.; Vijay, K.V. Genetic epidemiology of coronary artery disease: An Asian Indian perspective. *J. Genet.* **2015**, *94*, 539–549. [CrossRef]
80. Anderson, N.L.; Anderson, N.G. The human plasma proteome: History, character, and diagnostic prospects. *Mol. Cell. Proteom.* **2002**, *1*, 845–867. [CrossRef]
81. Smith, J.G.; Gerszten, R.E. Emerging affinity-based proteomic technologies for large-scale plasma profiling in cardiovascular disease. *Circulation* **2017**, *135*, 1651–1664. [CrossRef]
82. Ronsein, G.E.; Vaisar, T.; Davidson, W.S.; Bornfeldt, K.E.; Probstfield, J.L.; O'Brien, K.D.; Zhao, X.-Q.; Heinecke, J.W. Niacin Increases Atherogenic Proteins in High-Density Lipoprotein of Statin-Treated Subjects. *Arterioscler. Thromb. Vasc. Biol.* **2021**, *41*, 2330–2341. [CrossRef]

83. Stitziel, N.O.; Kanter, J.E.; Bornfeldt, K.E. Emerging Targets for Cardiovascular Disease Prevention in Diabetes. *Trends Mol. Med.* **2020**, *26*, 744–757. [CrossRef]
84. Zha, Y.; Lu, Y.; Zhang, T.; Yan, K.; Zhuang, W.; Liang, J.; Cheng, Y.; Wang, Y. CRISPR/Cas9-mediated knockout of APOC3 stabilizes plasma lipids and inhibits Atherosclerosis in rabbits. *Lipids Health Dis.* **2021**, *20*, 180. [CrossRef] [PubMed]
85. Bray, G.A.; Heisel, W.E.; Afshin, A.; Jensen, M.D.; Dietz, W.H.; Long, M.; Kushner, R.F.; Daniels, S.R.; Wadden, T.A.; Tsai, A.G.; et al. The science of obesity management: An Endocrine Society scientific statement. *Endocr. Rev.* **2018**, *39*, 79–132. [CrossRef] [PubMed]
86. Goff, D.C., Jr.; Lloyd-Jones, D.M.; Bennett, G.; Coady, S.; D'Agostino, R.B.; Gibbons, R.; Greenland, P.; Lackland, D.T.; Levy, D.; O'Donnell, C.J.; et al. 2013 ACC/AHA guideline on the assessment of cardiovascular risk: A report of the American College of Cardiology/American Heart Association task force on practice guidelines. *Circulation* **2014**, *129*, S49–S73. [CrossRef] [PubMed]
87. Stone, N.J.; Robinson, J.G.; Lichtenstein, A.H.; Merz, C.N.B.; Blum, C.B.; Eckel, R.H.; Goldberg, A.C.; Gordon, D.; Levy, D.; Lloyd-Jones, D.M.; et al. 2013 ACC/AHA guideline on the treatment of blood cholesterol to reduce atherosclerotic cardiovascular risk in adults: A report of the American College of Cardiology/American Heart Association task force on practice guidelines. *J. Am. Coll. Cardiol.* **2014**, *63*, 2889–2934. [CrossRef]
88. Lusis, A.J. Atherosclerosis. *Nature* **2000**, *407*, 233–241. [CrossRef]
89. Zhu, K.F.; Wang, Y.M.; Zhu, J.Z.; Zhou, Q.Y.; Wang, N.F. National prevalence of coronary heart disease and its relationship with human development index: A systematic review. *Eur. J. Prev. Cardiol.* **2016**, *23*, 530–543. [CrossRef]
90. Gaziano, T.A.; Bitton, A.; Anand, S.; Abrahams-Gessel, S.; Murphy, A. Growing epidemic of coronary heart disease in low- and middle-income countries. *Curr. Probl. Cardiol.* **2010**, *35*, 72–115. [CrossRef]
91. Xu, Z.; Yu, D.; Yin, X.; Zheng, F.; Li, H. Socioeconomic status is associated with global diabetes prevalence. *Oncotarget* **2017**, *8*, 44434–44439. [CrossRef]
92. Argent, A.C.; Balachandran, R.; Vaidyanathan, B.; Khan, A.; Kumar, R.K. Management of undernutrition and failure to thrive in children with congenital heart disease in low- and middle-income countries. *Cardiol. Young* **2017**, *27*, S22–S30. [CrossRef]
93. Mardones-Santander, F.; Rosso, P.; Stekel, A.; Ahumada, E.; Llaguno, S.; Pizarro, F.; Salinas, J.; Vial, I.; Walter, T. Effect of a milk-based food supplement on maternal nutritional status and fetal growth in underweight Chilean women. *Am. J. Clin. Nutr.* **1988**, *47*, 413–419. [CrossRef]
94. Krachler, M.; Lindschinger, M.; Eber, B.; Watzinger, N.; Wallner, S. Trace elements in coronary heart disease: Impact of intensi-fied lifestyle modification. *Biol. Trace Elem. Res.* **1997**, *60*, 175–185. [CrossRef] [PubMed]
95. Rovira, J.; Hernández-Aguilera, A.; Luciano-Mateo, F.; Cabré, N.; Baiges-Gaya, G.; Nadal, M.; Martín-Paredero, V.; Camps, J.; Joven, J.; Domingo, J.L. Trace elements and Paraoxonase-1 activity in lower extremity artery disease. *Biol. Trace Elem. Res.* **2018**, *186*, 74–84. [CrossRef]
96. Strain, J.J. Putative role of dietary trace elements in coronary heart disease and cancer. *Br. J. Biomed. Sci.* **1994**, *51*, 241–251. [PubMed]
97. Shokrzadeh, M.; Ghaemian, A.; Salehifar, E.; Aliakbari, S.; Saravi, S.S.; Ebrahimi, P. Serum zinc and copper levels in ischemic cardiomyopathy. *Biol. Trace Elem. Res.* **2009**, *127*, 116–123. [CrossRef] [PubMed]
98. Ilyas, A.; Shah, M.H. Abnormalities of selected trace elements in patients with coronary artery disease. *Acta Cardiol. Sin.* **2015**, *31*, 518–527.
99. Hughes, S.; Samman, S. The effect of zinc supplementation in humans on plasma lipids, antioxidant status and thrombogenesis. *J. Am. Coll. Nutr.* **2006**, *25*, 285–291. [CrossRef]
100. Meng, H.; Wang, Y.; Zhou, F.; Ruan, J.; Duan, M.; Wang, X.; Yu, Q.; Yang, P.; Chen, W.; Meng, F. Reduced Serum Zinc Ion Concentration Is Associated with Coronary Heart Disease. *Biol. Trace Elem. Res.* **2021**, *199*, 4109–4118. [CrossRef]
101. Dev, S.; Babitt, J.L. Overview of iron metabolism in health and disease. *Hemodial. Int.* **2017**, *21*, S6–S20. [CrossRef]
102. Ye, Q.; Chen, W.; Huang, H.; Tang, Y.; Wang, W.; Meng, F.; Wang, H.; Zheng, Y. Iron and zinc ions, potent weapons against multidrug-resistant bacteria. *Appl. Microbiol. Biotechnol.* **2020**, *104*, 5213–5227. [CrossRef]
103. Muckenthaler, M.U.; Rivella, S.; Hentze, M.W.; Galy, B. A red carpet for iron metabolism. *Cell* **2017**, *168*, 344–361. [CrossRef]
104. Cornelissen, A.; Guo, L.; Sakamoto, A.; Virmani, R.; Finn, A.V. New insights into the role of iron in inflammation and Atherosclerosis. *EBioMedicine* **2019**, *47*, 598–606. [CrossRef] [PubMed]
105. Eijkelkamp, B.A.; Hassan, K.A.; Paulsen, I.T.; Brown, M.H. Investigation of the human pathogen Acinetobacter baumannii under iron limiting conditions. *BMC Genom.* **2011**, *12*, 126. [CrossRef] [PubMed]
106. Sullivan, J.L. Iron and the sex difference in heart disease risk. *Lancet* **1981**, *1*, 1293–1294. [CrossRef]
107. Balla, G.; Jacob, H.S.; Eaton, J.W.; Belcher, J.D.; Vercellotti, G.M. Hemin: A possible physiological mediator of low-density lipoprotein oxidation and endothelial injury. *Arterioscler. Thromb.* **1991**, *11*, 1700–1711. [CrossRef] [PubMed]
108. Bouhlel, M.A.; Derudas, B.; Rigamonti, E.; Dièvart, R.; Brozek, J.; Haulon, S.; Zawadzki, C.; Jude, B.; Torpier, G.; Marx, N.; et al. PPARgamma activation primes human monocytes into alternative M2 macrophages with anti-inflammatory properties. *Cell Metab.* **2007**, *6*, 137–143. [CrossRef]
109. Jelani, Q.U.; Harchandani, B.; Cable, R.G.; Guo, Y.; Zhong, H.; Hilbert, T.; Newman, J.D.; Katz, S.D. Effects of serial phlebotomy on vascular endothelial function: Results of a prospective, double-blind, randomized study. *Cardiovasc. Ther.* **2018**, *36*, 1755–5922. [CrossRef]

110. Klingler, K.R.; Zech, D.; Wielckens, K. Haemochromatosis: Automated detection of the two-point mutations in the HFE gene: Cys282Tyr and His63Asp. *Clin. Chem. Lab. Med.* **2000**, *38*, 1225–1230. [CrossRef]
111. Aalbers, T.G.; Houtman, J.P. Relationships between trace elements and Atherosclerosis. *Sci. Total Environ.* **1985**, *43*, 255–283. [CrossRef]
112. Eshak, E.S.; Iso, H.; Yamagishi, K.; Maruyama, K.; Umesawa, M.; Tamakoshi, A. Associations between copper and zinc intakes from diet and mortality from cardiovascular disease in a large population-based prospective cohort study. *J. Nutr. Biochem.* **2018**, *56*, 126–132. [CrossRef]
113. Kodali, H.P.; Pavilonis, B.T.; Schooling, C.M. Effects of copper and zinc on ischemic heart disease and myocardial infarction: A Mendelian randomization study. *Am. J. Clin. Nutr.* **2018**, *108*, 237–242. [CrossRef]
114. Fan, Y.; Zhang, C.; Bu, J. Relationship between selected serum metallic elements and obesity in children and adolescents in the U.S. *Nutrients* **2017**, *9*, 104. [CrossRef] [PubMed]
115. Ades, P.A.; Savage, P.D. Obesity in coronary heart disease: An unaddressed behavioural risk factor. *Prev. Med.* **2017**, *104*, 117–119. [CrossRef] [PubMed]
116. Kalita, H.; Hazarika, A.; Devi, R. Withdrawal of high-carbohydrate, high-fat diet alters the status of trace elements to ameliorate metabolic syndrome in rats with type 2 diabetes mellitus. *Can. J. Diabetes* **2020**, *44*, 317–326. [CrossRef] [PubMed]
117. Shi, Y.; Zou, Y.; Shen, Z.; Xiong, Y.; Zhang, W.; Liu, C.; Chen, S. Trace elements, PPARs, and metabolic syndrome. *Int. J. Mol. Sci.* **2020**, *21*, 2612. [CrossRef]
118. Li, J.; Lo, K.; Shen, G.; Feng, Y.Q.; Huang, Y.Q. Gender difference in the association of serum selenium with all-cause and cardiovascular mortality. *Postgrad. Med.* **2020**, *132*, 148–155. [CrossRef]

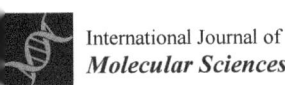

Review

Different Approaches in Therapy Aiming to Stabilize an Unstable Atherosclerotic Plaque

Michal Kowara and Agnieszka Cudnoch-Jedrzejewska *

Laboratory of Centre for Preclinical Research, Department of Experimental and Clinical Physiology, Medical University of Warsaw, 02-091 Warsaw, Poland; michal.kowara@wum.edu.pl
* Correspondence: agnieszka.cudnoch@wum.edu.pl

Abstract: Atherosclerotic plaque vulnerability is a vital clinical problem as vulnerable plaques tend to rupture, which results in atherosclerosis complications—myocardial infarctions and subsequent cardiovascular deaths. Therefore, methods aiming to stabilize such plaques are in great demand. In this brief review, the idea of atherosclerotic plaque stabilization and five main approaches—towards the regulation of metabolism, macrophages and cellular death, inflammation, reactive oxygen species, and extracellular matrix remodeling have been presented. Moreover, apart from classical approaches (targeted at the general mechanisms of plaque destabilization), there are also alternative approaches targeted either at certain plaques which have just become vulnerable or targeted at the minimization of the consequences of atherosclerotic plaque erosion or rupture. These alternative approaches have also been briefly mentioned in this review.

Keywords: atherosclerotic plaque; stabilization; vulnerable plaque; inflammation; macrophage; intravascular ultrasound; myocardial infarction; necrotic cores; cell death

Citation: Kowara, M.; Cudnoch-Jedrzejewska, A. Different Approaches in Therapy Aiming to Stabilize an Unstable Atherosclerotic Plaque. *Int. J. Mol. Sci.* **2021**, *22*, 4354. https://doi.org/10.3390/ijms22094354

Academic Editor: Eva Kassi

Received: 28 February 2021
Accepted: 14 April 2021
Published: 21 April 2021

Publisher's Note: MDPI stays neutral with regard to jurisdictional claims in published maps and institutional affiliations.

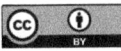

Copyright: © 2021 by the authors. Licensee MDPI, Basel, Switzerland. This article is an open access article distributed under the terms and conditions of the Creative Commons Attribution (CC BY) license (https://creativecommons.org/licenses/by/4.0/).

1. Introduction

Atherosclerotic plaque is the pathophysiological basis of ischemic heart disease–a widespread disease in both developed and developing countries [1]. A principal complication of ischemic heart disease is myocardial infarction, which constitutes the main cause of mortality worldwide [2]. Myocardial infarction is a consequence of the sudden occlusion of the coronary artery supplying the myocardial tissue, which is caused mainly (75% of the time) by atherosclerotic plaque rupture and thrombus generation [3–5]. This deficiency in the oxygen supply leads to myocardial cell damage and necrosis which compromises the entire heart activity and might result in ion current disturbances leading to life-threatening ventricular arrhythmias [6,7]. The development of atherosclerotic plaque is a long process composed of several stages (Figure 1).

Briefly, apo-B containing lipoproteins (especially LDL) pass through the endothelial layer of the arterial intima and accumulate within the subendothelial area where they are endocytosed by intimal macrophages. Simultaneously, local blood flow disturbances (non-linear flow) in atherosclerosis-susceptible regions (e.g., arterial branches) cause decreased shear stress that is detected by the endothelial cells in the process of mechanotransduction. These processes change the microenvironment of the arterial wall intima, which promotes subsequent alterations—foam cell generation, vascular smooth muscle cell migration, and their conversion from contractile into the synthetic phenotype, extracellular matrix remodeling, plaque growth, fibrous cap formation, and finally, necrotic core formation and calcifications [8,9]. In addition, Peter Libby emphasized the crucial role of the immune system in atherogenesis [10]. Many plaques develop into stable structures which manifest clinically as chronic coronary syndrome, but some of them undergo special ultrastructural alterations making them prone to rupture. Such plaques are called 'unstable' or 'vulnerable' [11]. According to the classic definition created by Virmani, vulnerable plaque is a thin-cap fibroatheroma (TCFA), characterized by a necrotic core presence with an overlying fibrous cap of thickness <65 μm [12]. The processes leading to plaque destabilization, i.e., apoptosis of VSMC within the fibrous cap, neovascularization, and necrotic core enlargement, are presented in Figure 2 [13].

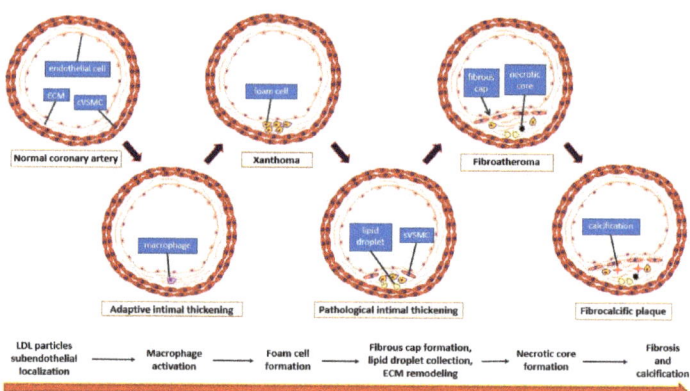

Figure 1. Stages of atherosclerotic plaque development (according to the Virmani classification [6]). cVSMC: vascular smooth muscle cell, contractile phenotype; sVSMC: vascular smooth muscle cell, synthetic phenotype; ECM: extracellular matrix.

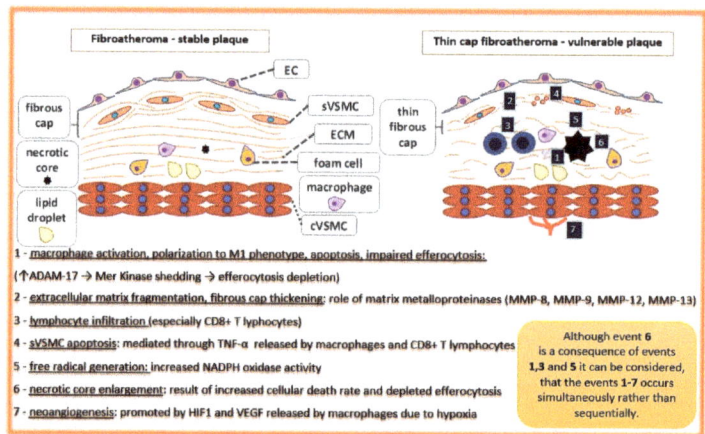

Figure 2. Pathophysiological processes and events leading to atherosclerotic plaque destabilization (events 1–7 in blue boxes). EC: endothelial cell; cVSMC: vascular smooth muscle cell, contractile phenotype; sVSMC: vascular smooth muscle cell, synthetic phenotype; ECM: extracellular matrix.

The occurrence of major cardiovascular adverse events (MACE—composite endpoint composed of death from cardiac causes, cardiac arrest, myocardial infarction, or rehospitalization because of unstable or progressive angina) relies on the presence of vulnerable plaques. A PROSPECT study on 697 patients with acute coronary syndrome treated with PCI revealed that the cumulative rate of MACE during a three-year follow-up referred to untreated, non-culprit lesions was significantly and independently correlated with the presence of thin-cap fibroatheroma on intravascular ultrasonography [14]. Therefore, therapies aimed at promoting atherosclerotic plaque stabilization would be warranted. However, because thin-cap fibroatheromas and stable fibroatheromas can transform into one another and the occurrence of vulnerable atherosclerotic plaque might be underestimated in clinical studies due to clinical silence, the optimal therapy aimed at stabilizing plaques should be concentrated on the promotion of molecular stabilizing pathways 'in general' rather than on the stabilization of certain atherosclerotic lesions (considered vulnerable on imaging) [15]. In this review, we summarize the crucial approaches towards plaque stabilization, and we present the clinical studies based on them.

2. General Considerations

Antiatherosclerotic properties are important features of certain drugs or chemical compounds. Indeed, a plethora of different substances—from precisely targeted molecules to traditional Chinese medicinal herbs, nutrients, or even gases such as hydrogen have been extensively investigated in search of their potentially beneficial impact on atherosclerotic plaques [16–19]. The animal models widely used in such investigations are genetically modified (ApoE−/− or LDL−/−) mice as well as WHHL (Watanabe-heritable hyperlipidemic) rabbits [20,21]. In such investigations, a vulnerable atherosclerotic plaque is obtained through dietary modification (i.e., high-fat diets containing high cholesterol) together with interventions such as angiotensin II infusion via an osmotic pump, cast placement around the common carotid artery, or balloon injury (in rabbits) [22,23]. Then, the animals are divided into a control group (receiving a saline solution) and the experimental group (receiving the study compound). When the study is finished, the vulnerable plaque indicators are assessed by immunohistochemical analysis in both animal groups. Although many preclinically investigated compounds have presented antiatherosclerotic features, only a minority of them have been proven to be clinically relevant. This situation occurs not only due to dissimilarities between the pathophysiology of atherosclerotic plaque development in animals and humans but also because of the difficulties in the design and performance of applicable clinical studies. Nevertheless, experiments with animal models make it possible to investigate different approaches towards plaque stabilization.

3. Approaches Directed at Specific Molecular Pathways

3.1. Approach towards Regulation of Metabolism

Knowledge about vulnerable atherosclerotic plaque development makes it possible to investigate whether therapies targeted at specific molecular pathways are able to stabilize it. One kind of such therapy is directed towards the modulation of metabolism. Oxidized low-density lipoproteins are considered to be crucial elements in the process of plaque initiation and progression; therefore, interventions aiming to decrease their level are considered plaque-stabilizing. Lipid-lowering agents, such as statins (hydroxymethylglutaryl-CoA synthase, i.e., cholesterol-synthesizing enzyme inhibitors), ezetimibe (an inhibitor of intestinal cholesterol absorption and Niemann-Pick C1-Like 1 antagonist), and alirocumab (antibody blocking proprotein convertase subtilisin/kexin type 9 and increasing LDL–LDLR recycling) improved atherosclerotic plaque stability in different animal models [21,24–26]. Contrary to the LDL particles, high-density lipoproteins (HDL) are considered atheroprotective because of reverse cholesterol transport promotion from lesional macrophages to the liver via interaction with the ATP-binding cassette transporter ABCA1 [27]. It has been demonstrated that recombinant HDL particles (especially Milano type rather than wild-type) promote plaque stability by decreasing intraplaque MMP-2 activity and the chemokine MCP-1 level when compared with a placebo in atherosclerotic New Zealand White rabbits [28]. The cholesteryl ester transfer protein (CETP) inhibitor anacetrapib, which increases HDL levels in serum, also presented similar antiatherosclerotic properties in mice [29]. However, even preclinical studies have demonstrated that LDL level reduction is more important in atherosclerotic plaque stabilization than an increase in HDL [30]. Apart from the lipids, glucose at higher concentrations also participates in the destabilization of atherosclerotic plaque. A study on diabetic ApoE−/− mice showed that hyperglycemia destabilizes the plaque via the inhibition of AMPKα and its target gene, prolyl-4-hydroxylase alpha 1 (P4Hα1), an enzyme participating in collagen synthesis [31]. In consequence, hypoglycemic medications are supposed to be plaque-stabilizing and are therefore antiatherosclerotic agents.

3.2. Approach towards Macrophages and Cellular Death Mechanisms

Macrophages contribute significantly to the process of atherosclerotic plaque destabilization. On the one hand, they orchestrate different, sometimes opposite, reactions and molecular pathways within the plaque microenvironment, promoting either plaque instability (M1 subpopulation) or plaque stability (M2 subpopulation) [32]. On the other hand, their conversion into lipid-laden foam cells and subsequent cellular death (in particular through necrosis or necroptosis, i.e., programmed necrosis) lead directly to necrotic core enlargement and plaque destabilization [33]. The situation is different when macrophages undergo typical programmed cellular death, i.e., apoptosis, which can be even atheroprotective in the initial phase of plaque development [34]. However, for plaque stability, it is necessary that the apoptotic bodies are robustly cleared through efferocytosis [35]. Another mechanism of cellular death that prevents plaque destabilization is autophagy, in which damaged organelles or cellular compartments are sequestrated into double-membrane structures called autophagosomes and then degraded by lysosomes [36]. Therefore, molecular pathways preventing macrophage conversion into foam cells or necrosis, as well as pathways promoting autophagy and appropriate clearance of apoptotic bodies (efferocytosis), may be atheroprotective. A study has demonstrated that ApoE−/− mice receiving arglabine, an NLRP3 antagonist which redirects macrophages towards autophagic pathways, presented a decreased level of IL-1β (a marker of inflammation) in plasma and reduced atherosclerotic lesions when compared with ApoE−/− mice from the control group [37]. For appropriate efferocytosis, a Mer Tyrosine Kinase (MerTK) expressed on the macrophage surface is required and pathways, which promote MerTK shedding from a membrane to the soluble form, impair this process. For instance, angiotensin II negatively affects efferocytosis through ADAM17 activation and subsequent MerTK shedding [38]. Apart from the aspects of cellular death, interventions preventing macrophage conversion into foam cells (such as inhibition of LOX-1, a receptor recognizing and internalizing oxLDL particles) as well as reverse cholesterol transport promotion in foam cells via LXRα receptor activation have been demonstrated to be atheroprotective in animal models [39–41].

3.3. Approach toward Inflammation and Immune Reactions

Vulnerable atherosclerotic plaques are characterized by a robust infiltration of different immune cells. Activation of lesional macrophages causes the production and secretion of diverse interleukins and chemokines, which subsequently drive immune cell infiltration [42,43]. Chemokines recruit neutrophils (CCL2) and T cells (CX3CL1, in more advanced lesions), whereas interleukins, such as IL-1β, activate those cells. Moreover, the immune cells transport through the endothelial layer (diapedesis) depend on adhesive molecules, such as ICAM-1 and VCAM-1. Significant augmentation of T cells (especially CD8+, i.e., cytotoxic T cells) has been observed within atherosclerotic plaque in vulnerable plaque specimens (derived from a biobank of human aortas covering the full spectrum of atherosclerotic disease) [44]. Therefore, antagonizing immune reactions responsible for the inflammatory state within the plaque would be an interesting therapeutic option [45]. As anticipated, inhibition of proinflammatory interleukins (such as IL-6) and chemokines (such as CXCL10) results in atherosclerotic plaque stabilization [46,47]. Interestingly, IL-1β inhibition over the entire time of plaque development in a mouse model resulted in a reduction in atherosclerotic plaque formation, but when such therapy was applied in mice with advanced lesions (from 18 to 24 weeks), not only was it not atheroprotective, but it also resulted in an increased number of macrophages within the plaque and abrogated beneficial remodeling [48,49]. This means that the entire system of interactions and reciprocal feedbacks during atherosclerotic plaque destabilization is very complex, and simple approaches (i.e., blocking factors that are considered to be proinflammatory) tend to be insufficient. For this reason, more general anti-inflammatory approaches are also used, for instance, colchicine, which has presented complex effects by inhibiting critical inflammatory signaling networks (inflammasome, proinflammatory cytokines, and adhesion molecules) [50,51]. Moreover, inflammatory mediators such as interleukins are under the control of transcription factors. For instance, an NF- B transcriptional factor is considered to be a crucial element of the inflammatory response, and many plaque-stabilizing effects induced by different substances are accompanied by NF-B suppression [52–54]. However, inflammatory pathways are also under the negative control of anti-inflammatory cytokines, and the promotion of anti-inflammatory pathways (e.g., genetic amplification of IL-37) presents a stabilizing effect on the plaque [55]. The cells responsible for the resolution of immune reactions are regulatory T cells (Tregs). It has been demonstrated in the ApoE−/− mouse model that pioglitazone (an antidiabetic drug belonging to the thiazolidinedione group) stabilized the atherosclerotic plaque, which was accompanied by an increase in the number of Tregs within the lesion [56]. Moreover, there is the innovative idea of using vaccines against atherosclerosis. In contrast to vaccines against infectious agents, vaccines against atherosclerosis aim to induce immune tolerance towards core antigens involved in atherosclerotic plaque development (such as ApoB-100 on oxLDL particles). The principal way to gain tolerance is Treg induction through the injections of peptides—fragments of the target antigen. An additional way for such vaccination is the generation of neutralizing autoantibodies, for instance, against PCSK9, which demonstrate antiatherosclerotic properties. These effects can be obtained with the use of special techniques such as the use of adjuvants, neoepitope development technologies, and vaccine platforms (e.g., Qβ bacteriophage virus-like particles) [57].

3.4. Approach towards Reactive Oxygen Species—Antioxidation Therapy

Reactive oxygen species play a pivotal role in atherosclerotic plaque progression and subsequent destabilization. They are generated mainly by enzymes, such as NADPH oxidases (NOX) localized within endothelial cells, fibroblasts, and vascular smooth muscle cells, and their expression is upregulated by proinflammatory factors such as IL-1β or Ang II [58,59]. First, reactive oxygen species cause lipid oxidation, which generates oxidized cholesterol derivatives such as 7-ketocholesterol (7-K) and 7β hydroxycholesterol (7β-OH). These compounds insert themselves into the cellular membrane and mediate a plethora of subsequent pathways inducing endothelial pump dysfunction, cell cycle blockade, and lysosomal or endoplasmic reticulum membrane damage in different cells (especially macrophages), leading to their apoptosis [60]. Second, reactive oxygen species cause direct damage to the DNA and promote mechanisms of cellular death in that way [61]. Moreover, oxidized cholesterol derivatives (27-hydroxycholesterol and aldehyde 4-hydroxynonenal) increase prostaglandin E production, which further enhances proinflammatory cytokines and matrix-degrading enzymes (especially matrix metalloproteinase 9), increasing the risk of atherosclerotic plaque rupture [62]. Reactive oxygen species are reciprocally linked with immune reactions. On the one hand, their production is under the control of proinflammatory cytokines such as TNF-α. On the other hand, the products of ROS activity, such as oxidized cholesterol derivatives, promote the expression of proinflammatory cytokines, e.g., IL-1β, TNF-α, IL-8, or chemokine MCP-1, as has been demonstrated in ApoE−/− mice lacking TNF-α and the human monocytic cell lines (U937 and THP-1) [63,64]. It is clear that the overproduction of reactive oxygen species is detrimental for the cells within the atherosclerotic plaque, and pathways induced by these agents may destabilize the plaque, leading to its rupture [65]. Therefore, pharmacological interventions leading to the neutralization of reactive oxygen species (either directly, in different mechanisms of antioxidation, or indirectly, by the abrogation of their generation) would be beneficial in atherosclerotic plaque stabilization. Interestingly, antioxidants are important food components, which leads to the idea that diet can be atheroprotective and plaque-stabilizing in that way. Indeed, many preclinical investigations on different nutrients have proven their stabilizing potential upon atherosclerotic plaque (such as soy isoflavones, vitamin E, carotenes, or xanthines) [66–69]. For example, ApoE−/− mice fed on blackberry extract rich with anthocyanin presented increased HDL levels and increased connective tissue content within the plaque, resulting in improved plaque stability when compared with the control group [70]. Moreover, the effect of stabilizing atherosclerotic plaques was also achieved by action on the controlling mechanisms; NOX2 (NADPH oxidase isoform 2, ROS generator) inhibition resulted in plaque stabilization, whereas Hsp70 (a protective chaperone) silencing resulted in plaque destabilization [71,72].

3.5. Approach towards Extracellular Matrix Remodeling and Neovascularization

It has to be emphasized that the entire plaque structure is based on scaffolding, i.e., an extracellular matrix (ECM) composed of collagens, elastin, proteoglycans, and fibronectin. These proteins constitute the connective tissue of the plaque. A fibrous cap, i.e., structure covering the plaque and maintaining its stability, is built up with vascular smooth muscle cells and macrophages embedded in collagen and elastin fibers. The appropriate, compact, and organized structure of the ECM component is crucial for plaque stability. Therefore, the influence on ECM protein synthesis or regulation by different methods (including miRNA) affects plaque stability [73–75]. The ECM structure is regulated by proteases—cathepsins, serine proteases, and metalloproteinases—matrix metalloproteinases (MMPs), α-disintegrin, metalloproteinases (ADAMs), and α-disintegrin and metalloproteinases with thrombospondin domains (ADAMTSs). Although all the proteases perform ECM protein hydrolysis, this site-specific hydrolysis results in different changes within the scaffold—some alterations lead towards ECM fragmentation, and other alterations lead towards strengthening restructuring [76,77]. Therefore, some proteases stabilize the plaque (like ADAM15), and other proteases destabilize it (such as virtually all MMPs, especially MMP-9) [78,79]. A histological study on human carotid artery specimens has revealed that a more vulnerable plaque phenotype correlated with an increased MMP-14 level and a decreased TIMP-3 (an inhibitor of tissue metalloproteinase) level [80]. Finally, vulnerable plaques are also characterized by neovascularization and proangiogenic factors (such as bFGF or CD137), which are supposed to play a role in plaque destabilization [81–84]. An optical coherence tomography study on 53 patients has shown an increase in intraplaque neovessel volume in vulnerable and ruptured plaques [85]. In consequence, therapies targeting intraplaque angiogenesis (e.g., axitinib—an inhibitor of VEGF receptor-1, -2, and -3) are considered to be plaque-stabilizing [86,87].

3.6. Specific Approaches—Summary

The abovementioned specific approaches are illustrated in Figure 3.

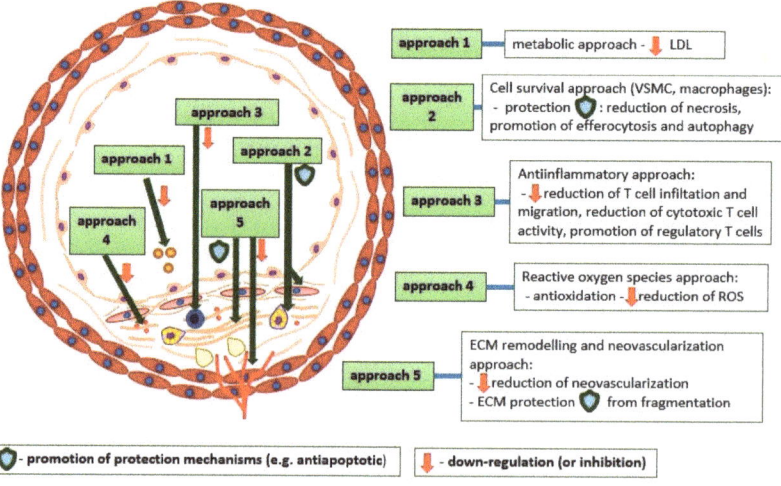

Figure 3. The approaches towards atherosclerotic plaque stabilization therapy and their molecular aspects.

Many different studies have already been conducted to explore specific approaches towards atherosclerotic plaque destabilization. Some examples of such preclinical studies have been presented in the text; others are presented in Table 1.

Table 1. Examples of atherosclerotic plaque stabilization treatment (five main approaches) in preclinical models and used drugs.

Approaches	Examples and Mechanisms	Investigated Drugs *
Metabolic approach	LDL lowering therapy: (a) Targeting HMG-CoA [21]; (b) Targeting cholesterol absorption [24]; (c) Enhancing LDL clearance [26].	(a) statins (e.g., lovastatin, rosuwastatin, atorvastatin, and pitavastatin); (b) ezetimibe; (c) PCSK9 inhibitors (alirocumab).
	Recombinant HDL particles [28]	75 mg/kg of apoA-I(Milano)
	Iron depletion → increased iron mobilization from macrophages [88,89]	Iron chelation therapy (deferasirox)
	MGL depletion → 2-AG ↑, CB2R activation [90]	N/A (genetic knock-out organisms used in this experiment)
Cell survival promotion approach	(a) Promotion of macrophage autophagy [38]; (b) Efficient efferocytosis of apoptotic bodies [36].	(a) trehalose (disaccharide); (b) AT1R blocker (losartan).
	(a) Inhibition of foam cell formation (e.g., LOX-1 inhibition) [40]; (b) Inhibition of endopasmatic reticulum (ER) stress [91].	(a) Different drugs which caused LOX-1 inhibition (e.g., Resveratrol, tanshinone II-A, and berberine); (b) 4-phenyl butyric acid (PBA)—a chemical chaperone).
	STAT6 upregulation → M2 macrophage polarization [92]	N/A (overexpression by recombinant pcDNA)
	Prevention from excessive PARP1 activation by severe DNA damage → prevention from ATP depletion [93]	For example, 3-Aminobenzamide (3-AB), doxycycline, thieno(2,3-c)isoquinolin-5-one (TIQ-A)
Anti-inflammatory approach	(a) Chemokine inhibition (e.g., CCL5 and CXCL10 via TWEAK blockade) [94]; (b) Cell adhesion molecule (e.g., VCAM-1) inhibition [95].	(a) anti-TWEAK mAb, maraviroc (CCR5 antagonist) [96]; (b) chalcone derivate (1m–6).
	(a) Proinflammatory cytokine (e.g., IL-6, IL-12, IL-17, IL-18) inhibition [46,97,98]; (b) Anti-inflammatory cytokine (such as IL-10, IL-37) promotion [55,99].	(a) For example, IL-6 neutralizing antibody (toclizumab); (b) For example, dietary nitrate (L-arginine).
	Cytotoxic CD8 + T lymphocyte (Tc) depletion [100]	CD8α or CD8β targeted monoclonal antibody
	Regulatory T lymphocyte (Treg) promotion [101]	For example, IL-2, mycophenolate mofetil, vitamin D, rapamycin, G-CSF
Reactive oxygen species approaches	Downregulation of ROS generators (e.g., NADPH oxidases NOX2) [71]	Nox2 inhibitor peptide (a chimeric 18-amino acid peptide)
	Attenuation of ROS derivative (e.g., 7β-OH) activity [60].	N/A (indirect methods like conjugation by glutathione)
	Promotion of ROS scavengers (such as HO-1 induced by Nrf transcriptional factor) [102]	N/A
	Direct ROS abruption (e.g., polyphenols) [103]	Different polyphenols (in this study–apple polyphenols)

Table 1. Cont.

Approaches	Examples and Mechanisms	Investigated Drugs *
ECM remodeling and neovascularization approach	Inhibition of matrix metalloproteinase (MMPs) synthesis and activity (especially MMP9) [104]	Ghrelin
	Promotion of collagen synthesis (e.g., by melatonin through Akt phosphorylation and subsequent P4Hα1 upregulation) [105]	Dietary nitrate treatment (KNO_3 or KNO_2)
	Influence on fibronectin (e.g., blockade of fibronectin-integrin α5 pathway) [106]	In vivo knockdown of phosphodiesterase 4D5 (siRNA)
	Inhibition of neovascularization (e.g., through bFGF blockade) [107]	K5 (a small molecule bFGF-inhibitor)

Abbreviations: MGL: monoglyceride lipase; 2-AG: 2-arachidonoylglycerol (endocannabinoid); PBA: 4-phenylbutyric acid; mAb: monoclonal antibody. * if applicable (in some studies, transgenic organisms were used to investigate specific cellular pathways).

4. An Integrated Approach

Atherosclerotic plaque destabilization is a complex process depending on many different pathways. Therefore, the concept that plaque-stabilizing therapy should target diverse pathways and pathophysiological processes simultaneously is reasonable. For instance, alkaloid berberine has a stabilizing effect on atherosclerotic plaques by the suppression of the ECM regulators MMP9 and EMMPRIN (MMP9 inducer), by autophagy promotion in macrophages, and by promoting antioxidative activity via PPARγ activation (the last effect observed in hyperhomocysteinemia mice) [108,109]. In fact, many agents considered primarily as 'specifically targeted' have turned out to be pleiotropic, e.g., lipid-lowering statins or hypoglycemic drugs. As an example, insulin has an anti-inflammatory and plaque-stabilizing effect via the PI3K-Akt pathway, which inhibits the TLR4 MyD88-NF-B signaling pathway, which was demonstrated using the RAW264.3 monocyte-macrophage lineage [110]. However, the essence of the integrated approach is to target key regulators—transcription factors or common elements of molecular pathways. Accurate examples are statins that inhibit mevalonic acid synthesis (by HMG-CoA blockade), causing subsequent inhibition of isoprenoid intermediates—farnesyl pyrophosphate (FPP) and geranylgeranyl pyrophosphate (GGPP) synthesis. These isoprenoid intermediates serve as lipid attachments necessary for the appropriate activity of small GTPases, especially Ras and Rho, which regulate many cellular pathways. The Rho protein activates Rho kinases (ROCK), which decrease eNOS synthesis and abolish the atheroprotective PI3K-Akt signaling pathway, whereas Rac1 (a member of the Rho subfamily) activates the nicotinamide adenine dinucleotide phosphate (NADPH) oxidase, which is responsible for reactive oxygen species (ROS) generation. As a result, statins induce anti-inflammatory effects (a decrease in proinflammatory cytokines, e.g., IL-6, IL-8, or MCP-1, and adhesive molecule expression, enhancement of Treg and reduction in Th17 lymphocyte differentiation), ECM stabilizing effects (through matrix metalloproteinases reduction), and antioxidative effects (inhibition of ROS generation) [111,112]. Another example of such an integrative approach is the targeting of lipoprotein-associated phospholipase A2 (Lp-PLA2) by its inhibitor, darapladib. Lp-PLA2 generates lysophosphatidic acid, which increases MMP9 production by the NF-B signaling pathway and simultaneously increases plaque inflammation (by mast cell activation and monocyte recruitment), leading to atherosclerotic plaque destabilization [113,114]. For this reason, Lp-PLA2 inhibition resulted in plaque stabilization in animal models [115]. The aforementioned approaches are addressed towards proteins that regulate diverse molecular pathways, but there is a different option—targeting epigenetic mechanisms driving gene expression. One such method is the usage of RNA interference—proteins are translated from their respective mRNA particles, which can be degraded by RISC complexes, composed of microRNA (miRNA) particles complementary to the corresponding mRNAs. MicroRNAs regulate virtually all stages of atherosclerotic plaque progression by downregulation of the corresponding mRNAs [116]. Some miRNA induces a stabilizing effect on the plaque structure, for instance, miR-520c-3p—a downregulator of RelA/p65 (NF-B subunit) or miR 181b-5p—a downregulator of NOTCH1 (a promoter of proinflammatory M1 macrophages) [117,118]. In contrast, an example of destabilizing miRNA is miR-124-3p [31,119]. Therefore, an application of agonists (agomirs) of stabilizing miRNAs or antagonists (antagomirs) of destabilizing miRNAs could prevent plaque vulnerability [120]. However, there is another method of an integrative approach promoting atherosclerotic plaque stability—the influence on gene expression through changes in chromatin compaction. DNA strands are wrapped onto nucleosomes built up from histones. Histone acetylation (performed by HATs—histone acetyltransferases) and histone deacetylation (performed by HDACs—histone deacetylases) regulate gene expression making them more or less accessible to RNA polymerase [121]. For instance, HDAC9 increases MMP-1 and MMP-2 expression and toll-like receptor (TLR) signaling at the histone level, and its deficiency or blockade results in inflammation resolution and plaque stabilization [122]. Sirtuins are regulators which also act as histone deacetylases. For example, SIRT2 exerts plaque-stabilizing effects by the inhibition of macrophage polarization towards the M1 phenotype and reduction in iNOS activity. These effects can be induced by Resveratrol, a SIRT2 agonist [123,124]. In summary, an integrative approach (the concept illustrated in Figure 4) makes it possible to have a wide range of effects upon the entire plaque and change its phenotype.

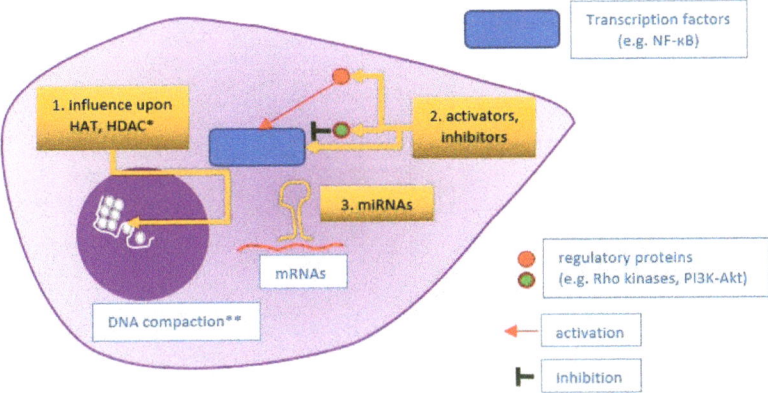

Figure 4. Idea of an integrative approach towards atherosclerotic plaque stabilization. 1. Influence upon mechanisms that are responsible for chromatin compaction and DNA accessibility for transcription machinery; 2. Activation or inhibition of transcription factors, regulating gene expression in the nucleus; 3. Influence upon miRNAs, i.e., particles that inhibit specific mRNA particles in the mechanism of complementarity. * HAT: histone acetyltransferase; HDAC: histone deacetylase; ** DNA compaction relies on nucleosome methylation or acetylation (regulated by HATs and HDACs).

5. Clinical Studies Conforming Plaque Stabilization

Numerous preclinical studies have confirmed the plaque-stabilizing effect of different approaches (as mentioned above). However, the promising results of studies on animal models have not been reflected in human clinical studies. There are several explanations for this, i.e., differences in the pathophysiological process of atherosclerotic plaque destabilization (guided by different genes) and in cellular subsets (such as the macrophage population) between laboratory animals and humans, different experimental conditions, and natural diversities in the human population [125–127]. Large clinical studies on medicines in the therapy of atherosclerosis particularly concentrate on clinical endpoints—especially mortality, mortality due to cardiovascular reasons, and MACE (a composite endpoint composed of mortality, myocardial infarction, stroke). From this point of view, a canakinumab (anti-IL-1β antibody) given to patients with a previous myocardial infarction (CANTOS study) caused a significant reduction in recurrent cardiovascular events (a dose of 150 mg once a month, relative risk 0.85; 95%CI, 0.74 to 0.98, $p = 0.021$) compared with a placebo [128]. Similarly, colchicine (0.5 mg a day) given to patients after a myocardial infarction caused a significant reduction in composite endpoint (RR 0.77; 95%CI, 0.61 to 0.96, $p = 0.02$) and a marked significant reduction in recurrent myocardial infarction (RR 0.26; 95%CI, 0.1 to 0.7) in comparison with a placebo, which was demonstrated in the COLCOT study [129]. In contrast, a study called STABILITY with darapladib conducted on patients with stable coronary artery disease (without prior myocardial infarction) failed to demonstrate a statistical significance between the darapladib and placebo groups in reference to composite endpoint and mortality, although it showed a slight but significant reduction in major coronary events (9.3% vs. 10.3%, $p = 0.045$) [130]. Similarly, the CETP inhibitor anacetrapib causing an HDL increase demonstrated a slight but significant reduction in major coronary events (REVEAL study) [131]. However, to verify whether a certain type of therapy results in atherosclerotic plaque stabilization, it is necessary to visualize the plaques in the coronary arteries and assess their stability exponents. Methods that enable such visualization are intravascular ultrasound (IVUS) and OCT (optical coherence tomography). Studies in which atherosclerotic plaques were assessed in the light of stability are presented in Table 2 [132].

Table 2. Clinical studies with outcomes referring to atherosclerotic plaque stabilization visualized with imaging methods (IVUS or OCT).

STUDY NAME	Treatment	No. of Investigated Patients (Period)	Clinical Outcome (MACE, Mortality)	Plaque Stabilization Effect (IVUS or OCT)
GAIN [133] [1]	Atorvastatin (20–80 mg) vs. placebo	65 and 66 (12 months)	Any ischemic event: 21.5% vs. 31.8% ($p = 0.184$)	IVUS: Larger hyperechogenicity index 42.2% vs. 10.1%, $p = 0.021$
REVERSAL [134] [2]	Atorvastatin 80 mg (intensive lipid-lowering) vs. Pravastatin 40 mg (moderate lipid-lowering)	253 and 249 (18 months)	Death: 0.3% vs. 0.3%—NS Myocardial infarction: 1.2% vs. 2.1%—NS	IVUS: Lower percent atheroma volume change 0.2% vs. 1.6%, $p < 0.001$
PRECISE-IVUS [37] [3]	Atorvastatin * + ezetimibe (10 mg) vs. Atorvastatin * alone	102 and 100 (9–12 months)	Cardiovascular events ** 11% vs. 14%—NS	IVUS: Change in normalized TAV −6.6% vs. −1.4%, $p < 0.001$
GLAGOV [135] [4]	Statin *** + PCSK9i (evolocumab 420 mg monthly) vs. Statin *** alone	423 and 423 (19 months)	Death: 0.6% vs. 0.8%—NS Non-fatal myocardial infarction: 2.1% vs 2.9%—NS	IVUS: Change in TAV −5.8% vs. −0.9%, $p < 0.001$
Christoph et al. [136]	Pioglitazone (30 mg) vs. Placebo	27 and 27 (9 months)	Insignificant differences, no MACE registered	VH-IVUS: Decrease in the necrotic core −1.3% vs. + 2.6%, $p = 0.008$
Tondapu et al. [137]	Rosuvastatin (10 mg) vs. Atorvastatin (20 mg)	24 and 19 (12 months)	Not applicable	OCT: Increased FCT **** 171.5 vs. 127.0 μm, $p = 0.03$; Decreased macrophages

[1] German Atorvastatin Intravascular Ultrasound Study Investigators; [2] Reversal of Atherosclerosis with Aggressive Lipid Lowering Study; [3] Plaque Regression With Cholesterol Absorption Inhibitor or Synthesis Inhibitor Evaluated by Intravascular Ultrasound; [4] Global Assessment of Plaque Regression With a PCSK9 Antibody as Measured by Intravascular Ultrasound. * Atorvastatin dose adequate for efficient lipid-lowering with target LDL < 70 mg/dL; ** Cardiovascular events—mainly revascularizations of de novo lesions, no cases of death during follow-up in this study; *** Statin dose adequate for efficient lipid lowering with target LDL < 80 mg/dL (or <60 mg/dL, in case of additional risk factors); **** similar baseline fibrous cap thickness in both groups (61.4 μm in rosuvastatin group and 60.8 μm in atorvastatin group); IVUS: intravascular ultrasound; VH-IVUS: virtual histology-intravascular ultrasound; OCT: optical coherence tomography; TAV: total atheroma volume; FCT: fibrous cap thickness.

6. Alternative Approaches

This review so far has presented approaches towards atherosclerotic plaque stabilization directed at general mechanisms—the enhancement of stabilizing pathways and the inhibition of destabilizing pathways. In this section, alternative approaches are discussed. As presented above, stable and vulnerable atherosclerotic plaques can transform into one another [15]. Nevertheless, approaches towards the stabilization of concrete and already developed unstable plaque are also under investigation. Examples of such therapies are photodynamic therapy (PDT), plasmonic photothermal therapy (PPTT), cytotoxic chemotherapy, and sonodynamic therapy (SDT) [16,138]. In PDT, administered photosensitizers accumulate within the atherosclerotic plaque (e.g., cross-linked dextran-coated iron oxide (CLIO) nanoparticles which accumulate in macrophages). Then, irradiation of the structure by NIR (near-infrared) causes free radical generation and a cytotoxic effect upon the macrophages (mainly from the M1 subset, dominating in a vulnerable structure), resulting in plaque stabilization. PPTT is quite similar to PDT, but in this method, photoabsorbers (e.g., gold nanoparticles) generate heat when irradiated by NIR. In cytotoxic chemotherapy, special agents are encapsulated in nanomedical liposomes (e.g., prednisolone phosphate) or other formulas such as hyaluronic acid-polypyrrole nanoparticles (e.g., doxorubicin), which make it possible for them to accumulate precisely within the plaque and exert their action. Finally, SDT compounds called sonosensitizers (such as curcumin) localize within the plaque and generate free radicals after exposure to ultrasound. Therefore, SDT is similar to PDT, but ultrasound waves penetrate more deeply than NIR. The principles of the abovementioned methods are illustrated in Figure 5.

Some clinical trials using the abovementioned methods in the therapy of atherosclerotic plaque have already been undertaken [139]. For instance, the NANOM-FIM trial has demonstrated that a group of patients who received silica-gold nanoparticles with subsequent PPTT presented a significantly higher probability of event-free survival than the control group (91.7% vs. 80%) who only received a drug-eluting stent [140]. Moreover, new discoveries such as quantum dots may enable high precision therapy with pre-selected cells introduced into the plaque [141].

In the discussion about approaches towards atherosclerotic plaque stabilization, it must be said that there is also a totally different option—not concentrating on plaque stabilization but rather on the minimization of the consequences of a plaque rupture. The idea of this approach is based on the hypothesis that it is difficult to precisely distinguish between stable and vulnerable atherosclerotic plaque, and microruptures or erosions might occur in many plaques considered to be stable. From that point of view, antithrombotic therapy could be crucial for the prevention of major cardiovascular events such as myocardial infarction because it inhibits clot generation and coronary artery obstruction in the case of a vulnerable plaque rupture or erosion [142]. Although aspirin (a 'classical' antithrombotic drug) has turned out to be beneficial in the primary prevention of myocardial infarction (ATT meta-analysis, 12% proportional reduction in serious cardiovascular events per year, $p = 0.0001$), it significantly increased the risk of major gastrointestinal and intracranial bleeding [143]. Therefore, the guidelines (similar to many ESC guidelines) consider aspirin to be a tool for secondary, but not primary, prevention of myocardial infarction.

Finally, approaches towards some pathways in atherosclerotic plaque destabilization still remain controversial, such as targeting pathways involved in plaque calcification (regulated by, for example, oncostatin M). Currently, it is supposed that although plaque macrocalcifications (as in fibrocalcific plaque) increase plaque stability, microcalcifications tend to destabilize the plaque [144].

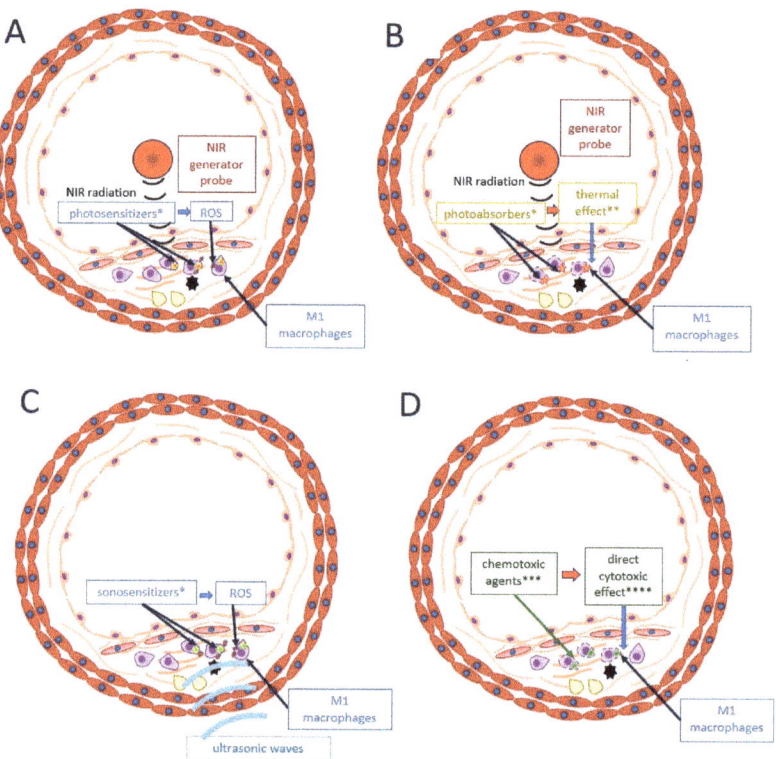

Figure 5. Alternative approaches towards atherosclerotic plaque stabilization targeted at concretely already developed vulnerable plaques. (**A**) photodynamic therapy (PDT); (**B**) plasmonic photothermal therapy (PPTT); (**C**) sonodynamic therapy; (**D**) cytotoxic chemotherapy. * photosensitizer, photoabsorber, or sonosensitizer previously injected into the organism, then accumulated within plaque macrophages; ** effects inducing apoptosis or other forms of cellular death; *** chemotoxic agents encapsulated in nanoformulas and targeted specifically to macrophages; **** apoptosis, necrosis, necroptosis. ROS: reactive oxygen species; NIR: near-infrared.

7. Conclusions

In summary, atherosclerotic plaque stabilization is a promising therapy for the reduction in cardiovascular disease burden. Although many interesting discoveries and approaches have already been discovered, there is still a lack of clinically proven methods that enable maintaining the stability of virtually all of the atherosclerotic plaques in a patient. Moreover, many aspects of plaque vulnerability are still controversial and are waiting for a more profound explanation.

Author Contributions: Conceptualization, M.K. and A.C.-J.; resources, M.K. and A.C.-J.; writing M.K.; supervision, A.C.-J. All authors have read and agreed to the published version of the manuscript.

Funding: This research received no external funding.

Conflicts of Interest: The authors declare no conflict of interest.

References

1. Malakar, A.K.; Choudhury, D.; Halder, B.; Paul, P.; Uddin, A.; Chakraborty, S. A review on coronary artery disease, its risk factors, and therapeutics. *J. Cell. Physiol.* **2019**, *234*, 16812–16823. [CrossRef] [PubMed]
2. Reed, G.W.; Rossi, J.E.; Cannon, C.P. Acute myocardial infarction. *Lancet* **2017**, *389*, 197–210. [CrossRef]
3. Frangogiannis, N.G. Pathophysiology of Myocardial Infarction. *Compr. Physiol.* **2015**, *5*, 1841–1875. [PubMed]

4. Tibaut, M.; Mekis, D.; Petrovic, D. Pathophysiology of Myocardial Infarction and Acute Management Strategies. *Cardiovasc. Hematol. Agents Med. Chem.* **2017**, *14*, 150–159. [CrossRef] [PubMed]
5. Kumar, A.; Cannon, C.P. Acute coronary syndromes: Diagnosis and management, part I. *Mayo Clin. Proc.* **2009**, *84*, 917–938. [CrossRef] [PubMed]
6. Aufderheide, T.P. Arrhythmias associated with acute myocardial infarction and thrombolysis. *Emerg. Med. Clin. N. Am.* **1998**, *16*, 583–600. [CrossRef]
7. Saleh, M.; Ambrose, J.A. Understanding myocardial infarction. *F1000Research* **2018**, *7*, 1378. [CrossRef] [PubMed]
8. Bentzon, J.F.; Otsuka, F.; Virmani, R.; Falk, E. Mechanisms of plaque formation and rupture. *Circ. Res.* **2014**, *114*, 1852–1866. [CrossRef] [PubMed]
9. Tabas, I.; Garcia-Cardena, G.; Owens, G.K. Recent insights into the cellular biology of atherosclerosis. *J. Cell Biol.* **2015**, *209*, 13–22. [CrossRef]
10. Geovanini, G.R.; Libby, P. Atherosclerosis and inflammation: Overview and updates. *Clin. Sci.* **2018**, *132*, 1243–1252. [CrossRef]
11. Khan, M.H.; Rochlani, Y.; Yandrapalli, S.; Aronow, W.S.; Frishman, W.H. Vulnerable Plaque: A Review of Current Concepts in Pathophysiology and Imaging. *Cardiol. Rev.* **2020**, *28*, 3–9. [CrossRef] [PubMed]
12. Virmani, R.; Burke, A.P.; Farb, A.; Kolodgie, F.D. Pathology of the vulnerable plaque. *J. Am. Coll. Cardiol.* **2006**, *47* (Suppl. 8), C13–C18. [CrossRef]
13. Silvestre-Roig, C.; de Winther, M.P.; Weber, C.; Daemen, M.J.; Lutgens, E.; Soehnlein, O. Atherosclerotic plaque destabilization: Mechanisms, models, and therapeutic strategies. *Circ. Res.* **2014**, *114*, 214–226. [CrossRef]
14. Stone, G.W.; Maehara, A.; Lansky, A.J.; de Bruyne, B.; Cristea, E.; Mintz, G.S.; Mehran, R.; McPherson, J.; Farhat, N.; Marso, S.P.; et al. A prospective natural-history study of coronary atherosclerosis. *N. Engl. J. Med.* **2011**, *364*, 226–235. [CrossRef]
15. Arbab-Zadeh, A.; Fuster, V. The myth of the "vulnerable plaque": Transitioning from a focus on individual lesions to atherosclerotic disease burden for coronary artery disease risk assessment. *J. Am. Coll. Cardiol.* **2015**, *65*, 846–855. [CrossRef]
16. Zhang, Y.; Koradia, A.; Kamato, D.; Popat, A.; Little, P.J.; Ta, H.T. Treatment of atherosclerotic plaque: Perspectives on theranostics. *J. Pharm. Pharmacol.* **2019**, *71*, 1029–1043. [CrossRef] [PubMed]
17. Yuan, R.; Shi, W.L.; Xin, Q.Q.; Chen, K.J.; Cong, W.H. Holistic Regulation of Angiogenesis with Chinese Herbal Medicines as a New Option for Coronary Artery Disease. *Evid. Based Complement. Alternat. Med.* **2018**, *2018*, 3725962. [CrossRef]
18. Song, G.; Tian, H.; Qin, S.; Sun, X.; Yao, S.; Zong, C.; Luo, Y.; Liu, J.; Yu, Y.; Sang, H.; et al. Hydrogen decreases atherosusceptibility in apolipoprotein B-containing lipoproteins and aorta of apolipoprotein E knockout mice. *Atherosclerosis* **2012**, *221*, 55–65. [CrossRef] [PubMed]
19. Tuttolomondo, A.; Simonetta, I.; Daidone, M.; Mogavero, A.; Ortello, A.; Pinto, A. Metabolic and Vascular Effect of the Mediterranean Diet. *Int. J. Mol. Sci.* **2019**, *20*, 4716. [CrossRef]
20. Veseli, B.E.; Perrotta, P.; De Meyer, G.R.A.; Roth, L.; Van der Donckt, C.; Martinet, W.; De Meyer, G.R.Y. Animal models of atherosclerosis. *Eur. J. Pharmacol.* **2017**, *816*, 3–13. [CrossRef]
21. Shiomi, M.; Koike, T.; Ito, T. Contribution of the WHHL rabbit, an animal model of familial hypercholesterolemia, to elucidation of the anti-atherosclerotic effects of statins. *Atherosclerosis* **2013**, *231*, 39–47. [CrossRef]
22. Hartwig, H.; Silvestre-Roig, C.; Hendrikse, J.; Beckers, L.; Paulin, N.; Van der Heiden, K.; Braster, Q.; Drechsler, M.; Daemen, M.J.; Lutgens, E.; et al. Atherosclerotic Plaque Destabilization in Mice: A Comparative Study. *PLoS ONE* **2015**, *10*, e0141019. [CrossRef]
23. Jain, M.; Frobert, A.; Valentin, J.; Cook, S.; Giraud, M.N. The Rabbit Model of Accelerated Atherosclerosis: A Methodological Perspective of the Iliac Artery Balloon Injury. *J. Vis. Exp.* **2017**. [CrossRef]
24. Gomez-Garre, D.; Munoz-Pacheco, P.; Gonzalez-Rubio, M.L.; Aragoncillo, P.; Granados, R.; Fernandez-Cruz, A. Ezetimibe reduces plaque inflammation in a rabbit model of atherosclerosis and inhibits monocyte migration in addition to its lipid-lowering effect. *Br. J. Pharmacol.* **2009**, *156*, 1218–1227. [CrossRef] [PubMed]
25. Muller-Wieland, D.; Kotzka, J.; Krone, W. Stabilization of atherosclerotic plaque during lipid lowering. *Curr. Opin. Lipidol.* **1997**, *8*, 348–353. [CrossRef]
26. Kuhnast, S.; van der Hoorn, J.W.; Pieterman, E.J.; van den Hoek, A.M.; Sasiela, W.J.; Gusarova, V.; Peyman, A.; Schafer, H.L.; Schwahn, U.; Jukema, J.W.; et al. Alirocumab inhibits atherosclerosis, improves the plaque morphology, and enhances the effects of a statin. *J. Lipid Res.* **2014**, *55*, 2103–2112. [CrossRef] [PubMed]
27. Ouimet, M.; Barrett, T.J.; Fisher, E.A. HDL and Reverse Cholesterol Transport. *Circ. Res.* **2019**, *124*, 1505–1518. [CrossRef]
28. Ibanez, B.; Giannarelli, C.; Cimmino, G.; Santos-Gallego, C.G.; Alique, M.; Pinero, A.; Vilahur, G.; Fuster, V.; Badimon, L.; Badimon, J.J. Recombinant HDL(Milano) exerts greater anti-inflammatory and plaque stabilizing properties than HDL(wild-type). *Atherosclerosis* **2012**, *220*, 72–77. [CrossRef] [PubMed]
29. Kuhnast, S.; van der Tuin, S.J.; van der Hoorn, J.W.; van Klinken, J.B.; Simic, B.; Pieterman, E.; Havekes, L.M.; Landmesser, U.; Luscher, T.F.; Willems van Dijk, K.; et al. Anacetrapib reduces progression of atherosclerosis, mainly by reducing non-HDL-cholesterol, improves lesion stability and adds to the beneficial effects of atorvastatin. *Eur. Heart J.* **2015**, *36*, 39–48. [CrossRef] [PubMed]
30. Van Craeyveld, E.; Gordts, S.C.; Nefyodova, E.; Jacobs, F.; De Geest, B. Regression and stabilization of advanced murine atherosclerotic lesions: A comparison of LDL lowering and HDL raising gene transfer strategies. *J. Mol. Med.* **2011**, *89*, 555–567. [CrossRef] [PubMed]

31. Liang, W.J.; Zhou, S.N.; Shan, M.R.; Wang, X.Q.; Zhang, M.; Chen, Y.; Zhang, Y.; Wang, S.X.; Guo, T. AMPKalpha inactivation destabilizes atherosclerotic plaque in streptozotocin-induced diabetic mice through AP-2alpha/miRNA-124 axis. *J. Mol. Med.* **2018**, *96*, 403–412. [CrossRef] [PubMed]
32. Barrett, T.J. Macrophages in Atherosclerosis Regression. *Arterioscler. Thromb. Vasc. Biol.* **2020**, *40*, 20–33. [CrossRef]
33. Kavurma, M.M.; Rayner, K.J.; Karunakaran, D. The walking dead: Macrophage inflammation and death in atherosclerosis. *Curr. Opin. Lipidol.* **2017**, *28*, 91–98. [CrossRef] [PubMed]
34. Babaev, V.R.; Yeung, M.; Erbay, E.; Ding, L.; Zhang, Y.; May, J.M.; Fazio, S.; Hotamisligil, G.S.; Linton, M.F. Jnk1 Deficiency in Hematopoietic Cells Suppresses Macrophage Apoptosis and Increases Atherosclerosis in Low-Density Lipoprotein Receptor Null Mice. *Arterioscler. Thromb. Vasc. Biol.* **2016**, *36*, 1122–1131. [CrossRef]
35. Linton, M.F.; Tao, H.; Linton, E.F.; Yancey, P.G. SR-BI: A Multifunctional Receptor in Cholesterol Homeostasis and Atherosclerosis. *Trends Endocrinol. Metab.* **2017**, *28*, 461–472. [CrossRef]
36. Evans, T.D.; Jeong, S.J.; Zhang, X.; Sergin, I.; Razani, B. TFEB and trehalose drive the macrophage autophagy-lysosome system to protect against atherosclerosis. *Autophagy* **2018**, *14*, 724–726. [CrossRef]
37. Abderrazak, A.; Couchie, D.; Mahmood, D.F.; Elhage, R.; Vindis, C.; Laffargue, M.; Mateo, V.; Buchele, B.; Ayala, M.R.; El Gaafary, M.; et al. Anti-inflammatory and antiatherogenic effects of the NLRP3 inflammasome inhibitor arglabin in ApoE2.Ki mice fed a high-fat diet. *Circulation* **2015**, *131*, 1061–1070. [CrossRef]
38. Zhang, Y.; Wang, Y.; Zhou, D.; Zhang, L.S.; Deng, F.X.; Shu, S.; Wang, L.J.; Wu, Y.; Guo, N.; Zhou, J.; et al. Angiotensin II deteriorates advanced atherosclerosis by promoting MerTK cleavage and impairing efferocytosis through the AT1R/ROS/p38 MAPK/ADAM17 pathway. *Am. J. Physiol. Cell Physiol.* **2019**, *317*, C776–C787. [CrossRef] [PubMed]
39. Feldmann, R.; Geikowski, A.; Weidner, C.; Witzke, A.; Kodelja, V.; Schwarz, T.; Gabriel, M.; Erker, T.; Sauer, S. Foam cell specific LXRalpha ligand. *PLoS ONE* **2013**, *8*, e57311. [CrossRef] [PubMed]
40. Kattoor, A.J.; Goel, A.; Mehta, J.L. LOX-1: Regulation, Signaling and Its Role in Atherosclerosis. *Antioxidants* **2019**, *8*, 218. [CrossRef] [PubMed]
41. Tian, K.; Ogura, S.; Little, P.J.; Xu, S.W.; Sawamura, T. Targeting LOX-1 in atherosclerosis and vasculopathy: Current knowledge and future perspectives. *Ann. N. Y. Acad. Sci.* **2019**, *1443*, 34–53. [CrossRef] [PubMed]
42. Weber, C.; Noels, H. Atherosclerosis: Current pathogenesis and therapeutic options. *Nat. Med.* **2011**, *17*, 1410–1422. [CrossRef]
43. Wolf, M.P.; Hunziker, P. Atherosclerosis: Insights into Vascular Pathobiology and Outlook to Novel Treatments. *J. Cardiovasc. Transl. Res.* **2020**, *13*, 744–757. [CrossRef]
44. van Dijk, R.A.; Duinisveld, A.J.; Schaapherder, A.F.; Mulder-Stapel, A.; Hamming, J.F.; Kuiper, J.; de Boer, O.J.; van der Wal, A.C.; Kolodgie, F.D.; V irmani, R.; et al. A change in inflammatory footprint precedes plaque instability: A systematic evaluation of cellular aspects of the adaptive immune response in human atherosclerosis. *J. Am. Heart Assoc.* **2015**, *4*, e001403. [CrossRef] [PubMed]
45. Sliva, J.; Charalambous, C.; Bultas, J.; Karetova, D. A new strategy for the treatment of atherothrombosis—Inhibition of inflammation. *Physiol. Res.* **2019**, *68* (Suppl. 1), S17–S30. [CrossRef] [PubMed]
46. Janssen, H.; Wagner, C.S.; Demmer, P.; Callies, S.; Solter, G.; Loghmani-khouzani, H.; Hu, N.; Schuett, H.; Tietge, U.J.; Warnecke, G.; et al. Acute perioperative-stress-induced increase of atherosclerotic plaque volume and vulnerability to rupture in apolipoprotein-E-deficient mice is amenable to statin treatment and IL-6 inhibition. *Dis. Model Mech.* **2015**, *8*, 1071–1080. [CrossRef] [PubMed]
47. Segers, D.; Lipton, J.A.; Leenen, P.J.; Cheng, C.; Tempel, D.; Pasterkamp, G.; Moll, F.L.; de Crom, R.; Krams, R. Atherosclerotic Plaque Stability Is Affected by the Chemokine CXCL10 in Both Mice and Humans. *Int. J. Inflam.* **2011**, *2011*, 936109. [CrossRef]
48. Gomez, D.; Baylis, R.A.; Durgin, B.G.; Newman, A.A.C.; Alencar, G.F.; Mahan, S.; St Hilaire, C.; Muller, W.; Waisman, A.; Francis, S.E.; et al. Interleukin-1beta has atheroprotective effects in advanced atherosclerotic lesions of mice. *Nat. Med.* **2018**, *24*, 1418–1429. [CrossRef]
49. Bhaskar, V.; Yin, J.; Mirza, A.M.; Phan, D.; Vanegas, S.; Issafras, H.; Michelson, K.; Hunter, J.J.; Kantak, S.S. Monoclonal antibodies targeting IL-1 beta reduce biomarkers of atherosclerosis in vitro and inhibit atherosclerotic plaque formation in Apolipoprotein E-deficient mice. *Atherosclerosis* **2011**, *216*, 313–320. [CrossRef] [PubMed]
50. Spartalis, M.; Spartalis, E.; Tzatzaki, E.; Tsilimigras, D.I.; Moris, D.; Kontogiannis, C.; Kaminiotis, V.V.; Paschou, S.A.; Chatzidou, S.; Siasos, G.; et al. The Beneficial Therapy with Colchicine for Atherosclerosis via Anti-inflammation and Decrease in Hypertriglyceridemia. *Cardiovasc. Hematol. Agents Med. Chem.* **2018**, *16*, 74–80. [CrossRef] [PubMed]
51. Cecconi, A.; Vilchez-Tschischke, J.P.; Mateo, J.; Sanchez-Gonzalez, J.; Espana, S.; Fernandez-Jimenez, R.; Lopez-Melgar, B.; Fernandez Friera, L.; Lopez-Martin, G.J.; Fuster, V.; et al. Effects of Colchicine on Atherosclerotic Plaque Stabilization: A Multimodality Imaging Study in an Animal Model. *J. Cardiovasc. Transl. Res.* **2020**, *14*, 150–160. [CrossRef]
52. Aguilar, E.C.; Leonel, A.J.; Teixeira, L.G.; Silva, A.R.; Silva, J.F.; Pelaez, J.M.; Capettini, L.S.; Lemos, V.S.; Santos, R.A.; Alvarez-Leite, J.I. Butyrate impairs atherogenesis by reducing plaque inflammation and vulnerability and decreasing NFkappaB activation. *Nutr. Metab. Cardiovasc. Dis.* **2014**, *24*, 606–613. [CrossRef] [PubMed]
53. Zhao, D.; Tong, L.; Zhang, L.; Li, H.; Wan, Y.; Zhang, T. Tanshinone II A stabilizes vulnerable plaques by suppressing RAGE signaling and NF-kappaB activation in apolipoprotein-E-deficient mice. *Mol. Med. Rep.* **2016**, *14*, 4983–4990. [CrossRef] [PubMed]
54. Shen, L.; Sun, Z.; Nie, P.; Yuan, R.; Cai, Z.; Wu, C.; Hu, L.; Jin, S.; Zhou, H.; Zhang, X.; et al. Sulindac-derived retinoid X receptor-alpha modulator attenuates atherosclerotic plaque progression and destabilization in ApoE(-/-) mice. *Br. J. Pharmacol.* **2019**, *176*, 2559–2572. [CrossRef]

55. Liu, J.; Lin, J.; He, S.; Wu, C.; Wang, B.; Liu, J.; Duan, Y.; Liu, T.; Shan, S.; Yang, K.; et al. Transgenic Overexpression of IL-37 Protects Against Atherosclerosis and Strengthens Plaque Stability. *Cell. Physiol. Biochem.* **2018**, *45*, 1034–1050. [CrossRef]
56. Tian, Y.; Chen, T.; Wu, Y.; Yang, L.; Wang, L.; Fan, X.; Zhang, W.; Feng, J.; Yu, H.; Yang, Y.; et al. Pioglitazone stabilizes atherosclerotic plaque by regulating the Th17/Treg balance in AMPK-dependent mechanisms. *Cardiovasc. Diabetol.* **2017**, *16*, 140. [CrossRef]
57. Kobiyama, K.; Saigusa, R.; Ley, K. Vaccination against atherosclerosis. *Curr. Opin. Immunol.* **2019**, *59*, 15–24. [CrossRef]
58. Lassegue, B.; Griendling, K.K. NADPH oxidases: Functions and pathologies in the vasculature. *Arterioscler. Thromb. Vasc. Biol.* **2010**, *30*, 653–661. [CrossRef] [PubMed]
59. Judkins, C.P.; Diep, H.; Broughton, B.R.; Mast, A.E.; Hooker, E.U.; Miller, A.A.; Selemidis, S.; Dusting, G.J.; Sobey, C.G.; Drummond, G.R. Direct evidence of a role for Nox2 in superoxide production, reduced nitric oxide bioavailability, and early atherosclerotic plaque formation in ApoE-/- mice. *Am. J. Physiol. Heart Circ. Physiol.* **2010**, *298*, H24–H32. [CrossRef]
60. Gargiulo, S.; Testa, G.; Gamba, P.; Staurenghi, E.; Poli, G.; Leonarduzzi, G. Oxysterols and 4-hydroxy-2-nonenal contribute to atherosclerotic plaque destabilization. *Free Radic. Biol. Med.* **2017**, *111*, 140–150. [CrossRef]
61. Martinet, W.; Knaapen, M.W.; De Meyer, G.R.; Herman, A.G.; Kockx, M.M. Elevated levels of oxidative DNA damage and DNA repair enzymes in human atherosclerotic plaques. *Circulation* **2002**, *106*, 927–932. [CrossRef]
62. Gargiulo, S.; Rossin, D.; Testa, G.; Gamba, P.; Staurenghi, E.; Biasi, F.; Poli, G.; Leonarduzzi, G. Up-regulation of COX-2 and mPGES-1 by 27-hydroxycholesterol and 4-hydroxynonenal: A crucial role in atherosclerotic plaque instability. *Free Radic. Biol. Med.* **2018**, *129*, 354–363. [CrossRef]
63. Prunet, C.; Montange, T.; Vejux, A.; Laubriet, A.; Rohmer, J.F.; Riedinger, J.M.; Athias, A.; Lemaire-Ewing, S.; Neel, D.; Petit, J.M.; et al. Multiplexed flow cytometric analyses of pro- and anti-inflammatory cytokines in the culture media of oxysterol-treated human monocytic cells and in the sera of atherosclerotic patients. *Cytometry A* **2006**, *69*, 359–373. [CrossRef] [PubMed]
64. Lamb, F.S.; Choi, H.; Miller, M.R.; Stark, R.J. TNFalpha and Reactive Oxygen Signaling in Vascular Smooth Muscle Cells in Hypertension and Atherosclerosis. *Am. J. Hypertens.* **2020**, *33*, 902–913. [PubMed]
65. Kohlgruber, S.; Upadhye, A.; Dyballa-Rukes, N.; McNamara, C.A.; Altschmied, J. Regulation of Transcription Factors by Reactive Oxygen Species and Nitric Oxide in Vascular Physiology and Pathology. *Antioxid. Redox Signal.* **2017**, *26*, 679–699. [CrossRef] [PubMed]
66. Yamagata, K. Soy Isoflavones Inhibit Endothelial Cell Dysfunction and Prevent Cardiovascular Disease. *J. Cardiovasc. Pharmacol.* **2019**, *74*, 201–209. [CrossRef]
67. Li, W.; Hellsten, A.; Jacobsson, L.S.; Blomqvist, H.M.; Olsson, A.G.; Yuan, X.M. Alpha-tocopherol and astaxanthin decrease macrophage infiltration, apoptosis and vulnerability in atheroma of hyperlipidaemic rabbits. *J. Mol. Cell. Cardiol.* **2004**, *37*, 969–978. [CrossRef] [PubMed]
68. Giordano, P.; Scicchitano, P.; Locorotondo, M.; Mandurino, C.; Ricci, G.; Carbonara, S.; Gesualdo, M.; Zito, A.; Dachille, A.; Caputo, P.; et al. Carotenoids and cardiovascular risk. *Curr. Pharm. Des.* **2012**, *18*, 5577–5589. [CrossRef]
69. Sozen, E.; Demirel, T.; Ozer, N.K. Vitamin E: Regulatory role in the cardiovascular system. *IUBMB Life* **2019**, *71*, 507–515. [CrossRef]
70. Farrell, N.; Norris, G.; Lee, S.G.; Chun, O.K.; Blesso, C.N. Anthocyanin-rich black elderberry extract improves markers of HDL function and reduces aortic cholesterol in hyperlipidemic mice. *Food Funct.* **2015**, *6*, 1278–1287. [CrossRef]
71. Quesada, I.M.; Lucero, A.; Amaya, C.; Meijles, D.N.; Cifuentes, M.E.; Pagano, P.J.; Castro, C. Selective inactivation of NADPH oxidase 2 causes regression of vascularization and the size and stability of atherosclerotic plaques. *Atherosclerosis* **2015**, *242*, 469–475. [CrossRef]
72. Zhang, H.L.; Jia, K.Y.; Sun, D.; Yang, M. Protective effect of HSP27 in atherosclerosis and coronary heart disease by inhibiting reactive oxygen species. *J. Cell. Biochem.* **2019**, *120*, 2859–2868. [CrossRef] [PubMed]
73. Holm Nielsen, S.; Jonasson, L.; Kalogeropoulos, K.; Karsdal, M.A.; Reese-Petersen, A.L.; Auf dem Keller, U.; Genovese, F.; Nilsson, J.; Goncalves, I. Exploring the role of extracellular matrix proteins to develop biomarkers of plaque vulnerability and outcome. *J. Intern. Med.* **2020**, *287*, 493–513. [CrossRef] [PubMed]
74. Kowara, M.; Cudnoch-Jedrzejewska, A.; Opolski, G.; Wlodarski, P. MicroRNA regulation of extracellular matrix components in the process of atherosclerotic plaque destabilization. *Clin. Exp. Pharmacol. Physiol.* **2017**, *44*, 711–718. [CrossRef] [PubMed]
75. Shami, A.; Goncalves, I.; Hultgardh-Nilsson, A. Collagen and related extracellular matrix proteins in atherosclerotic plaque development. *Curr. Opin. Lipidol.* **2014**, *25*, 394–399. [CrossRef] [PubMed]
76. Berg, G.; Barchuk, M.; Miksztowicz, V. Behavior of Metalloproteinases in Adipose Tissue, Liver and Arterial Wall: An Update of Extracellular Matrix Remodeling. *Cells* **2019**, *8*, 158. [CrossRef] [PubMed]
77. Newby, A.C. Proteinases and plaque rupture: Unblocking the road to translation. *Curr. Opin. Lipidol.* **2014**, *25*, 358–366. [CrossRef] [PubMed]
78. Li, T.; Li, X.; Feng, Y.; Dong, G.; Wang, Y.; Yang, J. The Role of Matrix Metalloproteinase-9 in Atherosclerotic Plaque Instability. *Mediat. Inflamm.* **2020**, *2020*, 3872367. [CrossRef]
79. Bultmann, A.; Li, Z.; Wagner, S.; Gawaz, M.; Ungerer, M.; Langer, H.; May, A.E.; Munch, G. Loss of protease activity of ADAM15 abolishes protective effects on plaque progression in atherosclerosis. *Int. J. Cardiol.* **2011**, *152*, 382–385. [CrossRef]

80. Johnson, J.L.; Jenkins, N.P.; Huang, W.C.; Di Gregoli, K.; Sala-Newby, G.B.; Scholtes, V.P.; Moll, F.L.; Pasterkamp, G.; Newby, A.C. Relationship of MMP-14 and TIMP-3 expression with macrophage activation and human atherosclerotic plaque vulnerability. *Mediat. Inflamm.* **2014**, *2014*, 276457. [CrossRef]
81. Sigala, F.; Savvari, P.; Liontos, M.; Sigalas, P.; Pateras, I.S.; Papalampros, A.; Basdra, E.K.; Kolettas, E.; Papavassiliou, A.G.; Gorgoulis, V.G. Increased expression of bFGF is associated with carotid atherosclerotic plaques instability engaging the NF-kappaB pathway. *J. Cell. Mol. Med.* **2010**, *14*, 2273–2280. [CrossRef] [PubMed]
82. Weng, J.; Wang, C.; Zhong, W.; Li, B.; Wang, Z.; Shao, C.; Chen, Y.; Yan, J. Activation of CD137 Signaling Promotes Angiogenesis in Atherosclerosis via Modulating Endothelial Smad1/5-NFATc1 Pathway. *J. Am. Heart Assoc.* **2017**, *6*, e004756. [CrossRef]
83. Guo, M.; Cai, Y.; Yao, X.; Li, Z. Mathematical modeling of atherosclerotic plaque destabilization: Role of neovascularization and intraplaque hemorrhage. *J. Theor. Biol.* **2018**, *450*, 53–65. [CrossRef]
84. Moreno, P.R.; Purushothaman, K.R.; Fuster, V.; Echeverri, D.; Truszczynska, H.; Sharma, S.K.; Badimon, J.J.; O'Connor, W.N. Plaque neovascularization is increased in ruptured atherosclerotic lesions of human aorta: Implications for plaque vulnerability. *Circulation* **2004**, *110*, 2032–2038. [CrossRef] [PubMed]
85. Taruya, A.; Tanaka, A.; Nishiguchi, T.; Matsuo, Y.; Ozaki, Y.; Kashiwagi, M.; Shiono, Y.; Orii, M.; Yamano, T.; Ino, Y.; et al. Vasa Vasorum Restructuring in Human Atherosclerotic Plaque Vulnerability: A Clinical Optical Coherence Tomography Study. *J. Am. Coll. Cardiol.* **2015**, *65*, 2469–2477. [CrossRef] [PubMed]
86. Perrotta, P.; Veseli, B.E.; Van der Veken, B.; Roth, L.; Martinet, W.; De Meyer, G.R.Y. Pharmacological strategies to inhibit intra-plaque angiogenesis in atherosclerosis. *Vasc. Pharmacol.* **2019**, *112*, 72–78. [CrossRef] [PubMed]
87. Van der Veken, B.; De Meyer, G.R.Y.; Martinet, W. Axitinib attenuates intraplaque angiogenesis, haemorrhages and plaque destabilization in mice. *Vasc. Pharmacol.* **2018**, *100*, 34–40. [CrossRef] [PubMed]
88. Sullivan, J.L. Macrophage iron, hepcidin, and atherosclerotic plaque stability. *Exp. Biol. Med.* **2007**, *232*, 1014–1020. [CrossRef] [PubMed]
89. Vinchi, F.; Porto, G.; Simmelbauer, A.; Altamura, S.; Passos, S.T.; Garbowski, M.; Silva, A.M.N.; Spaich, S.; Seide, S.E.; Sparla, R.; et al. Atherosclerosis is aggravated by iron overload and ameliorated by dietary and pharmacological iron restriction. *Eur. Heart J.* **2020**, *41*, 2681–2695. [CrossRef]
90. Vujic, N.; Schlager, S.; Eichmann, T.O.; Madreiter-Sokolowski, C.T.; Goeritzer, M.; Rainer, S.; Schauer, S.; Rosenberger, A.; Woelfler, A.; Doddapattar, P.; et al. Monoglyceride lipase deficiency modulates endocannabinoid signaling and improves plaque stability in ApoE-knockout mice. *Atherosclerosis* **2016**, *244*, 9–21. [CrossRef] [PubMed]
91. Erbay, E.; Babaev, V.R.; Mayers, J.R.; Makowski, L.; Charles, K.N.; Snitow, M.E.; Fazio, S.; Wiest, M.M.; Watkins, S.M.; Linton, M.F.; et al. Reducing endoplasmic reticulum stress through a macrophage lipid chaperone alleviates atherosclerosis. *Nat. Med.* **2009**, *15*, 1383–1391. [CrossRef] [PubMed]
92. Gong, M.; Zhuo, X.; Ma, A. STAT6 Upregulation Promotes M2 Macrophage Polarization to Suppress Atherosclerosis. *Med. Sci. Monit. Basic Res.* **2017**, *23*, 240–249. [CrossRef] [PubMed]
93. Henning, R.J.; Bourgeois, M.; Harbison, R.D. Poly(ADP-ribose) Polymerase (PARP) and PARP Inhibitors: Mechanisms of Action and Role in Cardiovascular Disorders. *Cardiovasc. Toxicol.* **2018**, *18*, 493–506. [CrossRef] [PubMed]
94. Fernandez-Laso, V.; Sastre, C.; Mendez-Barbero, N.; Egido, J.; Martin-Ventura, J.L.; Gomez-Guerrero, C.; Blanco-Colio, L.M. TWEAK blockade decreases atherosclerotic lesion size and progression through suppression of STAT1 signaling in diabetic mice. *Sci. Rep.* **2017**, *7*, 46679. [CrossRef] [PubMed]
95. Chen, L.W.; Tsai, M.C.; Chern, C.Y.; Tsao, T.P.; Lin, F.Y.; Chen, S.J.; Tsui, P.F.; Liu, Y.W.; Lu, H.J.; Wu, W.L.; et al. A chalcone derivative, 1m-6, exhibits atheroprotective effects by increasing cholesterol efflux and reducing inflammation-induced endothelial dysfunction. *Br. J. Pharmacol.* **2020**, *177*, 5375–5392. [CrossRef] [PubMed]
96. Cipriani, S.; Francisci, D.; Mencarelli, A.; Renga, B.; Schiaroli, E.; D'Amore, C.; Baldelli, F.; Fiorucci, S. Efficacy of the CCR5 antagonist maraviroc in reducing early, ritonavir-induced atherogenesis and advanced plaque progression in mice. *Circulation* **2013**, *127*, 2114–2124. [CrossRef] [PubMed]
97. Tang, X. Analysis of interleukin-17 and interleukin-18 levels in animal models of atherosclerosis. *Exp. Ther. Med.* **2019**, *18*, 517–522. [CrossRef]
98. Niessner, A.; Shin, M.S.; Pryshchep, O.; Goronzy, J.J.; Chaikof, E.L.; Weyand, C.M. Synergistic proinflammatory effects of the antiviral cytokine interferon-alpha and Toll-like receptor 4 ligands in the atherosclerotic plaque. *Circulation* **2007**, *116*, 2043–2052. [CrossRef]
99. Khambata, R.S.; Ghosh, S.M.; Rathod, K.S.; Thevathasan, T.; Filomena, F.; Xiao, Q.; Ahluwalia, A. Antiinflammatory actions of inorganic nitrate stabilize the atherosclerotic plaque. *Proc. Natl. Acad. Sci. USA* **2017**, *114*, E550–E559. [CrossRef]
100. Kyaw, T.; Winship, A.; Tay, C.; Kanellakis, P.; Hosseini, H.; Cao, A.; Li, P.; Tipping, P.; Bobik, A.; Toh, B.H. Cytotoxic and proinflammatory CD8+ T lymphocytes promote development of vulnerable atherosclerotic plaques in apoE-deficient mice. *Circulation* **2013**, *127*, 1028–1039. [CrossRef]
101. Ou, H.X.; Guo, B.B.; Liu, Q.; Li, Y.K.; Yang, Z.; Feng, W.J.; Mo, Z.C. Regulatory T cells as a new therapeutic target for atherosclerosis. *Acta Pharmacol. Sin.* **2018**, *39*, 1249–1258. [CrossRef]
102. Fiorelli, S.; Porro, B.; Cosentino, N.; Di Minno, A.; Manega, C.M.; Fabbiocchi, F.; Niccoli, G.; Fracassi, F.; Barbieri, S.; Marenzi, G.; et al. Activation of Nrf2/HO-1 Pathway and Human Atherosclerotic Plaque Vulnerability: An In Vitro and In Vivo Study. *Cells* **2019**, *8*, 356. [CrossRef]

103. Xu, Z.R.; Li, J.Y.; Dong, X.W.; Tan, Z.J.; Wu, W.Z.; Xie, Q.M.; Yang, Y.M. Apple Polyphenols Decrease Atherosclerosis and Hepatic Steatosis in ApoE-/- Mice through the ROS/MAPK/NF-kappaB Pathway. *Nutrients* **2015**, *7*, 7085–7105. [CrossRef]
104. Wang, L.; Chen, Q.; Ke, D.; Li, G. Ghrelin inhibits atherosclerotic plaque angiogenesis and promotes plaque stability in a rabbit atherosclerotic model. *Peptides* **2017**, *90*, 17–26. [CrossRef]
105. Li, H.; Li, J.; Jiang, X.; Liu, S.; Liu, Y.; Chen, W.; Yang, J.; Zhang, C.; Zhang, W. Melatonin enhances atherosclerotic plaque stability by inducing prolyl-4-hydroxylase alpha1 expression. *J. Hypertens.* **2019**, *37*, 964–971. [CrossRef]
106. Budatha, M.; Zhang, J.; Zhuang, Z.W.; Yun, S.; Dahlman, J.E.; Anderson, D.G.; Schwartz, M.A. Inhibiting Integrin alpha5 Cytoplasmic Domain Signaling Reduces Atherosclerosis and Promotes Arteriogenesis. *J. Am. Heart Assoc.* **2018**, *7*, e007501. [CrossRef]
107. Parma, L.; Peters, H.A.B.; Sluiter, T.J.; Simons, K.H.; Lazzari, P.; de Vries, M.R.; Quax, P.H.A. bFGF blockade reduces intraplaque angiogenesis and macrophage infiltration in atherosclerotic vein graft lesions in ApoE3*Leiden mice. *Sci. Rep.* **2020**, *10*, 15968. [CrossRef] [PubMed]
108. Huang, Z.; Wang, L.; Meng, S.; Wang, Y.; Chen, T.; Wang, C. Berberine reduces both MMP-9 and EMMPRIN expression through prevention of p38 pathway activation in PMA-induced macrophages. *Int. J. Cardiol.* **2011**, *146*, 153–158. [CrossRef] [PubMed]
109. Li, H.; He, C.; Wang, J.; Li, X.; Yang, Z.; Sun, X.; Fang, L.; Liu, N. Berberine activates peroxisome proliferator-activated receptor gamma to increase atherosclerotic plaque stability in Apoe(-/-) mice with hyperhomocysteinemia. *J. Diabetes Investig.* **2016**, *7*, 824–832. [CrossRef] [PubMed]
110. Yan, H.; Ma, Y.; Li, Y.; Zheng, X.; Lv, P.; Zhang, Y.; Li, J.; Ma, M.; Zhang, L.; Li, C. Insulin inhibits inflammation and promotes atherosclerotic plaque stability via PI3K-Akt pathway activation. *Immunol. Lett.* **2016**, *170*, 7–14. [CrossRef]
111. Kagami, S.; Owada, T.; Kanari, H.; Saito, Y.; Suto, A.; Ikeda, K.; Hirose, K.; Watanabe, N.; Iwamoto, I.; Nakajima, H. Protein geranylgeranylation regulates the balance between Th17 cells and Foxp3+ regulatory T cells. *Int. Immunol.* **2009**, *21*, 679–689. [CrossRef] [PubMed]
112. Oesterle, A.; Laufs, U.; Liao, J.K. Pleiotropic Effects of Statins on the Cardiovascular System. *Circ. Res.* **2017**, *120*, 229–243. [CrossRef] [PubMed]
113. Bot, M.; de Jager, S.C.; MacAleese, L.; Lagraauw, H.M.; van Berkel, T.J.; Quax, P.H.; Kuiper, J.; Heeren, R.M.; Biessen, E.A.; Bot, I. Lysophosphatidic acid triggers mast cell-driven atherosclerotic plaque destabilization by increasing vascular inflammation. *J. Lipid Res.* **2013**, *54*, 1265–1274. [CrossRef]
114. Gu, C.; Wang, F.; Zhao, Z.; Wang, H.; Cong, X.; Chen, X. Lysophosphatidic Acid Is Associated with Atherosclerotic Plaque Instability by Regulating NF-kappaB Dependent Matrix Metalloproteinase-9 Expression via LPA2 in Macrophages. *Front. Physiol.* **2017**, *8*, 266. [CrossRef]
115. Zhang, H.; Zhang, J.Y.; Sun, T.W.; Shen, D.L.; He, F.; Dang, Y.H.; Li, L. Amelioration of atherosclerosis in apolipoprotein E-deficient mice by inhibition of lipoprotein-associated phospholipase A2. *Clin. Investig. Med.* **2013**, *36*, E32–E41. [CrossRef]
116. Solly, E.L.; Dimasi, C.G.; Bursill, C.A.; Psaltis, P.J.; Tan, J.T.M. MicroRNAs as Therapeutic Targets and Clinical Biomarkers in Atherosclerosis. *J. Clin. Med.* **2019**, *8*, 2199. [CrossRef]
117. Wang, J.; Hu, X.; Hu, X.; Gao, F.; Li, M.; Cui, Y.; Wei, X.; Qin, Y.; Zhang, C.; Zhao, Y.; et al. MicroRNA-520c-3p targeting of RelA/p65 suppresses atherosclerotic plaque formation. *Int. J. Biochem. Cell Biol.* **2021**, *131*, 105873. [CrossRef] [PubMed]
118. An, T.H.; He, Q.W.; Xia, Y.P.; Chen, S.C.; Baral, S.; Mao, L.; Jin, H.J.; Li, Y.N.; Wang, M.D.; Chen, J.G.; et al. MiR-181b Antagonizes Atherosclerotic Plaque Vulnerability Through Modulating Macrophage Polarization by Directly Targeting Notch1. *Mol. Neurobiol.* **2017**, *54*, 6329–6341. [CrossRef]
119. Chen, W.; Yu, F.; Di, M.; Li, M.; Chen, Y.; Zhang, Y.; Liu, X.; Huang, X.; Zhang, M. MicroRNA-124-3p inhibits collagen synthesis in atherosclerotic plaques by targeting prolyl 4-hydroxylase subunit alpha-1 (P4HA1) in vascular smooth muscle cells. *Atherosclerosis* **2018**, *277*, 98–107. [CrossRef]
120. Loyer, X.; Mallat, Z.; Boulanger, C.M.; Tedgui, A. MicroRNAs as therapeutic targets in atherosclerosis. *Expert Opin. Ther. Targets* **2015**, *19*, 489–496. [CrossRef]
121. Yiew, K.H.; Chatterjee, T.K.; Hui, D.Y.; Weintraub, N.L. Histone Deacetylases and Cardiometabolic Diseases. *Arterioscler Thromb Vasc Biol.* **2015**, *35*, 1914–1919. [CrossRef]
122. Schiano, C.; Benincasa, G.; Franzese, M.; Della Mura, N.; Pane, K.; Salvatore, M.; Napoli, C. Epigenetic-sensitive pathways in personalized therapy of major cardiovascular diseases. *Pharmacol. Ther.* **2020**, *210*, 107514. [CrossRef]
123. Zhang, B.; Ma, Y.; Xiang, C. SIRT2 decreases atherosclerotic plaque formation in low-density lipoprotein receptor-deficient mice by modulating macrophage polarization. *Biomed. Pharmacother.* **2018**, *97*, 1238–1242. [CrossRef]
124. Pan, Y.; Zhang, H.; Zheng, Y.; Zhou, J.; Yuan, J.; Yu, Y.; Wang, J. Resveratrol Exerts Antioxidant Effects by Activating SIRT2 To Deacetylate Prx1. *Biochemistry* **2017**, *56*, 6325–6328. [CrossRef]
125. Pasterkamp, G.; van der Laan, S.W.; Haitjema, S.; Foroughi Asl, H.; Siemelink, M.A.; Bezemer, T.; van Setten, J.; Dichgans, M.; Malik, R.; Worrall, B.B.; et al. Human Validation of Genes Associated With a Murine Atherosclerotic Phenotype. *Arterioscler. Thromb. Vasc. Biol.* **2016**, *36*, 1240–1246. [CrossRef]
126. Willemsen, L.; de Winther, M.P. Macrophage subsets in atherosclerosis as defined by single-cell technologies. *J. Pathol.* **2020**, *250*, 705–714. [CrossRef] [PubMed]
127. Allahverdian, S.; Pannu, P.S.; Francis, G.A. Contribution of monocyte-derived macrophages and smooth muscle cells to arterial foam cell formation. *Cardiovasc. Res.* **2012**, *95*, 165–172. [CrossRef] [PubMed]

128. Ridker, P.M.; Everett, B.M.; Thuren, T.; MacFadyen, J.G.; Chang, W.H.; Ballantyne, C.; Fonseca, F.; Nicolau, J.; Koenig, W.; Anker, S.D.; et al. Antiinflammatory Therapy with Canakinumab for Atherosclerotic Disease. *N. Engl. J. Med.* **2017**, *377*, 1119–1131. [CrossRef] [PubMed]
129. Tardif, J.C.; Kouz, S.; Waters, D.D.; Bertrand, O.F.; Diaz, R.; Maggioni, A.P.; Pinto, F.J.; Ibrahim, R.; Gamra, H.; Kiwan, G.S.; et al. Efficacy and Safety of Low-Dose Colchicine after Myocardial Infarction. *N. Engl. J. Med.* **2019**, *381*, 2497–2505. [CrossRef] [PubMed]
130. White, H.D.; Held, C.; Stewart, R.; Tarka, E.; Brown, R.; Davies, R.Y.; Budaj, A.; Harrington, R.A.; Steg, P.G.; The Stability Investigators; et al. Darapladib for preventing ischemic events in stable coronary heart disease. *N. Engl. J. Med.* **2014**, *370*, 1702–1711.
131. Bowman, L.; Hopewell, J.C.; Chen, F.; Wallendszus, K.; Stevens, W.; Collins, R.; Wiviott, S.D.; Cannon, C.P.; Braunwald, E. HPS3/TIMI55-REVEAL Collaborative Group; et al. Effects of Anacetrapib in Patients with Atherosclerotic Vascular Disease. *N. Engl. J. Med.* **2017**, *377*, 1217–1227. [PubMed]
132. Daida, H.; Dohi, T.; Fukushima, Y.; Ohmura, H.; Miyauchi, K. The Goal of Achieving Atherosclerotic Plaque Regression with Lipid-Lowering Therapy: Insights from IVUS Trials. *J. Atheroscler. Thromb.* **2019**, *26*, 592–600. [CrossRef]
133. Schartl, M.; Bocksch, W.; Koschyk, D.H.; Voelker, W.; Karsch, K.R.; Kreuzer, J.; Hausmann, D.; Beckmann, S.; Gross, M. Use of intravascular ultrasound to compare effects of different strategies of lipid-lowering therapy on plaque volume and composition in patients with coronary artery disease. *Circulation* **2001**, *104*, 387–392. [CrossRef] [PubMed]
134. Nissen, S.E.; Tuzcu, E.M.; Schoenhagen, P.; Brown, B.G.; Ganz, P.; Vogel, R.A.; Crowe, T.; Howard, G.; Cooper, C.J.; Brodie, B.; et al. Effect of intensive compared with moderate lipid-lowering therapy on progression of coronary atherosclerosis: A randomized controlled trial. *JAMA* **2004**, *291*, 1071–1080. [CrossRef] [PubMed]
135. Nicholls, S.J.; Puri, R.; Anderson, T.; Ballantyne, C.M.; Cho, L.; Kastelein, J.J.; Koenig, W.; Somaratne, R.; Kassahun, H.; Yang, J.; et al. Effect of Evolocumab on Progression of Coronary Disease in Statin-Treated Patients: The GLAGOV Randomized Clinical Trial. *JAMA* **2016**, *316*, 2373–2384. [CrossRef]
136. Christoph, M.; Herold, J.; Berg-Holldack, A.; Rauwolf, T.; Ziemssen, T.; Schmeisser, A.; Weinert, S.; Ebner, B.; Said, S.; Strasser, R.H.; et al. Effects of the PPARgamma agonist pioglitazone on coronary atherosclerotic plaque composition and plaque progression in non-diabetic patients: A double-center, randomized controlled VH-IVUS pilot-trial. *Heart Vessel.* **2015**, *30*, 286–295. [CrossRef]
137. Thondapu, V.; Kurihara, O.; Yonetsu, T.; Russo, M.; Kim, H.O.; Lee, H.; Soeda, T.; Minami, Y.; Jang, I.K. Comparison of Rosuvastatin Versus Atorvastatin for Coronary Plaque Stabilization. *Am. J. Cardiol.* **2019**, *123*, 1565–1571. [CrossRef]
138. Geng, C.; Zhang, Y.; Hidru, T.H.; Zhi, L.; Tao, M.; Zou, L.; Chen, C.; Li, H.; Liu, Y. Sonodynamic therapy: A potential treatment for atherosclerosis. *Life Sci.* **2018**, *207*, 304–313. [CrossRef]
139. Yoo, S.W.; Oh, G.; Ahn, J.C.; Chung, E. Non-Oncologic Applications of Nanomedicine-Based Phototherapy. *Biomedicines* **2021**, *9*, 113. [CrossRef]
140. Kharlamov, A.N.; Tyurnina, A.E.; Veselova, V.S.; Kovtun, O.P.; Shur, V.Y.; Gabinsky, J.L. Silica-gold nanoparticles for atheroprotective management of plaques: Results of the NANOM-FIM trial. *Nanoscale* **2015**, *7*, 8003–8015. [CrossRef] [PubMed]
141. Scoville, D.K.; Nolin, J.D.; Ogden, H.L.; An, D.; Afsharinejad, Z.; Johnson, B.W.; Bammler, T.K.; Gao, X.; Frevert, C.W.; Altemeier, W.A.; et al. Quantum dots and mouse strain influence house dust mite-induced allergic airway disease. *Toxicol. Appl. Pharmacol.* **2019**, *368*, 55–62. [CrossRef] [PubMed]
142. Jia, H.; Dai, J.; Hou, J.; Xing, L.; Ma, L.; Liu, H.; Xu, M.; Yao, Y.; Hu, S.; Yamamoto, E.; et al. Effective anti-thrombotic therapy without stenting: Intravascular optical coherence tomography-based management in plaque erosion (the EROSION study). *Eur. Heart J.* **2017**, *38*, 792–800. [CrossRef] [PubMed]
143. Baigent, C.; Blackwell, L.; Collins, R.; Emberson, J.; Godwin, J.; Peto, R.; Buring, J.; Hennekens, C.; Kearney, P.; Antithrombotic Trialists' Collaboration; et al. Aspirin in the primary and secondary prevention of vascular disease: Collaborative meta-analysis of individual participant data from randomised trials. *Lancet* **2009**, *373*, 1849–1860. [PubMed]
144. Shioi, A.; Ikari, Y. Plaque Calcification During Atherosclerosis Progression and Regression. *J. Atheroscler. Thromb.* **2018**, *25*, 294–303. [CrossRef]

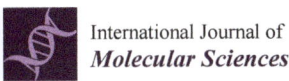

Article

Estrogen Receptor Subtypes Elicit a Distinct Gene Expression Profile of Endothelial-Derived Factors Implicated in Atherosclerotic Plaque Vulnerability

Narjes Nasiri-Ansari [1], Eliana Spilioti [1,2], Ioannis Kyrou [3,4,5,6], Vassiliki Kalotychou [7], Antonios Chatzigeorgiou [8], Despina Sanoudou [9,10,11], Karin Dahlman-Wright [12], Harpal S. Randeva [3,4], Athanasios G. Papavassiliou [1], Paraskevi Moutsatsou [1] and Eva Kassi [1,13,*]

1. Department of Biological Chemistry, Medical School, National and Kapodistrian University of Athens, 11527 Athens, Greece
2. Laboratory of Toxicological Control of Pesticides, Scientific Directorate of Pesticides' Control and Phytopharmacy, Benaki Phytopathological Institute, 14561 Athens, Greece
3. Warwickshire Institute for the Study of Diabetes, Endocrinology and Metabolism (WISDEM), University Hospitals Coventry and Warwickshire NHS Trust, Coventry CV2 2DX, UK
4. Warwick Medical School, University of Warwick, Coventry CV4 7AL, UK
5. Laboratory of Dietetics and Quality of Life, Department of Food Science and Human Nutrition, School of Food and Nutritional Sciences, Agricultural University of Athens, 11855 Athens, Greece
6. Centre for Sport, Exercise and Life Sciences, Research Institute for Health & Wellbeing, Coventry University, Coventry CV1 5FB, UK
7. Department of Internal Medicine, Laikon General Hospital, Medical School, National and Kapodistrian University of Athens, 11527 Athens, Greece
8. Department of Physiology, Medical School, National and Kapodistrian University of Athens, 11527 Athens, Greece
9. Clinical Genomics and Pharmacogenomics Unit, 4th Department of Internal Medicine, Attikon Hospital Medical School, National and Kapodistrian University of Athens, 11527 Athens, Greece
10. Center for New Biotechnologies and Precision Medicine, Medical School, National and Kapodistrian University of Athens, 11527 Athens, Greece
11. Biomedical Research Foundation of the Academy of Athens, 11527 Athens, Greece
12. Department of Biosciences and Nutrition, Novum, Karolinska Institute, SE-14183 Huddinge, Sweden
13. Endocrine Unit, 1st Department of Propaedeutic Internal Medicine, Laiko General Hospital, National and Kapodistrian University of Athens, 11527 Athens, Greece
* Correspondence: ekassi@med.uoa.gr; Tel.: +30-21-0746-2699; Fax: +30-21-0746-2703

Abstract: In the presence of established atherosclerosis, estrogens are potentially harmful. MMP-2 and MMP-9, their inhibitors (TIMP-2 and TIMP-1), RANK, RANKL, OPG, MCP-1, lysyl oxidase (LOX), PDGF-β, and ADAMTS-4 play critical roles in plaque instability/rupture. We aimed to investigate (i) the effect of estradiol on the expression of the abovementioned molecules in endothelial cells, (ii) which type(s) of estrogen receptors mediate these effects, and (iii) the role of p21 in the estrogen-mediated regulation of the aforementioned factors. Human aortic endothelial cells (HAECs) were cultured with estradiol in the presence or absence of TNF-α. The expression of the aforementioned molecules was assessed by qRT-PCR and ELISA. Zymography was also performed. The experiments were repeated in either ERα- or ERβ-transfected HAECs and after silencing p21. HAECs expressed only the GPR-30 estrogen receptor. Estradiol, at low concentrations, decreased MMP-2 activity by 15-fold, increased LOX expression by 2-fold via GPR-30, and reduced MCP-1 expression by 3.5-fold via ERβ. The overexpression of ERα increased MCP-1 mRNA expression by 2.5-fold. In a low-grade inflammation state, lower concentrations of estradiol induced the mRNA expression of MCP-1 (3.4-fold) and MMP-9 (7.5-fold) and increased the activity of MMP-2 (1.7-fold) via GPR-30. Moreover, p21 silencing resulted in equivocal effects on the expression of the abovementioned molecules. Estradiol induced different effects regarding atherogenic plaque instability through different ERs. The balance of the expression of the various ER subtypes may play an important role in the paradoxical characterization of estrogens as both beneficial and harmful.

Citation: Nasiri-Ansari, N.; Spilioti, E.; Kyrou, I.; Kalotychou, V.; Chatzigeorgiou, A.; Sanoudou, D.; Dahlman-Wright, K.; Randeva, H.S.; Papavassiliou, A.G.; Moutsatsou, P.; et al. Estrogen Receptor Subtypes Elicit a Distinct Gene Expression Profile of Endothelial-Derived Factors Implicated in Atherosclerotic Plaque Vulnerability. *Int. J. Mol. Sci.* **2022**, *23*, 10960. https://doi.org/10.3390/ijms231810960

Academic Editor: Claudio de Lucia

Received: 12 August 2022
Accepted: 14 September 2022
Published: 19 September 2022

Publisher's Note: MDPI stays neutral with regard to jurisdictional claims in published maps and institutional affiliations.

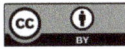

Copyright: © 2022 by the authors. Licensee MDPI, Basel, Switzerland. This article is an open access article distributed under the terms and conditions of the Creative Commons Attribution (CC BY) license (https://creativecommons.org/licenses/by/4.0/).

Keywords: atherosclerosis; plaque vulnerability; estrogen; estrogen receptors; GPR-30; endothelial cells; matrix metalloproteinases MMPs; MCP-1; p21

1. Introduction

Atherosclerosis is known to be the major cause of coronary artery disease (CAD), which remains amongst the most prevalent diseases and is the leading cause of death among women in developed countries, such as USA [1]. The prevalence of atherosclerosis was reported as 101.11/per 1000 individuals in 2015 [2] and it was rated as the second leading cause of death following cancer in Canada, with the economic burden of USD 66.6 billion CAD spent between 2005 and 2016 [3]. Atherosclerosis is a systematic inflammatory process which implicates cells of both the immune system and vessel walls. It is considered as the underlying cause of cardiovascular disease (CVD) mortality in both men and women, although, at younger ages, men are at a higher risk of CVD than women of the same age [4–6]. Compared to women of reproductive age, the risk of atherosclerosis is significantly increased in women after menopause due to prolonged estrogen deficiency [7,8]. The homeostasis of estrogens is strongly regulated by the balance between its synthesis and deactivation. Decreased circulating estrogen levels, along with estrogen sulfotransferase (SULT1E1), in diabetic postmenopausal women [9] may contribute to an increased risk of atherosclerosis development [9,10]. Interestingly, increased SULT1E1 expression has been found in the atheromatic plaque of both mice and humans, as compared to normal arteries [11]. Notably, SULT1E1 is a key enzyme known to catalyze the sulfation of estrogens, leading to its inactivation [9].

The exogenous administration of estrogen as a hormone-replacement therapy (HRT) is commonly prescribed for postmenopausal women in order to ameliorate the risk of estrogen deficiency-related diseases [12].

The atherogenic process evolves in different stages, starting with endothelium activation/dysfunction and ending with atherosclerotic plaque vulnerability and rupture [13]. Although plaque rupture remains the main plaque complication, other recently identified mechanisms, such as calcified nodules protruding into the artery lumen, have been associated with coronary thrombosis and sudden death [14].

Endothelium is the key vessel wall component involved in the initiation of the atherosclerotic process, while its possible role in the later stages has been widely hypothesized, since the major part of the luminal surface of the artery coated with advanced atherosclerotic plaque is still covered by the intact endothelium, although an area of endothelial denudation can also be detected [15]. It should be noted that the influence of estrogen is highly dependent not only on the cell type but also on its "environment", with atherogenic plaque representing a special environment containing an extracellular matrix (ECM) under the endothelial layer.

The beneficial actions of estrogen in various tissues and organs, including the cardiovascular system, have been widely recognized. Several observational studies have shown that estrogens provide protection against CVD during the postmenopausal period [7,16]. Concerning the role of phytoestrogens in atherosclerosis progression, the vast majority of clinical studies have shown that phytoestrogen supplementation exerts a rather modest beneficial effect in reducing the CVD risk profile of postmenopausal women, mostly through influencing the blood lipid profile and biomarkers of the endothelial function, while in women with an increased risk of atherosclerosis, a harmful effect on CIMT (carotid intima-media thickness) progression may be observed [17]. Data from animal studies indicated that the treatment of ovariectomized rats with fresh soy oil (phytoestrogen) resulted in the improvement of the atherosclerosis-related blood lipid profile [18], as well as the atherosclerotic plaque's inflammatory and antioxidant status [19]. However, it should be noted that the repetitive consumption of heated soy oil increased the serum parameters related to atherosclerosis in ovariectomized rats [18].

Moreover, randomized prospective controlled studies failed to confirm the benefits of hormone replacement therapy (HRT) in regard to the primary and secondary prevention of cardiovascular events in postmenopausal women. On the contrary, treatment with estrogen was found to potentially increase the risk of CAD, thus leading to a dramatic decrease in its use [20–23]. The discrepancy between observational and clinical trials may be related, among other factors, to cardiovascular comorbidities, the age at treatment initiation, and time since menopause—a hypothesis that has been referred as "the timing hypothesis". Thus, HRT appears to be relatively safe only in younger women who are asymptomatic for CVD and within 10 years away from menopause [23–25]. This suggests that, after the onset of atherosclerosis and in the presence of atherosclerotic plaque, estrogen may be potentially harmful. Although the protective effects of estrogens in the early stages of the atheromatosis process (endothelium activation/dysregulation) have been extensively investigated in both in vivo (animal models and clinical studies) and in vitro studies [24,26–29], data regarding their influences on factors implicated in the later stages of the atherosclerosis process which lead to the plaque vulnerability are limited. It has been hypothesized that the altered expression of estrogen receptors (ER) ERα, Erβ, and GPR-30 on the vascular wall, along with the atherosclerotic lesions following estrogen deprivation, is strongly involved [16,26,30–32].

During the stages of plaque rupture and/or erosion, among other factors, monocyte chemoattractant protein-1 (MCP-1) and inflammatory cytokines such as tumor necrosis factor-α (TNF-α) promote atherosclerotic plaque vulnerability through processes such as intimal thickening, ECM degradation, vascular mineralization, and calcification within the atheroma [33]. Recent data indicate the existence of a possible link between circulating MCP-1 levels and the risk of stroke and coronary artery disease [34–36]. Moreover, MCP-1 plaque levels have been associated with histopathological hallmarks of plaque vulnerability [36]. The metalloproteinases MMP-2 and MMP-9, as well as their inhibitors, TIMP-1 and TIMP-2, are both expressed in the endothelial cells [37,38].

Recent data point toward a close association of the expression and activity of matrix metalloproteinases (MMPs) with plaque stability and the consequent incident of cardiovascular complications, since they regulate the collagen degradation of the ECM [33,37–40]. The ratio between the expression and activity of MMPs and their inhibitors, known as the tissue inhibitors of metalloprotease (TIMPs), has been used as a critical indicator of CVD pathogenesis and atherosclerotic plaque instability in both human and animal studies [38,41]. Independently of the roles of TIMP on MMP inhibition, TIMP-2 mediates the G1 cell cycle arrest [42,43] by binding to human endothelial cells through $\alpha 3/\beta 1$, leading to decreased angiogenesis and cell proliferation [14,43]. Notably, the inhibition of cycle progression during the G1 phase of the cell cycle by the inactivation of cyclin-cyclin-dependent kinase (CDK) complexes contributes to reduced atherosclerotic plaque formation and neointimal thickening [44].

ECM proteins are also regulated by metalloproteinases with thrombospondin motifs, such as ADAMTS family members. ADMTS-4 has recently emerged as an important player in the atherosclerosis process [45]. Interestingly, in ADAMTS-4 knockout (KO) mice, a decrease in high fat diet-induced atherosclerosis and increased plaque stability were observed [46]. A positive correlation of serum levels of ADAMTS-4 with an increased risk of developing CAD has been proved in regard to various patient groups with different underlying diseases [45].

Platelet-derived growth factor-β (PDGF-β) is also expressed by endothelial cells and regulates the atherosclerosis progression and the plaque stability. Notably, AG1296, a potent tyrosine kinase inhibitor which can block the PDGF-PDGFR signaling pathway, was found to enhance plaque stability via, among other mechanisms, the reduction in the expression of MMP-2 and MMP-9 [47].

Lysyl oxidase (LOX) is also involved in the process of plaque vulnerability. Low LOX activity can lead to defective collagen cross-linking, which in turn can weaken the fibrous cap and favor the presence of soluble forms of collagen which are highly susceptible to metalloproteinase degradation. Indeed, higher levels of LOX have been detected in more stable plaques [48,49].

Moreover, plaque calcification—a lesion associated with coronary thrombosis, even in the absence of eroded or ruptured plaque—is directly linked to the imbalance between the receptor activator of the nuclear factor NFκB ligand (RANKL) and osteoprotegerin (OPG), which are also expressed in endothelial cells [50–52].

OPG, a secreted member of the TNF receptor family, is a decoy receptor for RANKL and inhibits the initiation of RANK signaling. Interestingly, OPG knockout mice displayed pronounced arterial calcification [53]. It has also been revealed that OPG exerts anti-apoptotic effects on endothelial cells, acting as an autocrine survival factor [54,55]. Since endothelial apoptosis precedes vascular calcification [56], OPG may exert its protective effect in vascular calcification through its anti-apoptotic action [57].

On the other hand, the overexpression of RANKL, which is also expressed in the endothelial cells, was found to elevate MMP-9 activation [52,58,59]. The aforementioned effect of RANKL is neutralized by OPG through the inhibition of the RANK/RANKL interaction [60]. The reduced OPG/RANKL ratio can indirectly increase metalloproteinase activity, leading to atherosclerotic plaque erosion and rupture [61]. Clinical studies have confirmed a strong association between OPG and soluble RANKL serum levels in CAD [62,63]. Moreover, OPG-induced LOX upregulation has been linked to the formation of stable fibrous caps in APOE knockout mice [64,65].

Recent studies have suggested the implication of the onco-suppressor p53 and its transcriptional target p21 in the atherogenesis process, as well as in plaque calcification [66,67]. The inactivation of p21 appears to exert atheroprotective effects by inhibiting lesion growth and the maintenance of atherosclerotic plaque stability [68]. Studies on tissues and organs affected by estrogen functions (both normal and neoplastic) have shown that estrogen regulates the expression of *p53* and *p21*; however, data regarding their estrogen-regulated expression in the vascular wall components that participate in the atherogenesis process are lacking [69–71].

While the protective effects of estrogens, with the crucial role of ERα, in the early stages of the atheromatosis process (endothelium activation/dysregulation) have been extensively investigated using both in vivo and in vitro approaches [8,72–74], data on estrogen's influences on factors implicated in the later stages of the atheromatosis process which lead to plaque vulnerability are limited. It has been hypothesized that the altered expression of estrogen receptors on the vascular wall, following estrogen deprivation, as well as the altered expression of estrogen receptors (ERα, Erβ, and GPR-30) in the atherosclerotic lesion, are implicated [26,31,32,75]. A previous study of the other types of cells besides those implicated in the atherosclerosis process (fibrochondrocytes) demonstrated that E_2 mediates MMP-9 overexpression through the activation of the ERα/ERK and NF-κB/ELK-1 signaling pathways [76]. Specifically, in the presence of E_2, ERα induces ERK phosphorylation, leading to the further activation of its downstream targets, such as NF-κB or ELK-1, and finally triggers MMP-9 overexpression. Interestingly, this effect was diminished in cells carrying mutations in the NF-κB or ELK-1 binding sites [76]. However, other studies have demonstrated that the effects of E_2 on NF-κB activity and MMP expression are cell-specific and, at least in part, depend on E_2 concentrations [77,78].

To this end, in this study, we aimed to investigate the effects of various concentrations of estradiol, either alone or after mimicking a low-grade inflammation state that occurs post-menopause in established atherosclerosis, on the expression of molecules involved in atherosclerosis plaque vulnerability (MCP-1, PDGF-β, ADAMTS-4, MMP-2, MMP-9, TIMP-1, TIMP-2, and OPG/RANK/RANKL expression) and MMP activity, using human aortic endothelial cells (HAECs), which offer the best in vitro model system for studying CVD. Moreover, we aimed to clarify whether these effects are mediated by the ERα, Erβ, or GPR-30 receptors. Finally, we delineated the role of p21 in the estrogen-mediated regulation of the expression of the aforementioned genes in the endothelial cells.

2. Result

2.1. The Incubation of HAEC Cells with Estradiol and TNF-α Had No Effect on Cell Viability

HAECs were treated with either 17β-estradiol (E$_2$) (10^{-10}–10^{-7} M) or TNF-α (2 ng/mL) for 24 h (24 h). A cell proliferation assay revealed that neither E$_2$ nor TNF-α had a significant impact on HAEC viability (Figure 1A).

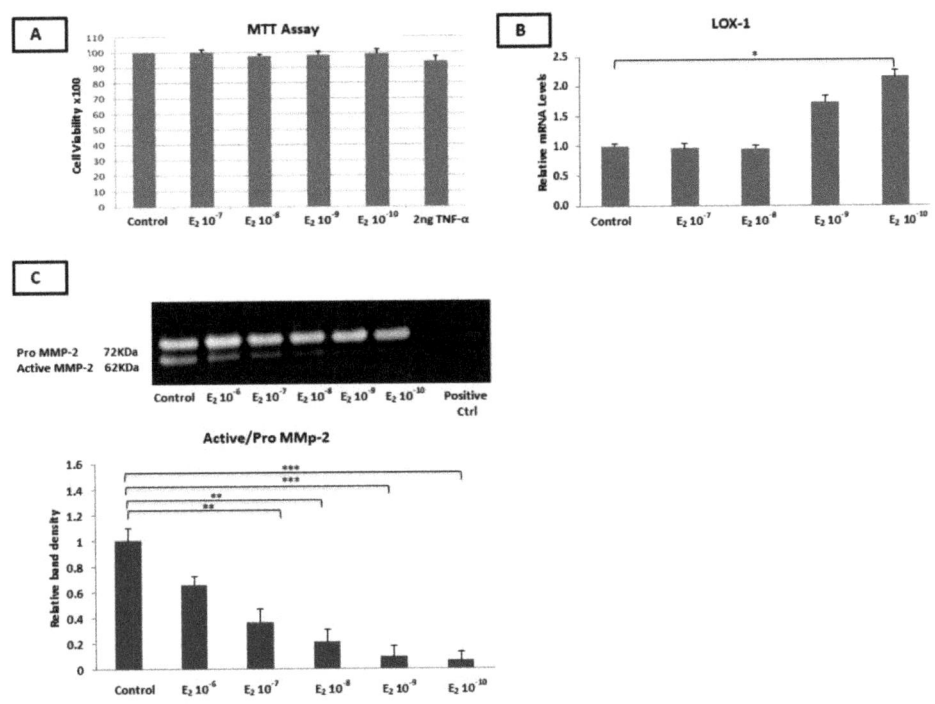

Figure 1. Effect of treatment with 10^{-10}–10^{-7} M E$_2$ on cell survival, atherosclerotic gene expression, and MMP-2 gelatinase activity. (**A**) MTT assay. Incubation of HAECs with 10^{-10}–10^{-7} M E$_2$ or 2 ng/mL TNF-α for 24 h had no significant effect on cell viability. (**B**) LOX-1 mRNA levels were significantly increased in the presence of 10^{-10} M E$_2$ over 24 h. (**C**) The ratio of active MMP-2/pro-MMP-2 was significantly reduced after 24 h of incubation with various concentrations of E$_2$. The graphical data are represented as mean ± SD of at least three independent experiments (*** $p < 0.001$, ** $p < 0.01$, * $p < 0.05$).

2.2. Estradiol Did Not Alter the mRNA Levels of RANK, OPG, and MCP-1 and the TIMP-1, TIMP-2, and MCP-1 Protein Levels

HAEC cells were incubated with E$_2$ (10^{-10}–10^{-7} M) for 6 h and 24 h.

The incubation of the cells with E$_2$ alone for 6 h had no significant effect on the expression of LOX, RANK, RANKL, OPG, MMP-2, MMP-9, TIMP-1, TIMP-2, PDGF-β, ADAMTS-4, and MCP-1 as compared to the untreated cells.

The incubation of the cells with E$_2$ for 24 h significantly increased the mRNA expression of LOX (10^{-10} M, $p < 0.05$) (Figure 1B), while the mRNA expression of the RANKL, MMP-2, MMP-9, TIMP-1, TIMP-2, OPG, PDGF-β, RANK, ADAMTS-4, and MCP-1 genes remained unchanged.

The protein levels of secreted TIMP-1, TIMP-2, and MCP-1 were not significantly altered after the incubation of the HAECs with various concentrations of E$_2$ for 6 h and 24 h, while the expression of secreted OPG was not detected under our experimental conditions, as assessed by ELISA.

2.3. Estradiol Reduced the MMP-2 Gelatinase Activity

The incubation of the HAECs with E_2 (10^{-10}–10^{-6} M) for 24 h resulted in a significant reduction in the active form of MMP-2 in a dose-dependent manner, with stronger effects at the lower concentrations of E_2 (10^{-7}–10^{-8} M, $p < 0.01$ and 10^{-9}–10^{-10} M, $p < 0.001$), compared to the untreated cells (Figure 1C) ($p < 0.05$).

2.4. Estradiol Altered the mRNA Expression of LOX-1, TIMP-1, MMP-9, and MCP-1 and MCP-1 Protein Levels under Inflammatory Conditions

In order to mimic the low-grade inflammation state that exists in postmenopausal women [79], we pre-incubated the endothelial cells with TNF-α for 24 h followed by co-incubation with E_2 for another 24 h. The RT-PCR analysis revealed a significant increase in the mRNA levels of MMP-9 (10^{-8} M, $p < 0.01$ and 10^{-9}–10^{-10} M, $p < 0.001$), TIMP-1 (10^{-10} M, $p < 0.05$), and both the mRNA (10^{-9} and 10^{-10} M, $p < 0.05$ and $p < 0.01$ respectively) and protein levels (10^{-7}–10^{-10} M, $p < 0.01$) of MCP-1 as compared to cells incubated with TNF-α alone (Figure 2A,B).

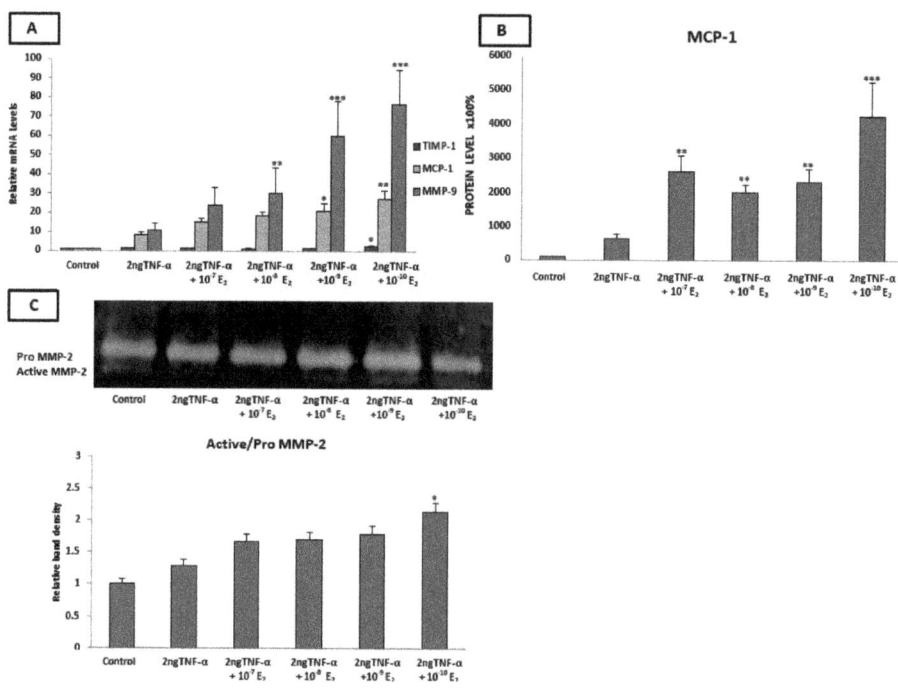

Figure 2. Effects of the pre-incubation of HAECs with 2 ng TNF-α followed by co-incubation of the cells with E_2 on the expression of genes and protein involved in plaque stability, as well as on MMP-2 gelatinase activity. (**A**) Pre-incubation of HAECs with 2 ng/mL TNF-α for 24 h followed by co-the incubation of cells with 10^{-10}–10^{-7} M E_2 for a further 24 h significantly increased the expression of TIMP-1, MCP-1, and MMP-9, as compared to cells incubated with TNF-α alone. (**B**) Pre-incubation of HAECs with 2 ng/mL TNF-α for 24 h followed by the co-incubation of cells with 10^{-10}–10^{-7} M E_2 for a further 24 h significantly increased the MCP-1 protein levels as compared to cells incubated with TNF-α alone. (**C**). The ratio of active MMP-2/pro-MMP-2 was significantly increased after 24 h incubation with 2 ng/mL TNF-α followed by the co-incubation of cells with 10^{-10} E_2. The graphical data are represented as mean ± SD of at least three independent experiments (*** $p < 0.001$, ** $p < 0.01$, * $p < 0.05$).

No significant effect was observed on the RANK, RANKL, MMP-2, ADAMTS-4, PDGF-β, and LOX mRNA levels, as well as on the TIMP-1,TIMP-2, and OPG protein levels.

2.5. Estradiol Induced MMP-2 Activity under Low-Grade Inflammatory Conditions

The matrix metalloproteinase activity was evaluated in cells pre-incubated with 2 ng TNF-α for 24 h and co-incubated with E_2 ($10^{-10}-10^{-7}$ M) for a further 24 h. As shown in Figure 2C, the incubation of cells with TNF-α alone induced MMP-2 activity as compared to untreated cells. A significant increase in MMP-2 activity was detected after the co-incubation of the cells with E_2 (10^{-10} M) as compared to cells incubated with TNF-α alone ($p < 0.05$). Notably, MMP-9 enzymatic activity was not detected in the presence of TNF-α using gelatin zymography.

2.6. HAECs Express the GPR30 Estrogen Receptor

Next, we aimed to investigate whether the observed changes in the expression of molecules implicated in the advanced stages of the atherosclerosis process upon treatment with E_2 were mediated through ERα-, Erβ-, or GPR-30-dependent pathways. Thus, the basal mRNA levels of ERα, Erβ, and GPR-30 were evaluated by qPCR. Interestingly, the HAECs expressed high levels of GPR-30 (Figure 3A), while the mRNA levels of ERα were faintly detected. ERβ mRNA levels were undetectable (Ct = 37) in the HAECs (Supplementary Figure S1). Furthermore, the ERα and ERβ proteins were not detected in the HAEC cells by western blot analysis (Supplementary Figure S1), while the GPR-30 protein was highly expressed (Figure 3A).

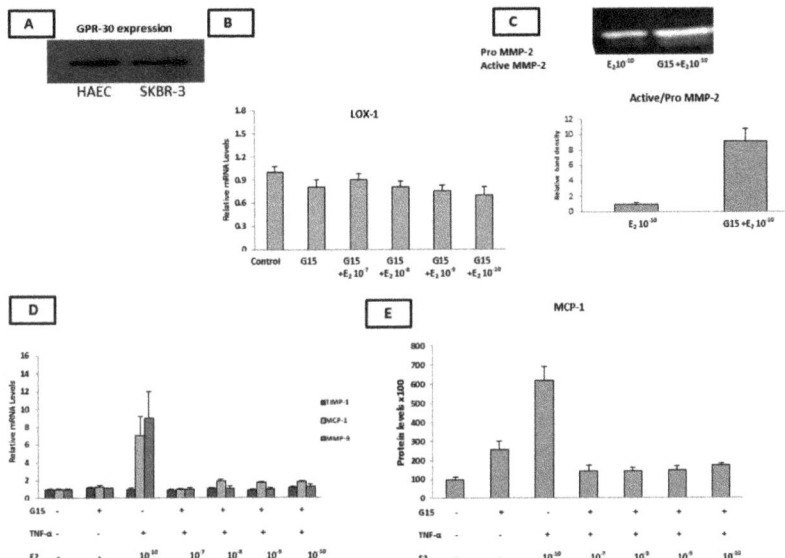

Figure 3. HAECs were co-incubated with G15 (GPR-30 antagonist) and various concentrations of E_2 in the presence/absence of low-grade inflammation (TNF-α). (**A**) GPR-30 protein levels were detected by western blotting in HAECs. (**B**) Co-incubation of HAECs with G15 and E_2 reversed the E_2-induced increase in LOX-1 mRNA levels (10^{-10} M of E_2). (**C**) Co-incubation of HAECs with G15 reversed the E_2-reduced active/proMMP-2 ratio (10^{-10} M of E_2). (**D**) Pre-incubation of cells with TNF-α followed by the co-incubation of cells with G15 and various concentrations of E_2 reversed the (TNF-α + E_2)-induced increase in TIMP-1, MCP-1, and MMP-9 mRNA levels. (**E**) Pre-incubation of cells with TNF-α followed by the co-incubation of cells with G15 and various concentrations of E_2 reversed the (TNF-α + E_2)-induced increase in MCP-1 protein levels. The graphical data are represented as mean ± SD of at least three independent experiments.

Notably, the Flag-ERβ MCF-7-tet-off breast cancer cell line was used as a positive control for the detection of both the ERα and ERβ mRNA levels, while SKBR-3 cells were used as a positive control for the detection of GPR-30.

2.7. G15 (GPR-30 Antagonist) Countered the Estradiol-Induced Expression of LOX, MCP-1,TIMP-1, MMP-9, and MCP-1 as Well as the Decreased MMP-2 Gelatinase Activity

Given that GPR-30 was the only ER expressed in our HAECs, we co-incubated cells with an E_2- and GPR-30-specific antagonist, G15 (10^{-6} M), in order to confirm that E_2 exerted its effects via GPR-30.

We found that G15 countered the effect of E_2 in inducing LOX mRNA expression (Figure 3B) and reversed the E_2-dependent reduction in the MMP-2 enzymatic activity in the HAECs (Figure 3C).

We then investigated the effect of G15 (10^{-6} M) on the observed changes in the expression of MCP-1, TIMP-1, and MMP-9 when the cells were pre-incubated with TNF-α (2 ng for 24 h) and co-incubated with various concentrations of E_2 (for a further 24 h). In the presence of G15, the mRNA levels of TIMP-1 (10^{-10} M of E_2) and MMP-9 (10^{-8}–10^{-10} M of E_2), as well as the mRNA and protein levels of MCP-1 (10^{-10}–10^{-7} M of E_2), which were increased after the co-incubation of the HAECs with TNF-α and E_2, reversed to the basal levels (Figure 3D,E).

These results indicate the E_2 (alone or in the presence of an inflammatory stimulus (TNF-α)) regulates the expression of the LOX-1 mRNA levels, MMP-2 gelatinase activity, and mRNA levels of LOX-1, MCP-1, MMP-9, TIMP-1, as well as the MCP-1 protein levels and MMP-2 gelatinase activity, respectively, through binding to GPR-30.

2.8. Estradiol Increased the Expression of MCP-1 and TIMP-1, as Well as MMP-2 Enzymatic Activity, through ERα

To determine the roles of the other two estrogen receptors (ERα and ERβ) in the regulation of molecules involved in the formation and stability of atherosclerotic plaque, we transfected HAECs with plasmids expressing either ERα or ERβ and their corresponding vectors, since both ERs were not expressed in the HAECs. Twenty-four hours after transfection with either plasmid, the transfection efficiency was evaluated by qPCR analysis (Supplementary Figure S1).

At twenty-four hours post-transfection, the ERα-transfected HAECs were incubated with E_2 (10^{-10}–10^{-7} M) for a further 24 h. The qPCR analysis revealed that E_2 significantly increased the expression of TIMP-1 and MCP-1 (10^{-7}–10^{-9} M of E_2 $p < 0.01$ and 10^{-10} M of E_2, $p < 0.05$ for both genes) in ERα-transfected HAECs (Figure 4A). These findings were confirmed at the protein level for MCP-1 only at the highest concentration of E_2 (10^{-7} M, $p < 0.01$) and for TIMP-1 at all concentration ranges of E_2 (10^{-7} M $p < 0.01$ and 10^{-8} M–10^{-10} M, $p < 0.05$) after 24 h of incubation (Figure 4B). No significant changes in the protein expression of TIMP-2 was detected after the incubation of the Erα-transfected HAECs with different concentrations of E_2.

Moreover, in ERα-transfected HAECs cells, the MMP-2 gelatinase activity was not altered upon incubation with various concentrations of E_2 (Figure 4C).

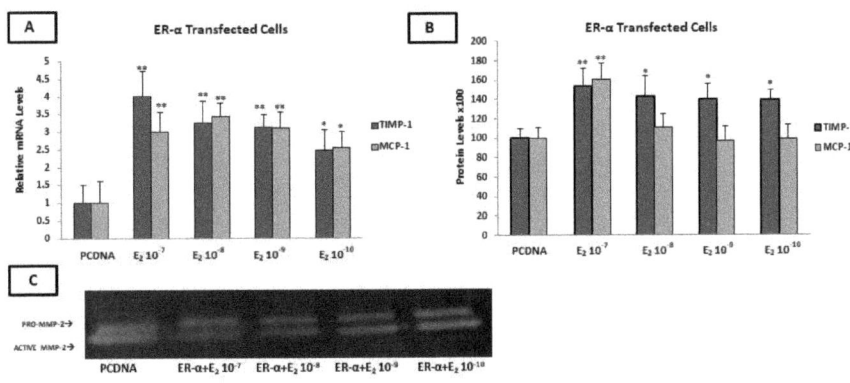
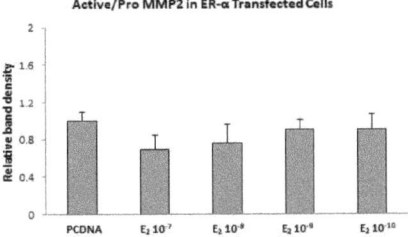

Figure 4. Effects of E_2 on the expression of factors involved in plaque stability in ERα-transfected HAECs. (**A**) Incubation of ER-transfected HAECs with E_2 induced an increase in the mRNA levels of TIMP-1 and MCP-1. (**B**) Incubation of ERα-transfected HAECs with E_2 induced an increase in TIMP-1 (at all concentrations of E_2) and MCP-1 (only at the concentration of 10^{-7} M of E_2) protein levels. (**C**) Incubation of ERα-transfected HAECs with E_2 had no effect on the MMP-2 gelatinase activity. The graphical data are represented as mean ± SD of at least three independent experiments (** $p < 0.01$, * $p < 0.05$).

2.9. Estradiol Reduced the PDGF-β mRNA Levels and MCP-1 Protein Levels through ERβ

As has already been mentioned, the applied HAECs did not express either of the two nuclear estrogen receptors. Therefore, we transfected cells with ERβ-GFP-tagged plasmid, and the transfection efficiency was determined by measuring the mRNA and protein levels of ERβ by both qPCR and western blot, respectively.

ERβ-transfected HAECs were incubated with E_2 ($10^{-10}-10^{-7}$ M) for 24 h. As shown in Figure 5A, E_2 significantly reduced the LOX and PDGF-β mRNA levels at concentrations of 10^{-10} M and $10^{-10}-10^{-9}$ M, respectively ($p < 0.05$), while no significant changes were observed in the MCP-1 mRNA levels.

The incubation of ERβ-transfected HAECs with E_2 ($10^{-10}-10^{-7}$ M) resulted in no significant changes in the mRNA levels of MMP-2, MMP-9, TIMP-1, TIMP-2, MCP-1, and ADAMST-4. The mRNA expression of OPG was undetectable after transfection with ERβ.

Interestingly, the ELISA demonstrated that the incubation of ERβ-transected HAECs with various concentrations ($10^{-10}-10^{-7}$ M) of E_2 resulted in a significant decrease in the MCP-1 protein levels (10^{-7} M of E_2 $p < 0.05$ and $10^{-8}-10^{-9}$ M of E_2 $p < 0.01$), with the more pronounced effect being exhibited at the lowest concentration of E_2 (10^{-10} M of E_2, $p < 0.001$). No significant changes in the protein expression of TIMP-1 and TIMP-2 were found after the incubation of the ERβ-transfected HAECs with different concentrations of E_2. Notably, OPG protein was not detected by ELISA in the cell supernatant (Figure 5B).

The incubation of ERβ-transfected cells with E_2 ($10^{-10}-10^{-7}$ M) did not change the MMP-2 enzymatic activity, as demonstrated by gelatin zymography. It is noteworthy that, under this condition, the MMP-9 pro-enzyme and active enzyme were not detected (Figure 5C).

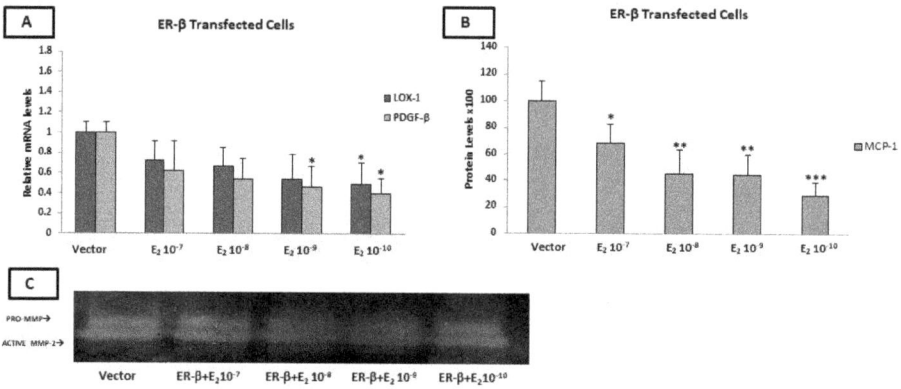

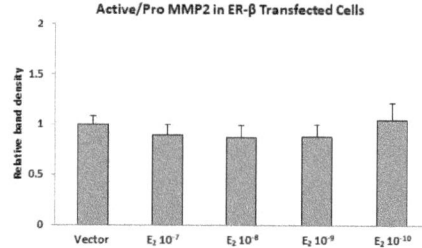

Figure 5. Effect of E_2 on the expression of factors involved in plaque stability in ERβ-transfected HAECs. (**A**) Incubation of ERβ-transfected HAECs with E_2 reduced the mRNA levels of LOX-1 (only at 10^{-10} M of E_2) and PDGF-β (10^{-9} and 10^{-10} M of E_2). (**B**) Incubation of ERβ-transfected HAECs with E_2 (10^{-7}–10^{-10} M) reduced MCP-1 protein levels. (**C**) Incubation of ERβ-transfected HAECs with E_2 had no effect on MMP-2 gelatinase activity. The graphical data are represented as mean ± SD of at least three independent experiments (*** $p < 0.001$, ** $p < 0.01$, * $p < 0.05$).

2.10. The p21 Silencing Reduced the Estradiol-Mediated Upregulation of MCP-1 and LOX-1, while It Increased the PDGF-β mRNA Levels

Previous studies have shown that the activation of GPR-30 leads to the upregulation of p21 [80,81]. The overexpression of p21 significantly reduced the expression of vascular cell adhesion molecule 1 (VCAM-1), inhibiting monocyte adhesion. These data suggest that p21 plays an important role in the process of atherogenesis [82]. However, data regarding the role of p21 in atherosclerosis plaque stability are lacking.

To this end, the expression of p21 was silenced in the HAECs using p21-siRNA. After p21 silencing, the cells were incubated with E_2 for 24 h. As shown in Figure 6A, significant reductions in the mRNA expression of MCP-1 (10^{-9} and 10^{-10} M of E_2, $p < 0.05$), LOX (10^{-9} and 10^{-10} M of E_2, $p < 0.05$), and ADAMST-4 (10^{-8} M of E_2, $p < 0.05$ and 10^{-10}–10^{-9} M of E_2, $p < 0.01$) were observed. On the contrary, the expression of PDGF-β was significantly increased after the incubation of the cells with E_2 (10^{-7} M, $p < 0.05$ and 10^{-8}–10^{-10} M, $p < 0.01$). No significant changes in the gene expression of MMP-2, MMP-9, TIMP-1, TIMP-2, and RANK were detected. The expression of OPG was undetectable by qPCR after p21 silencing.

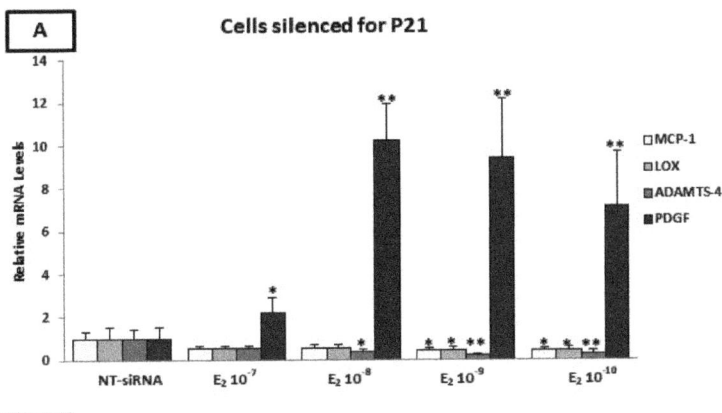
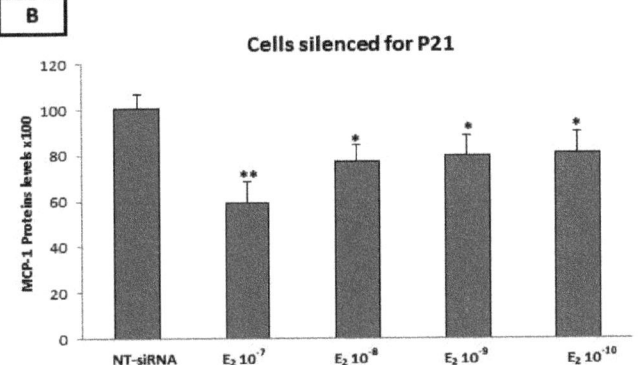

Figure 6. Effect of E$_2$ on the expression of factors involved in plaque stability in p21-silenced HAECs. (**A**) Incubation of p21-silenced cells with E$_2$ resulted in the induction of PDGF-β (10^{-10}–10^{-7} M of E$_2$) and reduction in MCP-1 (10^{-10}–10^{-9} M of E$_2$), LOX-1 (10^{-10}–10^{-8} M of E$_2$) and ADAMTS-4 (10^{-10} M of E$_2$) mRNA levels. (**B**) Incubation of p21-silenced cells with E$_2$ resulted in reduced MCP-1 protein levels (10^{-10}–10^{-7} M of E$_2$). The graphical data are represented as mean ± SD of at least three independent experiments (** $p < 0.01$, * $p < 0.05$).

2.11. Evaluation of MCP-1, TIMP-1, TIMP-2, and OPG Protein Levels by ELISA after p21 Silencing

The effects of p21 silencing on the protein levels of TIMP-1, TIMP-2, MCP-1, and OPG were evaluated by ELISA. The expression of MCP-1 was significantly reduced after the incubation of the cells with E$_2$ at concentrations of 10^{-7} M ($p < 0.01$) and 10^{-8}–10^{-10} M ($p < 0.05$) for 24 h, while no significant changes in the expression of TIMP-1 and TIMP-2 were detected (Figure 6B). Furthermore, the OPG protein remained undetectable in the cell supernatant, as revealed by ELISA.

3. Discussion

The timing hypothesis was first proposed by Thomas Clarkson in 1998 and later confirmed by the Early Versus Late Intervention Trial (ELITE) and Peking studies [83]. According to these studies, the administration of exogenous estrogen to women who have had a menopausal status for approximately ten years can exert adverse effects leading to CVD complications, indicating that, when atherosclerosis is already established, HRT does not provide cardiovascular protection [83]. In line with this hypothesis, both prospective randomized Women's Health Initiative (WHI) and ELITE studies demonstrated that HRT must be started within 5 to a maximum of 10 years of menopause in order to exert cardioprotective effects without adverse effects [83,84]. However, there are no data regarding the molecular mechanism of estrogen-induced adverse effects on established atherosclerosis. Our in vitro study was designed to investigate the "timing hypothesis" of estrogen replacement therapy at the molecular level and shed light on the specific roles of the different estrogen receptors in the advanced stages of atherosclerosis.

According to our findings, the incubation of HAECs with E_2 alone, at the lower concentration, increased the expression of LOX, while it exerted no significant effects on the expression of other molecules implicated in the advanced stages of atherosclerosis and plaque vulnerability, such as MMP-2, MMP-9, PDGF-β, TIMP-1, and MCP-1. A study by Sun et al. [85] showed that the incubation of HUVECs with a phytoestrogen, namely pseudoprotodioscin, resulted in a reduction in MCP-1 mRNA expression, an effect mediated by ERα. This inconsistency could be due to differences in the estrogen receptor profiles of our HAECs, which expressed only GPR-30.

We also demonstrated that E_2 decreased the MMP-2 activity. Interestingly, since our cells express only GPR-30, this favorable effect is exerted via this membrane receptor. Indeed, co-incubation with the antagonist G15 reversed the decrease in the MMP-2 activity.

In order to mimic the low-grade inflammation state that exists in postmenopausal women with atherosclerosis, we pre-incubated the endothelial cells with TNF-α at a low concentration [86,87] and then co-incubated them with E_2 at various concentrations, including the low concentrations found in the serum of women receiving estrogen replacement therapy.

Interestingly, under low-grade inflammation, E_2 at low concentrations (10^{-10} M) increased the mRNA and protein levels of MCP-1, which is a key player in atherosclerotic plaque formation and destabilization.

MCP-1 is one of the most widely studied chemokines involved in the atherosclerosis process and has been postulated to be a direct mediator of plaque instability [88]. Interestingly, the local gene silencing of MCP-1 expression turned a vulnerable plaque into a more stable plaque phenotype in ApoE(−/−) mice [89]. The elevated expression of MCP-1 has also been found in the unstable plaques of CVD symptomatic patients [90].

Notably, the co-incubation with the GPR-30 antagonist G15 totally reversed the stimulatory effect of E_2 on MCP-1 mRNA expression, implying that GPR-30 exerts unfavorable effects of E_2 on the molecules implicated in the vulnerability of atherosclerotic plaque under low-grade inflammation conditions.

A previous study investigating the effect of E_2 on MCP-1 expression in breast cancer cell lines reported that E_2 induced MCP-1 expression when the cells were pre-treated with TNF-α. Notably, these breast cancer cells expressed both GPR-30 and ERα [91]. On the other hand, in rat aortic smooth muscle cells (RASMCs), E_2 inhibited the stimulatory effect of TNF-α on MCP-1 expression via an ERβ-dependent mechanism [92,93]. Accordingly, herein, we found that ERβ mediates the MCP-1-lowering effects of E_2, albeit in the absence of inflammatory stimuli.

Our data showed that, in a low-grade inflammation state, E_2 also reduced LOX-1 expression, an effect mediated via GPR-30. Our current knowledge regarding the role of LOX in the formation, progression, and vulnerability of atherosclerosis plaque is limited and is mostly derived from in vitro studies. Interestingly, a study by Jover et al. revealed that the expression of LOX is linked to plaque stability. As such, low LOX activity could lead to defective collagen cross-linking, resulting in a weaker fibrous cap and plaque instability [48,49]. Previous studies on another type of cells (Ishikawa cells) demonstrated that, in the absence of TNF-α, E_2 induced LOX-1 expression, while in rat cardiac fibroblasts, it exerted the opposite effect, mediated mainly through ERβ [94,95].

Increased MMP activity is a known indicator of atherosclerotic plaque instability [38,96,97]. Elevated MMP-2 activity has been determined to be an independent mortality marker in patients with acute coronary syndrome [98]. Studies in ApoE-/- mice showed that MMP-2 activity also contributes to the calcification of advanced atherosclerotic lesions [78,79]. Herein, we showed that E_2 can reduce the activation of MMP-2 in a dose-dependent manner. More interestingly, low concentrations of E_2 showed a more potent effect on the attenuation of MMP-2 activity. A previous study conducted on smooth muscle cells (ASMC) isolated from B6 mice showed that E_2 reduced MMP-2 activity, indicating its favorable effects in the absence of inflammation [99]. Wingrove et al. demonstrated that the incubation of human coronary artery vascular smooth muscle (CAVSMC) cells with E_2 for 72 h resulted in a dose-dependent increase in the expression of pro-MMP-2, an effect that was reversed by the estrogen receptor antagonist tamoxifen [100]. In line with these findings, we found that the expression of pro-MMP-2 was also induced; however, the conversion of pro-MMP2 to active MMP2 was decreased upon treatment with E_2. Significantly, we found that, in a state resembling low-grade inflammation (such as established atherosclerosis), E_2 further increased the TNF-α-induced MMP-2 activation in HAECs, with the greatest effect at the lowest concentration.

The expression of MMP-9 was faintly detected in the presence of E_2 alone, while it was significantly elevated upon treatment of the HAECs with TNF-α alone, as expected [101,102]. Interestingly, we demonstrated that E_2 further promoted the TNF-α-induced MMP-9 expression in the HAECs. Zanger et al. demonstrated a significant increase in the MMP-9 plasma levels of 10 postmenopausal women with a history of established CAD when receiving oral HRT, which is of clinical relevance to our observation [103]. However, not all clinical studies point towards a harmful effect of oral hormone replacement therapy on the indices of plaque vulnerability [103,104]. This divergency could be attributed to differences in age, the duration of the post-menopausal period, and the existence (or not) of established CVD among the studies' participants.

It is known that the imbalance between MMPs and TIMPs is implicated in atherosclerotic plaque instability [105]. Reduced TIMP expression has been correlated with unstable plaques and acute coronary syndrome in humans [106]. Our results showed that E_2 increased the TNFα-induced expression of TIMP-1. However, this elevation did not exceed the MMP-9 overexpression, suggesting that, in the presence of inflammatory stimuli, E_2 increased the MMP-9/TIMP-1 expression ratio. In accordance with our in vitro model, the MMP-9/TIMP1 ratio was also significantly higher in women receiving estrogen replacement therapy compared to women not taking HRT [107].

All the abovementioned effects were mediated via GPR-30, since the HAECs used for our experiments expressed only this estrogen receptor. Previous studies demonstrated that estrogen can regulate MMP and TIMP expression by binding to either the classical estrogen receptors ERα and ERβ or its membrane-bound estrogen receptor GPER-30 [108]. However, GPR-30 seems to play a prominent role in the regulation of MMPs in the cardiovascular system [109,110]. As such, apigenin, a compound with strong estrogen-like effects, inhibited the MMP-9 expression in endothelial cells through GPR-30 [111], while the incubation of cardiac fibroblasts isolated from Sprague–Dawley rats with G1, an GPR-30 agonist, significantly increased the MMP-2 and reduced TIMP-1 expression [108].

Notably, previous studies demonstrated that estrogen can regulate MMP and TIMP expression by binding to either the classical estrogen receptors ERα and ERβ or its membrane-bound estrogen receptor GPR-30 [108]. To elucidate the specific role of the classical estrogen receptors in the regulation of the abovementioned factors implicated in the later stages of the atherosclerosis process, we transfected HAECs with either ERα or ERβ. Herein, we observed that the transfection of HAECs with either ERα or ERβ did not affect the MMP-2 and MMP-9 expression and gelatinase activity. Although the TIMP-1 and TIMP-2 mRNA levels were elevated significantly after the incubation of Erα-transfected cells with E_2 at lower concentrations, the protein levels of TMP-1 and TIMP-2 were not increased significantly, suggesting possible post-transcriptional modifications.

Moreover, the incubation of ERα-transfected HAECs with E_2 resulted in a marginal increase in the LOX-1 and MCP-1 expression. Studies on other estrogen-dependent tissues have shown that E_2 induces LOX mRNA expression in the uteri of WT mice, as compared to ERαKO mice, indicating the important role of ERα in estrogen-mediated LOX overexpression [112,113]. Moreover, ERα inhibition was found to reduce the MCP-1 expression in mesangial cells [114].

Our data also revealed that the incubation of Erβ-transfected cells with E_2 results in a reduced PDGF-β and LOX expression. There is evidence to suggest that ERβ reduces the expression and secretion of the pro-agiogenic factors PDGF-β in T47D breast cancer cells [115].

In line with our findings, Iorga et al. showed that DPN treatment, a selective Erβ agonist, in mice with advanced heart failure (HF) significantly reduces the LOX-1 mRNA expression in the ventricles as compared to untreated HF mice [94]. Moreover, the transfection of cells with ERβ resulted in a reduced MCP-1 protein expression, while it had no effect on the TIMP-1 and TIMP-2 protein levels. As shown by Kanda et al., E_2-bound ERβ restrains the expression of MCP-1 by inhibiting the Sp1 and AP-1 transcriptional activities in keratinocytes [116]. To our knowledge, the present study provides the first experimental evidence to support the regulatory roles of ERβ in PDGF-β and MCP-1 expression in the endothelial cells.

Divergent data exist regarding the role of p21 in the atherosclerosis process and plaque stability, which has been assumed as both proatherogenic and antiatherogenic according to animal studies. However, the majority of the literature points toward a favorable effect; thus, therapies that target p21WAF1 for inactivation, in the appropriate situation, may offer protection against atherosclerosis [66,68,117,118].

Given the equivocal role of p21 in the atherosclerosis process and the fact that E_2 can exert effects by regulating p21 expression [71], we also aimed to explore the effect of p21 silencing on the estrogen-induced changes in the expression of molecules involved in the later stages of atherosclerosis [68].

Our results illustrate that the incubation of HAECs with E_2 after p21 silencing results in reductions in the MCP-1, ADAMST-4 and LOX mRNA levels. It is noteworthy that, when p21 is expressed, a low concentration of E_2 exerts the opposite effects, inducing the expression of LOX-1 in HAECs. As addressed in the literature, p21 positively affects the expression of MCP-1 in endothelial cells [119]. Additionally, it has been shown that the activation of GPR-30 (via the G1 agonist) increases the expression of p21 in breast cancer cell lines [81]. Given that GPR-30 is the only estrogen receptor expressed in our cells, it appears that the increase in the LOX expression by E_2 is mediated by GPR-30 through p21, thus providing a possible explanation for the effect of p21 silencing, which resulted in reduced LOX expression. It should be noted that, in the literature thus far, there are no data regarding the regulation of LOX by p21 in human endothelial cells. Another notable finding of our study is that p21 silencing resulted in a significant increase in PDGF-β expression in HAECs upon treatment with E_2, which may contribute to plaque instability [120]. Based on these findings, it could be suggested that the expression of PDGF-β, LOX -1, and MCP-1 is regulated by estrogen through more than one mechanism, including a p21-dependent mechanism. Moreover, p21 silencing may change the balance of these multiple (counter-)regulatory mechanisms, thus resulting in either an atheroprotective effect by decreasing the expression of LOX-1, MCP-1, and ADAMTS-4 or an increased risk of atheromatic plaque rupture through the elevation of PDGF-β expression, depending on the actions that finally prevail.

Summarizing our data, in the absence of an inflammatory stimulus, E_2, at low concentrations resembling those in the serum of postmenopausal women receiving estrogen replacement therapy, exerts atheroprotective effects by mainly decreasing MMP-2 activity and increasing LOX expression via GPR-30 and by reducing MCP-1 protein expression via ERβ. The overexpression of ERα may result in E_2-induced plaque instability by increasing the MCP-1 protein expression and MMP-2 activity. Significantly, in a low-grade inflammation state, such as established atherosclerosis, E_2 promotes the destabilization of the atherosclerotic plaque by inducing the expression of molecules such as MCP-1 and MMP-9 and by increasing the activity of MMP-2 in the endothelial cells. These effects appear to be mediated via GPR-30. Moreover, p21 silencing results in equivocal effects on the expression of molecules involved in plaque vulnerability.

In conclusion, E_2 induced different effects regarding atheromatous plaque instability through different ERs. The balance of the expression of the various ER subtypes may play an important role in the paradoxical characterization of estrogens as both beneficial and harmful.

To the best of our knowledge, this is the first study to assess, in vitro, the interrelation between different expression profiles of estrogen receptors and their regulatory effects on the expression of endothelial-derived factors implicated in atherosclerotic plaque vulnerability, addressing, at the same time, the possible involvement of p21 in this process. The strengths of this study are: (1) the performance of our experiments using aortic (arterial) endothelial cells (HAECs), which offer the best endothelial in vitro model system for studying the progression of atherosclerosis; (2) the fact that we incubated our cells with concentrations of E_2 that resemble those observed in the serum of postmenopausal women receiving estrogen replacement therapy; and (3) the fact that we pre-incubated the aortic endothelial cells with TNF-α at concentrations that mimic the low-grade inflammation state observed in postmenopausal women with established atherosclerosis. The main limitation of our study is that we failed to assess (due to the HAECs' sensitivity to the double transfection procedure) the role of p21 in the expression profiles of endothelial-derived factors involved in plaque vulnerability in the presence of either ERα or Erβ or both.

Further in vitro studies on other cellular components (i.e., VSMCs, immune cells) participating in the later stages of the atherosclerosis process, as well as studies on atherosclerosis animal models mimicking the postmenopausal status, are needed in order to delineate the exact roles of estrogen and of each estrogen receptor subtype in the atherosclerotic inflammatory process, so as to develop specific ER agonists/antagonists with an improved benefit/risk ratio.

4. Materials and Methods

4.1. Cell Culture and Treatment

Human aortic endothelial cells (HAECs) were purchased from Lonza and cultured in M200 medium (Gibco; Thermo Fisher Scientific, Inc., Waltham, MA, USA) supplemented with 10% fetal bovine serum (Gibco; Thermo Fisher Scientific, Inc.), 10% low-serum growth supplement (Gibco; Thermo Fisher Scientific, Inc.), and antibiotics (1% penicillin/streptomycin (Invitrogen; Thermo Fisher Scientific, Inc., Waltham, MA, USA). Cells were cultured in a cell incubator, providing a humidified environment with 5% CO_2 and 95% air at 37 °C. Confluent four- to seven-passage HAECs were used in all the experiments.

4.2. MTT Assay

Endothelial cells were plated 16 h before treatment on a 96-well plate at a cell density of 1×10^4 cells per well. Cells were then incubated with various concentrations of E_2 ($10^{-10}-10^{-7}$ M) (Cat. No: E2758, Sigma-Aldrich, St. Louis, MO, USA) and 2 ng/mL TNF-α alone for 24 h. The percentage of viable cells was measured using 0.5 mg/mL thiazolyl blue tetrazolium bromide (MTT). After 3 h of incubation at 37 °C, the MTT solution was removed and 100 μL of isopropanol was added to each well to aid the crystal dissolution. The optical density (OD) values of the colorimetric changes were measured using an ELISA reader at 570 nm.

4.3. Transfection with Small Interfering RNA

The HAECs were transfected at a 70% confluence for 24 h with 20 nM small interfering (si) RNAs targeting human p21 (sc-29427, Santa Cruz Technology, Dallas, TX, USA) using Lipofectamine 2000 reagent (Invitrogen) according to the manufacturer's instructions. After 6 h, fresh medium was added, and the cells were incubated in full medium for further 24 h. Next, the cells were incubated with various concentrations of E_2 ($10^{-10}-10^{-7}$ M) for 24 h prior to analysis.

4.4. Transient Transfection Assays

Next, 1×10^5 HAEC were seeded in each well of the 12-well plate in 1 mL complete media. After 24 h, 1 µg/mL of the either ERα, ERβ, or a corresponding empty vector using DNA was introduced to the cells using AppliFect LowTox (A9027-applichem) transfection reagent according to the manufacturer's instructions. Briefly, the cells were incubated with the DNA/AppliFect LowTox mix for 4 h, and then the media was replaced with fresh media for a further 20 h. Twenty-four after the transfection, the media was switched to 5% charcoal stripped FBS (Gibco) phenol-free complete media for another 6 h, followed by the incubation of the cells with the various concentrations of E_2 (10^{-10}–10^{-7} M) for a further 24 h. The efficiency of the transfection was determined by qPCR and western blot analysis. All experiments were repeated a minimum of three times.

4.5. RNA Isolation and qPCR

The qRT-PCR was performed as previously described [121]. For the quantitative real-time PCR, HAEC cells were plated on 12-well plates 16 h prior to treatment with various concentrations of E_2 (10^{-10}–10^{-7} M) for periods of 6, 12, and 24 h. The cells were also pre-incubated with TNF-α (2 ng/mL) for 24 h in order to mimic the low-grade inflammation seen in atherosclerosis, and then co-incubated with various concentrations of E_2. At the end of the treatment, the cells were harvested and the total RNA was isolated from the HAECs using NucleoSpin® RNA Plus (Macherey-Nagel, Düren, Germany). The quality of the extracted mRNA was evaluated by nanodrop. A volume equal to 1000 ng of RNA was then reverse-transcribed using the LunaScript™ RT SuperMix Kit (New England Biolabs, Ipswich, MA, USA) in accordance with the manufacturer's instructions. Glyceraldehyde 3-phosphate dehydrogenase (GAPDH) was used as a normalization control. The mRNA levels of GAPDH, MMP2, MMP-9, TIMP-1, TIMP-2, MCP-1, OPG, RANK, RANKL, ADAMTS-4, lysyl oxidase (LOX), PDGF-,β and p21, as well as the presence of estrogen receptors ERα, Erβ, and GPR-30 in the HAEC cells, were evaluated using the SYBR Green-based quantitative real-time polymerase chain reaction (qRT-PCR) protocol on a CFX96 (Biorad). The 2−ΔΔCT method was used to determine the expression level. The sequence of the primers used in this study is listed in Table 1. All experiments were performed in triplicate.

Table 1. The sequences of primers used for the qRT-PCR analysis.

Primer	Forward	Reverse
MMP-2	5′-TGGCAAGTACGGCTTCTGTC-3′	5′-TTCTTGTCGCGGTCGTAGTC-3′
MMP-9	5′-TGCGCTACCACCTCGAACTT-3′	5′-GATGCCATTGACGTCGTCCT-3′
TIMP-1	5′-TGCGGATACTTCCACAGGTC-3′	5′-GCATTCCTCACAGCCAACAG-3′
TIMP-2	5′-AAGAGCCTGAACCACAGGTA-3′	5′-GAGCCGTCACTTCTCTTGAT-3′
MCP-1	5′-AATAGGAAGATCTCAGTGCA-3′	5′-TCAAGTCTTCGGAGTTTGGG-3′
OPG	5′-GGAACCCCAGAGCGAAATACA-3′	5′-CCTGAAGAATGCCTCCTCACA-3′
RANK	5′-CCCGTTGCAGCTCAACAAG-3′	5′-GCATTTGTCCGTGGAGGAA-3′
RANKL	5′-ACGCAGTGAAAACACAGTT-3′	5′-TGCCTCTGGCTGGAAACC-3′
LOX-1	5′-CCAGAGGAGAGTGGCTGAAG-3′	5′-CCAGGTAGCTGGGGTTTACA-3′
PDGF-β	5′-CCATTCCCGAGGAGCTTTATG-3′	5′-CAGCAGGCGTTGGAGATCAT-3′
P21	5′-ATGAAATTCACCCCCTTTCC-3′	5′-CCCTAGGCTGTGCTCACTTC-3′
ER-α	5′-TGGGCTTACTGACCAACCTG-3′	5′-CCTGATCATGGAGGGTCAAA-3′
ER-β	5′-AGAGTCCCTGGTGTGAAGCA-3′	5′-GACAGCGCAGAAGTGAGCATC-3′
GPR-30	5′-TCACGGGCCACATTGTCAACCTC	5′-GCTGAACCTCACATCTGACTGCTC
GAPDH	5′-GGGTGTGAACCATGAGAAGT-3′	5′-CATGCCAGTGAGCTTCCCGTT-3′
ADAMTS-4	5′-GACACTGGTGGTGGCAGATG-3′	5′-TCACTGTTAGCAGGTAGCGCTTTA-3′

4.6. SDS-PAGE and Western-Blot Analysis

The western blot analysis was performed as previously described [121]. Briefly, whole-cell lysates were prepared in lysis buffer (Cell-Signaling Technology, Boston, MA, USA). Samples containing 30 µg of protein were resolved using electrophoresis gels and transferred to a nitrocellulose membrane. The membranes were blocked for 1 h with 5% skimmed milk in PBS with 0.1% Tween 20 and subsequently incubated overnight at 4 °C with anti-ERα (sc-8002, Santa Cruz Technology, Dallas, TX, USA, 1:800), anti-ERβ (sc-390243, Santa Cruz Technology, Dallas, TX, USA, 1:800) anti-GPR30 (sc-48524-R, Santa Cruz Technology, 1:800), anti-p21 (Cell-Signaling, MA, USA, 1:500), and anti-β-actin (Millipore Corporation, Billerica, MA, USA, 1:5000) primary antibodies. The membranes were probed with secondary antibodies coupled with horseradish peroxidase goat anti-mouse IgG-HRP (31430, Thermo Scientific; 1:2500) and goat anti-rabbit IgG-HRP (AP132P, Millipore Corporation, Billerica, MA, USA, 1:2500) at room temperature (RT) for 1 h. The detection of the immunoreactive bands was performed using Clarity Western ECL Substrate (BioRad, Bio-Rad Laboratories Inc., Hercules, CA, USA). For this purpose, β-actin served as a loading control. The densitometric analysis was performed using Image J.

4.7. ELISA

Cell-secreted TIMP-1 (DTM100, R&D Systems, Minneapolis, MN, USA), TIMP-2 (DTM200, R&D Systems, Minneapolis, MN, USA), MCP-1 (DCP00, R&D Systems, Minneapolis, MN, USA), and OPG (RAB0484, Sigma-Aldrich, St. Louis, Missouri, USA) were measured with the respective ELISA kits containing pre-coated ELISA plates, and the assays were performed as described by the manufacturers. Briefly, 100 µL of cell culture supernatant or standard was incubated in each well for 3 h at RT. Then, the HRP-conjugated antibody was added and incubated for 1 h at RT, followed by aspiration and three washes. Next, horseradish peroxidase was added and incubated for 1 h, followed by aspiration and washes. 3,3′,5,5′-Tetramethylbenzidine substrate was added to each well and incubated for 30 min in a dark chamber. Stop solution was added, and the absorbency of all ELISAs was read at 450 nm with a plate reader (Bio-Rad® Microplate Absorbance Reader, Bio-Rad Laboratories Inc., Hercules, CA, USA).

4.8. Zymography

The gelatin zymography activity of MMP-2 was evaluated by measuring the gelatinolytic activities of pro-MMP-2 and active MMP-2. Equal numbers of HAECs (1×10^{-6} cells/well) were cultured in M200 medium for 24 h, and then either normal HAECs or cells transfected with ERα, ERβ, plasmid, or p21 siRNA were serum-starved for 16 h. Thereafter, the cells were incubated with various concentrations of E_2 (10^{-10}–10^{-7} M) alone (24 h) or pre-incubated with TNF-α (2 ng/mL) for 24 h and then co-incubated with various concentrations of E_2 for a further 24 h. At the end of the incubation time, the cell supernatant was collected and concentrated using Amicon Ultra centrifugal filters (30 kDa-Millipore). The protein concentrations were calculated by performing a Bradford assay. Pro-MMP-2 and active MMP-2 proteins in the conditioned media were separated without prior boiling by electrophoresis with 10% sodium dodecyl sulfatepolyacrylamide gels containing 0.1% (weight/volume) gelatin (Sigma-Aldrich). The gels were incubated with 2.5% Triton X-100 for 1 h at room temperature. The gels were then incubated at 37 °C in the developing buffer (Invitrogen) for 16 h. The gels were stained with 0.5% Coomassie Brilliant Blue (AppliChem, Darmstadt, Germany) and de-stained in a solution containing 40% methanol and 10% acetic acid. Clear zones against the blue background indicated the presence of gelatinolytic activity. The densitometrical analyses of the zymographic images were performed using image J software (NIH, Bethesda, MD, USA).

4.9. Statistical

Data are represented as mean ± SD. The statistical analysis was performed using Student's *t*-test with a two-tailed distribution. The statistical analysis of the real-time

PCR data was performed using the non-parametric test (Wilcoxon signed rank test). All statistical analyses were performed using GraphPad Prism 7 Software. In all conditions, the minimum level of significance was set at $p < 0.05$.

Supplementary Materials: The following supporting information can be downloaded at: https://www.mdpi.com/article/10.3390/ijms231810960/s1.

Author Contributions: N.N.-A. and E.S. performed all the experiments. V.K. performed part of the qPCR experiments. N.N.-A. and E.S. contributed to the writing of the manuscript. N.N.-A., V.K., D.S. and I.K. evaluated the results and contributed to the data analysis and preparation of figures. V.K, I.K. and A.C. contributed to the data evaluation and analysis. P.M., A.G.P., K.D.-W. and E.K. contributed to the interpretation of the results. A.G.P., H.S.R. and E.K. performed the critical review of the study's design. E.K. conceived the project idea, designed and supervised the experiments, and interpreted the results. E.K critically revised the manuscript with the contribution of N.N.-A. E.K. gave the final approval of the version to be published. All authors have read and agreed to the published version of the manuscript.

Funding: This work was funded by the "ARISTEIA" program (Program's code: 11897).

Institutional Review Board Statement: Not applicable.

Informed Consent Statement: Not applicable.

Data Availability Statement: Data are contained within the article and its Supplementary Materials.

Conflicts of Interest: The authors declare no conflict of interest.

References

1. Garcia, M.; Mulvagh, S.L.; Merz, C.N.; Buring, J.E.; Manson, J.E. Cardiovascular Disease in Women: Clinical Perspectives. *Circ. Res.* **2016**, *118*, 1273–1293. [CrossRef]
2. Kim, H.; Kim, S.; Han, S.; Rane, P.P.; Fox, K.M.; Qian, Y.; Suh, H.S. Prevalence and incidence of atherosclerotic cardiovascular disease and its risk factors in Korea: A nationwide population-based study. *BMC Public Health* **2019**, *19*, 1112. [CrossRef]
3. Chen, G.; Farris, M.S.; Cowling, T.; Pinto, L.; Rogoza, R.M.; MacKinnon, E.; Champsi, S.; Anderson, T.J. Prevalence of atherosclerotic cardiovascular disease and subsequent major adverse cardiovascular events in Alberta, Canada: A real-world evidence study. *Clin. Cardiol.* **2021**, *44*, 1613–1620. [CrossRef]
4. Sima, P.; Vannucci, L.; Vetvicka, V. Atherosclerosis as autoimmune disease. *Ann. Transl. Med.* **2018**, *6*, 116. [CrossRef]
5. Spring, B.; Moller, A.C.; Colangelo, L.A.; Siddique, J.; Roehrig, M.; Daviglus, M.L.; Polak, J.F.; Reis, J.P.; Sidney, S.; Liu, K. Healthy lifestyle change and subclinical atherosclerosis in young adults: Coronary Artery Risk Development in Young Adults (CARDIA) study. *Circulation* **2014**, *130*, 10–17. [CrossRef]
6. Barton, M. Cholesterol and atherosclerosis: Modulation by oestrogen. *Curr. Opin. Lipidol.* **2013**, *24*, 214–220. [CrossRef]
7. Stampfer, M.J.; Colditz, G.A.; Willett, W.C.; Manson, J.E.; Rosner, B.; Speizer, F.E.; Hennekens, C.H. Postmenopausal estrogen therapy and cardiovascular disease. Ten-year follow-up from the nurses' health study. *N. Engl. J. Med.* **1991**, *325*, 756–762. [CrossRef]
8. Meng, Q.; Li, Y.; Ji, T.; Chao, Y.; Li, J.; Fu, Y.; Wang, S.; Chen, Q.; Chen, W.; Huang, F.; et al. Estrogen prevent atherosclerosis by attenuating endothelial cell pyroptosis via activation of estrogen receptor alpha-mediated autophagy. *J. Adv. Res.* **2021**, *28*, 149–164. [CrossRef]
9. Fashe, M.; Yi, M.; Sueyoshi, T.; Negishi, M. Sex-specific expression mechanism of hepatic estrogen inactivating enzyme and transporters in diabetic women. *Biochem. Pharmacol.* **2021**, *190*, 114662. [CrossRef]
10. Fonseca, M.I.H.; da Silva, I.T.; Ferreira, S.R.G. Impact of menopause and diabetes on atherogenic lipid profile: Is it worth to analyse lipoprotein subfractions to assess cardiovascular risk in women? *Diabetol. Metab. Syndr.* **2017**, *9*, 22. [CrossRef]
11. Sato, A.; Watanabe, H.; Yamazaki, M.; Sakurai, E.; Ebina, K. Estrogen Sulfotransferase is Highly Expressed in Vascular Endothelial Cells Overlying Atherosclerotic Plaques. *Protein. J.* **2022**, *41*, 179–188. [CrossRef]
12. Fait, T. Menopause hormone therapy: Latest developments and clinical practice. *Drugs Context* **2019**, *8*, 212551. [CrossRef]
13. Hansson, G.K.; Libby, P. The immune response in atherosclerosis: A double-edged sword. *Nat. Rev. Immunol.* **2006**, *6*, 508–519. [CrossRef]
14. Seo, D.W.; Saxinger, W.C.; Guedez, L.; Cantelmo, A.R.; Albini, A.; Stetler-Stevenson, W.G. An integrin-binding N-terminal peptide region of TIMP-2 retains potent angio-inhibitory and anti-tumorigenic activity in vivo. *Peptides* **2011**, *32*, 1840–1848. [CrossRef]
15. Botts, S.R.; Fish, J.E.; Howe, K.L. Dysfunctional Vascular Endothelium as a Driver of Atherosclerosis: Emerging Insights Into Pathogenesis and Treatment. *Front. Pharmacol.* **2021**, *12*, 787541. [CrossRef]
16. Salaminia, S.; Mohsenzadeh, Y.; Motedayen, M.; Sayehmiri, F.; Dousti, M. Hormone Replacement Therapy and Postmenopausal Cardiovascular Events: A Meta-Analysis. *Iran. Red. Crescent. Med.* **2019**, *21*, e82298. [CrossRef]

17. Wolters, M.; Dejanovic, G.M.; Asllanaj, E.; Gunther, K.; Pohlabeln, H.; Bramer, W.M.; Ahrens, J.; Nagrani, R.; Pigeot, I.; Franco, O.H.; et al. Effects of phytoestrogen supplementation on intermediate cardiovascular disease risk factors among post-menopausal women: A meta-analysis of randomized controlled trials. *Menopause* **2020**, *27*, 1081–1092. [CrossRef]
18. Adam, S.K.; Das, S.; Soelaiman, I.N.; Umar, N.A.; Jaarin, K. Consumption of repeatedly heated soy oil increases the serum parameters related to atherosclerosis in ovariectomized rats. *Tohoku J. Exp. Med.* **2008**, *215*, 219–226. [CrossRef]
19. Hassan, H.A.; Abdel-Wahhab, M.A. Effect of soybean oil on atherogenic metabolic risks associated with estrogen deficiency in ovariectomized rats: Dietary soybean oil modulate atherogenic risks in overiectomized rats. *J. Physiol. Biochem.* **2012**, *68*, 247–253. [CrossRef]
20. Hulley, S.; Grady, D.; Bush, T.; Furberg, C.; Herrington, D.; Riggs, B.; Vittinghoff, E. Randomized trial of estrogen plus progestin for secondary prevention of coronary heart disease in postmenopausal women. Heart and Estrogen/progestin Replacement Study (HERS) Research Group. *JAMA* **1998**, *280*, 605–613. [CrossRef]
21. Kim, J.E.; Chang, J.H.; Jeong, M.J.; Choi, J.; Park, J.; Baek, C.; Shin, A.; Park, S.M.; Kang, D.; Choi, J.Y. A systematic review and meta-analysis of effects of menopausal hormone therapy on cardiovascular diseases. *Sci. Rep.* **2020**, *10*, 20631. [CrossRef] [PubMed]
22. Rossouw, J.E.; Anderson, G.L.; Prentice, R.L.; LaCroix, A.Z.; Kooperberg, C.; Stefanick, M.L.; Jackson, R.D.; Beresford, S.A.; Howard, B.V.; Johnson, K.C.; et al. Risks and benefits of estrogen plus progestin in healthy postmenopausal women: Principal results From the Women's Health Initiative randomized controlled trial. *JAMA* **2002**, *288*, 321–333. [CrossRef] [PubMed]
23. Mehta, J.; Kling, J.M.; Manson, J.E. Risks, Benefits, and Treatment Modalities of Menopausal Hormone Therapy: Current Concepts. *Front. Endocrinol.* **2021**, *12*, 564781. [CrossRef] [PubMed]
24. Denti, L. The hormone replacement therapy (HRT) of menopause: Focus on cardiovascular implications. *Acta Biomed.* **2010**, *81* (Suppl. S1), 73–76. [PubMed]
25. Hodis, H.N.; Mack, W.J. The timing hypothesis and hormone replacement therapy: A paradigm shift in the primary prevention of coronary heart disease in women. Part 1: Comparison of therapeutic efficacy. *J. Am. Geriatr. Soc.* **2013**, *61*, 1005–1010. [CrossRef]
26. Arnal, J.F.; Fontaine, C.; Billon-Gales, A.; Favre, J.; Laurell, H.; Lenfant, F.; Gourdy, P. Estrogen receptors and endothelium. *Arterioscler. Thromb. Vasc. Biol.* **2010**, *30*, 1506–1512. [CrossRef]
27. Nofer, J.R. Estrogens and atherosclerosis: Insights from animal models and cell systems. *J. Mol. Endocrinol.* **2012**, *48*, R13–R29. [CrossRef]
28. Trenti, A.; Tedesco, S.; Boscaro, C.; Trevisi, L.; Bolego, C.; Cignarella, A. Estrogen, Angiogenesis, Immunity and Cell Metabolism: Solving the Puzzle. *Int. J. Mol. Sci.* **2018**, *19*, 859. [CrossRef]
29. Lenfant, F.; Tremollieres, F.; Gourdy, P.; Arnal, J.F. Timing of the vascular actions of estrogens in experimental and human studies: Why protective early, and not when delayed? *Maturitas* **2011**, *68*, 165–173. [CrossRef]
30. Davezac, M.; Buscato, M.; Zahreddine, R.; Lacolley, P.; Henrion, D.; Lenfant, F.; Arnal, J.F.; Fontaine, C. Estrogen Receptor and Vascular Aging. *Front. Aging* **2021**, *2*, 727380. [CrossRef]
31. Arnal, J.F.; Lenfant, F.; Metivier, R.; Flouriot, G.; Henrion, D.; Adlanmerini, M.; Fontaine, C.; Gourdy, P.; Chambon, P.; Katzenellenbogen, B.; et al. Membrane and Nuclear Estrogen Receptor Alpha Actions: From Tissue Specificity to Medical Implications. *Physiol. Rev.* **2017**, *97*, 1045–1087. [CrossRef] [PubMed]
32. Kassi, E.; Spilioti, E.; Nasiri-Ansari, N.; Adamopoulos, C.; Moutsatsou, P.; Papanagiotou, A.; Siasos, G.; Tousoulis, D.; Papavassiliou, A.G. Vascular Inflammation and Atherosclerosis: The Role of Estrogen Receptors. *Curr. Med. Chem.* **2015**, *22*, 2651–2665. [CrossRef] [PubMed]
33. Shioi, A.; Ikari, Y. Plaque Calcification During Atherosclerosis Progression and Regression. *J. Atheroscler. Thromb.* **2018**, *25*, 294–303. [CrossRef] [PubMed]
34. Georgakis, M.K.; Gill, D.; Rannikmae, K.; Traylor, M.; Anderson, C.D.; Lee, J.M.; Kamatani, Y.; Hopewell, J.C.; Worrall, B.B.; Bernhagen, J.; et al. Genetically Determined Levels of Circulating Cytokines and Risk of Stroke. *Circulation* **2019**, *139*, 256–268. [CrossRef] [PubMed]
35. Georgakis, M.K.; Malik, R.; Bjorkbacka, H.; Pana, T.A.; Demissie, S.; Ayers, C.; Elhadad, M.A.; Fornage, M.; Beiser, A.S.; Benjamin, E.J.; et al. Circulating Monocyte Chemoattractant Protein-1 and Risk of Stroke: Meta-Analysis of Population-Based Studies Involving 17 180 Individuals. *Circ. Res.* **2019**, *125*, 773–782. [CrossRef] [PubMed]
36. Georgakis, M.K.; van der Laan, S.W.; Asare, Y.; Mekke, J.M.; Haitjema, S.; Schoneveld, A.H.; de Jager, S.C.A.; Nurmohamed, N.S.; Kroon, J.; Stroes, E.S.G.; et al. Monocyte-Chemoattractant Protein-1 Levels in Human Atherosclerotic Lesions Associate With Plaque Vulnerability. *Arterioscler. Thromb. Vasc. Biol.* **2021**, *41*, 2038–2048. [CrossRef]
37. Ho, F.M.; Liu, S.H.; Lin, W.W.; Liau, C.S. Opposite effects of high glucose on MMP-2 and TIMP-2 in human endothelial cells. *J. Cell Biochem.* **2007**, *101*, 442–450. [CrossRef]
38. Olejarz, W.; Lacheta, D.; Kubiak-Tomaszewska, G. Matrix Metalloproteinases as Biomarkers of Atherosclerotic Plaque Instability. *Int. J. Mol. Sci.* **2020**, *21*, 3946. [CrossRef]
39. Vacek, T.P.; Rehman, S.; Neamtu, D.; Yu, S.; Givimani, S.; Tyagi, S.C. Matrix metalloproteinases in atherosclerosis: Role of nitric oxide, hydrogen sulfide, homocysteine, and polymorphisms. *Vasc. Health Risk Manag.* **2015**, *11*, 173–183. [CrossRef]
40. Wang, X.; Khalil, R.A. Matrix Metalloproteinases, Vascular Remodeling, and Vascular Disease. *Adv. Pharmacol.* **2018**, *81*, 241–330. [CrossRef]

41. Nasiri-Ansari, N.; Dimitriadis, G.K.; Agrogiannis, G.; Perrea, D.; Kostakis, I.D.; Kaltsas, G.; Papavassiliou, A.G.; Randeva, H.S.; Kassi, E. Canagliflozin attenuates the progression of atherosclerosis and inflammation process in APOE knockout mice. *Cardiovasc. Diabetol.* **2018**, *17*, 106. [CrossRef] [PubMed]
42. Perez-Martinez, L.; Jaworski, D.M. Tissue inhibitor of metalloproteinase-2 promotes neuronal differentiation by acting as an anti-mitogenic signal. *J. Neurosci.* **2005**, *25*, 4917–4929. [CrossRef] [PubMed]
43. Seo, D.W.; Li, H.; Qu, C.K.; Oh, J.; Kim, Y.S.; Diaz, T.; Wei, B.; Han, J.W.; Stetler-Stevenson, W.G. Shp-1 mediates the antiproliferative activity of tissue inhibitor of metalloproteinase-2 in human microvascular endothelial cells. *J. Biol. Chem.* **2006**, *281*, 3711–3721. [CrossRef]
44. Wessely, R. Atherosclerosis and cell cycle: Put the brakes on! Critical role for cyclin-dependent kinase inhibitors. *J. Am. Coll. Cardiol.* **2010**, *55*, 2269–2271. [CrossRef]
45. Novak, R.; Hrkac, S.; Salai, G.; Bilandzic, J.; Mitar, L.; Grgurevic, L. The Role of ADAMTS-4 in Atherosclerosis and Vessel Wall Abnormalities. *J. Vasc. Res.* **2022**, *59*, 69–77. [CrossRef]
46. Kumar, S.; Chen, M.; Li, Y.; Wong, F.H.; Thiam, C.W.; Hossain, M.Z.; Poh, K.K.; Hirohata, S.; Ogawa, H.; Angeli, V.; et al. Loss of ADAMTS4 reduces high fat diet-induced atherosclerosis and enhances plaque stability in ApoE(-/-) mice. *Sci. Rep.* **2016**, *6*, 31130. [CrossRef] [PubMed]
47. Dong, M.; Zhou, C.; Ji, L.; Pan, B.; Zheng, L. AG1296 enhances plaque stability via inhibiting inflammatory responses and decreasing MMP-2 and MMP-9 expression in ApoE−/− mice. *Biochem. Biophys. Res. Commun.* **2017**, *489*, 426–431. [CrossRef]
48. Jover, E.; Silvente, A.; Marin, F.; Martinez-Gonzalez, J.; Orriols, M.; Martinez, C.M.; Puche, C.M.; Valdes, M.; Rodriguez, C.; Hernandez-Romero, D. Inhibition of enzymes involved in collagen cross-linking reduces vascular smooth muscle cell calcification. *FASEB J.* **2018**, *32*, 4459–4469. [CrossRef]
49. Martinez-Gonzalez, J.; Varona, S.; Canes, L.; Galan, M.; Briones, A.M.; Cachofeiro, V.; Rodriguez, C. Emerging Roles of Lysyl Oxidases in the Cardiovascular System: New Concepts and Therapeutic Challenges. *Biomolecules* **2019**, *9*, 610. [CrossRef]
50. Kim, M.S.; Day, C.J.; Morrison, N.A. MCP-1 is induced by receptor activator of nuclear factor-{kappa}B ligand, promotes human osteoclast fusion, and rescues granulocyte macrophage colony-stimulating factor suppression of osteoclast formation. *J. Biol. Chem.* **2005**, *280*, 16163–16169. [CrossRef]
51. Montecucco, F.; Steffens, S.; Mach, F. The immune response is involved in atherosclerotic plaque calcification: Could the RANKL/RANK/OPG system be a marker of plaque instability? *Clin. Dev. Immunol.* **2007**, *2007*, 75805. [CrossRef]
52. Rochette, L.; Meloux, A.; Rigal, E.; Zeller, M.; Cottin, Y.; Vergely, C. The Role of Osteoprotegerin and Its Ligands in Vascular Function. *Int. J. Mol. Sci.* **2019**, *20*, 705. [CrossRef] [PubMed]
53. Schoppet, M.; Preissner, K.T.; Hofbauer, L.C. RANK ligand and osteoprotegerin: Paracrine regulators of bone metabolism and vascular function. *Arterioscler. Thromb. Vasc. Biol.* **2002**, *22*, 549–553. [CrossRef] [PubMed]
54. Malyankar, U.M.; Scatena, M.; Suchland, K.L.; Yun, T.J.; Clark, E.A.; Giachelli, C.M. Osteoprotegerin is an alpha vbeta 3-induced, NF-kappa B-dependent survival factor for endothelial cells. *J. Biol. Chem.* **2000**, *275*, 20959–20962. [CrossRef] [PubMed]
55. Wang, Y.; Liu, Y.; Huang, Z.; Chen, X.; Zhang, B. The roles of osteoprotegerin in cancer, far beyond a bone player. *Cell Death Discov.* **2022**, *8*, 252. [CrossRef]
56. Boraldi, F.; Lofaro, F.D.; Quaglino, D. Apoptosis in the Extraosseous Calcification Process. *Cells* **2021**, *10*, 131. [CrossRef]
57. Ono, T.; Hayashi, M.; Sasaki, F.; Nakashima, T. RANKL biology: Bone metabolism, the immune system, and beyond. *Inflamm. Regen.* **2020**, *40*, 2. [CrossRef]
58. Omland, T.; Ueland, T.; Jansson, A.M.; Persson, A.; Karlsson, T.; Smith, C.; Herlitz, J.; Aukrust, P.; Hartford, M.; Caidahl, K. Circulating osteoprotegerin levels and long-term prognosis in patients with acute coronary syndromes. *J. Am. Coll. Cardiol.* **2008**, *51*, 627–633. [CrossRef]
59. Gu, J.H.; Tong, X.S.; Chen, G.H.; Liu, X.Z.; Bian, J.C.; Yuan, Y.; Liu, Z.P. Regulation of matrix metalloproteinase-9 protein expression by 1alpha, 25-(OH)(2)D(3) during osteoclast differentiation. *J. Vet. Sci.* **2014**, *15*, 133–140. [CrossRef]
60. Rochette, L.; Meloux, A.; Rigal, E.; Zeller, M.; Cottin, Y.; Vergely, C. The role of osteoprotegerin in the crosstalk between vessels and bone: Its potential utility as a marker of cardiometabolic diseases. *Pharmacol. Ther.* **2018**, *182*, 115–132. [CrossRef]
61. Sandberg, W.J.; Yndestad, A.; Oie, E.; Smith, C.; Ueland, T.; Ovchinnikova, O.; Robertson, A.K.; Muller, F.; Semb, A.G.; Scholz, H.; et al. Enhanced T-cell expression of RANK ligand in acute coronary syndrome: Possible role in plaque destabilization. *Arterioscler. Thromb. Vasc. Biol.* **2006**, *26*, 857–863. [CrossRef] [PubMed]
62. Kiechl, S.; Schett, G.; Schwaiger, J.; Seppi, K.; Eder, P.; Egger, G.; Santer, P.; Mayr, A.; Xu, Q.; Willeit, J. Soluble receptor activator of nuclear factor-kappa B ligand and risk for cardiovascular disease. *Circulation* **2007**, *116*, 385–391. [CrossRef] [PubMed]
63. Mohammadpour, A.H.; Shamsara, J.; Nazemi, S.; Ghadirzadeh, S.; Shahsavand, S.; Ramezani, M. Evaluation of RANKL/OPG Serum Concentration Ratio as a New Biomarker for Coronary Artery Calcification: A Pilot Study. *Thrombosis* **2012**, *2012*, 306263. [CrossRef] [PubMed]
64. Ovchinnikova, O.; Gylfe, A.; Bailey, L.; Nordstrom, A.; Rudling, M.; Jung, C.; Bergstrom, S.; Waldenstrom, A.; Hansson, G.K.; Nordstrom, P. Osteoprotegerin promotes fibrous cap formation in atherosclerotic lesions of ApoE-deficient mice-brief report. *Arterioscler. Thromb. Vasc. Biol.* **2009**, *29*, 1478–1480. [CrossRef]
65. Ovchinnikova, O.A.; Folkersen, L.; Persson, J.; Lindeman, J.H.; Ueland, T.; Aukrust, P.; Gavrisheva, N.; Shlyakhto, E.; Paulsson-Berne, G.; Hedin, U.; et al. The collagen cross-linking enzyme lysyl oxidase is associated with the healing of human atherosclerotic lesions. *J. Intern. Med.* **2014**, *276*, 525–536. [CrossRef]

66. Merched, A.J.; Chan, L. Absence of p21Waf1/Cip1/Sdi1 modulates macrophage differentiation and inflammatory response and protects against atherosclerosis. *Circulation* **2004**, *110*, 3830–3841. [CrossRef]
67. Secchiero, P.; Corallini, F.; Rimondi, E.; Chiaruttini, C.; di Iasio, M.G.; Rustighi, A.; Del Sal, G.; Zauli, G. Activation of the p53 pathway down-regulates the osteoprotegerin expression and release by vascular endothelial cells. *Blood* **2008**, *111*, 1287–1294. [CrossRef]
68. Suzuki, M.; Minami, A.; Nakanishi, A.; Kobayashi, K.; Matsuda, S.; Ogura, Y.; Kitagishi, Y. Atherosclerosis and tumor suppressor molecules (review). *Int. J. Mol. Med.* **2014**, *34*, 934–940. [CrossRef]
69. Berger, C.; Qian, Y.; Chen, X. The p53-estrogen receptor loop in cancer. *Curr. Mol. Med.* **2013**, *13*, 1229–1240. [CrossRef]
70. Chimento, A.; De Luca, A.; Avena, P.; De Amicis, F.; Casaburi, I.; Sirianni, R.; Pezzi, V. Estrogen Receptors-Mediated Apoptosis in Hormone-Dependent Cancers. *Int. J. Mol. Sci.* **2022**, *23*, 1242. [CrossRef]
71. Wright, J.W.; Stouffer, R.L.; Rodland, K.D. High-dose estrogen and clinical selective estrogen receptor modulators induce growth arrest, p21, and p53 in primate ovarian surface epithelial cells. *J. Clin. Endocrinol. Metab.* **2005**, *90*, 3688–3695. [CrossRef] [PubMed]
72. McRobb, L.S.; McGrath, K.C.Y.; Tsatralis, T.; Liong, E.C.; Tan, J.T.M.; Hughes, G.; Handelsman, D.J.; Heather, A.K. Estrogen Receptor Control of Atherosclerotic Calcification and Smooth Muscle Cell Osteogenic Differentiation. *Arterioscler. Thromb. Vasc. Biol.* **2017**, *37*, 1127–1137. [CrossRef] [PubMed]
73. Villablanca, A.C.; Tenwolde, A.; Lee, M.; Huck, M.; Mumenthaler, S.; Rutledge, J.C. 17beta-estradiol prevents early-stage atherosclerosis in estrogen receptor-alpha deficient female mice. *J. Cardiovasc. Transl. Res.* **2009**, *2*, 289–299. [CrossRef] [PubMed]
74. Fontaine, C.; Morfoisse, F.; Tatin, F.; Zamora, A.; Zahreddine, R.; Henrion, D.; Arnal, J.-F.; Lenfant, F.; Garmy-Susini, B. The Impact of Estrogen Receptor in Arterial and Lymphatic Vascular Diseases. *Int. J. Mol. Sci.* **2020**, *21*, 3244. [CrossRef] [PubMed]
75. Sun, T.; Cao, L.; Ping, N.N.; Wu, Y.; Liu, D.Z.; Cao, Y.X. Formononetin upregulates nitric oxide synthase in arterial endothelium through estrogen receptors and MAPK pathways. *J. Pharm. Pharmacol.* **2016**, *68*, 342–351. [CrossRef]
76. Ahmad, N.; Chen, S.; Wang, W.; Kapila, S. 17beta-estradiol Induces MMP-9 and MMP-13 in TMJ Fibrochondrocytes via Estrogen Receptor alpha. *J. Dent. Res.* **2018**, *97*, 1023–1030. [CrossRef]
77. Ghisletti, S.; Meda, C.; Maggi, A.; Vegeto, E. 17beta-estradiol inhibits inflammatory gene expression by controlling NF-kappaB intracellular localization. *Mol. Cell. Biol.* **2005**, *25*, 2957–2968. [CrossRef]
78. Hirano, S.; Furutama, D.; Hanafusa, T. Physiologically high concentrations of 17beta-estradiol enhance NF-kappaB activity in human T cells. *Am. J. Physiol. Regul. Integr. Comp. Physiol.* **2007**, *292*, R1465–R1471. [CrossRef]
79. Abu-Taha, M.; Rius, C.; Hermenegildo, C.; Noguera, I.; Cerda-Nicolas, J.M.; Issekutz, A.C.; Jose, P.J.; Cortijo, J.; Morcillo, E.J.; Sanz, M.J. Menopause and ovariectomy cause a low grade of systemic inflammation that may be prevented by chronic treatment with low doses of estrogen or losartan. *J. Immunol.* **2009**, *183*, 1393–1402. [CrossRef] [PubMed]
80. Chan, Q.K.; Lam, H.M.; Ng, C.F.; Lee, A.Y.; Chan, E.S.; Ng, H.K.; Ho, S.M.; Lau, K.M. Activation of GPR30 inhibits the growth of prostate cancer cells through sustained activation of Erk1/2, c-jun/c-fos-dependent upregulation of p21, and induction of G(2) cell-cycle arrest. *Cell Death Differ.* **2010**, *17*, 1511–1523. [CrossRef]
81. Wei, W.; Chen, Z.J.; Zhang, K.S.; Yang, X.L.; Wu, Y.M.; Chen, X.H.; Huang, H.B.; Liu, H.L.; Cai, S.H.; Du, J.; et al. The activation of G protein-coupled receptor 30 (GPR30) inhibits proliferation of estrogen receptor-negative breast cancer cells in vitro and in vivo. *Cell Death Dis.* **2014**, *5*, e1428. [CrossRef] [PubMed]
82. Obikane, H.; Abiko, Y.; Ueno, H.; Kusumi, Y.; Esumi, M.; Mitsumata, M. Effect of endothelial cell proliferation on atherogenesis: A role of p21(Sdi/Cip/Waf1) in monocyte adhesion to endothelial cells. *Atherosclerosis* **2010**, *212*, 116–122. [CrossRef] [PubMed]
83. Hodis, H.N.; Mack, W.J.; Henderson, V.W.; Shoupe, D.; Budoff, M.J.; Hwang-Levine, J.; Li, Y.; Feng, M.; Dustin, L.; Kono, N.; et al. Vascular Effects of Early versus Late Postmenopausal Treatment with Estradiol. *N. Engl. J. Med.* **2016**, *374*, 1221–1231. [CrossRef] [PubMed]
84. Naftolin, F.; Friedenthal, J.; Nachtigall, R.; Nachtigall, L. Cardiovascular health and the menopausal woman: The role of estrogen and when to begin and end hormone treatment. *F1000Research* **2019**, *8*, 1576. [CrossRef] [PubMed]
85. Sun, B.; Yang, D.; Yin, Y.Z.; Xiao, J. Estrogenic and anti-inflammatory effects of pseudoprotodioscin in atherosclerosis-prone mice: Insights into endothelial cells and perivascular adipose tissues. *Eur. J. Pharmacol.* **2020**, *869*, 172887. [CrossRef]
86. Kuntz, S.; Asseburg, H.; Dold, S.; Rompp, A.; Frohling, B.; Kunz, C.; Rudloff, S. Inhibition of low-grade inflammation by anthocyanins from grape extract in an in vitro epithelial-endothelial co-culture model. *Food Funct.* **2015**, *6*, 1136–1149. [CrossRef]
87. Lee, H.; Jee, Y.; Hong, K.; Hwang, G.S.; Chun, K.H. MicroRNA-494, upregulated by tumor necrosis factor-alpha, desensitizes insulin effect in C2C12 muscle cells. *PLoS ONE* **2013**, *8*, e83471. [CrossRef]
88. Deshmane, S.L.; Kremlev, S.; Amini, S.; Sawaya, B.E. Monocyte chemoattractant protein-1 (MCP-1): An overview. *J. Interferon. Cytokine Res.* **2009**, *29*, 313–326. [CrossRef]
89. Liu, X.L.; Zhang, P.F.; Ding, S.F.; Wang, Y.; Zhang, M.; Zhao, Y.X.; Ni, M.; Zhang, Y. Local gene silencing of monocyte chemoattractant protein-1 prevents vulnerable plaque disruption in apolipoprotein E-knockout mice. *PLoS ONE* **2012**, *7*, e33497. [CrossRef]
90. Cho, K.Y.; Miyoshi, H.; Kuroda, S.; Yasuda, H.; Kamiyama, K.; Nakagawara, J.; Takigami, M.; Kondo, T.; Atsumi, T. The phenotype of infiltrating macrophages influences arteriosclerotic plaque vulnerability in the carotid artery. *J. Stroke Cerebrovasc. Dis.* **2013**, *22*, 910–918. [CrossRef]
91. Ariazi, E.A.; Brailoiu, E.; Yerrum, S.; Shupp, H.A.; Slifker, M.J.; Cunliffe, H.E.; Black, M.A.; Donato, A.L.; Arterburn, J.B.; Oprea, T.I.; et al. The G protein-coupled receptor GPR30 inhibits proliferation of estrogen receptor-positive breast cancer cells. *Cancer Res.* **2010**, *70*, 1184–1194. [CrossRef] [PubMed]

92. Xing, D.; Feng, W.; Miller, A.P.; Weathington, N.M.; Chen, Y.F.; Novak, L.; Blalock, J.E.; Oparil, S. Estrogen modulates TNF-alpha-induced inflammatory responses in rat aortic smooth muscle cells through estrogen receptor-beta activation. *Am. J. Physiol. Heart Circ. Physiol.* **2007**, *292*, H2607–H2612. [CrossRef] [PubMed]
93. Xing, D.; Oparil, S.; Yu, H.; Gong, K.; Feng, W.; Black, J.; Chen, Y.F.; Nozell, S. Estrogen modulates NFkappaB signaling by enhancing IkappaBalpha levels and blocking p65 binding at the promoters of inflammatory genes via estrogen receptor-beta. *PLoS ONE* **2012**, *7*, e36890. [CrossRef] [PubMed]
94. Iorga, A.; Umar, S.; Ruffenach, G.; Aryan, L.; Li, J.; Sharma, S.; Motayagheni, N.; Nadadur, R.D.; Bopassa, J.C.; Eghbali, M. Estrogen rescues heart failure through estrogen receptor Beta activation. *Biol. Sex. Differ.* **2018**, *9*, 48. [CrossRef]
95. Zong, W.; Jiang, Y.; Zhao, J.; Zhang, J.; Gao, J.G. Estradiol plays a role in regulating the expression of lysyl oxidase family genes in mouse urogenital tissues and human Ishikawa cells. *J. Zhejiang Univ. Sci. B* **2015**, *16*, 857–864. [CrossRef] [PubMed]
96. Newby, A.C. Metalloproteinases and vulnerable atherosclerotic plaques. *Trends Cardiovasc. Med.* **2007**, *17*, 253–258. [CrossRef]
97. Stoneman, V.E.; Bennett, M.R. Role of apoptosis in atherosclerosis and its therapeutic implications. *Clin. Sci.* **2004**, *107*, 343–354. [CrossRef]
98. Dhillon, O.S.; Khan, S.Q.; Narayan, H.K.; Ng, K.H.; Mohammed, N.; Quinn, P.A.; Squire, I.B.; Davies, J.E.; Ng, L.L. Matrix metalloproteinase-2 predicts mortality in patients with acute coronary syndrome. *Clin. Sci.* **2009**, *118*, 249–257. [CrossRef]
99. Potier, M.; Karl, M.; Elliot, S.J.; Striker, G.E.; Striker, L.J. Response to sex hormones differs in atherosclerosis-susceptible and -resistant mice. *Am. J. Physiol. Endocrinol. Metab.* **2003**, *285*, E1237–E1245. [CrossRef]
100. Wingrove, C.S.; Garr, E.; Godsland, I.F.; Stevenson, J.C. 17beta-oestradiol enhances release of matrix metalloproteinase-2 from human vascular smooth muscle cells. *Biochim. Biophys. Acta* **1998**, *1406*, 169–174. [CrossRef]
101. Inoue, S.; Nakazawa, T.; Cho, A.; Dastvan, F.; Shilling, D.; Daum, G.; Reidy, M. Regulation of arterial lesions in mice depends on differential smooth muscle cell migration: A role for sphingosine-1-phosphate receptors. *J. Vasc. Surg.* **2007**, *46*, 756–763. [CrossRef]
102. Johnson, C.; Galis, Z.S. Matrix metalloproteinase-2 and -9 differentially regulate smooth muscle cell migration and cell-mediated collagen organization. *Arterioscler. Thromb. Vasc. Biol.* **2004**, *24*, 54–60. [CrossRef]
103. Zanger, D.; Yang, B.K.; Ardans, J.; Waclawiw, M.A.; Csako, G.; Wahl, L.M.; Cannon, R.O., 3rd. Divergent effects of hormone therapy on serum markers of inflammation in postmenopausal women with coronary artery disease on appropriate medical management. *J. Am. Coll. Cardiol.* **2000**, *36*, 1797–1802. [CrossRef]
104. Koh, K.K.; Ahn, J.Y.; Kang, M.H.; Kim, D.S.; Jin, D.K.; Sohn, M.S.; Park, G.S.; Choi, I.S.; Shin, E.K. Effects of hormone replacement therapy on plaque stability, inflammation, and fibrinolysis in hypertensive or overweight postmenopausal women. *Am. J. Cardiol.* **2001**, *88*, 1423–1426. [CrossRef]
105. Amin, M.; Pushpakumar, S.; Muradashvili, N.; Kundu, S.; Tyagi, S.C.; Sen, U. Regulation and involvement of matrix metalloproteinases in vascular diseases. *Front. Biosci.* **2016**, *21*, 89–118. [CrossRef]
106. Romero, J.R.; Vasan, R.S.; Beiser, A.S.; Polak, J.F.; Benjamin, E.J.; Wolf, P.A.; Seshadri, S. Association of carotid artery atherosclerosis with circulating biomarkers of extracellular matrix remodeling: The Framingham Offspring Study. *J. Stroke Cerebrovasc. Dis.* **2008**, *17*, 412–417. [CrossRef]
107. Lewandowski, K.C.; Komorowski, J.; Mikhalidis, D.P.; Bienkiewicz, M.; Tan, B.K.; O'Callaghan, C.J.; Lewinski, A.; Prelevic, G.; Randeva, H.S. Effects of hormone replacement therapy type and route of administration on plasma matrix metalloproteinases and their tissue inhibitors in postmenopausal women. *J. Clin. Endocrinol. Metab.* **2006**, *91*, 3123–3130. [CrossRef]
108. Wang, H.; Zhao, Z.; Lin, M.; Groban, L. Activation of GPR30 inhibits cardiac fibroblast proliferation. *Mol. Cell Biochem.* **2015**, *405*, 135–148. [CrossRef]
109. Hwang, J.; Hodis, H.N.; Hsiai, T.K.; Asatryan, L.; Sevanian, A. Role of annexin II in estrogen-induced macrophage matrix metalloproteinase-9 activity: The modulating effect of statins. *Atherosclerosis* **2006**, *189*, 76–82. [CrossRef]
110. Lappano, R.; De Marco, P.; De Francesco, E.M.; Chimento, A.; Pezzi, V.; Maggiolini, M. Cross-talk between GPER and growth factor signaling. *J. Steroid Biochem Mol. Biol.* **2013**, *137*, 50–56. [CrossRef]
111. Palmieri, D.; Perego, P.; Palombo, D. Apigenin inhibits the TNFalpha-induced expression of eNOS and MMP-9 via modulating Akt signalling through oestrogen receptor engagement. *Mol. Cell Biochem.* **2012**, *371*, 129–136. [CrossRef]
112. Voloshenyuk, T.G.; Larkin, K.; Fournett, A.; Gardner, J.D. Estrogen receptor dependence of lysyl oxidase expression and activity in cardiac fibroblasts. *FASEB J.* **2012**, *26*, 1059.16. [CrossRef]
113. Li, S.Y.; Yan, J.Q.; Song, Z.; Liu, Y.F.; Song, M.J.; Qin, J.W.; Yang, Z.M.; Liang, X.H. Molecular characterization of lysyl oxidase-mediated extracellular matrix remodeling during mouse decidualization. *FEBS Lett.* **2017**, *591*, 1394–1407. [CrossRef]
114. Dasgupta, S.; Eudaly, J. Estrogen receptor-alpha mediates Toll-like receptor-2 agonist-induced monocyte chemoattractant protein-1 production in mesangial cells. *Results Immunol.* **2012**, *2*, 196–203. [CrossRef]
115. Zhou, Y.; Liu, X. The role of estrogen receptor beta in breast cancer. *Biomark. Res.* **2020**, *8*, 39. [CrossRef]
116. Kanda, N.; Watanabe, S. 17Beta-estradiol inhibits MCP-1 production in human keratinocytes. *J. Investig. Dermatol.* **2003**, *120*, 1058–1066. [CrossRef]
117. Condorelli, G.; Aycock, J.K.; Frati, G.; Napoli, C. Mutated p21/WAF/CIP transgene overexpression reduces smooth muscle cell proliferation, macrophage deposition, oxidation-sensitive mechanisms, and restenosis in hypercholesterolemic apolipoprotein E knockout mice. *FASEB J.* **2001**, *15*, 2162–2170. [CrossRef]

118. Smith, R.C.; Branellec, D.; Gorski, D.H.; Guo, K.; Perlman, H.; Dedieu, J.F.; Pastore, C.; Mahfoudi, A.; Denefle, P.; Isner, J.M.; et al. p21CIP1-mediated inhibition of cell proliferation by overexpression of the gax homeodomain gene. *Genes. Dev.* **1997**, *11*, 1674–1689. [CrossRef]
119. Matsuda, S.; Umemoto, S.; Yoshimura, K.; Itoh, S.; Murata, T.; Fukai, T.; Matsuzaki, M. Angiotensin Activates MCP-1 and Induces Cardiac Hypertrophy and Dysfunction via Toll-like Receptor 4. *J. Atheroscler. Thromb.* **2015**, *22*, 833–844. [CrossRef]
120. Doi, T.; Yoshino, T.; Fuse, N.; Boku, N.; Yamazaki, K.; Koizumi, W.; Shimada, K.; Takinishi, Y.; Ohtsu, A. Phase I study of TAS-102 and irinotecan combination therapy in Japanese patients with advanced colorectal cancer. *Investig. New Drugs* **2015**, *33*, 1068–1077. [CrossRef]
121. Kassi, E.; Nasiri-Ansari, N.; Spilioti, E.; Kalotychou, V.; Apostolou, P.E.; Moutsatsou, P.; Papavassiliou, A.G. Vitamin D interferes with glucocorticoid responsiveness in human peripheral blood mononuclear target cells. *Cell Mol. Life Sci.* **2016**, *73*, 4341–4354. [CrossRef]

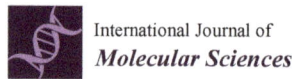
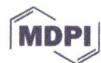

Article

Circulatory Rejuvenated EPCs Derived from PAOD Patients Treated by CD34⁺ Cells and Hyperbaric Oxygen Therapy Salvaged the Nude Mouse Limb against Critical Ischemia

Yin-Chia Chen [1,†], Jiunn-Jye Sheu [1,2,3,†], John Y. Chiang [4,5], Pei-Lin Shao [6], Shun-Cheng Wu [7,8,9], Pei-Hsun Sung [2,3,10], Yi-Chen Li [10], Yi-Ling Chen [2,3,10], Tien-Hung Huang [2,3,6,10], Kuan-Hung Chen [11] and Hon-Kan Yip [2,3,6,10,12,13,*]

[1] Division of Thoracic and Cardiovascular Surgery, Department of Surgery, Kaohsiung Chang Gung Memorial Hospital and Chang Gung University College of Medicine, Kaohsiung 83301, Taiwan; w780726@cgmh.org.tw (Y.-C.C.); cvsjjs@gmail.com (J.-J.S.)
[2] Institute for Translational Research in Biomedicine, Kaohsiung Chang Gung Memorial Hospital, Kaohsiung 83301, Taiwan; e12281@cgmh.org.tw (P.-H.S.); rylchen.msu@gmail.com (Y.-L.C.); tienhunghuang@gmail.com (T.-H.H.)
[3] Center for Shockwave Medicine and Tissue Engineering, Kaohsiung Chang Gung Memorial Hospital, Kaohsiung 83301, Taiwan
[4] Department of Computer Science and Engineering, National Sun Yat-Sen University, Kaohsiung 80424, Taiwan; chiang@cse.nsysu.edu.tw
[5] Department of Healthcare Administration and Medical Informatics, Kaohsiung Medical University, Kaohsiung 80756, Taiwan
[6] Department of Nursing, Asia University, Taichung 41354, Taiwan; m8951016@gmail.com
[7] Regenerative Medicine and Cell Therapy Research Center, Kaohsiung Medical University, Kaohsiung 80756, Taiwan; shunchengwu@hotmail.com
[8] Orthopaedic Research Center, Kaohsiung Medical University, Kaohsiung 80756, Taiwan
[9] Post-Baccalaureate Program in Nursing, Asia University, Taichung 41354, Taiwan
[10] Department of Cardiology, Department of Internal Medicine, Kaohsiung Chang Gung Memorial Hospital and Chang Gung University College of Medicine, Kaohsiung 83301, Taiwan; ryichenli@gmail.com
[11] Department of Anesthesiology, Kaohsiung Chang Gung Memorial Hospital and Chang Gung University College of Medicine, Kaohsiung 83301, Taiwan; amigofx35@gmail.com
[12] Department of Medical Research, China Medical University Hospital, China Medical University, Taichung 40402, Taiwan
[13] Division of Cardiology, Department of Internal Medicine, Xiamen Chang Gung Hospital, Xiamen 361028, China
* Correspondence: han.gung@msa.hinet.net
† These Authors contributed equally.

Received: 1 September 2020; Accepted: 13 October 2020; Published: 23 October 2020

Abstract: This study tested whether circulatory endothelial progenitor cells (EPCs) derived from peripheral arterial occlusive disease (PAOD) patients after receiving combined autologous CD34+ cell and hyperbaric oxygen (HBO) therapy (defined as rejuvenated EPCs) would salvage nude mouse limbs against critical limb ischemia (CLI). Adult-male nude mice ($n = 40$) were equally categorized into group 1 (sham-operated control), group 2 (CLI), group 3 (CLI-EPCs (6×10^5) derived from PAOD patient's circulatory blood prior to CD34$^+$ cell and HBO treatment (EPC^{Pr-T}) by intramuscular injection at 3 h after CLI induction) and group 4 (CLI-EPCs (6×10^5) derived from PAOD patient's circulatory blood after CD34$^+$ cell and HBO treatment (EPC^{Af-T}) by the identical injection method). By 2, 7 and 14 days after the CLI procedure, the ischemic to normal blood flow (INBF) ratio was highest in group 1, lowest in group 2 and significantly lower in group 4 than in group 3 ($p < 0.0001$). The protein levels of endothelial functional integrity (CD31/von Willebrand factor (vWF)/endothelial nitric-oxide synthase (eNOS)) expressed a similar pattern to that of INBF. In contrast, apoptotic/mitochondrial-damaged (mitochondrial-Bax/caspase-3/PARP/cytosolic-cytochrome-C) biomarkers and fibrosis (Smad3/TGF-ß) exhibited an opposite pattern, whereas the protein expressions of anti-fibrosis (Smad1/5 and BMP-2) and mitochondrial integrity (mitochondrial-cytochrome-C) showed an identical pattern of INBF (all $p < 0.0001$). The protein expressions of angiogenesis biomarkers (VEGF/SDF-1α/HIF-1α) were progressively increased from groups 1 to 3 (all $p < 0.0010$). The number of small vessels and endothelial cell surface markers (CD31$^+$/vWF$^+$) in the CLI area displayed an identical pattern of INBF (all $p < 0.0001$). CLI automatic amputation was higher in group 2 than in other groups (all $p < 0.001$). In conclusion, EPCs from HBO-C34+ cell therapy significantly restored the blood flow and salvaged the CLI in nude mice.

Keywords: critical limb ischemia; endothelial progenitor cells; nude mice; angiogenesis; hyperbaric oxygen therapy

1. Introduction

Peripheral arterial occlusive disease (PAOD), a high prevalence aging-associated chronic disease, not only incurs huge public healthcare costs but also causes unacceptably high morbidity and mortality worldwide. PAOD, one of the major manifestations of systemic atherosclerosis [1], has been established to affect 12% of the adult population and up to 20% of the elderly [2]. Patients with PAOD may develop critical limb ischemia (CLI) at the late stage of the disease process [2,3]. Undoubtedly, the CLI commonly occurs when arterial blood flow is greatly restricted, resulting in perfusion in capillary beds and inadequately sustained microvasculature. Ultimately, hypoxia and exhausted energy develop in the tissues and cells in the ischemic area [4,5]. Importantly, clinical studies have delineated that thousands of patients are asymptomatic prior to the development of CLI [6,7], which poses an obstacle to early diagnosis and early treatment for the purposes of slowing or abolishing disease progression and the development of unacceptable complications.

Treatment for the CLI, therefore, remains a formidable challenge to clinicians [8]. Without appropriate treatment, 5-year mortality of patients with asymptomatic PAOD is estimated for up to 19% of those diagnosed; and increases to 24% for patients with symptomatic PAOD [9]. Additionally, one-year mortality for CLI is identified for as many as 25% of those diagnosed [10]. Of particular importance is that patients with PAOD have a significantly elevated incidence of cardiovascular morbidity and mortality [9].

Failure in salvaging the critical limb can lead to limb loss and the high cost of patient care following amputation [11,12]. While surgical or endovascular revascularization is currently utilized for the treatment of CLI with an acceptable success rate [13–15], for those patients who are not candidates for surgical or endovascular intervention and those who failed the revascularization or bypass occlusion, the clinical outcomes remain dismal [13,14]. Accordingly, an alternative strategy for the treatment of CLI patients who are refractory to conventional therapy is urgently necessary.

Growing data have demonstrated that cell therapy effectively restored blood flow in the ischemic area, resulting in improved ischemic related organ dysfunction mainly through angiogenesis, neovascularization, anti-inflammation, immunomodulation and tissue regeneration in various disease entities [16–18]. Thus, cell therapy has emerged as an attractive modality for the treatment of ischemic heart and cerebral vascular diseases that has been reported to give promising results in animal model studies and clinical trials [16–20]. However, a majority of the clinical trials demonstrated that stem cell therapy, including those of autologous bone marrow-derived mononuclear cells or circulatory derived autologous endothelial progenitor cells (EPCs), did not offer additional benefits for salvaging the ischemic limb and improving the clinical outcomes [21,22]. This result could be mainly due to the coexisting serious atherosclerosis of small vessels [8,10] and severe dysfunctions of EPCs, capillary beds and microvasculature in this subgroup of patients [8]. Thus, improving the EPC function through culturing (i.e., rejuvenated EPCs) and increasing the permeability of microvasculature for EPC migration and homing in on the ischemic area could be an innovative approach for the treatment of CLI.

Hyperbaric oxygen (HBO) therapy is a traditional therapy for patients with ischemic PAOD [23]. It is proposed that the underlying mechanism of HBO therapy that is predominantly involved in improving ischemic PAOD is the increase of vascular wall permeability and production of hypoxia-inducible factor (HIF)-1α and stromal cell-derived factor (SDF)-1α that enhance the angiogenesis, circulatory EPCs level and blood flow in the ischemic area [24,25]. Unsatisfactorily, the overall limb salvage and progression of the ischemic process have not been significantly decreased in patients receiving HBO therapy [26]. This may be due to the diffusion of oxygen into the ischemic organ that creates a hyperbaric environment being extremely limited [27,28] in severe PAOD patients. Interestingly, our recent study demonstrates that HBO increases the number and function of circulatory EPCs [25]. This finding highlights that HBO may play an accessory role in: (1) promoting the mobilization of EPCs from bone marrow to the circulation; (2) enhancing the capillary/microvascular permeability; (3) augmenting the intrinsic and extrinsic EPCs crossing the vessel wall and homing in on the ischemic area; and (4) acting as a contributor for repairing endothelial functions in the ischemic area via increasing oxygen diffusion into the ischemia, increasing the likelihood of successfully salvaging the limbs of CLI patients.

Based on the aforementioned issues [16–28], we tested the hypothesis that treatment with EPCs derived from PAOD patients who received combined $CD34^+$ cell and HBO therapy (defined as rejuvenated EPCs) would offer additional benefits than either one therapy alone for protecting limbs against the CLI procedure in nude mouse.

2. Results

2.1. Ischemic/Normal Blood Flow (INBF) Ratio Measured by Laser Doppler Scan at Days 2, 7 and 14 after Left Femoral Artery Ligated and Totally Removed and Automatic Amputation of Distal Critical Ischemic Limb

To elucidate whether intramuscular administration of EPCs which were derived from PAOD patients prior to and after receiving combined therapy of HBO and $CD34^+$ cells would salvage the CLI animals, a laser Doppler scan was utilized for determining the INBF ratio in each group of animals. The result demonstrated that by days 2, 7 and 14 after the CLI procedure, the INBF was highest in group 1 (i.e., SC), lowest in group 2 (CLI only) and significantly lower in group 3 (CLI + EPCs which were derived from PAOD patient's circulatory blood prior to receiving combined HBO and $CD34^+$ cell treatment) than in group 4 (CLI + EPCs which were derived from PAOD patient's circulatory blood after receiving HBO therapy and $CD34^+$ cell treatment four times) (Figure 1A–O).

Additionally, by day 28 after the CLI procedure, we identified that the number of automatic amputations of distal ischemic limbs was significantly higher in groups 2 and 3 than in groups 1 and 4, but showed no significant difference between groups 2 and 3 or between 1 and 4, suggesting only rejuvenated EPCs effectively preserved the limb from the CLI procedure (Figure 1P).

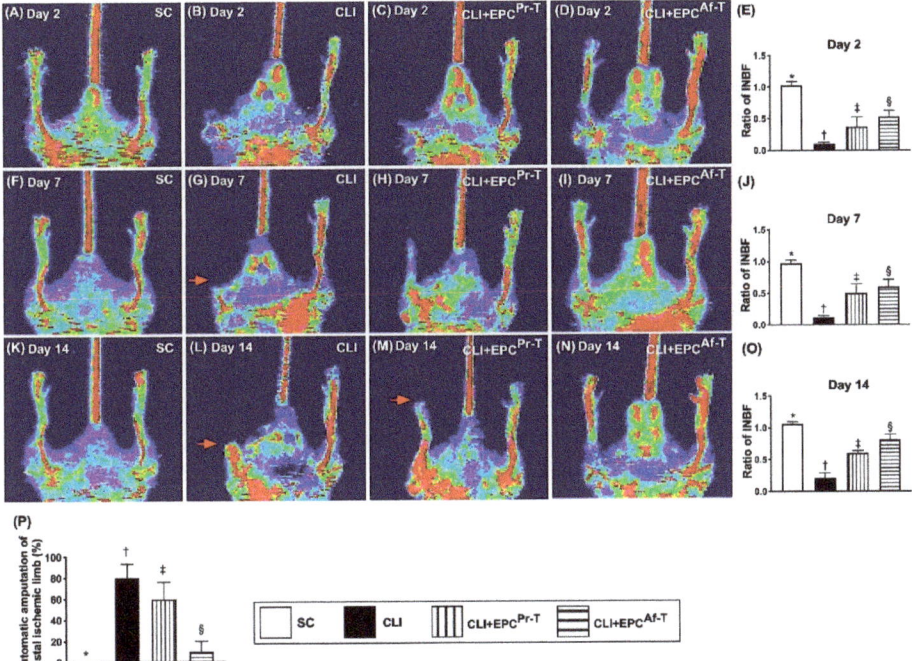

Figure 1. Ischemic/normal blood flow (INBF) ratio measured by laser Doppler scan at days 2, 7 and 14 after left femoral artery ligation. (**A–D**) Illustrating the laser Doppler finding of blood flow of right and left (CLI zone) limbs among the four groups at day 2 after CLI procedure; (**E**) Analytical result of ratio of INBF, * vs. other groups with different symbols (†, ‡, §), $p < 0.0001$; (**F–I**) Illustrating the laser Doppler finding of blood flow of right and left (CLI zone) limbs among the four groups at day 7 after CLI procedure; (**J**) Analytical result of ratio of INBF, * vs. other groups with different symbols (†, ‡, §), $p < 0.0001$; (**K–N**) Illustrating the laser Doppler finding of blood flow of right and left (CLI zone) limbs among the four groups at day 14 after CLI procedure; (**O**) Analytical result of ratio of INBF, * vs. other groups with different symbols (†, ‡, §), $p < 0.0001$; (**P**) Analytical result of percentage of automatic amputation of distal ischemic limb (red arrows) among the four groups by day 28 after CLI procedure, * vs. †, $p < 0.0001$. All statistical analyses are performed by one-way ANOVA, followed by the Bonferroni multiple comparison post hoc test ($n = 10$ for each group). Symbols (*, †, ‡, §) indicate significance (at 0.05 level). SC = sham-operated control; CLI = critical limb ischemia; EPCs = endothelial progenitor cells; EPC^{Pr-T} = EPCs derived from severe PAOD patient's circulatory blood prior to $CD34^+$ cell and HBO treatment; EPC^{Af-T} = EPCs derived from severe PAOD patient's circulatory blood after $CD34^+$ cell and HBO treatment; PAOD = peripheral arterial occlusive disease; HBO = hyperbaric oxygen.

2.2. The Protein Expressions of Endothelial Cell Functional Integrity in CLI Zone by Day 28 after CLI Procedure

To assess the impact of EPC therapy on protecting the integrity of endothelial cell integrity, the Western blot analysis of a quadriceps specimen, which was harvested from the ischemic zone, was performed. The result showed that the protein expressions of CD31, von Willebrand factor (vWF) and endothelial nitric-oxide synthase (eNOS), three indices of endothelial cell integrity, were highest in group 1, lowest in group 2 and significantly higher in group 4 than in group 3 (Figure 2).

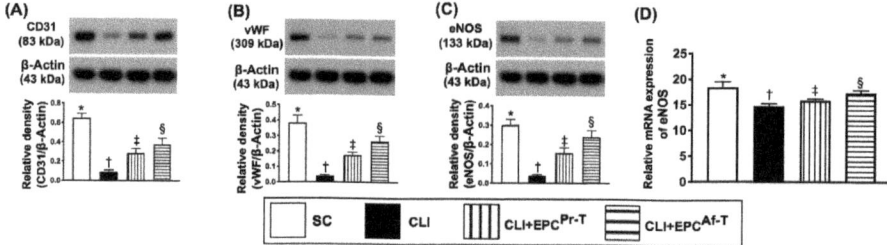

Figure 2. Protein expressions of endothelial cell functional integrity and gene expression of endothelial nitric-oxide synthase (eNOS) in CLI zone by day 28 after CLI procedure. (**A**) Protein expression of CD31, * vs. other groups with different symbols (†, ‡, §), $p < 0.0001$; (**B**) Protein expression of von Willebrand factor (vWF), * vs. other groups with different symbols (†, ‡, §), $p < 0.0001$; (**C**) Protein expression of eNOS, * vs. other groups with different symbols (†, ‡, §), $p < 0.0001$; (**D**) mRNA expression of eNOS, * vs. other groups with different symbols (†, ‡, §), $p < 0.0001$. All statistical analyses are performed by one-way ANOVA, followed by the Bonferroni multiple comparison post hoc test ($n = 6$ for each group). Symbols (*, †, ‡, §) indicate significance (at 0.05 level). SC = sham-operated control; CLI = critical limb ischemia; EPC = endothelial progenitor cells; EPC^{Pr-T} = EPCs derived from severe PAOD patient's circulatory blood prior to $CD34^+$ cell and HBO treatment; EPC^{Af-T} = EPCs derived from severe PAOD patient's circulatory blood after $CD34^+$ cell and HBO treatment; PAOD = peripheral arterial occlusive disease; HBO = hyperbaric oxygen.

2.3. Protein Expressions of Angiogenesis in CLI Zone by Day 28 after CLI Procedure

We further evaluated whether EPC therapy would enhance the angiogenesis in the CLI area by performing Western blot analysis for the typical angiogenesis biomarkers. The results showed that the protein expressions of CXCR4, SDF-1α, VEGF and HIF-1α, four indicators of angiogenesis, were significantly progressively increased from groups 1 to 4, suggesting an intrinsic response to ischemic stimulation that was augmented by EPC therapy (Figure 3).

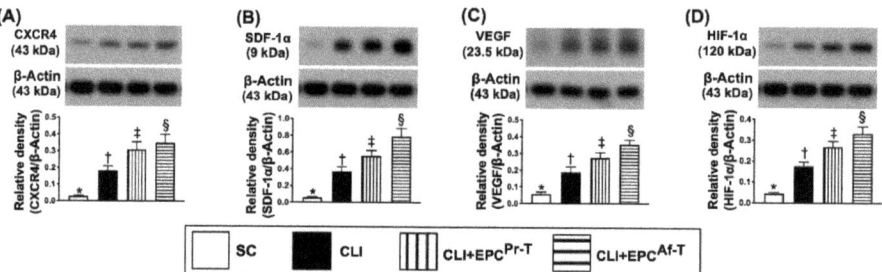

Figure 3. Protein expressions of angiogenesis factors in CLI zone by day 28 after CLI procedure. (**A**) Protein expression of CXCR4, * vs. other groups with different symbols (†, ‡, §), $p < 0.0001$; (**B**) Protein expression of stromal cell-derived factor (SDF)-1α, * vs. other groups with different symbols (†, ‡, §), $p < 0.0001$; (**C**) Protein expression of vascular endothelial growth factor (VEGF), * vs. other groups with different symbols (†, ‡, §), $p < 0.0001$; (**D**) Protein expression of hypoxia-inducible factor (HIF)-1α, * vs. other groups with different symbols (†, ‡, §), $p < 0.0001$. All statistical analyses are performed by one-way ANOVA, followed by the Bonferroni multiple comparison post hoc test ($n = 6$ for each group). Symbols (*, †, ‡, §) indicate significance (at 0.05 level). SC = sham-operated control; CLI = critical limb ischemia; EPC = endothelial progenitor cells; EPC^{Pr-T} = EPCs derived from severe PAOD patient's circulatory blood prior to $CD34^+$ cell and HBO treatment; EPC^{Af-T} = EPCs derived from severe PAOD patient's circulatory blood after $CD34^+$ cell and HBO treatment; PAOD = peripheral arterial occlusive disease; HBO = hyperbaric oxygen.

2.4. Protein Expressions of Fibrotic and Antifibrotic Biomarkers in CLI Zone by Day 28 after CLI Procedure

To test whether EPC therapy would attenuate the protein level of ischemia-related fibrosis in the quadriceps muscle, the Western blot analysis was performed. As we expected, the protein expressions of TGF-ß and Smad3, two indicators of fibrosis, were lowest in group 1, highest in group 2 and significantly lower in group 4 than in group 3 (Figure 4A,B). On the other hand, the protein expressions of Smad1/5 and BMP-2, two indicators of antifibrosis, displayed an opposite pattern of fibrosis among the four groups (Figure 4C,D).

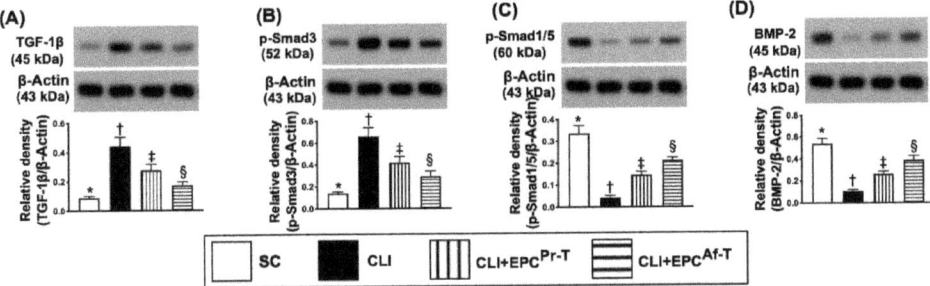

Figure 4. Protein expressions of fibrotic and antifibrotic biomarkers in CLI zone by day 28 after CLI procedure. (**A**) Protein expression of transforming growth factor (TGF)-ß, * vs. other groups with different symbols (†, ‡, §), $p < 0.0001$; (**B**) Protein expression of Smad3, * vs. other groups with different symbols (†, ‡, §), $p < 0.0001$; (**C**) Protein expression of Smad1/5, * vs. other groups with different symbols (†, ‡, §), $p < 0.0001$; (**D**) Protein expression of bone morphogenetic protein (BMP)-2, * vs. other groups with different symbols (†, ‡, §), $p < 0.0001$. All statistical analyses are performed by one-way ANOVA, followed by the Bonferroni multiple comparison post hoc test ($n = 6$ for each group). Symbols (*, †, ‡, §) indicate significance (at 0.05 level). SC = sham-operated control; CLI = critical limb ischemia; EPC = endothelial progenitor cells; EPC^{Pr-T} = EPCs derived from severe PAOD patient's circulatory blood prior to CD34$^+$ cell and HBO treatment; EPC^{Af-T} = EPCs derived from severe PAOD patient's circulatory blood after CD34$^+$ cell and HBO treatment; PAOD = peripheral arterial occlusive disease; HBO = hyperbaric oxygen.

2.5. Protein Expressions of Apoptotic, Mitochondrial-Damaged and Mitochondrial-Integrity Biomarkers in CLI Zone by Day 28 after CLI Procedure

Next, for the assessment of apoptotic biomarkers, we also performed the Western blot analysis. The results demonstrated that the protein expressions of mitochondrial Bax (mit-Bax), cleaved caspase 3 (c-Csp3) and cleaved poly (ADP-ribose) polymerase (c-PARP), three indicators of apoptosis and cytosolic cytochrome C (cyt-Cyto-C) and indicators of mitochondrial damage, were highest in group 2, lowest in group 1 and significantly higher in group 3 than in group 4 (Figure 5A–D), whereas the protein expression of mitochondrial cytochrome C (mit-Cyto-C), an indicator of mitochondrial integrity, exhibited an opposite pattern of apoptosis among the four groups (Figure 5E).

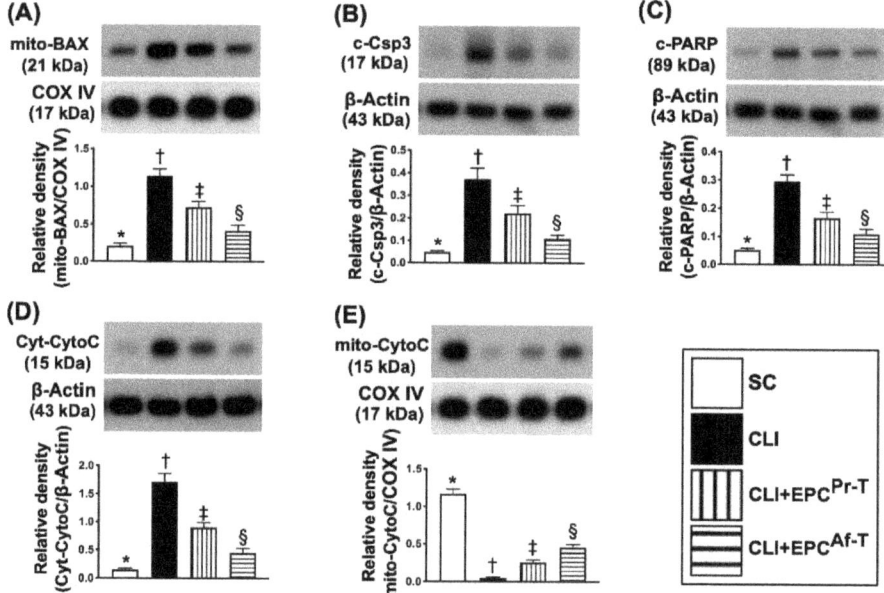

Figure 5. Protein expression of apoptotic, mitochondrial-damaged and mitochondrial-integrity biomarkers in CLI zone by day 28 after CLI procedure. (**A**) Protein expression of mitochondrial (mit-Bax), * vs. other groups with different symbols (†, ‡, §), $p < 0.0001$; (**B**) Protein expression of cleaved caspase 3 (c-Csp3), * vs. other groups with different symbols (†, ‡, §), $p < 0.0001$; (**C**) Protein expression of cleaved poly (ADP-ribose) polymerase 1 (c-PARP), * vs. other groups with different symbols (†, ‡, §), $p < 0.0001$; (**D**) Protein expression of cytosolic cytochrome C (cyt-Cyto-C), * vs. other groups with different symbols (†, ‡, §), $p < 0.0001$; (**E**) Protein expression of mitochondrial cytochrome C (mit-Cyto-C), * vs. other groups with different symbols (†, ‡, §), $p < 0.0001$. All statistical analyses are performed by one-way ANOVA, followed by the Bonferroni multiple comparison post hoc test ($n = 6$ for each group). Symbols (*, †, ‡, §) indicate significance (at 0.05 level). SC = sham-operated control; CLI = critical limb ischemia; EPC = endothelial progenitor cells; EPC^{Pr-T} = EPCs derived from severe PAOD patient's circulatory blood prior to $CD34^+$ cell and HBO treatment; EPC^{Af-T} = EPCs derived from severe PAOD patient's circulatory blood after $CD34^+$ cell and HBO treatment; PAOD = peripheral arterial occlusive disease; HBO = hyperbaric oxygen.

2.6. Cellular Expressions of Endothelial Cell and EPC Surface Markers in CLI Zone by Day 28 after CLI Procedure

To confirm the therapeutic impact of EPCs on the integrity of endothelial cells, we utilized the findings of immunofluorescent (IF) microscopy. The results exhibited that the cellular expressions of CD31 and vWF, two indicators of endothelial cell surface markers, were highest in group 1, lowest in group 2 and significantly higher in group 4 than in group 3 (Figure 6).

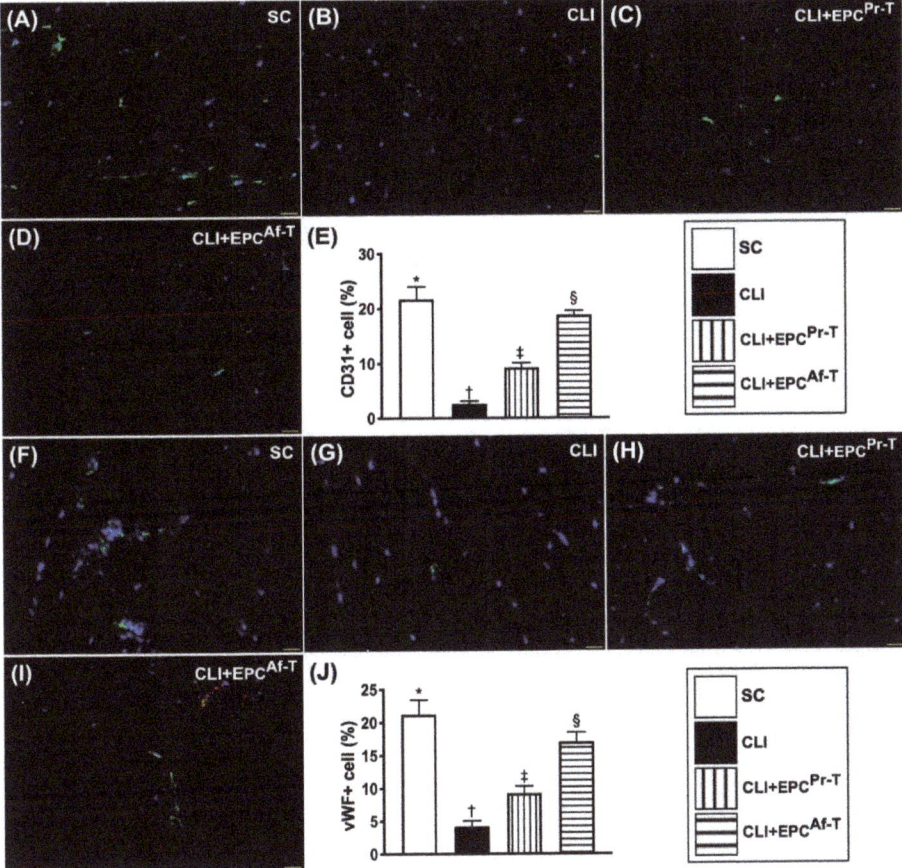

Figure 6. Cellular expressions of endothelial cell surface markers in CLI zone by day 28 after CLI procedure. (**A–D**) Illustrating the immunofluorescent (IF) microscopic finding (400×) for identification of CD31$^+$ cells (green color) in the CLI area; (**E**) Analytical result of number of CD31+ cells, * vs. other groups with different symbols (†, ‡, §), $p < 0.0001$; (**F–I**) Illustrating the IF microscopic finding (400×) for identification of von Willebrand factor (vWF)$^+$ cells (green color) in the CLI area; (**J**) Analytical result of the number of vWF+ cells, * vs. other groups with different symbols (†, ‡, §), $p < 0.0001$. Scale bars in right lower corner represent 20 µm. All statistical analyses are performed by one-way ANOVA, followed by Bonferroni multiple comparison post hoc testing ($n = 6$ for each group). Symbols (*, †, ‡, §) indicate significance (at 0.05 level). SC = sham-operated control; CLI = critical limb ischemia; EPC = endothelial progenitor cells; EPC^{Pr-T} = EPCs derived from severe PAOD patient's circulatory blood prior to CD34$^+$ cell and HBO treatment; EPC^{Af-T} = EPCs derived from severe PAOD patient's circulatory blood after CD34$^+$ cell and HBO treatment; PAOD = peripheral arterial occlusive disease; HBO = hyperbaric oxygen.

Additionally, we utilized the same method to further confirm the expressions of angiogenesis factors in the ischemic quadriceps muscle. The IF imaging study displayed that the cellular expressions of CXCR4 and SDF-1α, two indices of angiogenesis biomarkers, were progressively increased from groups 1 to 4, implicating an intrinsic response to ischemic stimulation that was upregulated by EPC therapy (Figure 7).

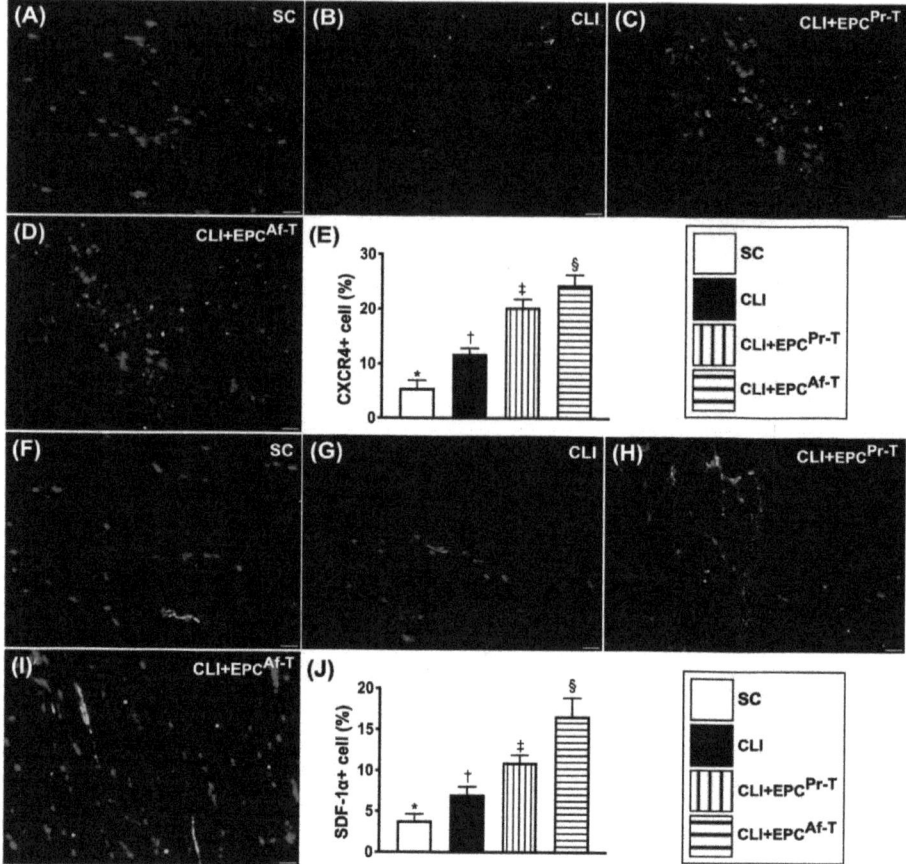

Figure 7. Cellular expressions of angiogenesis markers in CLI zone by day 28 after CLI procedure. (**A–D**) Illustrating the immunofluorescent (IF) microscopic finding (400×) for identification of CXCR4$^+$ cells (green color) in the CLI area; (**E**) Analytical result of number of CXCR4$^+$ cells, * vs. other groups with different symbols (†, ‡, §), $p < 0.0001$; (**F–I**) Illustrating the IF microscopic finding (400×) for identification of stromal cell-derived factor (SDF)-1α$^+$ cells (green color) in CLI area; (**J**) Analytical result of number of SDF-1α$^+$ cells, * vs. other groups with different symbols (†, ‡, §), $p < 0.0001$. All statistical analyses are performed by one-way ANOVA, followed by the Bonferroni multiple comparison post hoc test ($n = 6$ for each group). Symbols (*, †, ‡, §) indicate significance (at 0.05 level). SC = sham-operated control; CLI = critical limb ischemia; EPC = endothelial progenitor cells; EPC^{Pr-T} = EPCs derived from severe PAOD patient's circulatory blood prior to CD34$^+$ cell and HBO treatment; EPC^{Af-T} = EPCs derived from severe PAOD patient's circulatory blood after CD34$^+$ cell and HBO treatment; PAOD = peripheral arterial occlusive disease; HBO = hyperbaric oxygen.

2.7. Small Vessel Density in CLI Zone by Day 28 after CLI Procedure

As expected, the number of small vessels (i.e., ≤25 μm) in the ischemic area of quadriceps was highest in group 1, lowest in group 2 and significantly higher in group 4 than in group 3 (Figure 8).

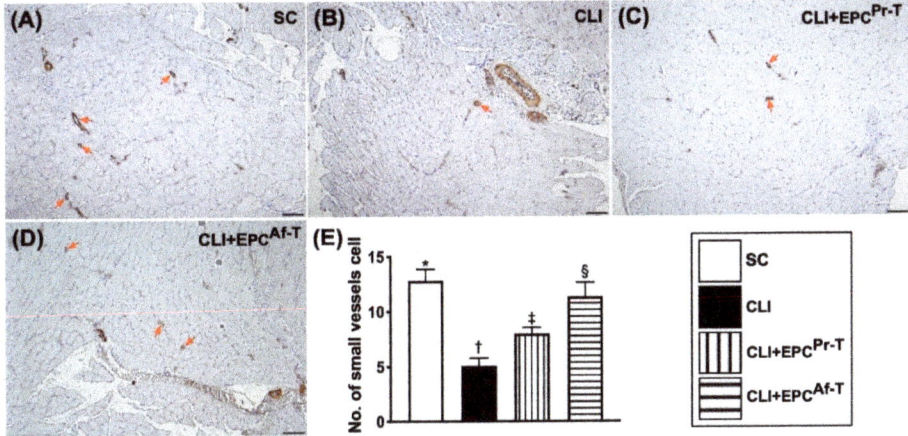

Figure 8. Small vessel density in CLI zone by day 28 after CLI procedure. (**A–D**) Illustrating the microscopic findings (100×) of alpha-smooth muscle actin (α-SMA) for identification of the number of small vessels (i.e., diameter ≤ 25.0 μM) (red arrows). (**E**) Analytic result of the number of small vessels, * vs. other groups with different symbols (†, ‡, §), $p < 0.0001$. All statistical analyses are performed by one-way ANOVA, followed by Bonferroni multiple comparison post hoc testing ($n = 6$ for each group). Symbols (*, †, ‡, §) indicate significance (at 0.05 level). SC = sham-operated control; CLI = critical limb ischemia; EPC = endothelial progenitor cells; EPC^{Pr-T} = EPCs derived from severe PAOD patient's circulatory blood prior to $CD34^+$ cell and HBO treatment; EPC^{Af-T} = EPCs derived from severe PAOD patient's circulatory blood after $CD34^+$ cell and HBO treatment; PAOD = peripheral arterial occlusive disease; HBO = hyperbaric oxygen.

2.8. Time Courses of Circulatory Endothelial Progenitor Cells among the Groups

To elucidate the serial changes of the circulating number of EPCs, flow cytometric analysis was performed for the peripheral blood mononuclear cells (PBMNCs). Time courses of flow cytometric analysis for identification of circulatory endothelial progenitor cells among the groups were showed in Supplementary Figure S1. The result showed that by day 0, the circulating number of c-kit/$CD31^+$, CD31/Sca-1+, KDR/$CD34^+$ and VE-Cadherin/$CD34^+$ cells, four indices of EPCs, did not differ among the four groups (Figure 9A–D). However, by day 4 and 15 after the CLI procedure, these parameters were progressively and significantly increased from groups 1 to 4, suggesting there was an intrinsic response to ischemic stimulation, which was further upregulated by EPC-HBO therapy (Figure 9E–L). An interesting finding was that the peak level of these circulating EPC biomarkers was reached by day 4 after the CLI procedure.

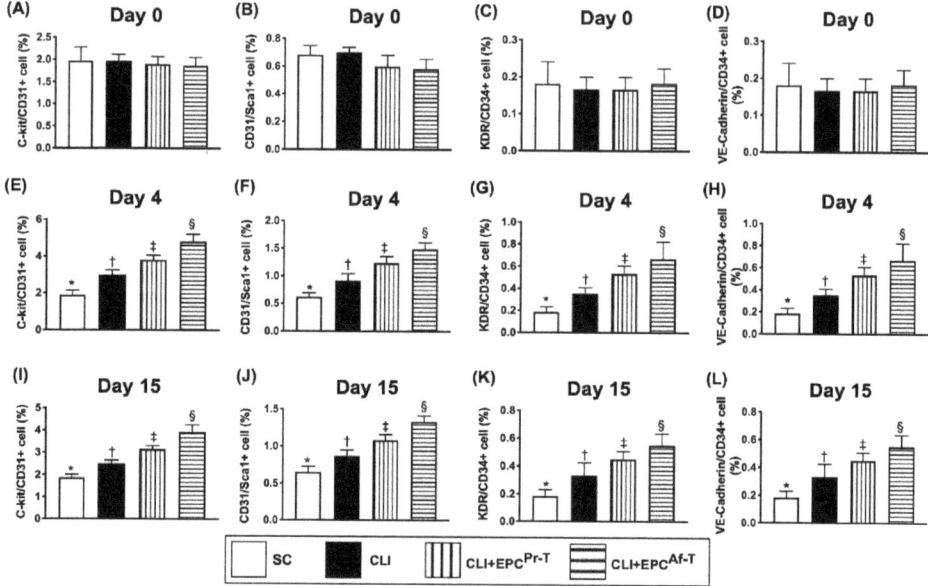

Figure 9. Illustrating the time courses of flow cytometric analysis of circulating levels of EPCs. (**A–D**) By day 0, the analytical of numbers of circulating levels of c-kit/CD31$^+$ (**A**), CD31/sca-1$^+$ (**B**), KDR/CD34$^+$ (**C**) and VE-Cadherin/CD34$^+$ (**D**) cells, all p value > 0.5; (**E–H**) By day 4, the analytical of numbers of circulating levels of c-kit/CD31$^+$ (**E**), CD31/sca-1$^+$ (**F**), KDR/CD34$^+$ (**G**) and VE-Cadherin/CD34$^+$ (**H**) cells, all p value < 0.0001; (**I–L**) By day 15, analytical of numbers of circulating levels of c-kit/CD31$^+$ (**I**), CD31/sca-1$^+$ (**J**), KDR/CD34$^+$ (**K**) and VE-Cadherin/CD34$^+$ (**L**) cells, all p value < 0.0001. All statistical analyses are performed by one-way ANOVA, followed by the Bonferroni multiple comparison post hoc test ($n = 6$ for each group). Symbols (*, †, ‡, §) indicate significance (at 0.05 level). SC = sham-operated control; CLI = critical limb ischemia; EPC = endothelial progenitor cells; EPC^{Pr-T} = EPCs derived from severe PAOD patient's circulatory blood prior to CD34$^+$ cell and HBO treatment; EPC^{Af-T} = EPCs derived from severe PAOD patient's circulatory blood after CD34$^+$ cell and HBO treatment; PAOD = peripheral arterial occlusive disease; HBO = hyperbaric oxygen.

3. Discussion

This study investigated the impact of cultured EPCs, which were derived from the circulatory blood of severe PAOD patients, on CLI nude mice and yielded several striking implications. First, this study found that the number of automatic amputation of distal limbs did not differ between the CLI group and EPC^{Pr-T} group, suggesting that EPCs derived from severe PAOD patients prior to being rejuvenated did not provide benefits for salvaging the distal part of the ischemic limb in nude mice. Second, the INBF value only showed weak statistical significance in the EPC^{Pr-T} group as compared with CLI only. These findings implicated that the EPC function was remarkably impaired in those of severe PAOD patients prior to receiving rejuvenation therapy. Third, on the other hand, the number of automatic amputations of distal portion of ischemic limbs was substantially reduced, whereas the INBF value was remarkably increased in EPC^{Af-T} (i.e., rejuvenated EPCs) animals than in those of EPC^{Pr-T} animals, highlighting that only those of rejuvenated EPCs effectively preserved the limb from the CLI procedure.

EPC therapy has been demonstrated to effectively enhance angiogenesis, restore the blood flow in the ischemic zone and improve ischemic related organ dysfunction by abundant data [16–20]. However, when the published data were carefully examined, we found that severe PAOD patients usually responded poorly to the EPC therapy [21,22], resulting in failure to save severe ischemic limbs in this high-risk subgroup of patients. An essential finding in the present study was that the therapeutic effect of EPCs which were derived from severe PAOD patients prior to $CD34^+$ cell and HBO therapy (i.e., non-rejuvenated EPCs) inadequately salvaged the nude mouse CLI, resulting in high incidence of automatic amputation and limb loss. Our findings, therefore, further support those of previous studies [21,22]. However, the results were inconsistent among the positive findings [16–20] and negative findings [21,22] of previous studies, and the findings of our study illustrated that some unidentified confounders might be present in these studies.

Undoubtedly, the fundamental pathological findings [8,10] demonstrate that the microvasculature of severe PAOD patients is always composed of severe thickness of intimal endothelial cell layer, a thickening and calcified medial layer and fibrosis of adventitia. Severe diffuse atherosclerotic changes in the arterioles and arteries, called "rusty vessels", also accompany the critical limitation of distal run of blood flow that is always observed in these patients [8]. Additionally, the EPCs function is always found to be severely impaired in this high-risk population of severe PAOD patients [25]. These essential issues could explain why the EPCs can never mobilize into microvasculature and penetrate into the endothelial layer and home in on the ischemic zone for angiogenesis.

Studies have proposed that the mechanistic basis of HBO therapy for improving critical limb ischemia/severe PAOD patients was mainly through increased vascular wall permeability, enhanced productions of HIF-1α and SDF-1α and augmented diffusion of oxygen into the ischemic area that, in turn, enhanced the circulatory level of EPCs, angiogenesis and restoration of blood flow in the ischemic area [24,25]. The most important finding in the present study was that as compared with CLI and EPC^{Pr-T} groups, the INBF value (i.e., an indicator of restored blood flow in the ischemic area) was substantially increased, whereas the automatic amputation of the distal ischemic limb was remarkably reduced in the EPC^{Af-T} group. These findings highlight that rejuvenated EPCs may serve as an innovative therapy for CLI/severe PAOD patients, especially those patients who are refractory to conventional therapy.

A principal finding in the present study was that, when we looked at the cellular-molecular levels, we found that the angiogenesis factor, neovascularization and the integrity of endothelial cells were markedly increased in EPC^{Af-T} animals compared to those of CLI and CLI-EPC^{Pr-T} animals. On the other hand, the fibrosis and apoptosis biomarkers in the ischemic quadriceps were notably lower in the former group than in the latter two groups. These findings could explain why the number of distal ischemic limb losses was remarkably lower, whereas the INBF value was remarkably increased in EPC^{Af-T} animals compared to those of CLI and CLI-EPC^{Pr-T} animals.

Study Limitation

This study contained limitations. First, in fact, the pathogenesis of the CLI model in nude mice was actually not identical to patient's acute limb ischemia/severe PAOD. Accordingly, the underlying mechanisms of CLI between these two species could not be identical. Second, we did not completely exclude the presence or absence of the immune reaction after the patient's EPCs were injected into the nude mice. Third, due to automatic amputation of distal ischemic limbs that occurred in the majority of CLI animals, we did not measure the INBF value by day 28 after the CLI procedure. Finally, although extensive works were done in the current study, the exactly mechanistic basis of xenogeneic EPC therapy for salvaging the nude mouse limbs from CLI is currently unclear. Perhaps, the proposed underlying mechanism in Figure 10 could, at least in part, provide useful information for further understanding this issue.

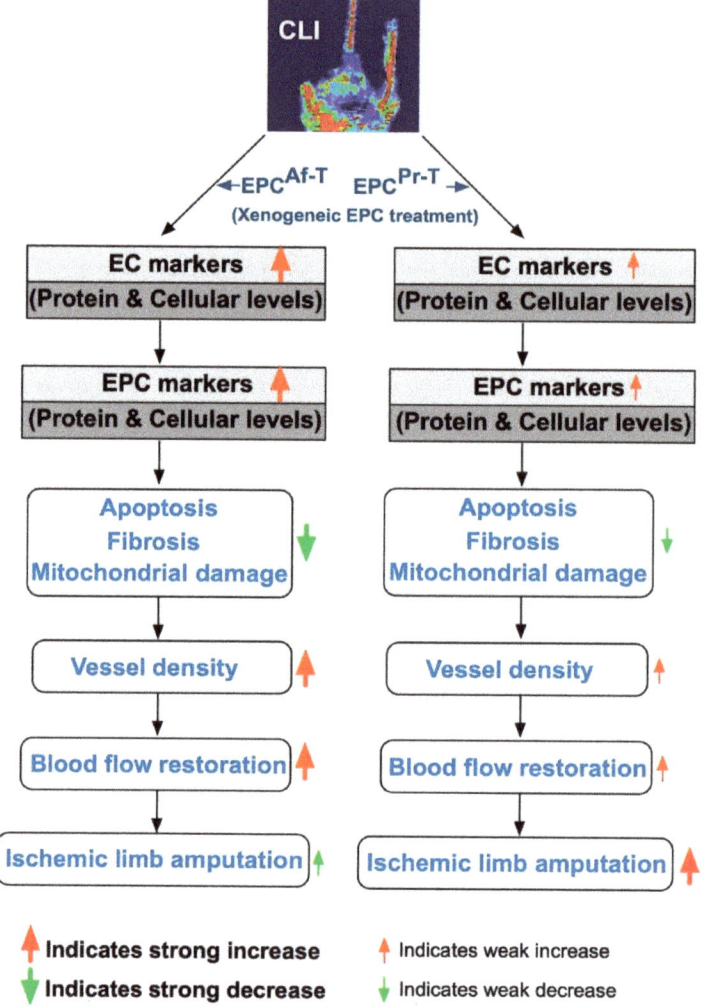

Figure 10. Illustrating the proposed underlying mechanism for rejuvenated xenogeneic EPCs effectively salvaging nude mouse limbs from CLI. CLI = critical limb ischemia; EPC = endothelial progenitor cells; EPC^{Pr-T} = EPCs derived from severe PAOD patient's circulatory blood prior to $CD34^+$ cell and HBO treatment; EPC^{Af-T} = EPCs derived from severe PAOD patient's circulatory blood after $CD34^+$ cell and HBO treatment.

4. Materials and Methods

4.1. Ethics and Study Design

The EPCs utilized in this animal model of CLI were derived from circulatory mononuclear cells of severe PAOD patients who were treated with HBO and autologous $CD34^+$ cells. This was a phase I clinical trial, which was approved by the Ministry of Health and Welfare, Taiwan, Republic of China (IRB No. 1076616554) and the Institutional Review Committee on Human Research at Chang Gung Memorial Hospital (IRB No. 201601217A0C602; date of approval 9 May 2018) in 2016. This phase I clinical trial was a prospective, randomized, open-label controlled trial to test the safety and efficacy of combined HBO and autologous circulatory CD34$^+$ cell treatment for patients with severe PAOD at a single medical center. The occlusive level of the arteries was below the ankle, where catheter-based or surgical intervention was inappropriate and ineffective to treat the ischemic area.

All the patients agreed to receive this alternative treatment. A written informed consent form was obtained from every patient before enrollment and treatment.

This study was designed to consecutively enroll study patients who had received optimal medical care. The patients were enrolled to either receive CD34$^+$ cells (2.5×10^7) in the most severe PAOD of the lower extremity (group 1) or serve as control subjects with only standard pharmacotherapy (group 2) (i.e., 1:1 randomization, $n = 10$ in each group). This study remains active for the enrollment of patients.

4.2. Procedure and Protocol for Isolation of Autologous CD34$^+$ Cells and Intra-Superficial Femoral Artery Infusion

The procedure and protocol for the isolation of circulatory CD34$^+$ cells were based on our previous reports [18]. In detail, prior to the isolation of peripheral blood-derived CD34$^+$ cells, granulocyte-colony stimulating factor (G-CSF) (5 µg/kg, every 12 h for eight doses) was subcutaneously given to each patient to augment the number of circulatory CD34$^+$ cells for subsequent collection via leukapheresis. After the last dose of G-CSF, the mononuclear cells isolated during leukapheresis were enriched for CD34$^+$ cells by using a commercially available device [COBE Spectra 6.1 (Terumo BCT Inc., Lakewood, CO, USA)] at 8:00 a.m. through a double-lumen catheter inserted into the right femoral vein. After a procedure time of about four hours, an adequate number of blood-derived CD34$^+$ cells were isolated (purified through fluorescence-activated cell sorting for CD34$^+$ cells) and ready for intra-renal artery transfusion.

After completing CD34$^+$ cell collection, the patients were immediately sent to the cardiac catheterization room to receiving the intra-superficial femoral arterial transfusion of CD34$^+$ cells into the target vessels below the ankle level.

4.3. Procedure and Protocol of Hyperbaric Oxygen Therapy

The procedure and protocol for hyperbaric oxygen therapy have been reported in our previous study [25]. The HBO therapy was performed for the patients in a sealed multi-place chamber at a pressure of 2.5 atmospheres absolute (ATA). Air pressure was gradually increased from 1 to 2.5 ATA over a 15 min duration. Oxygen of 100% medical-grade was inhaled through a plastic face mask for 25 min, followed by a 5 min break, for a total of 90 min per treatment. Air pressure was then decompressed from 2.5 ATA down to 1.0 ATA within 15 min to complete the treatment. HBO was performed daily, five times a week, for a total of 10–15 treatments.

All patients that received HBO therapy were safe without any complications, irrespective of recruitment from the hospitalization or outpatient department.

4.4. Ethics of Animal Model Study

All animal procedures were approved by the Institute of Animal Care and Use Committee at Kaohsiung Chang Gung Memorial Hospital (Affidavit of Approval of Animal Use Protocol No. 2017121301; date of approval 30 January 2018) and performed in accordance with the Guide for the Care and Use of Laboratory Animals.

Animals were housed in an Association for Assessment and Accreditation of Laboratory Animal Care International (AAALAC; Frederick, MD, USA)-approved animal facility in our hospital with controlled temperature and light cycles (24 °C and 12/12 light cycle).

4.5. Animal Model of CLI, Animal Grouping and Strategic Treatments

The procedure and protocol of CLI were based on our previous report [29]. Briefly, pathogen-free, adult male nude mice weighing 22–25 g (Charles River Technology, BioLASCO Taiwan Co., Ltd., Taiwan) in CLI groups were anesthetized by inhalation of 2.0% isoflurane. The nude mice were placed in a supine position on a warming pad at 37 °C with the left hind limbs shaved. Under sterile conditions, the left femoral artery, small arterioles, circumferential femoral artery and veins were exposed and ligated over their proximal and distal portions before removal. To avoid the presence of collateral circulation, the branches were removed altogether. For the laser Doppler study, 10 nude mice in each group were utilized and 6 nude mice in each group were used for cellular-molecular assessment. For animals that served as controls, only the arteries were isolated, without ligation.

For the purpose of the study, adult-male nude mice ($n = 40$) were equally categorized into group 1 (sham-operated control (i.e., SC)), group 2 (CLI), group 3 (CLI + EPCs, 6×10^5 cells, derived from severe PAOD patient's circulatory blood prior to CD34$^+$ cell and HBO treatment (EPCPr-T) by intramuscular injection at 3 h after CLI induction), and group 4 (CLI + EPCs, 6×10^5 cells, derived from severe PAOD patient's circulatory blood after CD34$^+$ cell and HBO treatment (EPC^{Af-T}, i.e., defined as rejuvenated EPCs) by intramuscular injection at 3 h after CLI induction).

4.6. Peripheral Blood Collected and Cultured for Endothelial Progenitor Cells

Peripheral blood was collected from four patients (i.e., one for two nude mice in the first two patients and one for three nude mice in the latter two patients) at 8:00 a.m. after the 5th HBO therapy and 24 h after EPC therapy to severe PAOD patients. The procedure and protocol for EPC culture were based on our previous reports [29,30] with some modification. In brief, the blood sampling was performed on day 21 (i.e., day 0 was the date of the 5th iteration of HBO therapy) prior to nude mouse CLI induction for xenogeneic transfusion. Isolated mononuclear cells from peripheral blood were cultured in a 100 mm diameter dish with 10 mL DMEM culture medium containing 10% FBS for 21 days. Flow cytometric analysis was performed for the identification of cellular characteristics (i.e., EPC surface markers) after cell labeling with appropriate antibodies on day 21 of cell cultivation prior to implantation.

4.7. Measurement of Blood Flow with Laser Doppler

The procedure and protocol were based on our previous reports [29]. In brief, animals in each group were anesthetized by inhalation of isoflurane (2.0%) on day 2, 7, 14 after CLI induction. The animals were placed supine on a warming pad (37 °C), and blood flow was detected in both inguinal areas by a laser Doppler scanner (moorLDLS, Moor Instruments, Axminster, UK). This instrument scans an area of skin, which is evaluated by the distance between the mirror and the skin. The laser beam penetrates the normal tissue and part of the incident light that is scattered by moving red blood cells (RBCs) in microvasculature/small arterioles, forming a frequency broadening that is finally investigated by a photodetector. The RBC velocities and concentration give rise to Doppler frequency shifts and account for the strength of the signal. The Doppler shift is thus proportional to a blood-flow related variable and is exhibited as an arbitrary perfusion unit (PU). The mean blood flow is computed to yield an average number of pixels. Accordingly, the ratio of blood flow (BF) in the left (ischemic (I)) leg to right (normal (N)) leg (i.e., INBF) was computed, resulting in a ratio of PU. By day 28, the animals in each group were euthanized, and the quadriceps muscles were collected for individual study.

4.8. Vessel Density in CLI Area

The procedure and protocol for vessel density has been described in our previous report [29]. In detail, the IHC staining of small blood vessels was performed with α-SMA (1:400) as the primary antibody at room temperature for 1 h, followed by washing with PBS thrice. Ten minutes after the addition of anti-mouse HRP-conjugated secondary antibodies, the tissue sections were washed with PBS thrice. Then, 3,3′-diaminobenzidine (DAB) (0.7 gm/tablet) (Sigma-Aldrich) was added, followed by washing with PBS thrice after one minute. Finally, hematoxylin was added as a counterstain for nuclei, followed by washing twice with PBS after one minute. The angiogenesis was analyzed only in regions of demonstrably ischemic-regenerating quadriceps muscle. Three quadricep sections were analyzed in each nude mouse. To avoid bias, three selected HPFs (200×) were analyzed in each section.

The mean number per HPF for each animal was then determined by the summation of all numbers divided by 9.

4.9. Western Blot Analysis

The procedure and protocol of western blot analysis was based on our previous reports [8,16,29,30]. In brief, equal amounts (30 μg) of protein extracts from ischemic quadriceps of the animals were loaded and separated by SDS-PAGE using 12% acrylamide gradients. The membranes were incubated with monoclonal antibodies against CD31 (1:1000, Abcam, Cambridge, UK), von Willebrand factor (vWF) (1:1000, Abcam), CXCR4 (1:1000, Abcam), VEGF (1:1000, Abcam), stromal cell-derived growth factor ((SDF)-1α) (1:1000, Cell Signaling), cytosolic cytochrome C (1:2000, BD), mitochondrial cytochrome C (1:1000, BD), endothelial nitric-oxide synthase (eNOS) (1:1000, Abcam), Bax (1:1000, Abcam), transforming growth factor ((TGF)-ß) (1:500, Abcam), phosphorylated (p)-Smad3 (1:1000, cell signaling), p-Smad1/5 (1:1000, cell signaling), bone morphogenetic protein (1:1000, Abcam), cleaved caspase 3 (c-Csp3) (1:1000, cell signaling), cleaved poly (ADP-ribose) polymerase (c-PARP) (1:1000, cell signaling) and hypoxic inducible factor ((HIF)-α) (1:1000, Abcam). Signals were detected with HRP-conjugated goat anti-mouse or goat anti-rabbit IgG. Proteins were transferred to nitrocellulose membranes, which were then incubated in the primary antibody solution (anti-DNP 1:150) for two hours, followed by incubation with a second antibody solution (1:300) for one hour at room temperature. The washing procedure was repeated eight times within 40 min. Immunoreactive bands were visualized by enhanced chemiluminescence (ECL; Amersham Biosciences, Little Chalfont, UK) and were then exposed to Biomax L film (Kodak, Rochester, NY, USA). For quantification, ECL signals were digitized using LabWorks software (UVP).

4.10. Immunohistochemical (IHC) and Immunofluorescent (IF) Staining

The procedure and protocols have been described by previous reports [8,16,29,30]. Briefly, sections were incubated with primary antibodies specifically against CD31 (1:200, BD Pharmingen, Franklin Lakes, NJ, USA), vWF (1:200, Abcam), CXCR4 (1:200, Abcam) and SDF-1α (1:100, Santa Cruz), while sections incubated with irrelevant antibodies served as controls. Three sections of kidney specimens from each rat were analyzed. For quantification, three random HPFs (400× for IHC and IF studies) were analyzed in each section. The mean number (expressed as a percentage) of positively-stained cells per HPF for each animal was first divided by the total positively DAPI-stained cells, then determined by the summation of all numbers divided by 9.

4.11. Statistical Analysis

Quantitative data were expressed as mean ± SD. Statistical analysis was adequately performed by ANOVA followed by the Bonferroni multiple comparison post hoc test. Statistical analysis was performed using SAS statistical software for Windows Version 8.2 (SAS Institute, Cary, NC, USA). A probability value of less than 0.05 was considered statistically significant.

5. Conclusions

In conclusion, our findings demonstrated that only rejuvenated EPC therapy could effectively restore the blood flow and salvage the critical ischemic limbs in the nude mouse model of CLI.

Supplementary Materials: The following are available online at http://www.mdpi.com/1422-0067/21/21/7887/s1, Figure S1: Figures of flow cytometric analysis for identification of circulating EPCs.

Author Contributions: Conceptualization, Y.-C.C. and J.-J.S.; validation, P.-H.S., K.-H.C. and Y.-L.C.; formal analysis and investigation, P.-L.S., S.-C.W., Y.-C.L., Y.-L.C., T.-H.H.; data curation, P.-H.S. and K.-H.C.; writing—original draft preparation, H.-K.Y.; writing—review and editing, J.Y.C.; supervision, H.-K.Y.; project administration and funding acquisition, J.-J.S. and H.-K.Y. All authors have read and agreed to the published version of the manuscript.

Funding: This study was funded by research grants from the National Science Council, Taiwan, Republic of China (MOST 107-2314-B-182A-070) and Kaohsiung Chang Gung Memorial Hospital (NMRPD1H0891).

Conflicts of Interest: The authors declare no conflict of interest.

References

1. Hiatt, W.R. Medical Treatment of Peripheral Arterial Disease and Claudication. *N. Engl. J. Med.* **2001**, *344*, 1608–1621. [CrossRef] [PubMed]
2. Hirsch, A.T.; Criqui, M.H.; Treat-Jacobson, D.; Regensteiner, J.G.; Creager, M.A.; Olin, J.W.; Krook, S.H.; Hunninghake, D.B.; Comerota, A.J.; Walsh, M.E.; et al. Peripheral Arterial Disease Detection, Awareness, and Treatment in Primary Care. *JAMA* **2001**, *286*, 1317–1324. [CrossRef] [PubMed]
3. Ouriel, K. Peripheral arterial disease. *Lancet* **2001**, *358*, 1257–1264. [CrossRef]
4. Dormandy, J.; Heeck, L.; Vig, S. The natural history of claudication: Risk to life and limb. *Semin. Vasc. Surg.* **1999**, *12*, 123–137. [PubMed]
5. Muluk, S.C.; Muluk, V.S.; Kelley, M.E.; Whittle, J.C.; Tierney, J.A.; Webster, M.W.; Makaroun, M.S. Outcome events in patients with claudication: A 15-year study in 2777 patients. *J. Vasc. Surg.* **2001**, *33*, 251–257. [CrossRef] [PubMed]
6. Dormandy, J.A.; Charbonnel, B.; A Eckland, D.J.; Erdmann, E.; Massi-Benedetti, M.; Moules, I.K.; Skene, A.M.; Tan, M.H.; Lefèbvre, P.J.; Murray, G.D.; et al. Secondary prevention of macrovascular events in patients with type 2 diabetes in the PROactive Study (PROspective pioglitAzone Clinical Trial In macroVascular Events): A randomised controlled trial. *Lancet* **2005**, *366*, 1279–1289. [CrossRef]
7. Rena, O.; Garavoglia, M.; Francini, M.; Bellora, P.; Oliaro, A.; Casadio, C. Solitary pericardial hydatid cyst. *J. Cardiovasc. Surg.* **2004**, *45*, 77–80.
8. Sheu, J.-J.; Lin, P.-Y.; Sung, P.-H.; Chen, Y.-C.; Leu, S.; Chen, Y.-L.; Tsai, T.-H.; Chai, H.-T.; Chua, S.; Chang, H.-W.; et al. Levels and values of lipoprotein-associated phospholipase A2, galectin-3, RhoA/ROCK, and endothelial progenitor cells in critical limb ischemia: Pharmaco-therapeutic role of cilostazol and clopidogrel combination therapy. *J. Transl. Med.* **2014**, *12*, 101. [CrossRef]
9. Diehm, C.; Allenberg, J.R.; Pittrow, D.; Mahn, M.; Tepohl, G.; Haberl, R.L.; Darius, H.; Burghaus, I.; Trampisch, H.J.; German Epidemiological Trial on Ankle Brachial Index Study Group. Mortality and Vascular Morbidity in Older Adults with Asymptomatic Versus Symptomatic Peripheral Artery Disease. *Circulation* **2009**, *120*, 2053–2061. [CrossRef]
10. Dormandy, J.; Heeck, L.; Vig, S. The fate of patients with critical leg ischemia. *Semin. Vasc. Surg.* **1999**, *12*, 142–147.
11. Norgren, L.; Hiatt, W.R.; Dormandy, J.A.; Nehler, M.R.; Harris, K.A.; Fowkes, F.G.; Group, T.I.W. Inter-Society Consensus for the Management of Peripheral Arterial Disease (TASC II). *J. Vasc. Surg.* **2007**, *45*, S5–S67. [CrossRef] [PubMed]
12. Bradbury, A.W.; Adam, D.J.; Bell, J.; Forbes, J.F.; Fowkes, F.G.R.; Gillespie, I.; Raab, G.; Ruckley, C.V. Multicentre randomised controlled trial of the clinical and cost-effectiveness of a bypass-surgery-first versus a balloon-angioplasty-first revascularisation strategy for severe limb ischaemia due to infrainguinal disease. The Bypass versus Angioplasty in Severe Ischaemia of the Leg (BASIL) trial. *Health Technol. Assess.* **2010**, *14*, 1–210. [CrossRef] [PubMed]
13. El-Sayed, H.F. Bypass surgery for lower extremity limb salvage: Vein bypass. *Methodist DeBakey Cardiovasc. J.* **2013**, *8*, 37–42. [CrossRef] [PubMed]
14. Vartanian, S.M.; Conte, M.S. Surgical Intervention for Peripheral Arterial Disease. *Circ. Res.* **2015**, *116*, 1614–1628. [CrossRef]
15. Thukkani, A.K.; Kinlay, S. Endovascular Intervention for Peripheral Artery Disease. *Circ. Res.* **2015**, *116*, 1599–1613. [CrossRef]
16. Leu, S.; Sun, C.-K.; Sheu, J.-J.; Chang, L.-T.; Yuen, C.-M.; Yen, C.-H.; Chiang, C.-H.; Ko, S.-F.; Pei, S.-N.; Chua, S.; et al. Autologous bone marrow cell implantation attenuates left ventricular remodeling and improves heart function in porcine myocardial infarction: An echocardiographic, six-month angiographic, and molecular—Cellular study. *Int. J. Cardiol.* **2011**, *150*, 156–168. [CrossRef]

17. Losordo, D.W.; Henry, T.D.; Davidson, C.; Lee, J.S.; Costa, M.A.; Bass, T.; Mendelsohn, F.; Fortuin, F.D.; Pepine, C.J.; Traverse, J.H.; et al. Intramyocardial, Autologous CD34+ Cell Therapy for Refractory Angina. *Circ. Res.* **2011**, *109*, 428–436. [CrossRef]
18. Lee, F.-Y.; Chen, Y.-L.; Sung, P.-H.; Ma, M.-C.; Pei, S.-N.; Wu, C.-J.; Yang, C.-H.; Fu, M.; Ko, S.-F.; Leu, S.; et al. Intracoronary Transfusion of Circulation-Derived CD34+ Cells Improves Left Ventricular Function in Patients With End-Stage Diffuse Coronary Artery Disease Unsuitable for Coronary Intervention. *Crit. Care Med.* **2015**, *43*, 2117–2132. [CrossRef]
19. Sung, P.-H.; Lee, F.-Y.; Tong, M.-S.; Chiang, J.Y.; Pei, S.-N.; Ma, M.-C.; Li, Y.-C.; Chen, Y.-L.; Wu, C.-J.; Sheu, J.-J.; et al. The Five-Year Clinical and Angiographic Follow-Up Outcomes of Intracoronary Transfusion of Circulation-Derived CD34+ Cells for Patients with End-Stage Diffuse Coronary Artery Disease Unsuitable for Coronary Intervention—Phase I Clinical Trial. *Crit. Care Med.* **2018**, *46*, e411–e418. [CrossRef]
20. Quyyumi, A.A.; Vasquez, A.; Kereiakes, D.J.; Klapholz, M.; Schaer, G.L.; Abdel-Latif, A.; Frohwein, S.; Henry, T.D.; Schatz, R.A.; Dib, N.; et al. PreSERVE-AMI: A Randomized, Double-Blind, Placebo-Controlled Clinical Trial of Intracoronary Administration of Autologous CD34+ Cells in Patients With Left Ventricular Dysfunction Post STEMI. *Circ. Res.* **2017**, *120*, 324–331. [CrossRef]
21. Peeters Weem, S.M.; Teraa, M.; de Borst, G.J.; Verhaar, M.C.; Moll, F.L. Bone Marrow derived Cell Therapy in Critical Limb Ischemia: A Meta-analysis of Randomized Placebo Controlled Trials. *Eur. J. Vasc. Endovasc. Surg.* **2015**, *50*, 775–783. [CrossRef]
22. Rigato, M.; Monami, M.; Fadini, G.P. Autologous Cell Therapy for Peripheral Arterial Disease: Systematic Review and Meta-Analysis of Randomized, Nonrandomized, and Noncontrolled Studies. *Circ. Res.* **2017**, *120*, 1326–1340. [CrossRef] [PubMed]
23. Slovut, D.P.; Sullivan, T.M. Critical limb ischemia: Medical and surgical management. *Vasc. Med.* **2008**, *13*, 281–291. [CrossRef]
24. Thom, S.R. Hyperbaric Oxygen: Its Mechanisms and Efficacy. *Plast. Reconstr. Surg.* **2011**, *127* (Suppl. 1), 131S–141S. [CrossRef] [PubMed]
25. Lin, P.Y.; Sung, P.H.; Chung, S.Y.; Hsu, S.L.; Chung, W.J.; Sheu, J.J.; Hsueh, S.K.; Chen, K.H.; Wu, R.W.; Yip, H.K. Hyperbaric Oxygen Therapy Enhanced Circulating Levels of Endothelial Progenitor Cells and Angiogenesis Biomarkers, Blood Flow, in Ischemic Areas in Patients with Peripheral Arterial Occlusive Disease. *J. Clin. Med.* **2018**, *7*, 548. [CrossRef] [PubMed]
26. Gorman, J.F.; Stansell, G.B.; Douglass, F.M. Limitations of Hyperbaric Oxygenation in Occlusive Arterial Disease. *Circulation* **1965**, *32*, 936–939. [CrossRef] [PubMed]
27. Manax, W.G.; Bloch, J.H.; Longerbeam, J.K.; Lillehei, R.C. Successful 24 Hour In Vitro Preservation of Canine Kidneys by the Combined Use of Hyperbaric Oxygenation and Hypothermia. *Surgery* **1964**, *56*, 275–282. [PubMed]
28. Schreml, S.; Szeimies, R.; Prantl, L.; Karrer, S.; Landthaler, M.; Babilas, P. Oxygen in acute and chronic wound healing. *Br. J. Dermatol.* **2010**, *163*, 257–268. [CrossRef]
29. Yeh, K.-H.; Sheu, J.-J.; Lin, Y.-C.; Sun, C.-K.; Chang, L.-T.; Kao, Y.-H.; Yen, C.-H.; Shao, P.-L.; Tsai, T.-H.; Chen, Y.-L.; et al. Benefit of combined extracorporeal shock wave and bone marrow-derived endothelial progenitor cells in protection against critical limb ischemia in rats*. *Crit. Care Med.* **2012**, *40*, 169–177. [CrossRef]
30. Chen, Y.-L.; Tsai, T.-H.; Wallace, C.G.; Chen, Y.-L.; Huang, T.-H.; Sung, P.-H.; Yuen, C.-M.; Sun, C.-K.; Lin, K.-C.; Chai, H.-T.; et al. Intra-carotid arterial administration of autologous peripheral blood-derived endothelial progenitor cells improves acute ischemic stroke neurological outcomes in rats. *Int. J. Cardiol.* **2015**, *201*, 668–683. [CrossRef]

Publisher's Note: MDPI stays neutral with regard to jurisdictional claims in published maps and institutional affiliations.

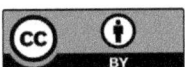

© 2020 by the authors. Licensee MDPI, Basel, Switzerland. This article is an open access article distributed under the terms and conditions of the Creative Commons Attribution (CC BY) license (http://creativecommons.org/licenses/by/4.0/).

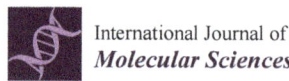

Article

Association of Soluble Suppression of Tumorigenesis-2 (ST2) with Endothelial Function in Patients with Ischemic Heart Failure

Stathis Dimitropoulos [1], Vasiliki Chara Mystakidi [1], Evangelos Oikonomou [1,2,*], Gerasimos Siasos [1,2], Vasiliki Tsigkou [1], Dimitris Athanasiou [1], Nikolaos Gouliopoulos [1], Evanthia Bletsa [1], Aimilios Kalampogias [1], Georgios Charalambous [1], Costas Tsioufis [1], Manolis Vavuranakis [2] and Dimitris Tousoulis [1]

[1] First Department of Cardiology, 'Hippokration' General Hospital, School of Medicine, National and Kapodistrian University of Athens, 11528 Athens, Greece; stakyp@yahoo.com (S.D.); xaram25@gmail.com (V.C.M.); ger_sias@hotmail.com (G.S.); bikytsigkoy@yahoo.gr (V.T.); dimitris.eathanasiou@yahoo.gr (D.A.); ngouliopoulos@yahoo.com (N.G.); evabletsa@gmail.com (E.B.); akalamp@gmail.com (A.K.); drcharalambous@yahoo.gr (G.C.); tsioufis@hippocratio.gr (C.T.); drtousoulis@hotmail.com (D.T.)
[2] Third Department of Cardiology, Medical School, National and Kapodistrian University of Athens, 15772 Athens, Greece; vavouran@otenet.gr
* Correspondence: boikono@gmail.com, Tel.: +30-210-7763488

Received: 14 October 2020; Accepted: 6 December 2020; Published: 9 December 2020

Abstract: Soluble suppression of tumorigenesis-2 (sST2) has been introduced as a marker associated with heart failure (HF) pathophysiology and status. Endothelial dysfunction is a component underlying HF pathophysiology. Therefore, we examined the association of arterial wall properties with sST2 levels in patients with HF of ischemic etiology. We enrolled 143 patients with stable HF of ischemic etiology and reduced left ventricular ejection fraction (LVEF) and 77 control subjects. Flow-mediated dilation (FMD) was used to evaluate endothelial function and pulse wave velocity (PWV) to assess arterial stiffness. Although there was no significant difference in baseline demographic characteristics, levels of sST2 were increased in HF compared to the control (15.8 (11.0, 21.8) ng/mL vs. 12.5 (10.4, 16.3) ng/mL; $p < 0.001$). In the HF group, there was a positive correlation of sST2 levels with age (rho = 0.22; $p = 0.007$) while there was no association of LVEF with sST2 (rho = −0.119; $p = 0.17$) nor with PWV (rho = 0.1; $p = 0.23$). Interestingly, sST2 was increased in NYHA III [20.0 (12.3, 25.7) ng/mL] compared to patients with NYHA II (15.0 (10.4, 18.2) ng/mL; $p = 0.003$) and inversely associated with FMD (rho = −0.44; $p < 0.001$) even after adjustment for possible confounders. In patients with chronic HF of ischemic etiology, sST2 levels are increased and are associated with functional capacity. There is an inverse association between FMD and sST2 levels, highlighting the interplay between the dysfunctional endothelium and HF pathophysiologic mechanisms.

Keywords: heart failure; soluble suppression of tumorigenesis-2; endothelial function; FMD

1. Introduction

The prevalence of heart failure (HF) worldwide is approximately 1% to 2% and it is estimated that it exceeds 10% in subjects over 70 years old [1,2]. Natriuretic peptides—b-type natriuretic peptide (BNP) and N terminal pro BNP (NTproBNP)—and cardiac troponins (Tn) I and T are found to be elevated in HF following increased myocardial wall stress, elevated filling pressures, subendocardial ischemia etc. [3,4]. Moreover, they are associated with prognosis and disease severity [4–6].

The European Society of Cardiology has already announced research on novel HF biomarkers so as to be used in clinical practice, as a multimarker approach is preferred over the old fashion single biomarker approach [7]. New biomarkers are those one of inflammation, oxidative stress, vascular dysfunction, and myocardial remodeling. They have been proposed as indices related to HF status, functional capacity, and prognosis [4,8,9]. Galectin-3 (Gal–3), soluble suppression of tumorigenesis-2 (sST2), and high-sensitivity cardiac troponin (hs–cTn) are mainly predictors of hospitalization and death in HF patients, and in addition to NPs can increase the prognostic value [10,11]. To this direction, sST2 has been introduced as a marker associated with acute decompensate heart failure, pro-inflammatory status, endothelial dysfunction, myocardial fibrosis. and adverse remodeling with prognostic capability [12]. Additionally, sST2 has a low biological variability and a low index of individuality (0.25), favorable characteristics that may be used for guiding therapy and monitoring HF patients [13–17].

Endothelial dysfunction is considered an initial step in the process of atherosclerosis and coronary artery disease progression and is considered as a component underlying HF pathophysiology. Endothelial dysfunction plays an important role in HF progression. It worsens the vasoconstriction and increases myocardial damage. Dysfunctional endothelium increases the afterload due to systemic and pulmonary vascular constriction. Myocardial perfusion is also impaired due to decreased coronary endothelium-dependent vasodilation [8,9,18].

Since ST2 is produced among other cells by endothelial cells of cardiac vasculature [19], in this study, we examined the association of arterial wall properties and endothelial function with sST2 levels in patients with HF of ischemic etiology.

2. Results

2.1. Demographic and Clinical Characteristics

As it is shown in Table 1, the mean age of the HF patients was 67 ± 12 years. From the HF patients 68% were categorized as NYHA class II. The median ejection fraction was 30% (25%, 40%). More than half of them (56%) had hypertension and 52% diabetes mellitus (DM).

Table 1. Study participants' demographic, clinical, and laboratory characteristics.

-	HF Group	Control Group	p-Value
Age (years)	67 ± 12	68 ± 10	0.45
Male gender (%)	85	81	0.439
BMI (kg/m^2)	28.2 ± 6.5	27.1 ± 3.5	0.055
DM (%)	52	37	0.02
Hypertension (%)	56	32	0.001
Hyperlipidemia (%)	60	20	0.08
NYHA 2 (%)	68	–	–
ACEI or ARB (%)	66	17	0.017
MRA (%)	58	3	<0.001
Diuretics (%)	77	13	<0.001
B-blockers (%)	88	29	<0.001
eGFR (mL/min)	78.5 (54.3, 108.8)	87.8 (71.1, 114.7)	0.48
Serum Urea (mg/dl)	44 (30, 69)	27 (24, 31)	<0.001
Serum Creatinine (mg/dl)	1.0 (0.9, 1.3)	0.8 (0.7, 1.0)	<0.001
NTproBNP (pg/mL)	140 (96, 290)	50 (32, 82)	0.001
TNFa (ng/mL)	2.4 (1.4, 2.7)	0.7 (0.6, 0.8)	<0.001
ICAM-1 (ng/mL)	276 (221, 315)	212 (175, 267)	<0.001
PWV (m/s)	8.7 (7.2, 10.6)	8.2 (7.4, 9.0)	0.01
FMD (%)	5.6 (3.2, 8.0)	6.1 (3.7, 8.3)	0.71
EF (%)	30 (25, 40)	55 (55, 60)	<0.001
sST2 (ng/mL)	15.8 (11.0, 21.8)	12.5 (10.4, 16.3)	<0.001

HF: Heart failure; BMI: Body Mass Index, DM: Diabetes Meletus, NYHA: New York Heart Association Classification, ACEI: Angiotensin Converting Enzyme Inhibitors, ARB: Angiotensin II Receptor Blockers, MRA: Mineralocorticoid Receptor Antagonists, eGFR: estimated Glomerular Filtration Rate, NTproBNP: N terminal pro hormone B-type Natriuretic Peptide, EF: Ejection Fraction, sST2: soluble Suppression of Tumorigenesis-2, TNFa: Tumor Necrosis Factor a, PWV: Pulse Wave Velocity, FMD: Flow-mediated Dilation; ICAM-1: Intracellular adhesion molecule 1.

In the control group, the mean age was 63 ± 10 years. As far as their medical history is concerned, 32% had hypertension, 37% had DM, and 20% had hyperlipidemia.

Between the two groups, there was no significant difference in age. The prevalence of DM (52% vs. 37%; $p = 0.02$) and hypertension (56% vs. 32%; $p = 0.001$) was higher in HF subjects compared to the control while there was no significant difference regarding the history of hyperlipidemia.

Significant differences between HF and control subjects were observed regarding treatment. The majority of HF subjects were under diuretics, angiotensin converting enzyme inhibitors (ACEIs), or angiotensin II receptor blockers (ARBs), and β–blockers.

Serum levels of urea and creatine was higher in subjects with HF compared to control. Serum ICAM-1 levels was higher in the HF group compared to the control group (276 (221, 315 ng/mL vs. 212 (175, 267) ng/mL, $p < 0.001$). NT pro-BNP in the HF group (140 (96, 290) pg/mL) was increased compared to the control group (50 (32, 82) pg/mL; $p < 0.001$). sST2 was higher in the HF group (15.8 (11.0, 21.8) ng/mL) compared to the control group (12.5 (10.4, 16.3) ng/mL; $p < 0.001$) (Figure 1).

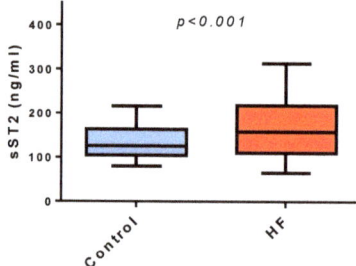

Figure 1. Serum levels of soluble Suppression of Tumorigenesis-2 are higher in the heart failure group compared to the control group. The Distribution of serum levels of soluble Suppression of Tumorigenesis-2 are shown with Box-plots sST2: Soluble Suppression of Tumorigenesis-2.

2.2. Factors Affecting sST2 Level in Subjects with Heart Failure

To examine how sST2 levels may be affected by various demographic, clinical, and laboratory factors, we examined in a univariate fashion the correlation of sST2 with multiple factors in the HF population.

2.3. Association of sST2 with Demographic Characteristics of Heart Failure Subjects

In subjects with HF, there was a positive correlation of sST2 with age (rho = 0.22; $p = 0.007$) but not with body mass index (rho = −0.094; $p = 0.42$). The sST2 levels did not differ between female and male subjects (15.4 (11.1, 18.7) ng/mL vs. 14.2 (10.3, 19.9) ng/mL; $p = 0.72$), between hypertensive and normotensive subjects (15.2 (10.9, 21.70 ng/mL vs. 12.9 (10.2, 17.4) ng/mL; $p = 0.08$), and between subjects with DM compared with normo-glycemic subjects (14.5 (10.6, 20.1) ng/mL vs. 13.5 (10.5, 18.7) ng/mL; $p = 0.45$) (Supplementary Figure S1A–E).

2.4. Association of sST2 with Clinical Characteristics in Subjects with Heart Failure

In subjects with HF, sST2 levels were not associated with LVEF (rho = −0.119; $p = 0.17$). Regarding the NYHA functional classification in the HF group, sST2 was higher in NYHA III (20.0 (12.3, 25.7) ng/mL) compared to patients with NYHA II (15.0 (10.4, 18.2) ng/mL; $p = 0.003$). The sST2 levels were not affected by the use or not of ACEI or ARB (15.1 (11.2, 22.9) ng/mL vs. 16.0 (7.8, 20.7) ng/mL; $p = 0.46$), by the use or not of mineralocorticoid receptor antagonist (MRA) (16.0 (9.9, 20.6) ng/mL vs. 12.9 (10.3, 18.5) ng/mL; $p = 0.77$), and by the use or not of β–blockers (14.8 (9.5, 21.8) ng/mL vs. 17.4 (11.2, 22.3) ng/mL; $p = 0.63$). sST2 levels were inversely associated with eGFR (rho = −1.75;

$p = 0.03$). sST2 was not associated with CRP (rho = 0.45; $p = 0.26$), TNFa (rho = −0.024; $p = 0.77$), ICAM–1 (rho = 0.02, $p = 0.84$), or NTproBNP (rho = 0.92; $p = 0.27$) (Supplementary Figure S1F–M).

sST2 was not associated with arterial stiffness—PWV (rho = 0.1; $p = 0.23$) (Figure 2A). Interestingly, sST2 was inversely associated with FMD (rho = −0.44; $p < 0.001$) (Figure 2B). To further test how sST2 levels are affected by endothelial function (FMD), independently from other confounders, we proceeded to a linear regression analysis in which we included all variables proved significant in the univariate analysis (Table 2). sST2 was, independently of other confounders, inversely associated with FMD in patients with HF of ischemic etiology, and for every increase in FMD by 1%, there is an anticipated decrease in sST2 levels by approximately 14 ng/mL.

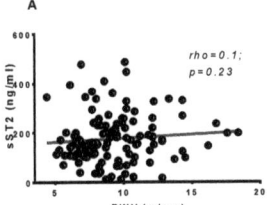 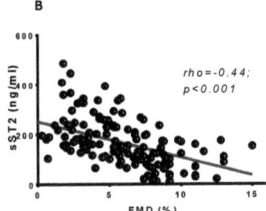

Figure 2. Levels of soluble suppression of Tumorigenesis-2 are inversely associated with FMD but not with PWV. (**A**) Scatter-dot of the association of PWV with soluble suppression of Tumorigenesis-2. (**B**) Scatter-dot of the association of FMD with soluble suppression of Tumorigenesis-2. sST2: Soluble Suppression of Tumorigenesis-2; PWV: Pulse wave velocity; FMD: Flow-mediated dilation.

Table 2. Multiple linear regression analysis for the association of sST2 (dependent variable) with several variable.

Variables	B Coefficient	95% CI	p-Value
Age (years)	1.35	−0.87, 3.55	0.22
Sex	29.91	−13.85, 73.68	0.17
eGFR	0.11	−0.56, 0.80	0.73
NYHA class	–	–	–
NYHA II	–	–	–
NYHA III	15.76	−2.09, 33.62	0.08
FMD (%)	−14.12	−20.02, −8.22	<0.001

eGFR: estimated Glomerular Filtration Rate, NYHA: New York Heart Association Classification, FMD: Flow-mediated dilation. For Sex, the reference category was set as female; For NYHA, the reference category was the NYHA 2 stage.

3. Discussion

In the present study, we examined the association between biomarkers of cardiovascular stress and interstitial fibrosis with vascular function in stable patients with systolic HF of ischemic etiology. We found that sST2, a novel HF biomarker associated with myocardial fibrosis, produced by either myocardial cells, fibroblasts or, endothelial cells, and prognosis [20–22] is correlated with FMD, which expresses the status and health of the endothelial cells layer, highlighting the key role of the endothelium in the progress of HF [8,9].

3.1. sST2 in Heart Failure

sST2 has been initially identified as a marker of myocyte stress [23]. sST2 assays are accurate with high repeatability [24], implying the possible use of sST2 as an additional clinical meaningful biomarker.

We identified a significant difference on sST2 levels between control and HF subjects, although there was significant overlap in the values observed in the two examined groups, which is in accordance with previous analytical studies on sST2 and the Framingham Heart Study [24,25]. Therefore, sST2 cannot be used in the etiologic diagnosis of dyspnea.

Beyond the role of sST2 as a surrogate of myocardial stress, sST2 is mainly produced by extracardiac tissues (i.e., alveolar cells, fibroblasts, vessel wall cells) [26–28]. As a response to the continuous stress stimulus, there is an upregulation in ST2 gene expression. Concerning sST2 release from alveolar epithelial cells, there is an association between the increase in alveolus thickness and the upregulation of sST2, which suggests a relationship between the severity of pulmonary edema congestion and alveolar strain with sST2 production [26]. Inflammatory and pro-fibrotic stimulus are also considered responsible for the activation of ST2 production and release in the circulation [26–28]. sST2 is a circulating receptor for interleukin 33 (Il-33). The connection between Il-33 and ST2 ligand provokes anti-inflammation and antithrombotic processes in the damaged heart. Therefore, sST2 is a decoy receptor of Il-33 and attenuates the beneficial effects of Il-33 connection to ST2 ligand, boosting inflammatory and thrombotic damage to the heart [29].

In our HF study population, we found that sST2 levels were associated with HF status and functional capacity of the patients as assessed with NYHA classification. Indeed, patients with functional impairment have been identified with higher values of sST2, although the levels of circulating sST2 were not associated with LVEF. These findings may be explained since in chronic HF, sST2 levels are mainly associated with LV diastolic dysfunction and increased left and right ventricular pressures, which are key determinants of the functional capacity of patients [30]. However, in our cohort of chronic HF patients, we did not identify any association of sST2 with NTproBNP levels. The lack of association can be attributed to the specific characteristics of our study population especially regarding the stable clinical condition for at least 3 months. Indeed, we excluded from the study subjects with recent decompensation or subjects not on optimal medical treatment and therefore with NT-pro-BNP levels at the lower rate.

Impaired renal function is a significant determinant of HF prognosis and is associated with myocardial fibrosis [31]. sST2 is associated with adverse prognosis in subjects with chronic kidney disease [31,32]. We found that in the HF population, sST2 was inversely associated with estimated GFR, implicating the cardiorenal axis and the bidirectional toxic effects of volume overload in the heart and kidneys.

3.2. sST2 and Vascular Wall Properties

Arterial wall properties constitute the second component of the cardiovascular system and have a key role in the cardiovascular homeostasis. They regulate vasomotor activity, arterial stiffness, afterload, and consequently cardiac function [33]. Impaired endothelial function has been proposed as a factor implicated in the development and progress of HF especially of ischemic etiology and several approaches may beneficially affect the endothelium in the concept of HF [34–36]. Systemic vasoconstrictor is observed in chronic HF settings and decreased endothelium-dependent vasodilatation may be the underlying pathophysiologic background contributing to a lower cardiac output state.

We found that in HF patients, there is an inverse association between endothelial function and sST2 levels. sST2 is produced among other cells by endothelial cells and alveolar epithelium [37]. The inverse association found in our study may be confirmatory that dysfunctional endothelium (under the stimulus of decrease shear stress, proinflammatory milieu, and oxidative stress) may lead to highly expressed levels of sST2, which in turn may have detrimental effects on cardiac function and remodeling. Indeed, even after adjustment for potential confounders associated with functional capacity, the health of the endothelial layer was a significant contributor of sST2 levels.

As opposed to endothelial function, we did not observe any association of sST2 levels with PWV and arterial stiffness a surrogate of arteriosclerosis in subjects with HF of ischemic etiology [38,39]. Although sST2 levels in patients with coronary artery disease have been associated with aortic stiffness, in our study population with stable chronic HF, we only identified a link between endothelial function and sST2 levels. In the same direction, we did not find an association between serum ICAM-1 levels and sST2 in our populations of HF subjects despite the well-described effects of adhesion molecules in endothelial dysfunction [40]. In HF, beyond the role of leukocytes and inflammatory milieu, underlying mechanisms may contribute to impairment of endothelium (i.e., low arterial shear stress, oxidative stress) [8].

3.3. Clinical Importance

Although sST2 levels cannot be used for diagnosis of HF, they are significantly associated with prognosis and functional capacity [41,42]. The association of endothelial function with sST2 levels emphasizes the role of the vascular system as an important determinant of functional capacity beyond left ventricle systolic performance. It may also imply a link between dysfunctional endothelium in the pulmonary circulation associated with congestion in patients with HF and emphasizes the systemic nature of HF syndrome, suggesting that treatment of underlying pathologic conditions may affect HF course.

3.4. Limitations

Although, in our study, we achieved a match case control population, the design of our study contains inherent limitations. Accordingly, we cannot conclude on the importance of ST2 on prognosis or diagnosis of HF. Moreover, based on our study findings, we cannot conclude on a straightforward association of ST2 levels with endothelial function and we cannot provide etiologic or pathophysiologic insights on the mechanisms underlying the link between ST2 and endothelial dysfunction in subjects with HF.

4. Methods

4.1. Study Population

In the period from June 2018 to March 2019, 143 patients with stable HF of ischemic etiology and reduced left ventricular ejection fraction (LVEF), as assessed by echocardiogram, were enrolled for the purpose of this study.

A group of 77 control subjects were also recruited from the outpatient cardiology department, where they were referred for preventive examination. All the recruited control patients had no symptoms or signs of heart failure and normal ejection fraction, had a normal physical examination, normal electrocardiogram, and a normal LVEF (>55%).

4.2. Data Collection and Biochemical Measurements

Demographics were collected in all subjects by the use of standard questionnaires and procedures. Clinical characteristics, and data regarding ECG, echocardiography, coronary angiography (in patients with HF of ischemic etiology), biochemistry, NTproBNP, high-sensitivity C–reactive protein (hsCRP), and pharmacotherapy were also collected.

Standard transthoracic echocardiographic examination was carried out in all subjects by the same expert using a vivid e-cardiovascular ultrasound system (General Electric, Milwaukee, WI, USA) equipped with a 2.0–3.6 MHz (harmonics) phased array transducer. Left ventricle ejection fraction was calculated by biplane Simpson's modified rule as previously described. All measurements were performed according to the recommendations of the American Society of Echocardiography and the European Association of Cardiovascular Imaging. The diagnosis of coronary artery disease was established by a history of myocardial infarction or by evidence of a coronary vessel luminal stenosis >75% as detected by coronography, either done in a previous hospitalization or in hospitalization during the enrollment of the patient in the study. Subjects finally enrolled in the study were under optimal medical treatment and under stable clinical status for at least three months prior to their entry in the study, as characterized by NYHA classification.

A fasting venous blood sample was taken from each individual by venipuncture between 8.00 and 10.00 a.m. Samples were centrifuged at 3000 rpm and serum/plasma was collected and stored at −80 °C until assayed. sST2 measured with a Presage™ ST2 Assay (Critical Diagnostics, San Diego, CA,

US). Calibration and standardization of these assays were performed according to the manufacturers' protocols. NTproBNP concentrations were measured quantitatively using a fluorescence immunoassay with a single-use device (Triage BNP Test; Biosite, Inc., San Diego, CA, USA). Tumor necrosis factor alpha (TNF-α) and intracellular adhesion molecule-1 (ICAM-1) levels in the serum were measured with enzyme link immunosorbent assays (ELISA). The Modification of Diet in Renal Disease study (MDRD) formula was used to estimate the glomerular filtration rate (eGFR).

Endothelial function was evaluated by estimating the flow-mediated dilation in the brachial artery [42]. In brief, after a 10-min rest, the right brachial artery was scanned in the longitudinal section, 5 cm above the antecubital fossa, using a Vivid e ultrasound system (General Electric, Milwaukee, WI, USA) equipped with a 5.0–13.0 MHz (harmonics) linear array ultrasound transducer. A pneumatic cuff placed distal to the ultrasound probe was then inflated to suprasystolic pressure on the forearm for 5 min to induce reactive hyperemia. After the release of the ischemia cuff, brachial artery diameter was measured manually with electronic calipers (as the average derived from multiple diameter measurements along a segment of the vessel) at the boundaries of the media–adventitia interfaces, every 15 s for 2 min, and FMD was defined as the % change of vessel diameter from rest to the maximum diameter following cuff release. The same examiner throughout the study conducted examinations. The same observer who was blinded to the image sequence assignment proceeded to all measurements of brachial artery diameter. Endothelium-independent dilation (EID) was defined as the % change of vessel diameter from rest to the maximum diameter post sublingual nitrate given.

Arterial stiffness was evaluated in all patients with pulse wave velocity (PWV) measurements. Carotid-femoral pulse wave velocity (PWV), which is considered to be an index of aortic stiffness, was calculated from measurements of the pulse transit time and the distance traveled between 2 recording sites (PWV = distance in meters divided by transit time in seconds) by using a well-validated noninvasive device (SphygmoCor; AtCor Medical, Sydney, NSW, Australia). Two different pulse waves were obtained at 2 sites (at the base of the neck for the common carotid and over the right femoral artery) with the transducer. Distance was defined as the distance from the suprasternal notch to the femoral artery minus the distance from the carotid artery to the suprasternal notch [38,42].

4.3. Bioethics

All subjects were informed about the aims of the study and gave their written informed consent. The study was approved by the local ethics committee of our institution (15 July 2014) and was carried out in accordance with the Declaration of Helsinki (1989).

4.4. Statistical Analysis

All variables were tested for normal distribution of the data using the P–P plots and Shapiro–Wilk test. Data are expressed as means ± standard deviation, when normally distributed otherwise, as median with interquartile range. Data not normally distributed were logarithmically transformed to improve normality and log-transformed data were used if normality was achieved. Differences between groups of subjects were tested with a t-test and chi square test for continuous and categorical variables, respectively. Spearman correlation was used to test for an association between continuous variables. A linear regression model was applied to test the association of FMD on sST2 independently from other established confounders (i.e., age, sex) or variables proved significant in the univariate analysis. Statistical analysis was performed using SPSS version 25 (IBM SPSS Statistics Version 25.0. Armonk, NY, USA).

5. Conclusion

In patients with chronic HF of ischemic etiology, sST2 levels are increased and are associated with functional capacity and renal impairment. There is an inverse association between FMD and sST2 levels, highlighting the interplay between dysfunctional endothelium interstitial fibrosis and the HF pathophysiologic mechanism as they can be evaluated by circulating sST2 levels.

Supplementary Materials: Supplementary materials can be found at http://www.mdpi.com/1422-0067/21/24/9385/s1, Figure S1: Multi-panel figure (A–K) showing how sST2 levels are associated with continuous and categorical variables in the heart failure group.

Author Contributions: S.D.: Methodology, investigation, data curation, formal analysis, writing—original draft preparation V.C.M.: Methodology, investigation, data curation, software, formal analysis, writing—original draft preparation, writing—review and editing E.O.: Conceptualization, investigation, data curation, Methodology, software, validation, writing—review and editing G.S.: Conceptualization, software, supervision, data collection V.T.: software, formal analysis, resources, data collection review D.A.: software, investigation, resources, data collection, review N.G.: software, investigation, resources, data collection, draft the manuscript E.B.: Methodology, software, investigation, data collection, draft the manuscript A.K.: investigation, resources, data curation, data collection, draft the manuscript G.C.: investigation, supervision, data collection, draft the manuscript C.T.: validation, writing—review and editing, supervision, investigation, review the manuscript M.V.: Conceptualization, validation, writing—review and editing, supervision D.T.: Conceptualization, validation, writing—review and editing, supervision. All authors have read and agreed to the published version of the manuscript.

Funding: This research received no external funding.

Conflicts of Interest: The authors declare no conflict of interest.

Abbreviations

sST2	Soluble Suppression of Tumorigenesis-2
HF	Heart failure
LVEF	Left ventricular ejection fraction
FMD	Flow mediated dilation
PWV	pulse wave velocity
BNP	b–type natriuretic peptide
NTproBNP	N terminal pro BNP
Tn	cardiac troponins
DM	diabetes mellitus
ACEI	Angiotensin Converting Enzyme Inhibitors
ARB	Angiotensin II Receptor Blockers
ECG	electrocardiogram
hsCRP	sensitivity C–reactive protein
BMI	Body Mass Index
NYHA	New York Heart Association Classification
MRA	Mineralocorticoid Receptor Antagonists
eGFR	estimated Glomerular Filtration Rate
EF	Ejection Fraction
TNFa	Tumor Necrosis Factor a
ICAM-1	Intracellular adhesion molecule 1

References

1. Mosterd, A.; Hoes, A.W. Clinical epidemiology of heart failure. *Heart* **2007**, *93*, 1137–1146. [CrossRef] [PubMed]
2. Redfield, M.M.; Jacobsen, S.J.; Burnett, J.C., Jr.; Mahoney, D.W.; Bailey, K.R.; Rodeheffer, R.J. Burden of systolic and diastolic ventricular dysfunction in the community: Appreciating the scope of the heart failure epidemic. *JAMA* **2003**, *289*, 194–202. [CrossRef]
3. Wettersten, N.; Maisel, A. Role of Cardiac Troponin Levels in Acute Heart Failure. *Card. Fail. Rev.* **2015**, *1*, 102–106. [CrossRef] [PubMed]
4. Yancy, C.W.; Jessup, M.; Bozkurt, B.; Butler, J.; Casey, D.E., Jr.; Colvin, M.M.; Drazner, M.H.; Filippatos, G.S.; Fonarow, G.C.; Givertz, M.M.; et al. 2017 ACC/AHA/HFSA Focused Update of the 2013 ACCF/AHA Guideline for the Management of Heart Failure: A Report of the American College of Cardiology/American Heart Association Task Force on Clinical Practice Guidelines and the Heart Failure Society of America. *J. Am. Coll. Cardiol.* **2017**, *70*, 776–803. [CrossRef] [PubMed]

5. Anguita, M.; Comin, J.; Almenar, L.; Crespo, M.; Delgado, J.; Gonzalez-Costello, J.; Hernandez-Madrid, A.; Manito, N.; Perez de la Sota, E.; Segovia, J.; et al. Comments on the ESC Guidelines for the diagnosis and treatment of acute and chronic heart failure 2012. A report of the Task Force of the Clinical Practice Guidelines Committee of the Spanish Society of Cardiology. *Rev. Esp. Cardiol. (Engl. Ed.)* **2012**, *65*, 874–878. [CrossRef]
6. Di Angelantonio, E.; Chowdhury, R.; Sarwar, N.; Ray, K.K.; Gobin, R.; Saleheen, D.; Thompson, A.; Gudnason, V.; Sattar, N.; Danesh, J. B-type natriuretic peptides and cardiovascular risk: Systematic review and meta-analysis of 40 prospective studies. *Circulation* **2009**, *120*, 2177–2187. [CrossRef] [PubMed]
7. Ponikowski, P.; Voors, A.A.; Anker, S.D.; Bueno, H.; Cleland, J.G.F.; Coats, A.J.S.; Falk, V.; Gonzalez-Juanatey, J.R.; Harjola, V.P.; Jankowska, E.A.; et al. 2016 ESC Guidelines for the Diagnosis and Treatment of Acute and Chronic Heart Failure. *Rev. Esp. Cardiol. (Engl. Ed.)* **2016**, *69*, 1167. [CrossRef]
8. Giannitsi, S.; Bougiakli, M.; Bechlioulis, A.; Naka, K. Endothelial dysfunction and heart failure: A review of the existing bibliography with emphasis on flow mediated dilation. *JRSM Cardiovasc. Dis.* **2019**, *8*, 2048004019843047. [CrossRef] [PubMed]
9. Lam, C.S.; Brutsaert, D.L. Endothelial dysfunction: A pathophysiologic factor in heart failure with preserved ejection fraction. *J. Am. Coll. Cardiol.* **2012**, *60*, 1787–1789. [CrossRef]
10. Chow, S.L.; Maisel, A.S.; Anand, I.; Bozkurt, B.; de Boer, R.A.; Felker, G.M.; Fonarow, G.C.; Greenberg, B.; Januzzi, J.L., Jr.; Kiernan, M.S.; et al. Role of Biomarkers for the Prevention, Assessment, and Management of Heart Failure: A Scientific Statement From the American Heart Association. *Circulation* **2017**, *135*, e1054–e1091. [CrossRef]
11. Villacorta, H.; Maisel, A.S. Soluble ST2 Testing: A Promising Biomarker in the Management of Heart Failure. *Arq. Bras. Cardiol.* **2016**, *106*, 145–152. [CrossRef]
12. Fraser, C.G. Inherent biological variation and reference values. *Clin. Chem. Lab. Med.* **2004**, *42*, 758–764. [CrossRef] [PubMed]
13. Meijers, W.C.; van der Velde, A.R.; Muller Kobold, A.C.; Dijck-Brouwer, J.; Wu, A.H.; Jaffe, A.; de Boer, R.A. Variability of biomarkers in patients with chronic heart failure and healthy controls. *Eur. J. Heart Fail.* **2016**, *19*, 357–365. [CrossRef] [PubMed]
14. Piper, S.; deCourcey, J.; Sherwood, R.; Amin-Youssef, G.; McDonagh, T. Biologic Variability of Soluble ST2 in Patients with Stable Chronic Heart Failure and Implications for Monitoring. *Am. J. Cardiol.* **2016**, *118*, 95–98. [CrossRef]
15. Wu, A.H.; Wians, F.; Jaffe, A. Biological variation of galectin-3 and soluble ST2 for chronic heart failure: Implication on interpretation of test results. *Am. Heart J.* **2013**, *165*, 995–999. [CrossRef] [PubMed]
16. Oikonomou, E.; Siasos, G.; Tsigkou, V.; Bletsa, E.; Panoilia, M.E.; Oikonomou, I.N.; Simanidis, I.; Spinou, M.; Papastavrou, A.; Kokosias, G.; et al. Coronary Artery Disease and Endothelial Dysfunction: Novel Diagnostic and Therapeutic Approaches. *Curr. Med. Chem.* **2020**, *27*, 1052–1080. [CrossRef]
17. Demyanets, S.; Kaun, C.; Pentz, R.; Krychtiuk, K.A.; Rauscher, S.; Pfaffenberger, S.; Zuckermann, A.; Aliabadi, A.; Groger, M.; Maurer, G.; et al. Components of the interleukin-33/ST2 system are differentially expressed and regulated in human cardiac cells and in cells of the cardiac vasculature. *J. Mol. Cell. Cardiol.* **2013**, *60*, 16–26. [CrossRef]
18. Parikh, R.H.; Seliger, S.L.; Christenson, R.; Gottdiener, J.S.; Psaty, B.M.; deFilippi, C.R. Soluble ST2 for Prediction of Heart Failure and Cardiovascular Death in an Elderly, Community-Dwelling Population. *J. Am. Heart Assoc.* **2016**, *5*. [CrossRef]
19. Song, Y.; Li, F.; Xu, Y.; Liu, Y.; Wang, Y.; Han, X.; Fan, Y.; Cao, J.; Luo, J.; Sun, A.; et al. Prognostic value of sST2 in patients with heart failure with reduced, mid-range and preserved ejection fraction. *Int. J. Cardiol.* **2020**, *304*, 95–100. [CrossRef]
20. Borovac, J.A.; Glavas, D.; Susilovic Grabovac, Z.; Supe Domic, D.; Stanisic, L.; D'Amario, D.; Kwok, C.S.; Bozic, J. Circulating sST2 and catestatin levels in patients with acute worsening of heart failure: A report from the CATSTAT-HF study. *ESC Heart Fail.* **2020**, 2818–2828. [CrossRef]
21. Braunwald, E. Biomarkers in heart failure. *N. Engl. J. Med.* **2008**, *358*, 2148–2159. [CrossRef]
22. Mueller, T.; Jaffe, A.S. Soluble ST2–analytical considerations. *Am. J. Cardiol.* **2015**, *115*, 8B–21B. [CrossRef]
23. Coglianese, E.E.; Larson, M.G.; Vasan, R.S.; Ho, J.E.; Ghorbani, A.; McCabe, E.L.; Cheng, S.; Fradley, M.G.; Kretschman, D.; Gao, W.; et al. Distribution and clinical correlates of the interleukin receptor family member soluble ST2 in the Framingham Heart Study. *Clin. Chem.* **2012**, *58*, 1673–1681. [CrossRef] [PubMed]

24. Pascual-Figal, D.A.; Perez-Martinez, M.T.; Asensio-Lopez, M.C.; Sanchez-Mas, J.; Garcia-Garcia, M.E.; Martinez, C.M.; Lencina, M.; Jara, R.; Januzzi, J.L.; Lax, A. Pulmonary Production of Soluble ST2 in Heart Failure. *Circ. Heart Fail.* **2018**, *11*, e005488. [CrossRef] [PubMed]
25. AbouEzzeddine, O.F.; McKie, P.M.; Dunlay, S.M.; Stevens, S.R.; Felker, G.M.; Borlaug, B.A.; Chen, H.H.; Tracy, R.P.; Braunwald, E.; Redfield, M.M. Suppression of Tumorigenicity 2 in Heart Failure With Preserved Ejection Fraction. *J. Am. Heart Assoc.* **2017**, *6*. [CrossRef] [PubMed]
26. Truong, Q.A.; Januzzi, J.L.; Szymonifka, J.; Thai, W.E.; Wai, B.; Lavender, Z.; Sharma, U.; Sandoval, R.M.; Grunau, Z.S.; Basnet, S.; et al. Coronary sinus biomarker sampling compared to peripheral venous blood for predicting outcomes in patients with severe heart failure undergoing cardiac resynchronization therapy: The BIOCRT study. *Heart Rhythm* **2014**, *11*, 2167–2175. [CrossRef] [PubMed]
27. Kakkar, R.; Lee, R.T. The IL-33/ST2 pathway: Therapeutic target and novel biomarker. *Nat. Rev. Drug Discov.* **2008**, *7*, 827–840. [CrossRef]
28. deFilippi, C.; Daniels, L.B.; Bayes-Genis, A. Structural heart disease and ST2: Cross-sectional and longitudinal associations with echocardiography. *Am. J. Cardiol.* **2015**, *115*, 59B–63B. [CrossRef]
29. Han, X.; Zhang, S.; Chen, Z.; Adhikari, B.K.; Zhang, Y.; Zhang, J.; Sun, J.; Wang, Y. Cardiac biomarkers of heart failure in chronic kidney disease. *Clin. Chim. Acta* **2020**, *510*, 298–310. [CrossRef]
30. Wang, Z.; Chen, Z.; Yu, H.; Ma, X.; Zhang, C.; Qu, B.; Zhang, W.; Chen, X. Superior prognostic value of soluble suppression of tumorigenicity 2 for the short-term mortality of maintenance hemodialysis patients compared with NT-proBNP: A prospective cohort study. *Ren. Fail.* **2020**, *42*, 523–530. [CrossRef]
31. Madsen, L.H.; Ladefoged, S.; Corell, P.; Schou, M.; Hildebrandt, P.R.; Atar, D. N-terminal pro brain natriuretic peptide predicts mortality in patients with end-stage renal disease in hemodialysis. *Kidney Int.* **2007**, *71*, 548–554. [CrossRef]
32. Oikonomou, E.; Siasos, G.; Zaromitidou, M.; Hatzis, G.; Mourouzis, K.; Chrysohoou, C.; Zisimos, K.; Mazaris, S.; Tourikis, P.; Athanasiou, D.; et al. Atorvastatin treatment improves endothelial function through endothelial progenitor cells mobilization in ischemic heart failure patients. *Atherosclerosis* **2015**, *238*, 159–164. [CrossRef] [PubMed]
33. Oikonomou, E.; Vogiatzi, G.; Karlis, D.; Siasos, G.; Chrysohoou, C.; Zografos, T.; Lazaros, G.; Tsalamandris, S.; Mourouzis, K.; Georgiopoulos, G.; et al. Effects of omega-3 polyunsaturated fatty acids on fibrosis, endothelial function and myocardial performance, in ischemic heart failure patients. *Clin. Nutr.* **2019**, *38*, 1188–1197. [CrossRef] [PubMed]
34. Tousoulis, D.; Oikonomou, E.; Siasos, G.; Chrysohoou, C.; Zaromitidou, M.; Kioufis, S.; Maniatis, K.; Dilaveris, P.; Miliou, A.; Michalea, S.; et al. Dose-dependent effects of short term atorvastatin treatment on arterial wall properties and on indices of left ventricular remodeling in ischemic heart failure. *Atherosclerosis* **2013**, *227*, 367–372. [CrossRef]
35. Aimo, A.; Januzzi, J.L., Jr.; Bayes-Genis, A.; Vergaro, G.; Sciarrone, P.; Passino, C.; Emdin, M. Clinical and Prognostic Significance of sST2 in Heart Failure: JACC Review Topic of the Week. *J. Am. Coll. Cardiol.* **2019**, *74*, 2193–2203. [CrossRef]
36. The Reference Values for Arterial Stiffness' Collaboration. Determinants of pulse wave velocity in healthy people and in the presence of cardiovascular risk factors: 'establishing normal and reference values'. *Eur. Heart J.* **2010**, *31*, 2338–2350. [CrossRef] [PubMed]
37. Takae, M.; Yamamoto, E.; Tokitsu, T.; Oike, F.; Nishihara, T.; Fujisue, K.; Sueta, D.; Usuku, H.; Motozato, K.; Ito, M.; et al. Clinical Significance of Brachial-Ankle Pulse Wave Velocity in Patients with Heart Failure with Reduced Left Ventricular Ejection Fraction. *Am. J. Hypertens.* **2019**, *32*, 657–667. [CrossRef]
38. Tousoulis, D.; Charakida, M.; Stefanadis, C. Endothelial function and inflammation in coronary artery disease. *Heart* **2006**, *92*, 441–444. [CrossRef]
39. Yucel, O.; Gul, I.; Zararsiz, A.; Demirpence, O.; Yucel, H.; Cinar, Z.; Zorlu, A.; Yilmaz, M.B. Association of soluble ST2 with functional capacity in outpatients with heart failure. *Herz* **2018**, *43*, 455–460. [CrossRef]
40. Aimo, A.; Januzzi, J.L., Jr.; Vergaro, G.; Richards, A.M.; Lam, C.S.P.; Latini, R.; Anand, I.S.; Cohn, J.N.; Ueland, T.; Gullestad, L.; et al. Circulating levels and prognostic value of soluble ST2 in heart failure are less influenced by age than N-terminal pro-B-type natriuretic peptide and high-sensitivity troponin T. *Eur J. Heart Fail.* **2020**. [CrossRef]

41. Tousoulis, D.; Antoniades, C.; Stefanadis, C. Evaluating endothelial function in humans: A guide to invasive and non-invasive techniques. *Heart* **2005**, *91*, 553–558. [CrossRef]
42. Rajzer, M.W.; Wojciechowska, W.; Klocek, M.; Palka, I.; Brzozowska-Kiszka, M.; Kawecka-Jaszcz, K. Comparison of aortic pulse wave velocity measured by three techniques: Complior, SphygmoCor and Arteriograph. *J. Hypertens.* **2008**, *26*, 2001–2007. [CrossRef] [PubMed]

Publisher's Note: MDPI stays neutral with regard to jurisdictional claims in published maps and institutional affiliations.

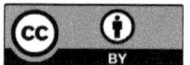 © 2020 by the authors. Licensee MDPI, Basel, Switzerland. This article is an open access article distributed under the terms and conditions of the Creative Commons Attribution (CC BY) license (http://creativecommons.org/licenses/by/4.0/).

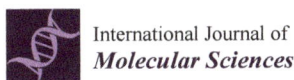

Article

Dapagliflozin Does Not Modulate Atherosclerosis in Mice with Insulin Resistance

Alida Taberner-Cortés [1], Ángela Vinué [1], Andrea Herrero-Cervera [1], María Aguilar-Ballester [1], José Tomás Real [1,2,3,4], Deborah Jane Burks [4,5], Sergio Martínez-Hervás [1,2,3,4] and Herminia González-Navarro [1,4,*]

1. Health Research Institute Clinic Hospital of Valencia-INCLIVA, 46010 Valencia, Spain; altacor@doctor.upv.es (A.T.-C.); m.angela.vinue@uv.es (Á.V.); anhecer@alumni.uv.es (A.H.-C.); abama4@alumni.uv.es (M.A.-B.); jose.t.real@uv.es (J.T.R.); sergio.martinez@uv.es (S.M.-H.)
2. Endocrinology and Nutrition Service, Clinic Hospital of Valencia, 46010 Valencia, Spain
3. Department of Medicine, University of Valencia, 46010 Valencia, Spain
4. CIBERDEM (Diabetes and Associated Metabolic Diseases), 28029 Madrid, Spain; dburks@cipf.es
5. CIPF Principe Felipe Research Center, 46012 Valencia, Spain
* Correspondence: herminia.gonzalez@uv.es; Tel.: +34-96-386-4403

Received: 1 October 2020; Accepted: 1 December 2020; Published: 3 December 2020

Abstract: Type 2 diabetes mellitus (T2DM) increases morbimortality in humans via enhanced susceptibility to cardiovascular disease (CVD). Sodium-glucose co-transporter 2 inhibitors (SGLT2i) are drugs designed for T2DM treatment to diminish hyperglycaemia by reducing up to 90% of renal tube glucose reabsorption. Clinical studies also suggest a beneficial action of SGLT2i in heart failure and CVD independent of its hypoglycaemiant effect. In the present study, we explored the effect of SGLT2i dapagliflozin (DAPA) in the metabolism and atherosclerosis in *Apoe−/−Irs2+/−* mice, which display accelerated atherosclerosis induced by insulin resistance. DAPA treatment of *Apoe−/−Irs2+/−* mice, which were fed a high-fat, high-cholesterol diet, failed to modify body weight, plasma glucose or lipid. Carbohydrate metabolism characterisation showed no effect of DAPA in the glucose tolerance test (GTT) despite augmented insulin levels during the test. In fact, decreased C-peptide levels in DAPA-treated mice during the GTT suggested impaired insulin release. Consistent with this, DAPA treatment of *Apoe−/−Irs2+/−* isolated islets displayed lower glucose-stimulated insulin secretion compared with vehicle-treated islets. Moreover, insulin-signalling experiments showed decreased pAKT activation in DAPA-treated adipose tissue indicating impaired insulin signalling in this tissue. No changes were seen in lesion size, vulnerability or content of macrophages, vascular smooth muscle cells, T cells or collagen. DAPA did not affect circulating inflammatory cells or cytokine levels. Hence, this study indicates that DAPA does not protect against atherosclerosis in insulin-resistant mice in hypercholesterolemic conditions.

Keywords: type 2 diabetes; SGLT2i; glucose metabolism; insulin resistance; atherosclerosis

1. Introduction

Type 2 diabetes mellitus (T2DM) produces a high morbidity and mortality rate worldwide, mostly by increasing the risk of cardiovascular disease (CVD) [1,2]. CVD is caused by complications of atherosclerosis, a chronic inflammatory disease. Atheroma lesions stem from dysfunction in the endothelial layer that facilitates the accumulation of lipoproteins and immune cells in the subendothelial space of vascular vessel walls. These incipient atheroma plaques can progress to different-stage lesions, a process that is modulated by the adaptive and innate immune system. The later stages of atherosclerosis are characterised by an unbalanced interplay of immune cells that leads to an unresolved inflammatory process. Excessive inflammation and cellular death events generate clinically critic unstable plaques prone to rupture and can precipitate acute thromboembolic events [3].

Insulin resistance (IR), a primary characteristic of T2DM that may develop up to ten years before disease onset, triggers a series of mechanisms in several vascular cell types that accelerate unstable plaque formation [2]. Consequently, treatments with drugs that restore cellular and tissular insulin sensitivity could potentially reduce CVD complications in T2DM [4]. In support of this, clinical trials designed to examine the safety of newly designed T2DM drugs on heart failure (HF) and CVD have underlined the pleiotropic actions of several anti-diabetic agents [4,5]. Specifically, various investigations have shown that sodium–glucose co-transporter 2 inhibitors (SGLT2i) have beneficial mechanisms against HF and CVD [6]. In this sense, peritoneal macrophages from diabetic *Apoe−/−* and *db/db* mice treated with SGLT2i displayed lower foam cell formation through reduced expression of lectin-like ox-LDL receptor-1 (Lox-1), acyl-coenzyme A:cholesterol acyltransferase 1 (ACAT1) and ATP-binding cassette transporter A1 (ABCA1) [7]. SGLT2i alleviate endothelial and vascular smooth muscle cell (VSMC) dysfunction [8]. In diabetic *Apoe−/−* mice, inflammatory mediators VCAM, Mcp1 and NFκB were reduced by dapagliflozin treatment [9], empagliflozin lowered TNFα and IL6 levels [10], and canagliflozin decreased expression of VCAM and Mcp1 [11]. On the other hand, cardiomyofibroblasts from *ob/ob* mice treated with DAPA showed decreased Nlrp3 inflammasome and inflammatory mediators by an AMPK-dependent mechanism independent of the glucose-lowering effect through SGLT2 [12].

Under normal conditions, apical SGLT2, located in the epithelial cells of the proximal renal tubes, reabsorbs glucose and sodium which enter into the blood through basal GLUT2 transporter [13,14]. Hence, selective inhibition of SGLT2 improves T2DM by reducing glucose and sodium reabsorption by up to 90%. The main consequence of this process is that the glucose and sodium are excreted into the urine, with unique hypoglycaemic and natriuretic effects [6,14]. Nonetheless, human clinical trials have demonstrated that SGLT2i reduces body weight, blood pressure, arterial stiffness, visceral adiposity and albuminuria independently by its glucose-lowering effect [5,6]. Treatment of T2DM patients with empagliflozin added to standard drug treatment diminished incidence of CV outcomes and deaths in the EMPA-REG study [15]. Similarly, the CANVAS clinical trial, which analysed T2DM patients with chronic kidney disease treated with canagliflozin, reported a significant decrease in CVD events and kidney failure [16,17]. In line with these clinical trials, in the DECLARE–TIMI 58 trial, dapagliflozin treatment reduced the rate of hospitalisation for heart failure and of death by CVD [18]. These studies point towards safe use of SGLT2i to prevent HF, not only in T2DM but also in subjects without T2DM that have shown positive results [5,19].

In the present study, we investigated the potential benefit of a selective SGLT2i, dapagliflozin (DAPA), in atherosclerosis in *Apoe−/−Irs2+/−* mice. This is a mouse model that, under atherogenic dietary conditions, displays IR and accelerated atherosclerosis but not hyperglycaemia or hypertension, hence a highly suitable model to evaluate the impact of the drug on atherosclerosis independently from its unique hypoglycaemic and natriuretic effects.

2. Results

2.1. Metabolic Characterisation of Apoe−/−Irs2+/− Mice Treated with DAPA or Vehicle

As expected, there was a significant increase in body weight (BW) in vehicle- and dapagliflozin(DAPA)-treated *Apoe−/−Irs2+/−* mice after receiving the atherogenic diet (Figure 1a) both in females and males. No differences were observed in BW between DAPA- and vehicle-treated mice. Similarly, fasting glucose levels remained unchanged between vehicle- and DAPA-treated male and female *Apoe−/−Irs2+/−* mice (Figure 1b). Fasting insulin levels were diminished in female DAPA-treated *Apoe−/−Irs2+/−* mice (Figure 1c, right panel) compared with vehicle-treated female controls. No changes were observed in male mice (Figure 1c, left panel). DAPA-treatment of *Apoe−/−Irs2+/−* mice did not alter fasting plasma levels of total-, apoB- and HDL-cholesterol or triacylglycerol (Figure 1d–g).

Hepatic analysis also revealed no effect of DAPA-treatment on triacylglycerol content in *Apoe−/−Irs2+/−* mice (Figure S1a,b, see section on supplementary data given at the end of this article) and absence of hepatic lipid droplets (Figure S1c).

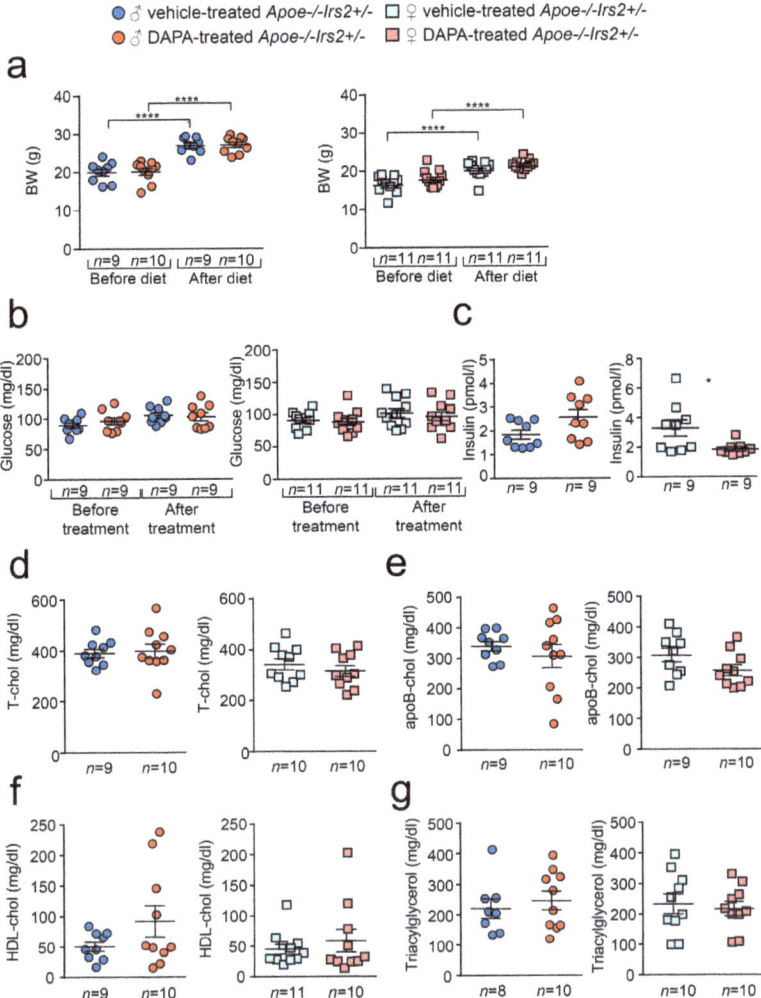

Figure 1. Effect of DAPA treatment in *Apoe−/−Irs2+/−* mice. (**a**) Body weight (BW) before and after atherogenic diet in male (left panel) and female (right panel) vehicle-treated and DAPA-treated *Apoe−/−Irs2+/−* mice. (**b**) Fasting plasma glucose levels in male (left panel) and female (right panel) vehicle-treated and DAPA-treated *Apoe−/−Irs2+/−* mice. (**c**) Fasting insulin levels in male (left panel) and female (right panel) vehicle- and DAPA-treated mice after treatment. (**d**) Total-cholesterol, (**e**) apoB-cholesterol, (**f**) HDL-cholesterol and (**g**) triacylglycerol levels in male (left panel) and female (right panel) DAPA- and vehicle-treated *Apoe−/−Irs2+/−* mice. Data are represented as individual points with mean ± sem. The statistical analysis for normal distribution was D'Agostino–Pearson and for differences was two-way ANOVA followed by Bonferroni's post-hoc test (**a**,**b**), Student's *t*-test (**c**,**f**, left panel), (**d**,**e**) and (**g**, right panel), and Mann–Whitney U test (**c**,**f**, right panel) and (**g**, left panel). **** $p < 0.0001$. * $p < 0.05$.

Next, we performed a more detailed characterisation of carbohydrate metabolism. Glucose tolerance measured as the area under the curve (AUC$_{glucose}$) parameter of the GTT was similar in both vehicle and DAPA-treated *Apoe−/−Irs2+/−* mice in both sexes (Figure 2a,b, right panels). The insulin release during the GTT, determined as AUC$_{insulin}$ at 120 min, was also indistinguishable between vehicle- and DAPA-treated *Apoe−/−Irs2+/−* male and female mice (Figure 2c,d, right panels). Insulin release at 30 min, AUC$_{insulin}$ 30 min (Figure 2c, middle panel) was higher in DAPA-treated male mice compared with vehicle-treated *Apoe−/−Irs2+/−* male controls. Moreover, C-peptide levels were reduced in DAPA-treated *Apoe−/−Irs2+/−* mice (Figure 2e, left panel) measured as AUC$_{c-peptide}$ at 120 min (Figure 2e right panel) indicating that the insulin increase was due to impaired clearance rather than higher pancreatic secretion. Consistent with this, glucose stimulated insulin secretion assay, in isolated islets from *Apoe−/−Irs2+/−* mice, demonstrated diminished insulin secretion index in DAPA-treated islets (Figure 2f) compared with vehicle-treated islet controls. Thus, these results suggest that DAPA impairs insulin action in sensitive tissues and insulin secretion by islets.

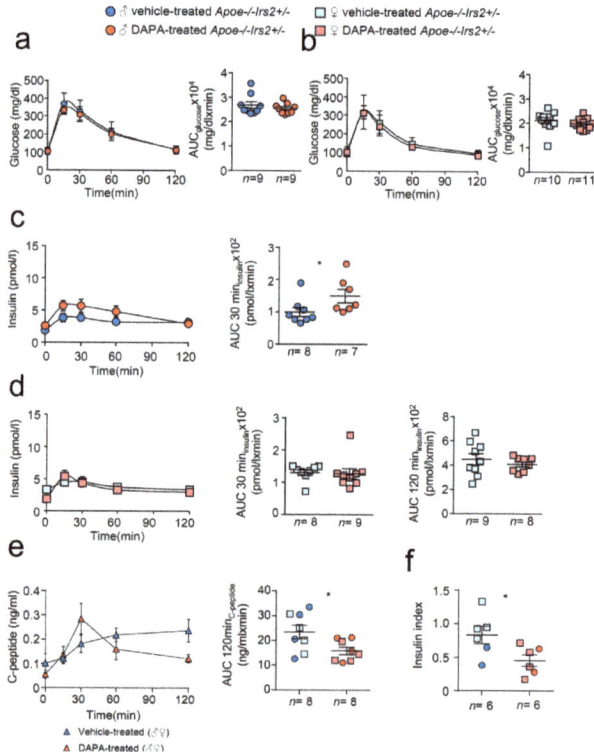

Figure 2. Metabolic characterisation of vehicle-treated and DAPA-treated *Apoe−/−Irs2+/−* mice. Glucose levels during the glucose tolerance test (GTT) and the area under the curve (AUC$_{glucose}$) generated from the glucose curve during the test for male (**a**) and female (**b**) vehicle- and DAPA-treated mice. Plasmatic insulin levels stimulated by the glucose infusion during the GTT and the AUC$_{insulin}$ calculated at 30 and 120 min of the test for (**c**) male and (**d**) female vehicle- and DAPA-treated mice. (**e**) C-peptide levels during the insulin tolerance test (ITT) and the corresponding AUC$_{c-peptide}$ in 4-hour-fasted mice. (**f**) Insulin secretion index obtained from the glucose-stimulated insulin secretion assay in isolated islets from *Apoe−/−Irs2+/−* mice treated with DAPA or vehicle. The statistical analysis for normal distribution was D'Agostino–Pearson (**a–f**) and Kolmogorov–Smirnov test (**f**) and for differences Student's *t*-test (**d**, right panel) and (**e,f**) and Mann–Whitney U test (**a–d**, left panel) (**a–c**) and (**d**, left panel). * $p < 0.05$.

To better analyse insulin action in DAPA-treated *Apoe−/−Irs2+/−* mice, insulin sensitivity and signalling were explored. Insulin sensitivity assessed by the insulin tolerance test (ITT) and measured by the AUC$_{glucose}$ revealed no effect of DAPA in *Apoe−/−Irs2+/−* mice neither in males (Figure 3a) or in females (Figure 3b). However, analysis of the insulin-signalling pathway activation in vitro showed decreased pAKT/AKT protein ratio levels in DAPA-treated adipose tissue explants (Figure 3c).

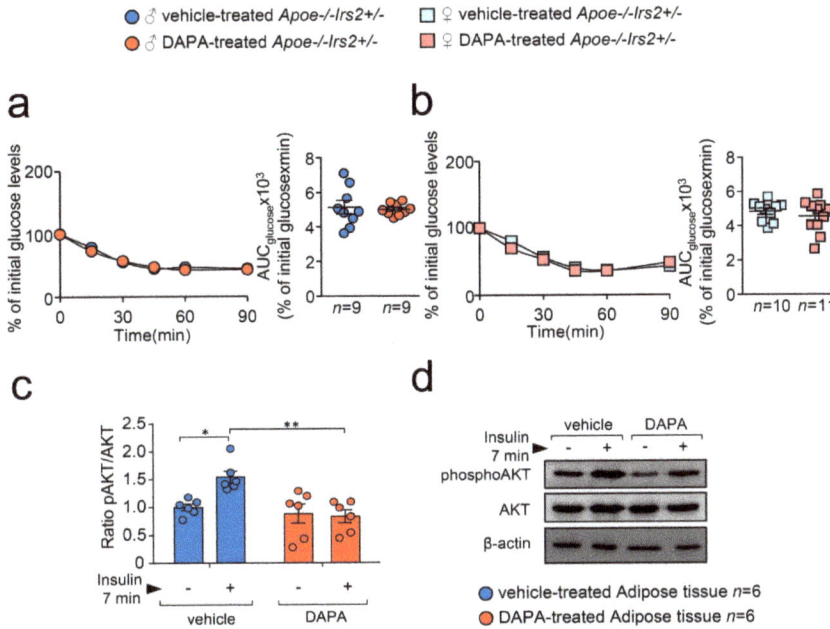

Figure 3. DAPA treatment effect on insulin sensitivity and signalling pathway. Glucose levels during the ITT and the corresponding AUC$_{glucose}$ in 4-hour-fasted (**a**) male and (**b**) female *Apoe−/−Irs2+/−* mice. (**c**) Quantification of phosphorylated(activated)-AKT1/2 (pAKT1/2)/AKT1/2 ratios in insulin-stimulated adipose tissue explants pretreated with vehicle or DAPA 1 µM. β-actin is shown as a sample loading control. Phosphorylated forms were normalised to total protein levels and were relativised to the unstimulated sample. (**d**) Representative blots are depicted on the right of the quantification. Statistical analysis tests for normal distribution were the D'Agostino–Pearson omnibus (**a**,**b**) and Kolmogorov–Smirnov test (**c**) and for differences, the Student's *t*-test (**a**,**b**) and two-way ANOVA followed by Tukey's multiple comparison test (**c**). * $p < 0.05$; ** $p < 0.01$.

These results indicate that DAPA does not have a beneficial effect on carbohydrate metabolism in *Apoe−/−Irs2+/−* mice and might even exert detrimental effects on insulin signalling and insulin secretion in certain conditions.

2.2. DAPA Treatment in Atherogenic Diet-Fed Apoe−/−Irs2+/− Mice Does Not Affect Atherosclerosis Lesion Size or Plaque Stability

En face atheroma lesion size determination in whole–mounted aortas showed no effect of DAPA-treatment in aortic arches or thoracic aortas of *Apoe−/−Irs2+/−* mice compared with vehicle-treated controls regardless of sex (Figure 4a–e). Atherosclerosis development determinations in cross-sections revealed similar sizes in male and female DAPA- and vehicle-treated *Apoe−/−Irs2+/−* mice in the three regions analysed, aortic root (Figure 4f–h), ascending aorta (Figure 4i–k), and aorta (Figure 4l–n).

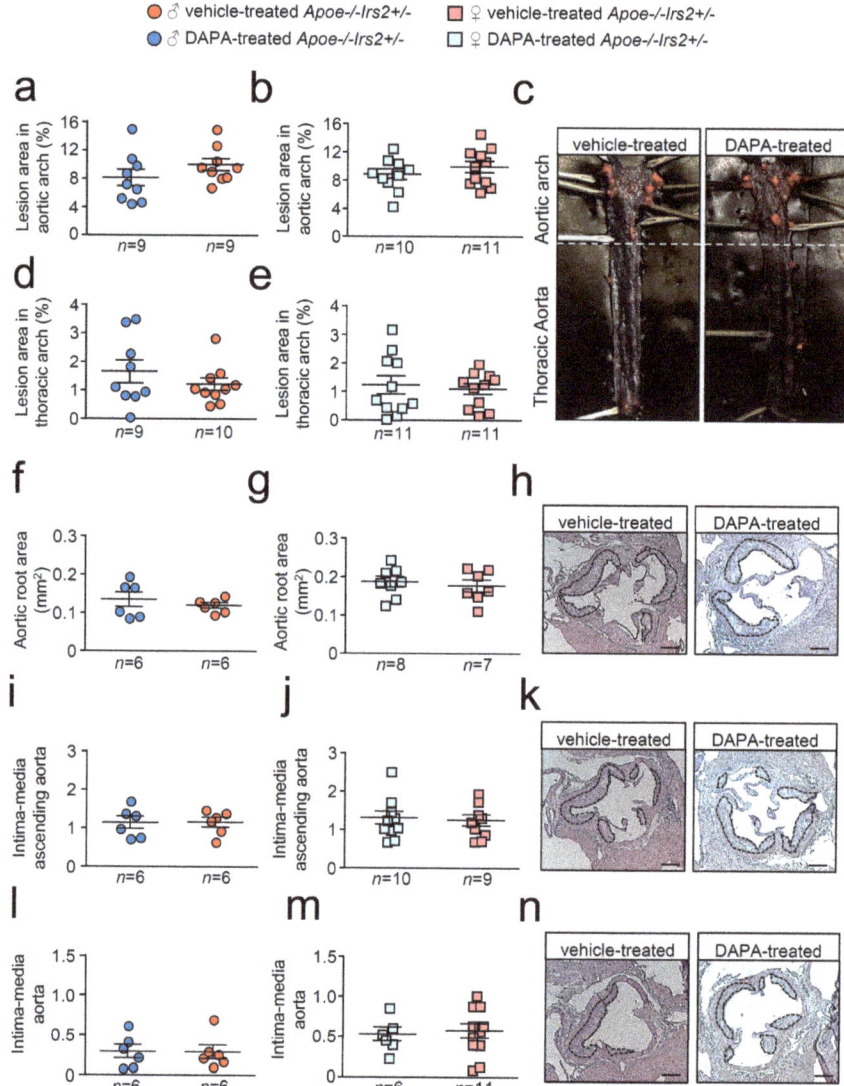

Figure 4. Atherosclerotic lesion size analysis in vehicle- and DAPA-treated *Apoe−/−Irs2+/−* mice. Atherosclerosis analysis in (**a,b**) the aortic arch and (**d,e**) the thoracic aorta of whole-mounted oil-red-O-stained aortas from both vehicle- and DAPA-treated male and female mice. Lesion size determinations in cross-sections of (**f,g**) the aortic root, in (**i,j**) the ascending aorta, and in (**l,m**) the aorta displayed as absolute area (**f,g**) and as an intima-media ratio (**i,j,l,m**). (**c**) Representative photographs of whole-mounted aortas. Magnification 0.17. Representative images of haematoxylin/eosin-stained cross-sections of the aortic root (**h**), ascending aorta (**k**) and aorta (**n**). The limits of the lesion are indicated by the dashed lines. Scale bar: 200 µm. The statistical analysis for normality was D'Agostino–Pearson omnibus test and for differences was the Student's *t*-test (**a,b,d,j**) and the Mann–Whitney U test (**e–g,i,l,m**).

Further analysis of the atheroma cellular composition and parameters of plaque stability was next performed. Macrophage, vascular smooth muscle cells (VSMCs), and T lymphocyte absolute and relative contents were undistinguishable between male and female DAPA- and vehicle-treated *Apoe−/−Irs2+/−* mice (Figure 5a–i).

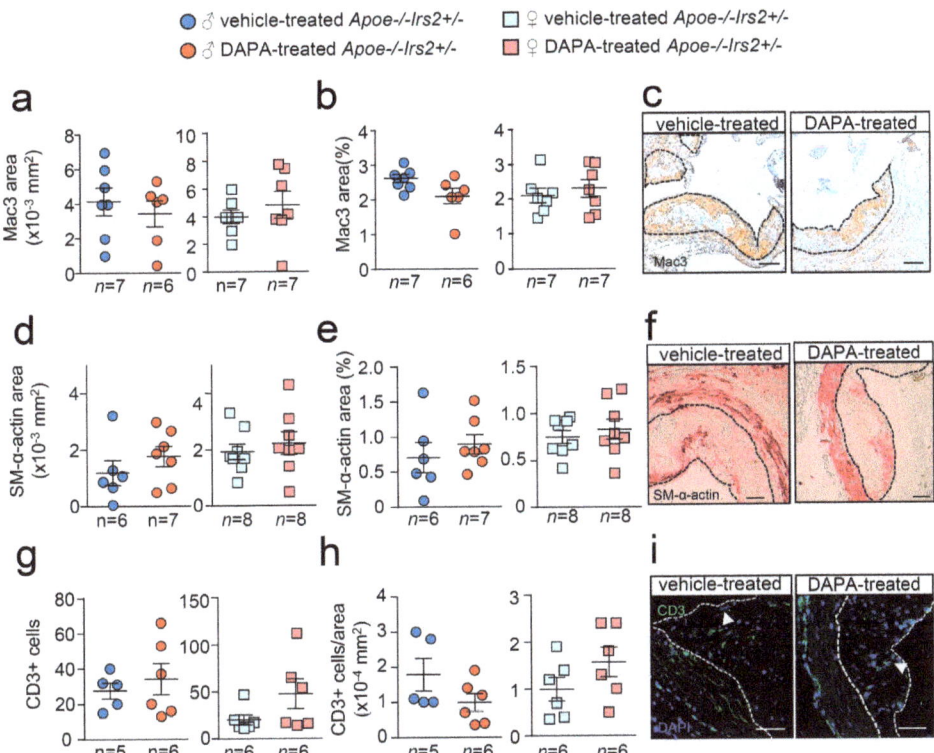

Figure 5. Effect of DAPA in atheroma plaque characteristics of *Apoe−/−Irs2+/−* mice. (**a,b**) Macrophage and (**d,e**) vascular smooth muscle cell (VSMC) content in aortic cross-sections from vehicle- and DAPA-treated male (left panels) and female mice (right panels), determined as Mac3+ and SM-α-actin+ areas measured as absolute area (in mm^2) (**a,d**) and as percentage of the positive-stained area relative to lesion area (**b,e**). Scale bar: 100 µm. Number of T lymphocytes in lesions of aortic cross-sections detected as CD3+ cells and depicted as (**g**) absolute cell number and as (**h**) cell number relative to lesion area (in mm^2) in both sexes from vehicle- and DAPA-treated mice. Scale bar: 50 µm. Photomicrographs next to the quantifications (**c,f,i**) show representative images of the immunostainings. White arrows in (**i**) point to CD3+ cells. The limits of the lesion are indicated by the dashed lines. The statistical analysis for normal distribution was the D'Agostino–Pearson omnibus test (**d,e**) and Kormokov–Smirnov was performed using Student's *t*-test (**d,e**. right panels) and Mann–Whitney U test (**a,b,g,h**) and (**d,e**, left panels).

Similarly, examination of collagen content, necrotic core area, fibrous cap thickness and elastic fibre's area failed to show differences between treatments (Figure 6a–f). Thus, DAPA treatment in *Apoe−/−Irs2+/−* mice on a 2-month atherogenic diet does not influence atherosclerosis development or plaque stability parameters.

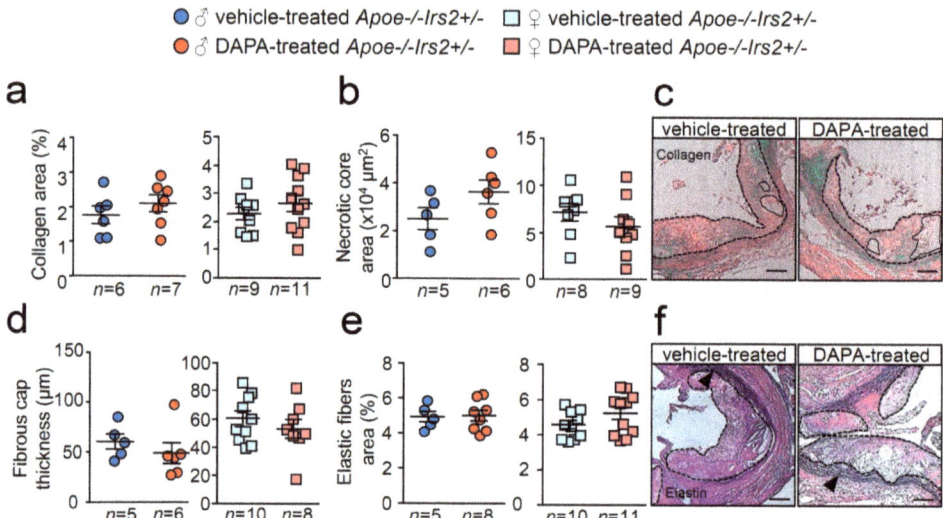

Figure 6. Effect of DAPA in atheroma plaque characteristics of *Apoe−/−Irs2+/−* mice. (**a**) Collagen content (in percentage), (**b**) necrotic core area (in μm^2) and (**d**) fibrous cap thickness (in μm) determined in Masson trichrome stained lesions from vehicle- and DAPA-treated male (left panels) and female (right panels) mice. (**e**) Elastin fibres' area assessed in Verhoeff-Van Gieson cross-sections and displayed as percentage of area relative to lesion area in male and female mice. Representative images of Masson trichrome (**c**,**f**) Verhoeff-Van Gieson stainings. Black arrows in (**f**) point to elastic fibre's breaks in the media. The dashed lines delineate the limits of the lesion and solid lines delineate the limits of representative necrotic cores. Scale bar: 100 μm. The statistical analysis for normal distribution was Kolmogorov–Smirnov test and for differences was the Student's *t*-test (**a**,**b**,**d**,**e**, right panels) and Mann–Whitney U test (**a**,**b**,**d**,**e**, left panels).

2.3. DAPA Treatment Effect in Inflammation in Apoe−/−Irs2+/− Mice Fed an Atherogenic Diet

Some investigations have suggested a role for gliflozins in inflammation and in heart failure through monocyte/macrophage polarisation and, in light of this, inflammatory parameters were studied.

Compared with vehicle-treated *Apoe−/−Irs2+/−* mice, DAPA-treated mice did not show differences in the circulating plasma levels of MCP1 or TNFα (Figure 7a,b). Analysis of circulating leukocytes showed similar percentages of lymphocytes, monocytes, and neutrophils between DAPA- and vehicle-treated *Apoe−/−Irs2+/−* male and female mice (Figure 7c,d). Monocyte subpopulations analysis did not detect changes in the proinvasive and proinflammatory Ly6C^{hi} subsets or in the pro-resolving Ly6C^{low} monocyte subpopulations in DAPA-treated *Apoe−/−Irs2+/−* mice compared with vehicle-treated controls (Figure 7e,f).

Likewise, T CD3+ CD4+ and CD8+ lymphocytes populations (Figure S2a,d,g) and their activated subpopulations CD3+CD69+, CD4+CD69+ and CD8+CD69+ (Figure S2b,e,h) remained unchanged. Circulating CD4+CD25+Foxp3+ Treg cell analysis showed also similar levels in DAPA- and vehicle-treated *Apoe−/−Irs2+/−* mice (Figure S2j).

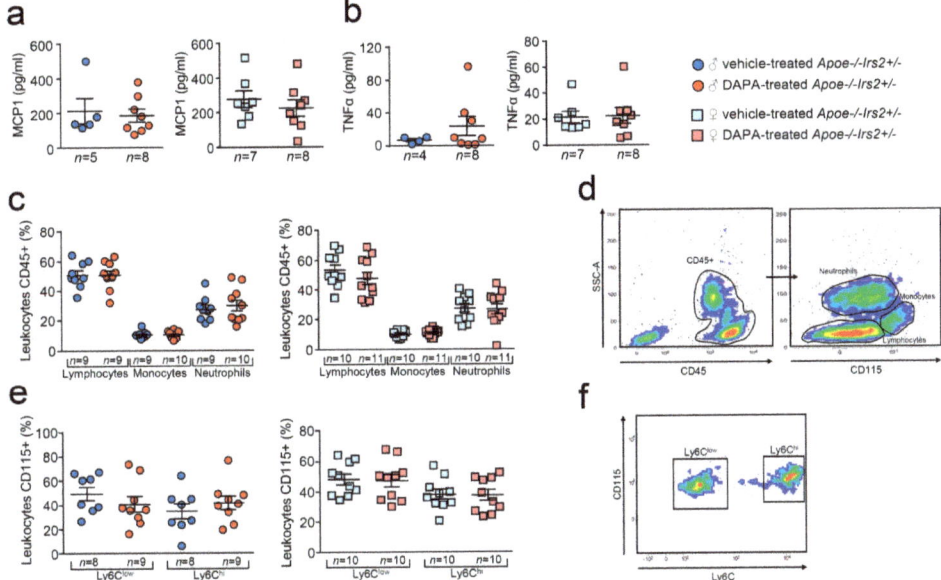

Figure 7. Effect of dapagliflozin in inflammatory mediators and cells in *Apoe−/−Irs2+/−* mice. Circulating plasma levels of (**a**) MCP1 and (**b**) TNFα proinflammatory cytokines. (**c**) Circulating levels (in percentage) of lymphocytes, monocytes and neutrophils in the CD45+ population, identified by morphology and CD115 monocyte marker. (**d**) Representative cytometry plots of the gating strategy used for the flow cytometry analysis in the different leukocyte populations. (**e**) Circulating levels of monocyte subpopulations (in percentage) identified as CD45+CD115+Ly6C^{low} pro-resolving and as CD45+CD115+Ly6C^{hi} invasive monocyte subsets in male and female mouse blood. (**f**) Representative cytometry plots of the gating strategy used for monocyte subsets in blood samples. The statistical analyses for normal distribution were Kolmogorov–Smirnov test (**a,b**) and D'Agostino–Pearson test (**c,e**) and for differences were Mann–Whitney U test (**a,b**) and Student's *t*-test (**c,e**).

2.4. Effect of DAPA in Apoe−/−Irs2+/− Mouse Macrophages

A recent investigation has shown that DAPA attenuates myocardial infarction through macrophage phenotype modulation [20], therefore, the effects of DAPA and DAPA conditioned media (DAPACM) and their respective vehicle controls were evaluated in in vitro *Apoe−/−Irs2+/−* murine-derived macrophages.

Cytokine expression analysis revealed diminished mRNA levels of *Mcp1* in DAPA-treated (Figure 8a) macrophages compared with vehicle-treated cells without changes in *Tnfa* (Figure 8b) or *Il6* (Figure 8c) expression. Consistent with the in vivo data, cytokine gene expression in macrophages was not altered by the treatment with media containing DAPA-treated mouse plasma, DAPACM, compared with that in macrophages treated with vehicleCM derived from vehicle-treated mice (Figure 8a–c). Analysis of surface macrophage markers showed no differences in the activation marker *Cd11c* among treatments (Figure S3a). DAPA-treated macrophages displayed diminished expression of the *Cd206* macrophage marker compared with controls (Figure S3b) but remained unchanged between DAPACM and vehicleCM treatments (Figure S3b). Consistent with the results in macrophages treated with conditioned media, the content of macrophage markers iNOS and ARGI in atheroma lesions was similar between DAPA- and vehicle-treated *Apoe−/−Irs2+/−* mice (Figure 8d,e).

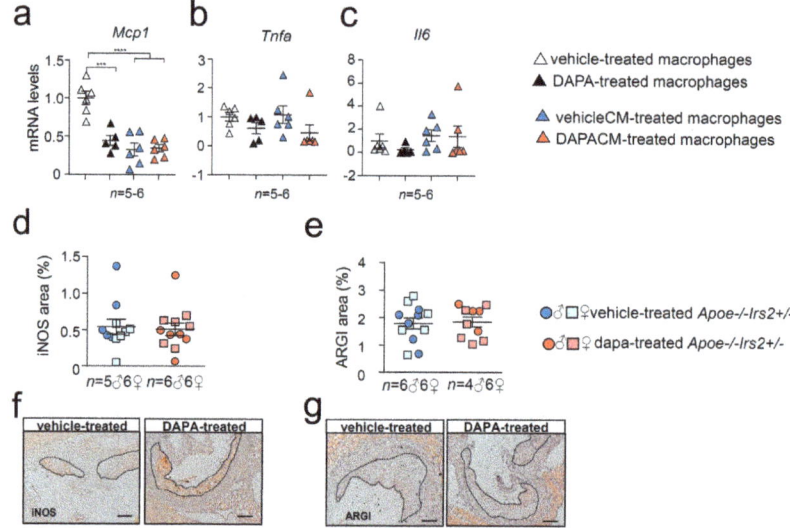

Figure 8. Effect of DAPA in *Apoe−/−Irs2+/−* mouse macrophage phenotype. mRNA expression of proinflammatory (**a**) *Mcp1*, (**b**) *Tnfa* and (**c**) *Il6* cytokines in *Apoe−/−Irs2+/−* macrophages treated with vehicle (vehicle-treated), 1μM of DAPA (DAPA-treated) or with conditioned media containing 10% of plasma from vehicle-treated mice (vehicleCM) or with conditioned media containing 10% of plasma from DAPA-treated mice (DAPACM). (**d**) iNOS and (**e**) ARGI lesional content in aortic cross-sections from vehicle- and DAPA-treated male and female mice, determined as percentage of positive stained area relative to lesion area. Representative images of the (**f**) iNOS, and (**g**) ARGI, stainings used for the quantifications are shown. Scale bar: 100 μm. The lesion is limited by dashed lines. The statistical analysis for normal distribution was Kolmogorov–Smirnov test and for differences was one-way ANOVA followed by Tukey's multiple comparison test (panel **a**), Kruskal–Wallis followed by Dunn's multiple comparison test (panels **b**,**c**) and Mann–Whitney U test (panels **d**,**e**). *** $p < 0.001$; **** $p < 0.0001$.

3. Discussion

T2DM is a major risk factor for developing atherosclerosis, the main cause of CVD. Human clinical trials have shown that anti-diabetic drug SGLT2i protects against CVD and HF in T2DM beyond its glucose-lowering effects. Several anti-diabetic agents control atherosclerosis development by restoring the homeostasis altered by IR in atheroma lesional cells, a key feature of T2DM. Therefore, in the present study we evaluated the potential of SGLT2i DAPA in restraining atherosclerosis in IR conditions. To this end, we investigated the effect of DAPA on *Apoe−/−Irs2+/−* mice, which, under cholesterol-enriched atherogenic diet conditions, display accelerated atherosclerosis, IR and hypercholesterolemia. Treatment of *Apoe−/−Irs2+/−* mice with DAPA did not result in changes in BW or fasting plasma glucose compared with vehicle-treated controls. Fasting insulin was increased in DAPA-treated females but not in males. Similarly, no differences in the levels of cholesterol (total, apoB- and HDL-cholesterol) or triacylglycerol were observed between vehicle- and DAPA-treated mice. Carbohydrate metabolism characterisation revealed no effect of DAPA on glucose tolerance or insulin sensitivity tests. Notwithstanding this, analysis of insulin release during the GTT demonstrated increased insulin levels but lower C-peptide release in DAPA-treated *Apoe−/−Irs2+/−* mice indicating abnormal insulin clearance. Further analysis showed impaired insulin secretion of isolated pancreatic islets treated with DAPA. In addition, impaired insulin signalling in adipose tissue explants pretreated with DAPA was observed suggesting a detrimental effect on insulin action in this tissue. Atherosclerosis lesion determinations in whole-mounted aorta and heart cross-sections did not show differences between vehicle and DAPA-treated mice. No effect of DAPA was observed in cellular and collagen contents or in plaque vulnerability parameters within atheroma lesions. Likewise, DAPA did not affect circulating immune system cells or plasmatic cytokine levels in vivo, although in macrophages resulted in a decrease in *Mcp1* and *Cd206* expression compared to vehicle-treated macrophages. Altogether this indicates that DAPA treatment in vivo does not protect against atherosclerosis in *Apoe−/−Irs2+/−* mice and it seems to interfere with islet insulin secretion and adipose tissue insulin-signalling. These data suggest that DAPA might not be effective against atherosclerotic complications associated with IR or prediabetic states.

SGLT2i has been widely demonstrated to exert protective effects in metabolism by reducing plasmatic hyperglycaemia and increasing glucosuria and natriuresis. Weight loss due to urinary loss of calories, improved renal function and blood pressure are direct consequences of SGLT2i [21,22]. Moreover, in T2DM subjects, empagliflozin treatment improved insulin β cell function and insulin sensitivity [23] while DAPA only ameliorated muscle insulin sensitivity [24]. In our study, with a mouse model exhibiting IR but no other T2DM features, which also had hyperlipidaemia due to a high-fat, high-cholesterol diet, DAPA treatment during the glucose challenge did not change glucose levels, despite increased insulin plasmatic concentration. Blood insulin levels are determined by pancreatic islet secretion but also by its plasmatic clearance. In fact, the observed decreased C-peptide release suggested impaired insulin secretion from pancreatic islets. Consistent with the latter, isolated pancreatic islets from *Apoe−/−Irs2+/−* mice treated with DAPA exhibited diminished insulin secretion index. Hence, the defective blood glucose lowering effect of the circulating insulin in DAPA-treated mice indicated otherwise defective clearance. Of note, defective insulin clearance and degradation are observed in subjects with T2DM frequently due to abnormal insulin–insulin receptor (INSR) internalisation and recycling in insulin-sensitive tissues, including liver, skeletal muscle, adipose tissue and kidney [25,26]. Consistent with defective INSR downstream signalling, experiments in adipose tissue demonstrated impaired insulin-pathway activation, shown by a reduction in phosphoAKT protein levels. Our results suggest that DAPA might affect metabolism by interfering with insulin-signalling in adipose tissue. Notwithstanding, given that the major contributors to insulin clearance are hepatic and skeletal muscle, further research must be conducted to demonstrate the hypothesis. Altogether, our study suggests that DAPA treatment in IR mice in hyperlipidaemic conditions might have limited effects.

In addition, DAPA did not alter atherosclerosis or inflammatory parameters in our mouse model. Preclinical investigations have shown that DAPA does not act on atherosclerosis in *Apoe−/−* mice, but significantly diminished lesion size in hyperglycaemic conditions without IR. Thus DAPA decreased atheroma size in streptozotozin (STZ)-induced hyperglycaemic and diabetic *Apoe−/−* mice through reduction in hyperglycaemia-induced foam cell formation [7]. On the other hand, empagliflozin treatment decreased atheroma plaques of *Apoe−/−* mice fed a carbohydrate- (43%) and fat- (41%) rich Western diet [10]. Although the authors suggested that IR improvement was the precipitant of atherosclerosis reduction, empagliflozin treatment also decreased carbohydrate-induced hyperglycaemia, which could help mitigate atherosclerosis development. In agreement with this, DAPA reduced atherosclerosis in STZ-induced diabetic *Ldlr−/−* [27] and *Apoe−/−* [28] mice. Consistent with these studies, empagliflozin [29] and canagliflozin [30] ameliorated endothelial dysfunction and atheroma lesion development in STZ-induced diabetic *Apoe−/−* mice. Empagliflozin also facilitated regression of atherosclerosis in STZ-induced hyperglycaemic mice whose atherosclerosis was induced by *Ldlr−* and *Srb1−* antisense oligonucleotide injection [31]. Altogether, these studies cast doubt on the beneficial actions of SGLTi in the absence of hyperglycaemia and suggest that anti-atherogenic effects are exerted by decreasing glucose levels independently of insulin action.

Among SGLT2i mechanisms [32], polarisation towards a non-invasive and pro-resolving phenotype of macrophages via increased signal transducer and activator of transcription 3 (STAT3) activity-dependent mechanism has been reported [20]. Notably, we have previously demonstrated that glucagon-like peptide 1 receptor (GLP1R) agonists decrease plaque size and vulnerability in *Apoe−/−Irs2+/−* mice by inducing a protective circulating immune cell phenotype, and by inducing polarisation of lesional macrophage to an anti-inflammatory phenotype [33]. Studies in the present investigation showed that in vitro treatment of macrophages with DAPA reduced expression of proinflammatory *Mcp1* cytokine and macrophage marker *Cd206*. However, here DAPA did not show an in vivo impact on either circulating immune cells or lesional macrophage content or markers (iNOS and ARGI). Therefore, our results show that although DAPA might have potential beneficial effects on macrophages in vitro, these are irrelevant for in vivo macrophage phenotype modulation and for atherosclerosis development in our experimental setting, characterised by the absence of hyperglycaemia.

In summary, our study indicates that DAPA treatment fails to alter glucose levels or atherosclerosis development in *Apoe−/−Irs2+/−* mice, which develop hypercholesterolemia and IR but not hyperglycaemia. Moreover, DAPA reduced glucose-stimulated insulin secretion from islets, insulin clearance in vivo and insulin-signalling in adipose tissue. The present investigation suggests that DAPA might not exert beneficial effects in atheroma vascular disease in IR and hypercholesterolemic conditions.

4. Materials and Methods

4.1. Mice, Diets and Drug Treatments

Apoe−/− and *Irs2+/−* mice were crossed to generate *Apoe−/−Irs2+/−* mice (C57BL/6J background, $n = 21$ male and $n = 22$ female). Mice had free access to water, were under temperature and humidity-controlled conditions (22 ± 2 °C, $55 \pm 10\%$) and with 12h light–dark cycles (8:00–20:00 h) in a conventional animal facility. Mice were maintained on a regular chow diet (Teklad Global Rodent Diets 6.5% fat; Tekland, Envigo, Barcelona, Spain) and at 8 weeks of age were placed on an atherogenic diet (10.8% fat, 0.75% cholesterol, S4892-E010, Ssniff, Soest, Germany) which is a Paigen-based diet with modifications as described before [34] for 8 weeks. For the last 6 weeks, mice were randomly assigned to receive daily treatment with dapagliflozin ($n = 11$ female $n = 11$ male; p.o. 3 mg/kg/day in 120 µL) or with vehicle [35] (carboxymethyl cellulose) ($n = 10$ female $n = 11$ male). Dose, timing of treatment, route of administration and drug concentration for delivery was based on previous investigations [33,35]. All animal procedures were approved by the Animal Ethics Committee of INCLIVA and University of Valencia (5/25/2017, procedure A1484231073016, administration approval 2017/VSC/PEA/00081) and complied with the 2010/63/EU European Parliament directive.

4.2. Plasmatic Biochemical Determinations and Metabolic Assays

Plasma was obtained from whole blood with ethylenediaminetetra-acetic acid (EDTA) of overnight-fasted mice. Analysis included triacylglycerol, total cholesterol, apoB-cholesterol, HDL-cholesterol (Wako Diagnostics, Mountain View, CA, USA) as previously described [36]. Glucose tolerance tests (GTTs) (2 g/Kg of body weight, BW, of glucose) and insulin tolerance tests (ITTs) (0.5 U/Kg of BW Humulina, Lilly, Alcobendas, Spain) were performed in overnight- and 4-h-fasted mice, respectively. Glucose levels were measured at different time points using a glucometer (Ascensia Elite, Bayer, Leverkusen, Germany). Fasting basal insulin and insulin-release and C-peptide levels during the GTT were measured using an anti-mouse insulin and C-peptide ELISA kit (CrystalChem, Zaandam, The Netherlands) as reported [36].

4.3. Pancreatic Islet Isolation and Glucose-Stimulated Insulin Secretion Assay

For islet isolation, *Apoe−/−Irs2+/−* mice were infused with Krebs buffer (127 mM NaCl, 5 mM KCl, 3 mM $CaCl_2$, 1.5 mM $MgCl_2$, 24 mM $NaHCO_3$, 6 mM Hepes, 2 mg/mL glucose, 0.1% albumin, equilibrated with 5% CO_2 in O_2) and the pancreas was dissected and digested with collagenase-NB8 (1 mg/mL, Serva, Heidelberg, Germany) at 37 °C in a shaking water bath for 20 min. Islets were handpicked under stereoscope as described [37]. Insulin secretion was evaluated by a glucose-stimulated insulin secretion assay at low (2.8 mmol/L) and high (16.7 mmol/L) glucose concentrations in KRBH buffer (140 mM NaCl, 2.5 mM KCl, 2.5 mM $CaCl_2$, 1 mM $MgCl_2$, 20 mM Hepes, 2 mg/mL glucose, 0.1% albumin). Four assays (5 islets each) were performed per condition and insulin concentrations were measured by ELISA. The glucose stimulated insulin secretion index was calculated as the ratio between high glucose-stimulated insulin release and the low glucose-stimulated insulin secretion normalised each by the insulin content of the islets.

4.4. Liver Triacylglycerol Content and Histochemical Staining

Triacylglycerol hepatic content was determined by tissue digestion and saponification in ethanolic potassium hydroxide, followed by enzymatic measurement of glycerol content (Free Glycerol Reagent, Sigma, St. Louis, MO, USA). For examination of lipid droplets in hepatic tissue, paraffin-embedded tissue sections were stained with haematoxylin–eosin and analysed as described [36].

4.5. Insulin Signalling Experiments in Adipose Tissue and Protein Analysis by Western Blot

Epididymal visceral fat pads from *Irs2+/−* mice were minced into 2–3 mm^3 and incubated 24 h at 100 mg/mL in 6 well-plates with DMEM-P/S/A-10%FBS media in a humidified 5% CO_2 atmosphere. Explants were washed with PBS1X twice and incubated with DMEM-P/S/A-0.1%FBS media for 24 h in the presence of DAPA 1 µM or media with vehicle as control adipose tissue. Explants were then stimulated 7 min with insulin (200 nM, Sigma, St. Louis, MO, USA) or vehicle and then snap-frozen in liquid N_2 for insulin-signalling pathway analysis by Western blot as described [38]. Briefly, protein extracts were obtained by homogenising adipose tissue in the presence of ice-cold fat lysis buffer (Hepes 50 mM, pH 7.5, NaCl 150 mM, Triton 1% vol/vol, glycerol 10% vol/vol) supplemented with Complete Mini cocktail, PhosSTOP (Roche, Mannheim, Germany), beta-glycerophosphate 50 mM (Sigma), 2 mM phenylmethylsulfonyl fluoride (PMSF, Roche) and 200 µM Na_3VO_4 (Sigma). Protein extracts (50 µg) were prepared with Laemmli buffer (5 min 95 °C) and subjected to 12% *w/v* polyacrylamide gel electrophoresis and Western blot as described. The following primary (1/200) and secondary (1/2000) antibodies were used to detect the proteins: pAKT (4058, Cell Signalling, Beverly, MA, USA), AKT1/2 (sc1619, Santa Cruz Biotech Dallas, TX, USA) and β-actin (A5441, Sigma, St. Louis, MO, USA), anti-mouse IgG-HRP (P0447, Dako), donkey anti-goat IgG-HRP (sc2056, Santa Cruz Biotech, Dallas, TX, USA) and goat anti-rabbit IgG-HRP (P0448, Dako Agilent, Santa Clara, CA, USA). The immunocomplexes were detected with an ECL Plus detection kit (ThermoFisher, Waltham, MA, USA). All antibodies for Western blot were acquired and used after checking that validation was performed by manufacturer company.

4.6. Atheroma Lesion Analysis

To quantify atheroma lesion size, aortas and hearts of mice were dissected and fixed with 4% paraformaldehyde/PBS (vol/vol). Lesion extension was assessed by an *en face* analysis of whole-mounted aortas stained with oil red-O (Sigma) using morphometric analysis (Fiji, ImageJ-win64, NIH, Bethesda, MD, USA). Hearts were paraffin-embedded, sectioned for haematoxylin/eosin staining and analysed for atheroma lesion size measured as lesion area (mm^2) in the aortic root and as the intima–media ratio in two regions of the ascending aorta [40].

4.7. Histopathological Characterisation of Atheroma Lesions

Collagen content, necrotic core area, and fibrous cap thickness of atheromas were determined in sections stained with Masson's trichrome staining. Elastic fibres were analysed in aortic cross-sections stained with Verhoeff-Van Gieson staining. For plaque instability, fibrous cap thickness (in µm) and necrotic core area (measured as $µm^2$) were determined. The fibrous caps were defined as regions above the necrotic cores and were later identified as non-stained acellular areas [39]. Macrophages in lesions were detected by immunohistochemistry in cross-sections treated for peroxidase inactivation (H_2O_2 0.3%) and blocking with horse serum (5%) followed by incubation overnight at 4 °C with an anti-Mac-3 antibody (1/200, Santa Cruz Biotechnology, Santa Cruz, CA, USA) and biotin-conjugated goat anti-rat secondary antibody incubation 1 h at room temperature (1/300, Santa Cruz). For inducible nitric oxide synthase (iNOS) and arginase I (ARGI) analysis, aortic cross-sections underwent antigen retrieval (citrate buffer, 10 mM, pH 6.5 high pressure and temperature), peroxidase inactivation (H_2O_2 3%), blocking with horse serum (5%), incubation overnight at 4 °C with primary antibodies (rabbit anti-MMP-9, 1/200 dilution, (UPSTATE-Millipore, Billerica, MA, USA), anti-iNOS antibody 1/100 dilution (Abcam, Cambridge, UK) and anti-arginase I 1/50 dilution (Sigma, St. Louis, MO, USA)), and incubation with a biotinylated anti-rabbit secondary antibody (1/500 dilution, Santa Cruz). Immunocomplexes were detected with streptavidin-HRP (ab7403, Abcam, Cambridge, UK) and then developed with DAB substrate. Counterstaining was done with haematoxylin and slides were mounted with EUKITT (Deltalab, Barcelona, Spain). Lesional VSMCs were detected using an anti-SMα-actin monoclonal alkaline phosphatase-conjugated antibody (1/20 dilution, Sigma) and Fast Red substrate (Sigma). Slides were mounted with glycerol gelatin (Sigma) [33]. All images were captured with a Leica DMD108 microscope coupled to a camera (Leica, Wetzlar, Germany). T-lymphocytes in atheromas were detected by immunofluorescence with a polyclonal anti-human CD3 antibody (1/75 dilution, Dako, Santa Clara, CA, USA) and Alexa Fluor®-488 anti-rabbit IgG secondary antibody (1/200 dilution, Invitrogen, Madrid, Spain). Slides were mounted with Slow-Fade Gold reagent (Invitrogen) and analysed with an inverted fluorescent microscope (DMI3000B, Leica). All antibodies used were validated using negative controls by omission of primary antibodies.

4.8. Enzyme-Linked ImmunoSorbent Assay (ELISA) of Cytokines

Circulating levels of cytokines were determined in isolated plasma from heparinised mouse blood (10U heparin/mL) using the specific cytokine DuoSet ELISA kits (R&D Systems, Minneapolis, MN, USA).

4.9. Circulating Leukocyte Analysis by Flow Cytometry

To characterise circulating leukocytes by flow cytometry, 10 µL of heparinised whole blood was incubated for 30 min at RT with CD45-FITC (BD Biosciences, Franklin Lakes, NJ, USA) to identify leukocytes. Lymphocytes and neutrophils were identified by complexity and morphology, whereas monocytes were gated based on the CD115-APC marker (Biolegend, San Diego, CA, USA). Ly6C-PerCP (BD Biosciences, San Diego, CA, USA) and CD115-APC (Biolegend, San Diego, CA, USA) were used for Ly6C^{low} and Ly6C^{hi}-monocyte subsets identification. For circulating lymphocytes analysis, 10 µL of heparinised whole blood was incubated with 5 µL Brilliant Stain Buffer (BD Biosciences, San Diego, CA, USA) followed by CD4-BV421, CD8a-BV510, CD3e-APC, or CD69-PE antibodies (BD Biosciences, San Diego, CA, USA). Mouse Tregs were identified using Kit FoxP3 Staining Buffer Set and with anti-CD25-APC, anti-Foxp3-PE, and anti-CD4-VioBlue (all from Miltenyi, Bergisch Gladbach, Germany). The samples were incubated with FACS Lysing solution (BD Biosciences) for 10 min before flow cytometry analysis (FACSVerse or FACS Fortessa Flow cytometer, BD Biosciences, San Diego, CA, USA).

4.10. Experiments with Bone Marrow-Derived Macrophages

Murine bone marrow-derived macrophages were obtained from the femoral and tibial bone marrow of mice sacrificed by cervical dislocation. Bone marrow cells were differentiated for 5–6 days with 10% FBS/DMEM (Lonza, Basel, Switzerland) supplemented with 10% L929-cell conditioned medium (LCM: as a source of macrophage colony-stimulating factor) [40]. For the last 24 h, macrophages were treated with 0.5%FBS/DMEM medium supplemented with vehicle, 1 µm of DAPA, 10% of plasma from DAPA-treated mice (Dapagliflozin-conditioned media, DAPACM) or 10% of plasma from vehicle-treated mice (vehicle-conditioned media, vehicleCM). Cytokine gene expression was analysed by qPCR.

4.11. Gene Expression Analysis by Quantitative Real-Time PCR

RNA (0.5–1 µg) from murine macrophages was obtained using TRIzol Reagent (Invitrogen), which was reverse-transcribed with the Maxima First Strand cDNA Synthesis kit and amplified with Luminaris Color HiGreen High ROX qPCR Master Mix (Thermo Scientific, Waltham, MA, USA) on a thermal Cycler 7900 FastSystem. Results were analysed with the provided software (Applied Biosystems, Foster city, CA, USA). mRNA levels were normalised to cyclophilin expression and relativised to controls. The primer sequences can be found in Supplementary Data Table S1.

4.12. Statistical Analysis

Quantitative variables are shown as single data points and mean ± sem. All data obtained were analysed unless these data were out of range of the standard curve or if samples were lost during the experimentation. Data were analysed for normal distribution using the D'Agostino–Pearson omnibus, Shapiro–Wilk test or Kolmogorov–Smirnov test. Differences were evaluated with the Student´s *t*-test, Mann–Whitney U test, two-way ANOVA followed by Bonferroni or Tukey's post hoc test, one-way ANOVA followed by Bonferroni or Tukey's multiple comparison test (more than two groups), or Kruskal–Wallis followed by Dunn's multiple comparison test (more than two groups) (GraphPadPrism Software Inc., La Jolla, CA, USA). Statistical significance was set at $p \leq 0.05$. Male and female data were displayed separately.

5. Conclusions

Altogether, our study indicates that in mice with IR but without hyperglycaemia or other characteristics of T2DM, DAPA treatment does not restrain atherosclerosis, and could have detrimental effects.

Supplementary Materials: Supplementary materials can be found at http://www.mdpi.com/1422-0067/21/23/9216/s1.

Author Contributions: A.T.-C. acquired and analysed the in vivo data, participated in the interpretation of results and helped to write the manuscript. A.H.-C. and M.A.-B. performed, islets, insulin-signalling, flow cytometry and macrophage experiments, interpreted the data and helped in the writing of the manuscript. Á.V. acquired in vivo data and critically revised the manuscript. D.J.B., S.M.-H. and J.T.R. participated in the study design and critically revised the manuscript. H.G.-N. conceived and designed the study, supervised data acquisition, interpreted the results, and wrote the manuscript. H.G.-N. is the guarantor of this work. All authors approved the final version of the manuscript. All authors have read and agreed to the published version of the manuscript.

Funding: This research was funded by Carlos III Health Institute, grant numbers PI16/00091 to H.G.-N. and PI19/00169 to H.G.-N. and S.M.-H. and the European Regional Development Fund (FEDER). H.G.-N. was an investigator in the Miguel Servet program from Carlos III Health Institute, grant number CP16/0013, and GenT Investigator of Excellence from Generalitat Valenciana, grant number CDEI-04-20-B. S.M.-H. is an investigator from the "Juan Rodes" program from Carlos III Health Institute, grant number JR18/00051. Á.V. received salary support from Proyecto Paula and A.H.-C. from Generalitat Valenciana, grant number APOTIP/2018/021. This work was also supported by CIBERDEM, grant number CB07/08/0043, a Carlos III Health Institute initiative.

Acknowledgments: We thank G. Herrera (INCLIVA, Spain) for assistance with the flow cytometry, A. Díaz (University of Valencia, Spain) for animal care and P. Rentero and S. Blesa for help with expression studies and analysis (INCLIVA, Spain). We also thank G. Hurtado for help with immunohistochemistry (University of Valencia, Spain).

Conflicts of Interest: The authors declare no conflict of interest.

Abbreviations

Apoe	apolipoprotein E
ARG	arginase I
AUC	area under the curve
BW	body weight
CVD	cardiovascular disease
DAPA	dapagliflozin
EDTA	ethylenediaminetetra-acetic acid
ELISA	enzyme-linked immunosorbent assay
GTT	glucose tolerance test
HF	heart failure
iNOS	inducible nitric oxide synthase
IR	insulin resistance
IRS2	insulin receptor substrate 2
ITT	insulin tolerance test
MMP9	matrix metallopeptidase 9
qPCR	quantitative polymerase chain reaction
SGLT2	sodium-glucose transporter 2
SGLT2i	sodium-glucose transporter 2 inhibitor
STAT	signal transducer and activator of transcription
STZ	streptozotocin
T2DM	type 2 diabetes mellitus
VSMC	vascular smooth muscle cells

References

1. *GLOBAL REPORT ON DIABETES WHO Library Cataloguing-in-Publication Data Global Report on Diabetes*; WHO Press: Geneva, Switzerland, 2016; ISBN 9789241565257.
2. Di Pino, A.; DeFronzo, R.A. Insulin Resistance and Atherosclerosis: Implications for Insulin Sensitizing Agents. *Endocr. Rev.* **2019**, 1447–1467. [CrossRef] [PubMed]
3. Libby, P.; Buring, J.E.; Badimon, L.; Hansson, G.K.; Deanfield, J.; Bittencourt, M.S.; Tokgözoğlu, L.; Lewis, E.F. Atherosclerosis. *Nat. Rev. Dis. Prim.* **2019**, *5*, 1–18. [CrossRef] [PubMed]
4. Scheen, A.J. Cardiovascular effects of new oral glucose-lowering agents DPP-4 and SGLT-2 inhibitors. *Circ. Res.* **2018**, *122*, 1439–1459. [CrossRef] [PubMed]
5. Zannad, F.; Ferreira, J.P.; Pocock, S.J.; Anker, S.D.; Butler, J.; Filippatos, G.; Brueckmann, M.; Ofstad, A.P.; Pfarr, E.; Jamal, W.; et al. SGLT2 inhibitors in patients with heart failure with reduced ejection fraction: A meta-analysis of the EMPEROR-Reduced and DAPA-HF trials. *Lancet* **2020**. [CrossRef]
6. Lytvyn, Y.; Bjornstad, P.; Udell, J.A.; Lovshin, J.A.; Cherney, D.Z.I. Sodium Glucose Cotransporter-2 Inhibition in Heart Failure. *Circulation* **2017**, *136*, 1643–1658. [CrossRef]
7. Terasaki, M.; Hiromura, M.; Mori, Y.; Kohashi, K.; Nagashima, M.; Kushima, H.; Watanabe, T.; Hirano, T. Amelioration of hyperglycemia with a sodium-glucose cotransporter 2 inhibitor prevents macrophage-driven atherosclerosis through macrophage foam cell formation suppression in type 1 and type 2 diabetic mice. *PLoS ONE* **2015**, *10*, e0143396. [CrossRef]
8. Lee, D.M.; Battson, M.L.; Jarrell, D.K.; Hou, S.; Ecton, K.E.; Weir, T.L.; Gentile, C.L. SGLT2 inhibition via dapagliflozin improves generalized vascular dysfunction and alters the gut microbiota in type 2 diabetic mice. *Cardiovasc. Diabetol.* **2018**, *17*, 62. [CrossRef]
9. Gaspari, T.; Spizzo, I.; Liu, H.B.; Hu, Y.; Simpson, R.W.; Widdop, R.E.; Dear, A.E. Dapagliflozin attenuates human vascular endothelial cell activation and induces vasorelaxation: A potential mechanism for inhibition of atherogenesis. *Diabetes Vasc. Dis. Res.* **2018**, *15*, 64–73. [CrossRef]
10. Han, J.H.; Oh, T.J.; Lee, G.; Maeng, H.J.; Lee, D.H.; Kim, K.M.; Choi, S.H.; Jang, H.C.; Lee, H.S.; Park, K.S.; et al. The beneficial effects of empagliflozin, an SGLT2 inhibitor, on atherosclerosis in ApoE −/− mice fed a western diet. *Diabetologia* **2017**, *60*, 364–376. [CrossRef]

11. Nasiri-Ansari, N.; Dimitriadis, G.K.; Agrogiannis, G.; Perrea, D.; Kostakis, I.D.; Kaltsas, G.; Papavassiliou, A.G.; Randeva, H.S.; Kassi, E. Canagliflozin attenuates the progression of atherosclerosis and inflammation process in APOE knockout mice. *Cardiovasc. Diabetol.* **2018**, *17*, 106. [CrossRef]
12. Ye, Y.; Bajaj, M.; Yang, H.C.; Perez-Polo, J.R.; Birnbaum, Y. SGLT-2 Inhibition with Dapagliflozin Reduces the Activation of the Nlrp3/ASC Inflammasome and Attenuates the Development of Diabetic Cardiomyopathy in Mice with Type 2 Diabetes. Further Augmentation of the Effects with Saxagliptin, a DPP4 Inhibitor. *Cardiovasc. Drugs Ther.* **2017**, *31*, 119–132. [CrossRef] [PubMed]
13. Alicic, R.Z.; Neumiller, J.J.; Johnson, E.J.; Dieter, B.; Tuttle, K.R. Sodium–glucose cotransporter 2 inhibition and diabetic kidney disease. *Diabetes* **2019**, *68*, 248–257. [CrossRef] [PubMed]
14. Lovshin, J.A.; Cherney, D.Z. Sodium transport in diabetes: Two sides to the coin. *Nat. Rev. Nephrol.* **2019**, *15*, 125–126. [CrossRef] [PubMed]
15. Zinman, B.; Wanner, C.; Lachin, J.M.; Fitchett, D.; Bluhmki, E.; Hantel, S.; Mattheus, M.; Devins, T.; Johansen, O.E.; Woerle, H.J.; et al. Empagliflozin, Cardiovascular Outcomes, and Mortality in Type 2 Diabetes. *N. Engl. J. Med.* **2015**, *373*, 2117–2128. [CrossRef]
16. Neal, B.; Perkovic, V.; Mahaffey, K.W.; de Zeeuw, D.; Fulcher, G.; Erondu, N.; Shaw, W.; Law, G.; Desai, M.; Matthews, D.R. Canagliflozin and Cardiovascular and Renal Events in Type 2 Diabetes. *N. Engl. J. Med.* **2017**, *377*, 644–657. [CrossRef]
17. Perkovic, V.; Jardine, M.J.; Neal, B.; Bompoint, S.; Heerspink, H.J.L.; Charytan, D.M.; Edwards, R.; Agarwal, R.; Bakris, G.; Bull, S.; et al. Canagliflozin and Renal Outcomes in Type 2 Diabetes and Nephropathy. *N. Engl. J. Med.* **2019**, *380*, 2295–2306. [CrossRef]
18. Wiviott, S.D.; Raz, I.; Bonaca, M.P.; Mosenzon, O.; Kato, E.T.; Cahn, A.; Silverman, M.G.; Zelniker, T.A.; Kuder, J.F.; Murphy, S.A.; et al. Dapagliflozin and Cardiovascular Outcomes in Type 2 Diabetes. *N. Engl. J. Med.* **2019**, *380*, 347–357. [CrossRef]
19. McMurray, J.J.V.; DeMets, D.L.; Inzucchi, S.E.; Køber, L.; Kosiborod, M.N.; Langkilde, A.M.; Martinez, F.A.; Bengtsson, O.; Ponikowski, P.; Sabatine, M.S.; et al. A trial to evaluate the effect of the sodium–glucose co-transporter 2 inhibitor dapagliflozin on morbidity and mortality in patients with heart failure and reduced left ventricular ejection fraction (DAPA-HF). *Eur. J. Heart Fail.* **2019**, *21*, 665–675. [CrossRef]
20. Lee, T.M.; Chang, N.C.; Lin, S.Z. Dapagliflozin, a selective SGLT2 Inhibitor, attenuated cardiac fibrosis by regulating the macrophage polarization via STAT3 signaling in infarcted rat hearts. *Free Radic. Biol. Med.* **2017**, *104*, 298–310. [CrossRef]
21. Lim, V.G.; Bell, R.M.; Arjun, S.; Kolatsi-Joannou, M.; Long, D.A.; Yellon, D.M. SGLT2 Inhibitor, Canagliflozin, Attenuates Myocardial Infarction in the Diabetic and Nondiabetic Heart. *JACC Basic Transl. Sci.* **2019**, *4*, 15–26. [CrossRef]
22. Beitelshees, A.L.; Leslie, B.R.; Taylor, S.I. Sodium–glucose cotransporter 2 inhibitors: A case study in translational research. *Diabetes* **2019**, *68*, 1109–1120. [CrossRef] [PubMed]
23. Ferrannini, E.; Muscelli, E.; Frascerra, S.; Baldi, S.; Mari, A.; Heise, T.; Broedl, U.C.; Woerle, H.J. Metabolic response to sodium-glucose cotransporter 2 inhibition in type 2 diabetic patients. *J. Clin. Investig.* **2014**, *124*, 499–508. [CrossRef] [PubMed]
24. Merovci, A.; Solis-Herrera, C.; Daniele, G.; Eldor, R.; Vanessa Fiorentino, T.; Tripathy, D.; Xiong, J.; Perez, Z.; Norton, L.; Abdul-Ghani, M.A.; et al. Dapagliflozin improves muscle insulin sensitivity but enhances endogenous glucose production. *J. Clin. Investig.* **2014**, *124*, 509–514. [CrossRef] [PubMed]
25. Chen, Y.; Huang, L.; Qi, X.; Chen, C. Insulin receptor trafficking: Consequences for insulin sensitivity and diabetes. *Int. J. Mol. Sci.* **2019**, *20*, 5007. [CrossRef] [PubMed]
26. Duckworth, W.C.; Bennett, R.G.; Hamel, F.G. Insulin Degradation: Progress and Potential*. *Endocr. Rev.* **1998**, *19*, 608–624. [CrossRef] [PubMed]
27. Al-Sharea, A.; Murphy, A.J.; Huggins, L.A.; Hu, Y.; Goldberg, I.J.; Nagareddy, P.R. SGLT2 inhibition reduces atherosclerosis by enhancing lipoprotein clearance in Ldlr −/− type 1 diabetic mice. *Atherosclerosis* **2018**, *271*, 166–176. [CrossRef]
28. Leng, W.; Ouyang, X.; Lei, X.; Wu, M.; Chen, L.; Wu, Q.; Deng, W.; Liang, Z. The SGLT-2 Inhibitor Dapagliflozin Has a Therapeutic Effect on Atherosclerosis in Diabetic ApoE -/- Mice. *Mediat. Inflamm.* **2016**, *2016*, 6305735. [CrossRef]

29. Ganbaatar, B.; Fukuda, D.; Shinohara, M.; Yagi, S.; Kusunose, K.; Yamada, H.; Soeki, T.; Hirata, K.-i.; Sata, M. Empagliflozin ameliorates endothelial dysfunction and suppresses atherogenesis in diabetic apolipoprotein E-deficient mice. *Eur. J. Pharmacol.* **2020**, *875*, 173040. [CrossRef]
30. Rahadian, A.; Fukuda, D.; Salim, H.M.; Yagi, S.; Kusunose, K.; Yamada, H.; Soeki, T.; Sata, M. Canagliflozin Prevents Diabetes-Induced Vascular Dysfunction in ApoE-Deficient Mice. *J. Atheroscler. Thromb.* **2020**, 1–11. [CrossRef]
31. Pennig, J.; Scherrer, P.; Gissler, M.C.; Anto-Michel, N.; Hoppe, N.; Füner, L.; Härdtner, C.; Stachon, P.; Wolf, D.; Hilgendorf, I.; et al. Glucose lowering by SGLT2-inhibitor empagliflozin accelerates atherosclerosis regression in hyperglycemic STZ-diabetic mice. *Sci. Rep.* **2019**, *9*, 1–12. [CrossRef]
32. Chin, K.L.; Ofori-Asenso, R.; Hopper, I.; Von Lueder, T.G.; Reid, C.M.; Zoungas, S.; Wang, B.H.; Liew, D. Potential mechanisms underlying the cardiovascular benefits of sodium glucose cotransporter 2 inhibitors: A systematic review of data from preclinical studies. *Cardiovasc. Res.* **2019**, *115*, 266–276. [CrossRef] [PubMed]
33. Vinué, Á.; Navarro, J.; Herrero-Cervera, A.; García-Cubas, M.; Andrés-Blasco, I.; Martínez-Hervás, S.; Real, J.T.; Ascaso, J.F.; González-Navarro, H. The GLP-1 analogue lixisenatide decreases atherosclerosis in insulin-resistant mice by modulating macrophage phenotype. *Diabetologia* **2017**, *60*, 1801–1812. [CrossRef] [PubMed]
34. González-Navarro, H.; Abu Nabah, Y.N.; Vinué, Á.; Andrés-Manzano, M.J.; Collado, M.; Serrano, M.; Andrés, V. p19ARF Deficiency Reduces Macrophage and Vascular Smooth Muscle Cell Apoptosis and Aggravates Atherosclerosis. *J. Am. Coll. Cardiol.* **2010**, *55*, 2258–2268. [CrossRef]
35. Ortega, R.; Collado, A.; Selles, F.; Gonzalez-Navarro, H.; Sanz, M.-J.J.; Real, J.T.; Piqueras, L. SGLT-2 (Sodium-Glucose Cotransporter 2) Inhibition Reduces Ang II (Angiotensin II)-Induced Dissecting Abdominal Aortic Aneurysm in ApoE (Apolipoprotein E) Knockout Mice. *Arterioscler. Thromb. Vasc. Biol.* **2019**, *39*, 1614–1628. [CrossRef] [PubMed]
36. Herrero-Cervera, A.; Vinué, Á.; Burks, D.J.; González-Navarro, H. Genetic inactivation of the LIGHT (TNFSF14) cytokine in mice restores glucose homeostasis and diminishes hepatic steatosis. *Diabetologia* **2019**, *62*, 2143–2157. [CrossRef]
37. Andrés-Blasco, I.; Herrero-Cervera, A.; Vinué, Á.; Martínez-Hervás, S.; Piqueras, L.; Sanz, M.J.; Burks, D.J.; González-Navarro, H. Hepatic lipase deficiency produces glucose intolerance, inflammation and hepatic steatosis. *J. Endocrinol.* **2015**, *227*, 179–191. [CrossRef]
38. Martínez-Hervás, S.; Vinué, Á.; Nú, L.; Andrés-Blasco, I.; Piqueras, L.; Tomás Real, J.; Francisco Ascaso, J.; Jane Burks, D.; Jesú Sanz, M.; González-Navarro, H. Insulin resistance aggravates atherosclerosis by reducing vascular smooth muscle cell survival and increasing CX 3 CL1/CX 3 CR1 axis. *Cardiovasc. Res.* **2014**. [CrossRef]
39. Andrés-Blasco, I.; Vinué, A.; Herrero-Cervera, A.; Martinez-Hervás, S.; Nuñez, L.; Piqueras, L.; Ascaso, J.F.; Sanz, M.J.; Burks, D.J.; González-Navarro, H. Hepatic lipase inactivation decreases atherosclerosis in insulin resistance by reducing LIGHT/lymphotoxin β-receptor pathway. *Thromb. Haemost.* **2016**, *116*, 379–393. [CrossRef]
40. González-Navarro, H.; Vinué, Á.; Sanz, M.J.; Delgado, M.; Pozo, M.A.; Serrano, M.; Burks, D.J.; Andrés, V. Increased dosage of Ink4/Arf protects against glucose intolerance and insulin resistance associated with aging. *Aging Cell* **2013**, *12*, 102–111. [CrossRef]

Publisher's Note: MDPI stays neutral with regard to jurisdictional claims in published maps and institutional affiliations.

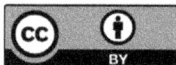

© 2020 by the authors. Licensee MDPI, Basel, Switzerland. This article is an open access article distributed under the terms and conditions of the Creative Commons Attribution (CC BY) license (http://creativecommons.org/licenses/by/4.0/).

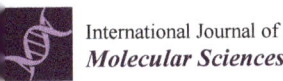

International Journal of *Molecular Sciences*

Review

Atrial Fibrillation: Pathogenesis, Predisposing Factors, and Genetics

Marios Sagris [1,*], Emmanouil P. Vardas [1,2], Panagiotis Theofilis [1], Alexios S. Antonopoulos [1], Evangelos Oikonomou [1,3] and Dimitris Tousoulis [1]

1. 1st Cardiology Clinic, 'Hippokration' General Hospital, School of Medicine, National and Kapodistrian University of Athens, 11528 Athens, Greece; vardas.man@gmail.com (E.P.V.); panos.theofilis@hotmail.com (P.T.); alexios.antonopoulos@cardiov.ox.ac.uk (A.S.A.); boikono@gmail.com (E.O.); drtousoulis@hotmail.com (D.T.)
2. Department of Cardiology, General Hospital of Athens "G. Gennimatas", 11527 Athens, Greece
3. 3rd Department of Cardiology, "Sotiria" Thoracic Diseases Hospital of Athens, University of Athens Medical School, 11527 Athens, Greece
* Correspondence: masagris1919@gmail.com; Tel.: +30-213-2088099; Fax: +30-213-2088676

Abstract: Atrial fibrillation (AF) is the most frequent arrhythmia managed in clinical practice, and it is linked to an increased risk of death, stroke, and peripheral embolism. The Global Burden of Disease shows that the estimated prevalence of AF is up to 33.5 million patients. So far, successful therapeutic techniques have been implemented, with a high health-care cost burden. As a result, identifying modifiable risk factors for AF and suitable preventive measures may play a significant role in enhancing community health and lowering health-care system expenditures. Several mechanisms, including electrical and structural remodeling of atrial tissue, have been proposed to contribute to the development of AF. This review article discusses the predisposing factors in AF including the different pathogenic mechanisms, sedentary lifestyle, and dietary habits, as well as the potential genetic burden.

Keywords: atrial fibrillation; pathogenesis; oxidative stress; predisposing factors; diets; Mediterranean diet; genetics

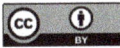

1. Introduction

Over the past hundred years, atrial fibrillation (AF) is the arrhythmia that has been studied the most among all other heart rhythm disorders, leading to valuable conclusions [1]. The prevalence of AF ranges from 2% in the general population to 10–12% in those aged 80 and older [2]. It is the most common arrhythmia in humans, and incidence increases with advancing age [2]. According to the Global Burden of Disease, the estimated prevalence of AF is up to 33.5 million individuals, as it affects 2.5–3.5% of populations in several countries [3]. Atrial fibrosis has emerged as a significant pathophysiological component, with links to AF recurrences, resistance to medication, and complications [3]. Studies on the histological as well as electrophysiological aspects of the disease have led to its better understanding, improving the therapeutic possibilities and effectively, the quality of life of patients [1]. However, crucial questions regarding the formation and perpetuation of the disease remain unanswered. In this article, an update is presented on the emerging data connecting oxidative stress and inflammation to unfavorable atrial structural and electrical remodeling [4]. Moreover, it is epidemiologically proven that AF is correlated to several factors that either individually or in combination promote the initial development of the arrhythmia and the episodes that characterize the disease [5,6]. Undoubtedly, aging constitutes the primary factor responsible for the pathogenesis of the arrhythmia [5]. Additionally, arterial hypertension, obesity, diabetes mellitus and genetic factors have also been confirmed by the Framingham studies to be significant predisposing factors of the disease, while multiple dietary components seem to play a protective role reducing the occurrence of AF [7–9]. The present review summarizes the role of specific risk factors and pathophysiological mechanism in the development and perpetuation of the arrhythmia.

2. Fibrosis

Several mechanisms have been postulated to play a role in the development of AF, through both the electrical and structural remodeling of the atrial tissue. Among them, fibrosis has been studied thoroughly, confirming its significant role in this process.

Fibrosis refers to the increased deposition of extracellular matrix proteins in the myocardial interstitial tissue due to the excessive proliferation of fibroblasts in response to pathological conditions. Fibroblasts are responsible for the structural support and maintenance of the homogeneity of the cardiac tissue. During the fibrotic process, fibroblasts differentiate to myofibroblasts, cells that have been studied for their effect on reducing conduction velocity in the myocardium, promoting an arrythmogenic substrate [10].

Fibroses can been classified into two distinct types, reparative and interstitial fibrosis:

1. Reparative fibrosis refers to the replacement of necrotic myocardial cells by fibrotic tissue [9,11].
2. Interstitial fibrosis can be sub-classified into:
    (a) Reactive fibrosis, which indicates the deposition of extracellular matrix (ECM) in the interstitial and perivascular space without the replacement of the damaged cells [9,11];
    (b) Infiltrative interstitial fibrosis, which refers to the deposition of glycosphingolipids or insoluble proteins in the interstitial space, as seen in amyloidosis or Fabry disease respectively [12].

The two different types of fibrosis may coexist.

2.1. Cellular Mediators of Atrial Fibrosis

Several cellular subtypes have been investigated for their effect in the fibrotic process and the subsequent promotion of atrial fibrillation. Among them, fibroblasts have been established as the main cellular effectors of atrial fibrosis [13]. Fibroblasts are small, spindle-shaped cells of mesenchymal origin, accounting for 10–15% of all cardiac tissue cells. [14] They are metabolically active cells, regulating the synthesis and turnover of the ECM, thus preserving the architectural integrity of the cardiac tissue. Multiple communication pathways have been established between fibroblasts and cardiomyocytes, altering the latter's electrophysiological properties. Under various pathological conditions and stress indicators, a phenotypic conversion of fibroblasts to alpha-smooth-muscle actin (αSMA) expressing myofibroblasts, takes place.

In detail, the activation and differentiation of local cardiac fibroblasts is dependent on multiple neurohumoral and mechanical profibrotic stress stimuli. Among the biochemical signals that have been identified to induce fibroblast differentiation, TGFβ has a prominent role in this process through both a canonical (SMAD-dependent) and non-canonical (SMAD-independent) pathway, which mediates the transcription of myofibroblast genes [15,16]. Additionally, angiotensin II (AngII) and endothelin 1 (ET-1), which bind to the G-protein-coupled receptors (GPCR) presented by cardiac fibroblasts, have been established as fibrotic mediators through the activation of a signaling cascade that promotes fibrotic gene transcription [17]. The activation and differentiation of fibroblasts is further enhanced when mechanical forces are applied that generate a more tensile and rigid matrix. The mechanisms that have been proposed to be responsible for the tension-based induction of myofibroblasts rely either on the activation of stretch-sensitive transient receptor potential (TRP) channels, which further activate factors such as TGFβ, or the force-mediated activation of p38 from the contractile signals of the cytoskeleton [18]. In conjunction with the aforementioned traditional fibroblast activation pathways, recent studies have brought to light significant mitochondrial, as well as cellular, metabolic components that promote the formation of myofibroblasts. Mitochondria act as key regulators in the fibroblast activation process by reducing their Ca^{2+} uptake in response to the profibrotic signals, a process that further enhances the cytosolic Ca^{2+} signaling pathway. Additionally, the profibrotic stressors induce the production of mitochondrial ROS, which activate factors such as p38 and ERK1/2, known for augmenting the transcription of fibrotic genes [19]. Lastly, various cellular metabolic functions have been highlighted over the past few years among the main drivers of myofibroblast formation. In particular, an increase in the rate of glutaminolysis in fibroblasts is considered crucial for their activation, while alterations in glycolysis with the subsequent increase in lactate production have been proposed as essential mechanisms for the promotion of the myofibroblast differentiation program [20]. Myofibroblast actions include recruiting inflammatory cells, promoting wound contraction, and secreting an excessive amount of ECM proteins such as collagen type I, III and IV; periostin; and fibronectin, leading to fibrosis [21,22].

In addition to fibroblasts, multiple inflammatory cells have been shown to be involved in the pro-fibrotic process. Studies have demonstrated the principal role that macrophages have in the regulation of fibrosis. Resident macrophages, originating from yolk sac-derived erythromyeloid progenitors (EMPs), populate the healthy myocardium, promoting its homeostasis. During the event of cardiac injury, multiple blood-borne monocytes infiltrate the myocardium and differentiate to macrophages [23]. Monocyte-derived macrophages express broad heterogeneity, enabling them to exert different functions, such as the production of multiple pro-fibrotic growth factors (IL-10, TGF-β, IGF-1, and PDGF), pro-inflammatory cytokines (IL-6, TNF-α, ROS), and proteases that contribute to matrix remodelling [23].

Likewise, following myocardial injury, T-cells populate the cardiac tissue in response to cytokine signalling. T-cells are then differentiated into either CD4+ (Th1, Th2) or CD8+ cytotoxic T cells, which exert distinct functions. In the immediate post-insult period, Th1 and CD8+ cells are the main residents of the myocardium [24]. These cells have been recognised for their anti-fibrotic functions, as they release mediators, such as IFN-γ and protein-10, which inhibit the action of the pro-fibrotic TGF-β. Additionally, INF-γ interferes with the activation of Th2 cells by impacting the production of IL4 and IL13 [24]. Progressing into the chronic injury period, Th2 cells overtake Th1 cells as the principal CD4+ cell phenotype in the myocardial tissue. In contrast to the latter, Th2 cells exhibit significant pro-fibrotic activity. This is performed mainly by secreting IL4 and IL13, molecules that stimulate collagen secretion either by enabling TFG-β or by recruiting monocytes in the lesion site [24].

Another component of the innate immunity, mast cells, have established their role as modulators for cardiac fibrosis. Studies have demonstrated that, under conditions of cardiac ischemia and pressure overload, mast cells multiplicate and degranulate pre-formed inflammatory and fibrotic (e.g.,TGF-β1, TNF, IL-1) mediators. Mast cells present in the cardiac tissue represent the connective tissue phenotype and contain both chymase and tryptase. Shiota et al. conducted a study that identified a 5.2-fold increase in chymase activity in hamsters with chronic pressure-overloaded hearts [25]. Multiple studies have proven the pro-fibrotic effect of increased chymase activity in cardiac remodelling by promoting the formation of angiotensin-II [26–28]. The increased levels of tryptase in fibrotic hearts have been shown to mediate fibroblast proliferation and differentiation to myofibroblasts. The mechanism responsible has been attributed to the stimulation of protease activated receptor-2 (PAR-2) in fibroblasts and the subsequent phosphorylation of extracellular signal-regulated protein kinases 1 and 2 (ERK $\frac{1}{2}$), which promotes the differentiation of fibroblasts to myofibroblasts [29]. Lastly, the role of histamine produced by mast cells has been thoroughly studied, establishing its significance in cardiac fibrosis. The detrimental role of histamine in cardiac fibrosis has been proven in an animal experiment, wherein a lack of histamine induced a response in H_2-receptor-deficient mice and reduced myocardial apoptosis and fibrosis [30]. Nevertheless, multiple anti-inflammatory and anti-fibrotic mediators are also among the degranulation products of mast cells, raising controversy over the exact function of mast cells in the process of tissue remodelling [31] (Figure 1).

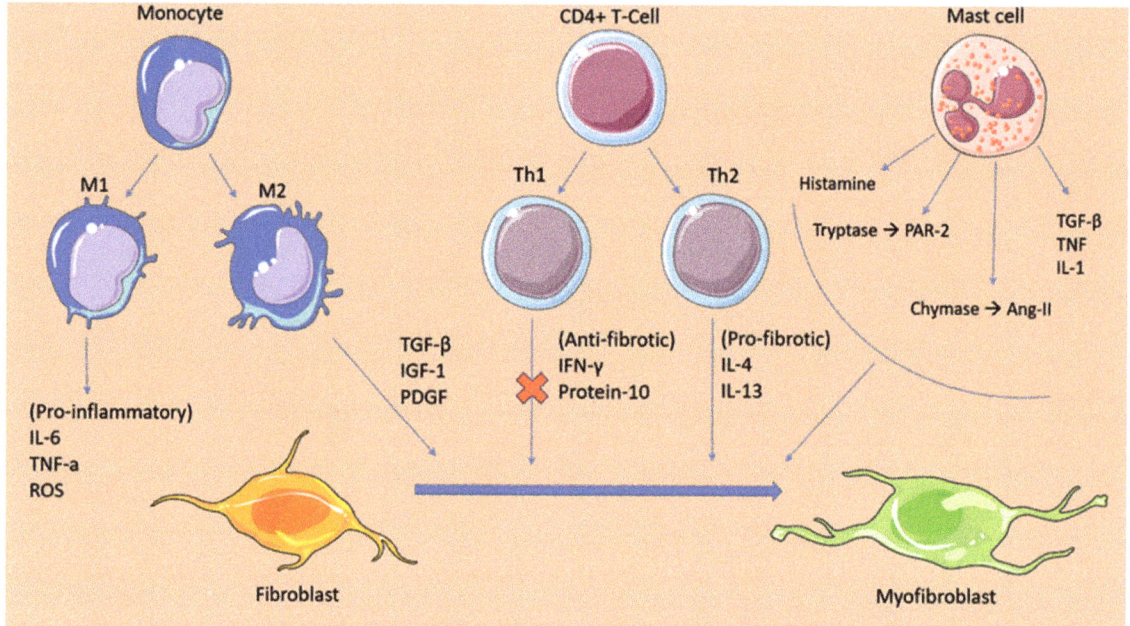

Figure 1. This graphical abstract summarizes the cellular mediators of atrial fibrosis. Following an insult, inflammatory mediators signal immune cells such as monocytes, CD4+ T-cells, and mast cells to infiltrate the atrial myocardium. These cells promote tissue fibrosis by secreting pro-fibrotic factors and regulatory molecules that enhance the activation and differentiation of fibroblasts to myofibroblasts. Additionally, the figure depicts the anti-fibrotic mediators that are secreted by Th1 cells in the early-insult stage and that are gradually overhauled by the products of pro-fibrotic Th2 cells. TGFβ, transforming growth factor beta; TNFα, tumor necrosis factor alpha; PDGF, platelet-derived growth factor; IL-1, interleukin 1; IL-4, interleukin 4; IL-6, interleukin 6; IL-10, interleukin 10; ROS, reactive oxygen species; IFNγ, interferon gamma; IGF-1, Insulin-like growth factor 1; Th1, t helper type 1; Th2, t helper type 2; PAR-2, protease activated receptor 2; Ang-II, angiotensin.

2.2. Fibrotic Mechanisms Inducing Atrial Fibrillation

Fibrosis has been established as a significant factor maintaining atrial fibrillation. There has been increased data associating the atrial remodelling induced by fibrosis with the promotion of AF. It has been proposed that the increased population of fibroblasts/myofibroblasts present in the fibrotic tissue and the increased deposition of ECM disrupt the myocardial bundles continuity, interfering with the gap-junction formation among cardiomyocytes. This event leads to conduction abnormalities, slowing conduction velocity and eventually forming unidirectional conduction blocks [32]. Moreover, as mentioned previously, myofibroblasts form communication channels with cardiomyocytes, altering their electrophysiological properties, giving rise to focal firing and re-entrant circuits.

Over the last 10 years, several clinical studies have been conducted to confirm the aforementioned mechanisms. Researchers from the Cardiovascular Research institute in Maastricht performed epicardial mapping in 24 patients with long-standing persistent AF, undergoing cardiac surgery, in an attempt to uncover the spatiotemporal characteristics of the fibrillatory process underlying the disease. The study confirmed the intra-atrial conduction disturbances with the presence of block lines running in parallel to the muscular bundles [33]. Additionally, a significant contribution in understanding the pathophysiology underlining the relationship between atrial fibrosis and arrhythmogenesis was made by Sebastien P.J Krul, et al., who studied the effect of interstitial fibrosis on conduction velocity [34]. Researchers obtained 35 atrial appendages during AF surgery and recorded the activation time as well as the longitudinal (CVl) and transverse (CVt) conduction velocity (CV). The results demonstrated that the thick interstitial fibrotic strands were directly associated with an increase in the longitudinal CV in contrary to the transverse CV, which was not affected [34]. However, a greater extent of transverse activation delay was observed because of the presence of activation block areas leading to a pattern of zig-zag conduction. This study points at the quality rather than the quantity of the fibrotic tissue as responsible for the formation of an arrhythmogenic substrate, with re-entry circuits enabling the perpetuation of atrial fibrillation [34]. To further verify the driver mechanisms of AF, Hansen et al. performed a simultaneous mapping of the sub-endocardial and sub-epicardial activation patterns, and then integrated these data to an MRI-produced atrial model, in an attempt to visualize the AF drivers. The researchers confirmed the presence of longitudinal conduction blocks in agreement with the epicardial mapping study and, in addition, proved that fibrosis due to cardiac diseases disrupts the myocardial architecture, promoting a structural substrate for re-entrant AF drivers [35].

3. Oxidative Stress

Over recent years, oxidative stress has been investigated as a potential essential mechanism in the development of AF. Reactive oxygen species (ROS) constitute the normal byproducts generated through the metabolism of oxygen. These molecules have been proven to have a multifaceted effect on the cells present in the heart tissue. Tahhan et al. recently revealed that the prevalence and incidence of AF were related to the redox potentials of glutathione (E_hGSH) and cysteine, markers of oxidative stress. The study concluded that the prevalence of AF was 30% higher for each 10% increase in E_hGSH, while the same alteration resulted in a 40% increase in the risk of incident AF [36]. The molecular processes underpinning atrial fibrillation development have been the subject of multiple clinical studies. Research evidence suggest that excessive ROS can directly affect ion channels and the propagation of action potential [37]. Hydrogen peroxide provokes trigger activity through the enhancement of late Na+ current, inducing early afterdepolarization (EAD) and delayed afterdepolarization (DAD). Moreover, ROS can induce a downregulation of the total Na+ current, an event that promotes the formation of reentry circuits. It is also worth mentioning that ROS can directly upregulate the L-type Ca^{2+} current and promote EADs by altering the intracellular calcium balance [37]. Recent experimental evidence suggests that the oxidation of ryanodine receptor 2 (RYR2) induces the intracellular release of Ca^{2+} from the sarcoplasmic reticulum, promoting the establishment of atrial fibrillation [38]. The generation of ROS in the myocardium has been attributed to many enzymatic sources. Among them, NADPH oxidase (NOX) has proven to have a critical role in the progress of AF. In studies performed in animal models, superoxide and H_2O_2 produced from activated NOX2 and NOX4 isoforms lead to myocyte apoptosis, fibrosis, and inflammation, which further promote atrial fibrillation perpetuation. One proposed mechanism through which ROS could exert their pro-arrhythmic function is by the oxidation of calmodulin-dependent protein kinase II (CaMKII) [39]. Oxidized CaMKII mediate the phosphorylation of the RYR2, leading to calcium overload and the formation of multiple wavelets triggering atrial fibrillation emergence [40]. In addition to the electrical remodeling stimulated by the mechanisms described, ROS have also been demonstrated to contribute to atria structural remodeling. Researchers from Slovakia showed that hydroxyl radicals can alter the myofibrillar protein structure and function, promoting myocardial injury and further contributing to the formation of a fertile substrate for the development of arrhythmias [5,41].

4. Inflammation

Inflammation has been linked to the onset and maintenance of atrial fibrillation, according to accumulating evidence. Inflammation contributes to the atrial remodelling involving both structural and electrophysiological alterations that form the basis for the disease. A large-scale prospective study involving 24,734 women participants investigated the association of inflammatory markers such as CRP, fibrinogen, and intercellular adhesion molecule 1 (sICAM-1) with the incidence of AF. The results suggested that inflammation is a strong indicator for the incidence of AF with the median plasma levels of the biomarkers being independently correlated with the development of the disease in patients [42]. That suggestion was further confirmed when scientists from Greece observed that the levels of high-sensitivity C-reactive protein (hs-CRP) are directly linked with the recurrence of AF after cardioversion and that the restoration of sinus rhythm (SR) resulted in a gradual decrease of hs-CRP [43], while Rotter et al. reported that CRP levels in individuals with AF declined following effective ablation [44,45]. Additionally, in a recent study, Yao C. et al. demonstrated that, in patients with atrial fibrillation, the activity of NLRP3 (NOD-, LRR-, and pyrin domain-containing protein 3) inflammasome in atrial cardiomyocytes was considerably enhanced. The upregulation of the NLRP3 inflammasome promotes the release of damage-associated molecular patterns (DAMPs), which lead to the activation of cardiac fibroblasts, cells that, as described earlier, are the main effectors of cardiac fibrosis [13].

Advances in the field of cardiology over the last years have led to the identification of many cellular and molecular mechanisms that suggest inflammation is responsible for the pathogenesis of AF. Under inflammatory stress, angiotensin II stimulates the production of proinflammatory cytokines (e.g., IL-6, IL-8, TNF-α) and the recruitment of immune cells. The role of AngII has also been established in the fibrosis and structural remodelling of the cardiac tissue through the activation of the MAPK-mediators of AngII/AT1R and the subsequent expression of the pro-fibrotic TGFβ1, which promotes fibroblast differentiation. Furthermore, increased pressure overload, as well as several gene polymorphisms in renin and angiotensin, mediate the formation of angiotensin II and the activation of angiotensin II receptors. Angiotensin II has been linked with the activation of NOX and the subsequent oxidation-related calcium-handling abnormalities, resulting in the electric remodelling of the atria. Additionally, NOX is a potent stimulator of the transcription factor nuclear factor-κB (NF-κB), which directly affects the sodium channel promoter regions, leading to a downregulation of the sodium channels and the promotion of AF mechanics [46,47]. The RAAS system mechanism lying behind AF development reflects the theory that atrial fibrillation begets atrial fibrillation. This notion can be justified by recent evidence suggesting that AngII not only causes inflammation but also that inflammation can promote AngII production through hs-CRP and TNF-a. These molecules, which are pronounced in inflammatory states, seem to have an upregulatory effect on the AT1R, further promoting this vicious cycle [48].

When associating inflammation with the occurrence of atrial fibrillation, it is important to mention the culprit of coronary artery disease in this phenomenon. Coronary heart disease has been associated with the development of atrial fibrillation through various mechanisms [49]. Among them, inflammation constitutes the most important determinant of atrial fibrillation presentation, second only to atrial infarction and the subsequent tissue fibrosis. Following the event of myocardial ischemia, local as well as systemic inflammation arises, which causes the release of various inflammatory factors such as IL-6 and CRP, which have been independently associated with the development of atrial fibrillation [50]. It has been proposed that IL-6 exerts its proarrhythmic effect by inducing atrial remodelling. Increased serum levels of IL-6 were associated by Psychari SN et al. with an increased left atrial size. The dilatation of the left atrium is believed to result from the stimulating effect of IL-6 on matrix-metalloproteinase-2 (MMP2), a protease that has been implicated in atrial remodeling [51]. Moreover, it has been demonstrated that inflammation induced by myocardial infarction can promote atrial remodeling through the activation of Toll-like receptors (TLR), factors of the innate immune system. Particularly, TLR 2 and TLR 4 mRNA expression is significantly enhanced in patients following MI, while elevated TLR-2 levels have been associated with increased left atrial size [52,53].

Of great importance when relating inflammation with AF, is the prothrombotic state present in the disease. A high CRP level has been related to the formation of thrombi in the left atrium [54]. Research has established the mechanisms of thrombogenesis in inflammation. During an inflammatory state, innate immune cells activation and the release of inflammatory ligands are upregulated. IL-2, IL-6, IL-8, TNF-a, and MCP-1 production is enhanced by the activated immune cells resulting in the synthesis of tissue factor (TF), von Willebrand factor (vWF), and P-selectin [55]. These molecules mediate platelet agglutination, as well as monocyte-endothelial cell attachment. This event combined with the endothelial damage induced in the atrium of a patient affected by AF severely increases the risk of thrombus formation [56–58] (Table 1).

Table 1. Differences in concentrations of inflammatory proteins in patients with and without atrial fibrillation.

Protein	Protein Serum Levels Difference	Atrial Tissue Levels Difference	Predictor for AF
CRP	NA	NA	Yes
MCP-1	+	+	No
MPO	NA	+	No
TGF-β	NA	+	No
TNF	NA	+	No
HSP-27	+	+	NA
HSP-70	-	-	NA
IL-1	NA	NA	NA
IL-6	NA	+	No
IL-8	+	+	NA
IL-10	NA	+	NA

Abbreviations: AF = atrial Fibrillation, IL = interleukin, CRP = C-reactive protein, TNF = tumor necrosis factor, HSP = heat shock protein, TGF = transforming growth factor, MPO = myeloperoxidase, MCP-1 = monocyte chemoattractant protein, NA = not applicable, (+) = There is a difference in concentration; (-) = There is no difference in concentration.

5. Sedentary Lifestyle

Over the last decade, efforts have been made to prove the association between behavioral lifestyle and AF incidence [59,60]. Said, M. A et al. noted that a log-additive effect on the risk of developing cardiovascular diseases was present when the health habits and the individual genetic background were considered in a large population [60]. The American Heart Association (AHA) recently established the concept of the American Heart Association's Life's Simple 7 (LS7) metrics based on four healthy behavior metrics (non-smoking, normal weight, moderate physical activity, and a healthy diet) and three health factors (normal cholesterol, blood pressure, and fasting blood glucose [FBG]) [61,62]. Yang, Y. et al. and a MESA study showed that the subgroup with 3 to 7 ideal components from the optimal LS7 status had low risk of AF (57~59% reduced risk), while adherence to the optimal LS7 status reduced the risk even more [62,63]. As a result of extended, uninterrupted sitting, sedentary lifestyles cause negative alterations in blood insulin and glucose levels. Insulin resistance is linked to endothelial dysfunction due to a mismatch between the phosphatidylinositol 3-kinase (PI3K) and mitogen-activated protein kinase (MAPK) signaling pathways [64]. In an insulin-resistant condition, PI3K signaling is diminished, resulting in lower nitric oxide availability, but MAPK signaling is unchanged, resulting in increased endothlin-1 synthesis, endothelial cell death, and inflammation [64,65].

The way that weight reduction affects AF incidence and symptoms was analyzed in a randomized observational trial of 248 patients [66]. When compared to the control group, the intervention group lost significantly more weight (14.3 vs. 3.6 kg) and had significantly lower atrial fibrillation symptom burden scores, symptom severity scores, number of episodes (2.5 vs. no change), and cumulative duration (692-min decline and 419-min increase) [66]. As far as the benefits in cardiac remodeling are concerned, interventricular septal thickness (1.1 and 0.6 mm) and the left atrial area (3.5 and 1.9 cm) were reduced in the intervention and control groups, respectively. AF was associated with worse postoperative outcomes, in particularly in patients with carotid artery disease, revealing high stroke/death risk [66–68]. Previous research discovered that increased self-reported sitting is related with increased levels of adipokines, C-reactive protein and low-grade inflammation, a result that was independent of physical activity levels [64]. Increased reactive oxygen species (ROS) production inside the arterial wall may be responsible for vascular remodeling, promoting smooth muscle cell proliferation and generating endothelial dysfunction. The formation of ROS has been linked to sedentary lifestyle while being viewed as a significant component in the etiology of cardiovascular disease, notably due to the production of superoxide, which is related with endothelial function deficits and hypertension [69]. These findings suggest that targeting ideal cardiovascular health and weight reduction may limit the incidence and the severity of AF [66,68].

6. Dietary Habits

6.1. Alcohol-Resveratrol

Of interest is the effect of multiple dietary components in the pathogenesis or treatment of AF. High levels of alcohol intake were associated with increased occurrence of AF, while moderate consumption lead more males than females to AF [70]. More specifically, Larson et al. present the risk ratios among drinkers of <1 drink/week (12 g alcohol/drink), in a cohort study with 7245 AF cases. The results were the same regardless of the inclusion of binge drinkers: a hazard ratio of 1.01 for 1 to 6 drinks/week, 1.07 for 7 to 14 drinks/week, 1.14 for 15 to 21 drinks/week, and 1.39 for >21 drinks/week [70]. The findings note that even moderate alcohol consumption could potentially lead to AF. Low level of alcohol is still a debateable issue as a risk factor for AF in a large amount of studies. Ariansen I. et al. show that the consumption of up to ten alcoholic beverages per week appears to be harmless, while higher consumption constitutes a predisposing factor for AF [71,72].

Although reduced alcohol intake has to be a rational treatment target for patients with AF, resveratrol, a bioactive polyphenol, found in red wine, grapes, seeds, and peanuts has recently attracted scientific attention as a cardioprotective nutritional supplement due to its antioxidant and vascular effects [73,74]. In AF, resveratrol presents antiarrhythmic qualities as it potentially operates as an inhibitor of both intracellular calcium release and pathogenic signaling cascades, preventing calcium excess and maintaining cardiomyocyte contractile function. Attempts have been made to generate novel resveratrol derivatives for the treatment of arrhythmias [73,74].

6.2. Caffeine

Caffeine is a methylxanthine that has been considered a potential arrhythmiogenic substance. Caffeine is contained in coffee, tea, cola, and energy drinks and has neurohormonal and sympathetic nervous system effect. Previous studies note that moderate coffee consumption decreases the risk of heart failure, coronary heart disease, stroke, DM type 2, and all-cause mortality from cardiovascular disease, as compared to non-consumers [75,76]. As far as AF incidence is concerned, a dose-response is presented from 6 prospective cohort studies. Studies show a 11% reduction for low doses and 16% for high doses of caffeine consumption, while the AF incidence decreases by 6% for every 300 mg/d increment in habitual caffeine intake [77]. The risk of AF was greater in people who consumed fewer than two cups of coffee per day (12-oz cup of coffee ~140 mg of caffeine) compared to people with higher consumption. On the other hand, the likelihood of AF incidence declined when caffeine consumption exceeded 436 mg/day [77]. The Physicians Health Study highlights that men who reported drinking 1 to 3 cups of coffee every day have a decreased incidence of AF. Specifically, rare/never coffee consumption is associated with a hazard ratio for AF at around 1.0, $\leq$1 cup/week at 0.85, 2 to 4 cups/week at 1.07, 5 to 6 cups/week at 0.93, 1 cup/day at 0.85, 2 to 3 cups/day at 0.86 (0.76–0.97), and 4+ cups/day 0.96 [78]. An innovative study of Casiglia E. et al. observed 1475 unselected men and women and stratified them into three groups of caffeine intake, after genotyping for the $-163C > A$

polymorphism of the CYP1A2 gene, regulating caffeine metabolism. With a larger caffeine intake, AF was considerably reduced in the third tertile (>320 mg/day) than in the first and the second, while no interaction was proven between slow caffeine metabolism and AF occurrence [79,80].

6.3. Mediterranean Diet

An increasing body of research suggests that the Mediterranean diet (Med-Diet) is useful in both the primary and secondary prevention of cardiovascular risk. This is achieved by the reduction of oxidation stress by the leading Med-Diet habits [81,82]. Patients with vascular events have lower glutathione peroxidase 3 (GPx3) levels compared to those without events; the Med-Diet favorably stimulates the antioxidant activity of GPx3 in AF, resulting in a reduced vascular event rate, while no differences regarding superoxide dismutase (SOD) activity have been found [83]. Pastori et al. showed significant reduction in AF's vascular events in patients with adherence to the Med-Diet. More specifically, the group of patients with AF and higher adherence to Med-Diet had by far the fewest vascular events (5.3%) in comparison to the low-adherence group (23.4%) and the intermediate-adherence group (8.4%). These findings show that the downregulation of soluble NOX2-derived peptide (sNOX2-dp) and the decreased excretion of F2-isoprostanes (F2-IsoP) have a strong relationship with adherence to the Med-Diet and could lead to a reduction of cardiovascular events in AF patients, through an antioxidant effect [83]. Pignatelli P. and Pastori D. et al. present that platelet function in AF patients may be affected by increased adherence to the Med-Diet through the reduction of the urinary excretion of 11-dehydro-TxB2 or 11-dehydrothromboxane B2 produced from the breakdown of thromboxane A2- and the negative effect to gut-derived lipopolysaccharides (LPS), which may contribute to major adverse cardiovascular events [84,85].

6.4. Virgin Oil—Magnesium—Lean Fish

A Mediterranean diet combined with extra virgin olive oil may lower the incidence of AF by the decrease of inflammatory markers—such as C-reactive protein or interleukin-6- and by its strong anti-oxidant effects. Magnesium has antiarrhythmic capabilities due to its tendency to modulate cardiac excitability by inhibiting calcium ion entrance into cells. According to a Mendelian randomization research, genetically greater blood magnesium levels may be related with a lower incidence of AF. This observation may have therapeutic implications because blood magnesium levels can be increased by supplementation and dietary recommendations,—boosting intake of green leafy vegetables—and intravenous administration [86,87]. As far as the effect of dietary intake of saturated fatty acids on the development of AF is concerned, when total n-3 polyunsaturated fatty acids replaced dietary saturated fatty acids, there was a slight rise in AF occurrences in males but not in women. Replacing saturated fatty acids with monounsaturated or long chain polyunsaturated -n-6 polyunsaturated- fatty acids was not associated with the risk of AF [88,89]. In the same pattern, the intake of total fish, fatty fish (herring/mackerel and salmon/whitefish/char), and long-chain omega-3 polyunsaturated fatty acids has no contribution in the occurrence of AF. In contrast, the group of patients who consume lean fish (cod/saithe/fish fingers) in a frequency of ≥3 servings/week presents a lower risk of AF than the group of never consumers [90,91] (Figure 2).

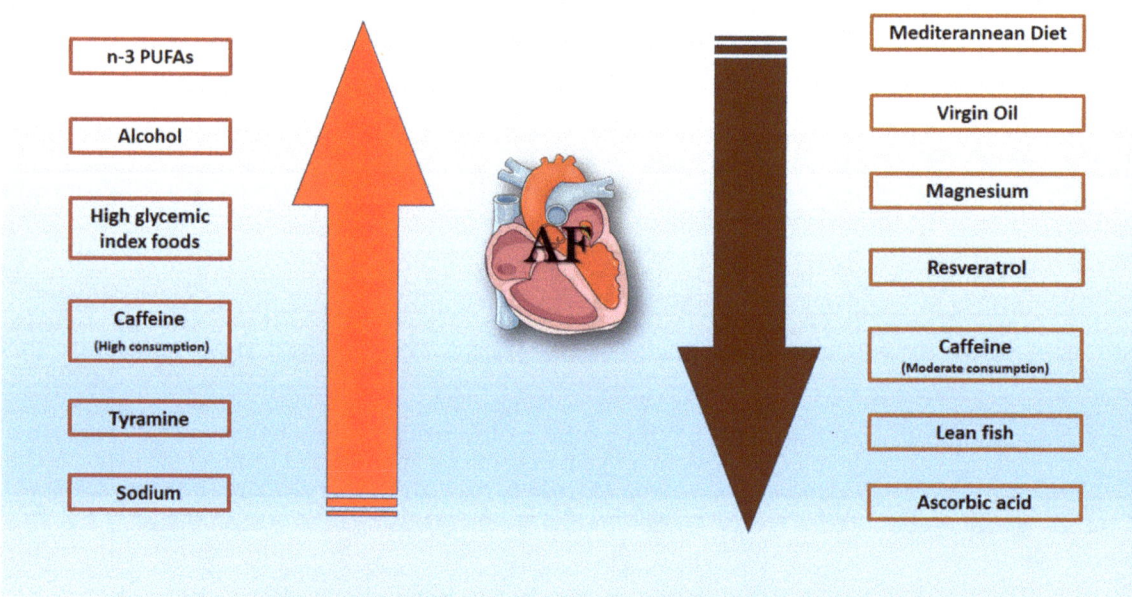

Figure 2. Graphical illustration of daily dietary habits that reduce (brown arrow) or increase (red arrow) the incidence of atrial fibrillation. n-3 PUFAs; polyunsaturated fatty acids.

7. Genetic Factors

Over the last decade, the identification of genes related to AF is a domain that has garnered much media and scientific attention. Ion-channel mutations provide important information on the processes driving AF; therefore, many methodologies and classic Mendelian genetics have been utilized to determine the potential family foundation. As far as the K^+ channel genes are concerned, the genes whose mutations increase the risk of AF occurrence are ABCC9 (I KATP), HCN4 (I f), KCNA5 (I Kur), KCND3 (I Ks), KCNE1 (IKs), KCNE2 (IKs), KCNE3 (IKs), KCNE4 (IKs), KCNE5 (IKs), KCNH2 (IKr), KCNJ2 (I K1), KCNJ5 (I KAch), KCNJ8 (I KATP), KCNN3 (IAHP), and KCNQ1 (IKs) [92]. The underlying mechanism is the higher K^+ current reducing refractoriness and encouraging re-entry while decreasing automaticity [2]. It has been found that rare mutations in the gap junctional protein-coding gene GJA5 and in the nuclear pore complex (nucleoporin) Nup155 could cause AF and sudden death even at a young age. These cases of AF are likely to be caused by the re-entry mechanism. Equally important is the suggestion that loss-of-function mutations delay repolarization and promote Ca^{2+} mediated after depolarization triggers AF. The above-mentioned phenomenon could be caused by: (a) the variants SCN1B, SCN2B, SCN3B, SCN4B, SCN5A, and SCN10A of Na+ channel genes; (b) junctophilin mutation (E169K), which was found to enhance the RyR2 Ca^{2+} leak, leading to the juvenile onset of AF; (c) a single nucleotide polymorphism (SNP) in CASR, which encodes a Ca^{+2}-sensing receptor that detects extracellular calcium ion levels and regulates calcium homeostasis [92]. The AFGen research uncovered 17 distinct susceptibility signals for AF at 14 different genetic locations; these include KCNN3, PRRX1, CAV1, SYNE2, C9orf3, HCN4, and MYOZ1 [2,92,93].

Various studies attempt to analyze the frequencies of single-nucleotide polymorphisms (SNPs) in genes whose protein products are involved in the pathogenesis of AF. Genome-wide association (GWAS) in the Japanese population identified that rs2200733, rs10033464 (located in the PITX2), and rs6584555 (located in the NURL1) were associated with AF [94]. In previous studies in Japan, six more loci were associated with AF: at 1q24 in PRRX1 (rs593479), 4q25 near PITX2 (rs2634073), 7q31 in CAV1 (rs1177384), 10q25 in NURL1 (rs6584555), 12q24 in CUX2 (rs649002), and 16q22 in ZFHX3 (rs12932445) [95]. The most significant finding was revealed in the study of Low S.K et al., in which different genetic factors lead to AF between Japanese and European population. Variants of KCND3, PPFIA4, SLC1A4-CEP68, HAND2, NEBL, and SH3PXD2A genes detected with five to six new loci differing between the two populations [96]. Korea Genome Epidemiology Study found two novel genetic loci on chromosomes 1q32.1/PPFIA4 (rs11579055) and 4q34.1/HAND2 (rs8180252), which were associated with the early-onset of AF. The loci on chromosome 4 has association with a previously proven gene in a European population. The found loci encode proteins involved in cell-to-cell communication, hypoxia, or long non-coding RNA [97].

Of scientific interest are the results of the GWAS on the variants of the transcription factor PITX2 [98,99]. The secretive protein is expressed in the adult left atrium, and, in early life, it is responsible for the regulation of the right–left differentiation of the embryonic heart, thorax, and aorta. The p.Met207Val variant produces a 3.1-fold increase in PITX2c transactivation activity in HeLa cells when compared to the wild-type equivalent. When the variant was expressed in contribution with wild-type PITX2c, an increase of arrhythmogenic mRNA levels of KCNH2 (2.6-fold), SCN1B (1.9-fold), GJA5 (3.1-fold), GJA1 (2.1-fold), and KCNQ1 in the homozygous form (1.8-fold) was revealed [98,100]. These genes encode for the IKr channel α subunit, the β-1 Na+ channel subunit, connexin 40, connexin 43, and the IKs channel α subunit, respectively [98–100]. Recent studies reveal that miRNAs can influence gene expression in hypertrophy and arrhythmia, as well as the numerous genes implicated in AF, making them viable molecular targets that may give greater clinical assistance. miR-21 and miR-133 seem to be involved in the structural remodeling of the atrium via enhanced fibrosis [101]. Differences in concentrations of miRNAs such as miR-21 between serum plasma and atrial tissue have been observed [101]. Studies have shown that miR-133b, miR-328, and miR-499 functionally control the ion regulating the activity of Ca^{2+} and K^+ channels [102]. Their concentrations were higher in the bloodstream of patients with acute new-onset AF and chronic AF rather than those without or with well-controlled AF [103,104]. Consequently, it is necessary to perform further studies on the strong genetic background of AF and the early detection of miRNA polymorphisms. SNPs can also improve the diagnosis and management of the AF patients as potential biomarkers (Table 2).

Table 2. Genetic mutations that are implicated in atrial fibrillation.

Gene of	Polymorphism-Mutation	Action
ABCC9 (I KATP)		
KCNA5 (I Kur)		
HCN4 (I f)		
KCND3 (I Ks)		
KCNE1 (IKs)		
KCNE2 (IKs)		
KCNE3 (IKs)	Potassium (K^+) channel genes	The increased K^+ current abbreviates refractoriness and promotes re-entry, while tending to reduce automaticity
KCNE4 (IKs)		
KCNE5 (IKs)		
KCNH2 (IKr)		
KCNJ2 (I K1)		
KCNJ5 (I KAch)		
KCNJ8 (I KATP)		
KCNN3 (IAHP)		
KCNQ1 (IKs)		

Table 2. Cont.

Gene of	Polymorphism-Mutation	Action
SCN1B SCN2B SCN3B SCN4B SCN5A SCN10A	Sodium (Na$^+$) channel genes	Delay repolarization and promote Ca^{+2} mediated after depolarization
GJA5	Mutations in the gap junctional protein	Re-entry mechanism
NUP155	Nuclear pore complex (nucleoporin) Nup155	Re-entry mechanism
E169K	Junctophilin mutation	Delay repolarization and promote Ca^{+2} mediated after depolarization enhancing RyR2 Ca^{+2} leak
CASR	rs1801725	Delay repolarization and promote Ca^{+2} mediated after depolarization
PITX2	rs2200733 rs10033464 rs2634073	PITX2 deficiency results in electrical and structural remodelling
NURL1	rs6584555 rs6584555	Undefined
PRRX1	rs593479	Undefined
CAV1	rs1177384	Undefined
CUX2	rs649002	Undefined
ZFHX3	rs12932445	Undefined

8. Prevention-Conclusions

Physicians might always estimate the AF risk for patients with burdened health profile (age, hypertension, diabetes, obesity etc.) via the multiple scales that have been introduced. Obesity, excessive alcohol use, and obstructive sleep apnoea are all known to contribute to unfavourable LA remodelling and AF risk [105,106]. As such, lifestyle and dietary modifications including weight loss, alcohol reduction, and cardiometabolic risk factor management would be a cornerstone for AF prevention [105,107]. The medical prescription of medications other than anti-inflammatory agents, such as angiotensin-converting enzyme inhibitors, angiotensin receptor blockers, and aldosterone antagonists, can all help to reduce LA enlargement, atrial fibrosis, and TGF-β indicators, as well as atrial dysfunction. These are the most widely used drugs for AF and have to be considered for patients with a history of heart failure [108,109]. The novel SGLT-2 inhibitors reveal beneficial effects in systolic heart failure included improved cardiac energy metabolism, the prevention of inflammation, oxidative stress, adverse cardiac remodelling, less LA enlargement, fibrosis, atrial mitochondrial dysfunction, inflammation, and AF inducibility [110].

As far as the recognition of potential paroxysmal AF is considered, new strategies with smart watches and other devices can detect events better than a traditional 24-h ambulatory ECG recording [111,112]. Rapid progress has been made in identifying the genetic basis for this common condition. For individuals with a remarkable family history of AF or cardiomyopathy, DNA sequencing for potential genetic loci that are associated with AF would be beneficial [113]. The correction of unfavourable stressors can result in decreased atrial size and a reduction of electrophysiological anomalies in a scenario of established pathological atrial enlargement, owing to continuous increases in volume or pressure load. As such, clinicians' high awareness of the field is the key point for the early identification of AF events, while the development of early prevention strategies and screening programs can be organized for patients with poor medical status [111].

Based on the above facts, it has become clear that fibrosis, inflammation, and oxidative stress, as well as behavioural and genetic factors, contribute decisively to the development of atrial fibrillation. Undoubtedly, the aforementioned risk factors, primarily the evolving atrial myopathy, form a fertile substrate for the establishment of anisotropic conduction properties in the atrial myocardium, the fragmentation of the electrical activity, and eventually, the development of atrial fibrillation.

Author Contributions: Conceptualization, M.S., P.T., E.P.V.; methodology, M.S., E.P.V.; bioinformatics, M.S., P.T. and A.S.A.; analysis, M.S., D.T.; data curation, D.T., E.O.; writing—original draft preparation, M.S. and E.P.V. writing—review and editing, M.S., P.T., E.P.V. and D.T. All authors have read and agreed to the published version of the manuscript.

Funding: This research received no external funding.

Institutional Review Board Statement: The study was conducted according to the guidelines of the Declaration of Helsinki and ap-proved by the Institutional Review Board of the KAISER FOUNDATION RESEARCH IN-STITUTE and the NATIONAL CANCER INSTITUTE.

Informed Consent Statement: Participants were included in the study unless they chose the "optout" option as described in the Material and Methods section.

Data Availability Statement: Not applicable.

Conflicts of Interest: The authors declare no conflict of interest.

References

1. Lau, D.H.; Linz, D.; Sanders, P. New Findings in Atrial Fibrillation Mechanisms. *Card Electrophysiol. Clin.* **2019**, *11*, 563–571. [CrossRef] [PubMed]
2. Staerk, L.; Sherer, J.A.; Ko, D.; Benjamin, E.J.; Helm, R.H. Atrial Fibrillation: Epidemiology, Pathophysiology, and Clinical Outcomes. *Circ. Res.* **2017**, *120*, 1501–1517. [CrossRef] [PubMed]
3. Morin, D.P.; Bernard, M.L.; Madias, C.; Rogers, P.A.; Thihalolipavan, S.; Estes, N.A., 3rd. The State of the Art: Atrial Fibrillation Epidemiology, Prevention, and Treatment. *Mayo Clin. Proc.* **2016**, *91*, 1778–1810. [CrossRef] [PubMed]
4. Jalife, J.; Kaur, K. Atrial remodeling, fibrosis, and atrial fibrillation. *Trends Cardiovasc. Med.* **2015**, *25*, 475–484. [CrossRef] [PubMed]
5. Sagris, M.; Antonopoulos, A.S.; Theofilis, P.; Oikonomou, E.; Siasos, G.; Tsalamandris, S.; Antoniades, C.; Brilakis, E.S.; Kaski, J.C.; Tousoulis, D. Risk factors profile of young and older patients with Myocardial Infarction. *Cardiovasc. Res.* **2021**. [CrossRef] [PubMed]
6. Diavati, S.; Sagris, M.; Terentes-Printzios, D.; Vlachopoulos, C. Anticoagulation Treatment in Venous Thromboembolism: Options and Optimal Duration. *Curr. Pharm. Des.* **2021**. [CrossRef]
7. Siasos, G.; Skotsimara, G.; Oikonomou, E.; Sagris, M.; Vasiliki-Chara, M.; Bletsa, E.; Stampouloglou, P.; Theofilis, P.; Charalampous, G.; Tousoulis, D. Antithrombotic Treatment in Diabetes Mellitus: A Review of the Literature about Antiplatelet and Anticoagulation Strategies Used for Diabetic Patients in Primary and Secondary Prevention. *Curr. Pharm. Des.* **2020**, *26*, 2780–2788. [CrossRef]
8. Mahmood, S.S.; Levy, D.; Vasan, R.S.; Wang, T.J. The Framingham Heart Study and the epidemiology of cardiovascular disease: A historical perspective. *Lancet* **2014**, *383*, 999–1008. [CrossRef]
9. Nattel, S. Molecular and Cellular Mechanisms of Atrial Fibrosis in Atrial Fibrillation. *JACC Clin. Electrophysiol.* **2017**, *3*, 425–435. [CrossRef]
10. Spencer, T.M.; Blumenstein, R.F.; Pryse, K.M.; Lee, S.-L.; Glaubke, D.A.; Carlson, B.E.; Elson, E.L.; Genin, G.M. Fibroblasts Slow Conduction Velocity in a Reconstituted Tissue Model of Fibrotic Cardiomyopathy. *ACS Biomater. Sci. Eng.* **2017**, *3*, 3022–3028. [CrossRef] [PubMed]
11. Burstein, B.; Nattel, S. Atrial fibrosis: Mechanisms and clinical relevance in atrial fibrillation. *J. Am. Coll. Cardiol.* **2008**, *51*, 802–809. [CrossRef] [PubMed]
12. Hinderer, S.; Schenke-Layland, K. Cardiac fibrosis—A short review of causes and therapeutic strategies. *Adv. Drug Deliv. Rev.* **2019**, *146*, 77–82. [CrossRef]
13. Yao, C.; Veleva, T.; Scott, L., Jr.; Cao, S.; Li, L.; Chen, G.; Jeyabal, P.; Pan, X.; Alsina, K.M.; Abu-Taha, I.D.; et al. Enhanced Cardiomyocyte NLRP3 Inflammasome Signaling Promotes Atrial Fibrillation. *Circulation* **2018**, *138*, 2227–2242. [CrossRef]
14. Nattel, S. Electrical coupling between cardiomyocytes and fibroblasts: Experimental testing of a challenging and important concept. *Cardiovasc. Res.* **2018**, *114*, 349–352. [CrossRef]
15. Davis, J.; Burr, A.R.; Davis, G.F.; Birnbaumer, L.; Molkentin, J.D. A TRPC6-Dependent Pathway for Myofibroblast Transdifferentiation and Wound Healing In Vivo. *Dev. Cell* **2012**, *23*, 705–715. [CrossRef]

16. Hoyles, R.K.; Derrett-Smith, E.C.; Khan, K.; Shiwen, X.; Howat, S.L.; Wells, A.U.; Abraham, D.J.; Denton, C.P. An Essential Role for Resident Fibroblasts in Experimental Lung Fibrosis Is Defined by Lineage-Specific Deletion of High-Affinity Type II Transforming Growth Factor β Receptor. *Am. J. Respir. Crit. Care Med.* **2011**, *183*, 249–261. [CrossRef] [PubMed]
17. Leask, A. Potential Therapeutic Targets for Cardiac Fibrosis. *Circ. Res.* **2010**, *106*, 1675–1680. [CrossRef]
18. Davis, J.; Molkentin, J.D. Myofibroblasts: Trust your heart and let fate decide. *J. Mol. Cell Cardiol.* **2014**, *70*, 9–18. [CrossRef]
19. Lu, H.; Tian, A.; Wu, J.; Yang, C.; Xing, R.; Jia, P.; Yang, L.; Zhang, Y.; Zheng, X.; Li, Z. Danshensu Inhibits β-Adrenergic Receptors-Mediated Cardiac Fibrosis by ROS/p38 MAPK Axis. *Biol. Pharm. Bull.* **2014**, *37*, 961–967. [CrossRef] [PubMed]
20. Gibb, A.A.; Lazaropoulos, M.P.; Elrod, J.W. Myofibroblasts and Fibrosis. *Circ. Res.* **2020**, *127*, 427–447. [CrossRef]
21. Pellman, J.; Zhang, J.; Sheikh, F. Myocyte-fibroblast communication in cardiac fibrosis and arrhythmias: Mechanisms and model systems. *J. Mol. Cell Cardiol.* **2016**, *94*, 22–31. [CrossRef]
22. Theofilis, P.; Sagris, M.; Antonopoulos, A.S.; Oikonomou, E.; Tsioufis, C.; Tousoulis, D. Inflammatory Mediators of Platelet Activation: Focus on Atherosclerosis and COVID-19. *Int. J. Mol. Sci.* **2021**, *22*, 1170. [CrossRef]
23. Kim, P.; Chu, N.; Davis, J.; Kim, D.H. Mechanoregulation of Myofibroblast Fate and Cardiac Fibrosis. *Adv. Biosyst* **2018**, *2*. [CrossRef]
24. Zaidi, Y.; Aguilar, E.G.; Troncoso, M.; Ilatovskaya, D.V.; DeLeon-Pennell, K.Y. Immune regulation of cardiac fibrosis post myocardial infarction. *Cell Signal.* **2021**, *77*, 109837. [CrossRef] [PubMed]
25. Shiota, N.; Jin, D.; Takai, S.; Kawamura, T.; Koyama, M.; Nakamura, N.; Miyazaki, M. Chymase is activated in the hamster heart following ventricular fibrosis during the chronic stage of hypertension. *FEBS Lett.* **1997**, *406*, 301–304. [CrossRef]
26. Ahmad, S.; Varagic, J.; Westwood, B.M.; Chappell, M.C.; Ferrario, C.M. Uptake and Metabolism of the Novel Peptide Angiotensin-(1-12) by Neonatal Cardiac Myocytes. *PLoS ONE* **2011**, *6*, e15759. [CrossRef] [PubMed]
27. Balcells, E.; Meng, Q.C.; Walter, H.; Johnson, J.; Oparil, S.; Dell'Italia, L.J. Angiotensin II formation from ACE and chymase in human and animal hearts: Methods and species considerations. *Am. J. Physiol. Heart Circ. Physiol.* **1997**, *273*, H1769–H1774. [CrossRef]
28. Shimizu, M.; Tanaka, R.; Fukuyama, T.; Aoki, R.; Orito, K.; Yamane, Y. Cardiac Remodeling and Angiotensin II-Forming Enzyme Activity of the Left Ventricle in Hamsters with Chronic Pressure Overload Induced by Ascending Aortic Stenosis. *J. Vet. Med Sci.* **2006**, *68*, 271–276. [CrossRef] [PubMed]
29. McLarty, J.L.; Meléndez, G.C.; Brower, G.L.; Janicki, J.S.; Levick, S.P. Tryptase/Protease-Activated Receptor 2 Interactions Induce Selective Mitogen-Activated Protein Kinase Signaling and Collagen Synthesis by Cardiac Fibroblasts. *Hypertension* **2011**, *58*, 264–270. [CrossRef] [PubMed]
30. Zeng, Z.; Shen, L.; Li, X.; Luo, T.; Wei, X.; Zhang, J.; Cao, S.; Huang, X.; Fukushima, Y.; Bin, J.; et al. Disruption of histamine H2 receptor slows heart failure progression through reducing myocardial apoptosis and fibrosis. *Clin. Sci.* **2014**, *127*, 435–448. [CrossRef] [PubMed]
31. Morgan, L.G.; Levick, S.P.; Voloshenyuk, T.G.; Murray, D.B.; Forman, M.F.; Brower, G.L.; Janicki, J.S. A novel technique for isolating functional mast cells from the heart. *Inflamm Res.* **2008**, *57*, 241–246. [CrossRef]
32. Nattel, S. How does fibrosis promote atrial fibrillation persistence: In silico findings, clinical observations, and experimental data. *Cardiovasc. Res.* **2016**, *110*, 295–297. [CrossRef] [PubMed]
33. Allessie, M.A.; de Groot, N.M.; Houben, R.P.; Schotten, U.; Boersma, E.; Smeets, J.L.; Crijns, H.J. Electropathological substrate of long-standing persistent atrial fibrillation in patients with structural heart disease: Longitudinal dissociation. *Circ. Arrhythm Electrophysiol.* **2010**, *3*, 606–615. [CrossRef] [PubMed]
34. Krul, S.P.; Berger, W.R.; Smit, N.W.; van Amersfoorth, S.C.; Driessen, A.H.; van Boven, W.J.; Fiolet, J.W.; van Ginneken, A.C.; van der Wal, A.C.; de Bakker, J.M.; et al. Atrial fibrosis and conduction slowing in the left atrial appendage of patients undergoing thoracoscopic surgical pulmonary vein isolation for atrial fibrillation. *Circ. Arrhythm Electrophysiol.* **2015**, *8*, 288–295. [CrossRef]
35. Hansen, B.J.; Zhao, J.; Csepe, T.A.; Moore, B.T.; Li, N.; Jayne, L.A.; Kalyanasundaram, A.; Lim, P.; Bratasz, A.; Powell, K.A.; et al. Atrial fibrillation driven by micro-anatomic intramural re-entry revealed by simultaneous sub-epicardial and sub-endocardial optical mapping in explanted human hearts. *Eur. Heart J.* **2015**, *36*, 2390–2401. [CrossRef]
36. Samman Tahhan, A.; Sandesara, P.B.; Hayek, S.S.; Alkhoder, A.; Chivukula, K.; Hammadah, M.; Mohamed-Kelli, H.; O'Neal, W.T.; Topel, M.; Ghasemzadeh, N.; et al. Association between oxidative stress and atrial fibrillation. *Heart Rhythm.* **2017**, *14*, 1849–1855. [CrossRef]
37. Sovari, A.A.; Dudley, S.C., Jr. Reactive oxygen species-targeted therapeutic interventions for atrial fibrillation. *Front. Physiol.* **2012**, *3*, 311. [CrossRef] [PubMed]
38. Xie, W.; Santulli, G.; Reiken, S.R.; Yuan, Q.; Osborne, B.W.; Chen, B.-X.; Marks, A.R. Mitochondrial oxidative stress promotes atrial fibrillation. *Sci. Rep.* **2015**, *5*, 11427. [CrossRef]
39. Yoo, S.; Aistrup, G.; Shiferaw, Y.; Ng, J.; Mohler, P.J.; Hund, T.J.; Waugh, T.; Browne, S.; Gussak, G.; Gilani, M.; et al. Oxidative stress creates a unique, CaMKII-mediated substrate for atrial fibrillation in heart failure. *JCI Insight* **2018**, *3*. [CrossRef] [PubMed]
40. Shan, J.; Xie, W.; Betzenhauser, M.; Reiken, S.; Chen, B.X.; Wronska, A.; Marks, A.R. Calcium leak through ryanodine receptors leads to atrial fibrillation in 3 mouse models of catecholaminergic polymorphic ventricular tachycardia. *Circ. Res.* **2012**, *111*, 708–717. [CrossRef] [PubMed]
41. Babusikova, E.; Kaplan, P.; Lehotsky, J.; Jesenak, M.; Dobrota, D. Oxidative modification of rat cardiac mitochondrial membranes and myofibrils by hydroxyl radicals. *Gen. Physiol. Biophys.* **2004**, *23*, 327–335.

42. Conen, D.; Ridker, P.M.; Everett, B.M.; Tedrow, U.B.; Rose, L.; Cook, N.R.; Buring, J.E.; Albert, C.M. A multimarker approach to assess the influence of inflammation on the incidence of atrial fibrillation in women. *Eur. Heart J.* **2010**, *31*, 1730–1736. [CrossRef] [PubMed]
43. Kallergis, E.M.; Manios, E.G.; Kanoupakis, E.M.; Mavrakis, H.E.; Kolyvaki, S.G.; Lyrarakis, G.M.; Chlouverakis, G.I.; Vardas, P.E. The role of the post-cardioversion time course of hs-CRP levels in clarifying the relationship between inflammation and persistence of atrial fibrillation. *Heart* **2008**, *94*, 200–204. [CrossRef]
44. Rotter, M.; Jaïs, P.; Vergnes, M.-C.; Nurden, P.; Takahashi, Y.; Sanders, P.; Rostock, T.; Hocini, M.; Sacher, F.; Haïssaguerre, M. Decline in C-Reactive Protein After Successful Ablation of Long-Lasting Persistent Atrial Fibrillation. *J. Am. Coll. Cardiol.* **2006**, *47*, 1231–1233. [CrossRef]
45. Mouselimis, D.; Tsarouchas, A.S.; Pagourelias, E.D.; Bakogiannis, C.; Theofilogiannakos, E.K.; Loutradis, C.; Fragakis, N.; Vassilikos, V.P.; Papadopoulos, C.E. Left atrial strain, intervendor variability, and atrial fibrillation recurrence after catheter ablation: A systematic review and meta-analysis. *Hellenic J. Cardiol.* **2020**, *61*, 154–164. [CrossRef]
46. Gao, G.; Dudley, S.C., Jr. Redox regulation, NF-kappaB, and atrial fibrillation. *Antioxid Redox Signal.* **2009**, *11*, 2265–2277. [CrossRef] [PubMed]
47. Theofilis, P.; Sagris, M.; Oikonomou, E.; Antonopoulos, A.S.; Siasos, G.; Tsioufis, C.; Tousoulis, D. Inflammatory Mechanisms Contributing to Endothelial Dysfunction. *Biomedicines* **2021**, *9*, 781. [CrossRef] [PubMed]
48. Satou, R.; Penrose, H.; Navar, L.G. Inflammation as a Regulator of the Renin-Angiotensin System and Blood Pressure. *Curr. Hypertens. Rep.* **2018**, *20*, 100. [CrossRef]
49. Liang, F.; Wang, Y. Coronary heart disease and atrial fibrillation: A vicious cycle. *Am. J. Physiol. Heart Circ. Physiol.* **2021**, *320*, H1–H12. [CrossRef] [PubMed]
50. Aronson, D.; Boulos, M.; Suleiman, A.; Bidoosi, S.; Agmon, Y.; Kapeliovich, M.; Beyar, R.; Markiewicz, W.; Hammerman, H.; Suleiman, M. Relation of C-reactive protein and new-onset atrial fibrillation in patients with acute myocardial infarction. *Am. J. Cardiol.* **2007**, *100*, 753–757. [CrossRef]
51. Marcus, G.M.; Whooley, M.A.; Glidden, D.V.; Pawlikowska, L.; Zaroff, J.G.; Olgin, J.E. Interleukin-6 and atrial fibrillation in patients with coronary artery disease: Data from the Heart and Soul Study. *Am. Heart J.* **2008**, *155*, 303–309. [CrossRef]
52. Zhang, P.; Shao, L.; Ma, J. Toll-Like Receptors 2 and 4 Predict New-Onset Atrial Fibrillation in Acute Myocardial Infarction Patients. *Int. Heart J.* **2018**, *59*, 64–70. [CrossRef]
53. Xu, Y.; Sharma, D.; Du, F.; Liu, Y. The role of Toll-like receptor 2 and hypoxia-induced transcription factor-1α in the atrial structural remodeling of non-valvular atrial fibrillation. *Int. J. Cardiol.* **2013**, *168*, 2940–2941. [CrossRef] [PubMed]
54. Maehama, T.; Okura, H.; Imai, K.; Saito, K.; Yamada, R.; Koyama, T.; Hayashida, A.; Neishi, Y.; Kawamoto, T.; Yoshida, K. Systemic inflammation and left atrial thrombus in patients with non-rheumatic atrial fibrillation. *J. Cardiol.* **2010**, *56*, 118–124. [CrossRef] [PubMed]
55. Kaski, J.C.; Arrebola-Moreno, A.L. Inflamación y trombosis en la fibrilación auricular. *Rev. Esp. Cardiol.* **2011**, *64*, 551–553. [CrossRef]
56. Shantsila, E.; Lip, G.Y. The role of monocytes in thrombotic disorders. Insights from tissue factor, monocyte-platelet aggregates and novel mechanisms. *Thromb. Haemost.* **2009**, *102*, 916–924. [CrossRef] [PubMed]
57. Nair, G.M.; Nery, P.B.; Redpath, C.J.; Birnie, D.H. The Role Of Renin Angiotensin System In Atrial Fibrillation. *J. Atr. Fibrillation* **2014**, *6*, 972. [CrossRef] [PubMed]
58. Sagris, M.; Theofilis, P.; Antonopoulos, A.S.; Tsioufis, C.; Oikonomou, E.; Antoniades, C.; Crea, F.; Kaski, J.C.; Tousoulis, D. Inflammatory Mechanisms in COVID-19 and Atherosclerosis: Current Pharmaceutical Perspectives. *Int. J. Mol. Sci.* **2021**, *22*, 6607. [CrossRef]
59. Liu, K.; Daviglus, M.L.; Loria, C.M.; Colangelo, L.A.; Spring, B.; Moller, A.C.; Lloyd-Jones, D.M. Healthy lifestyle through young adulthood and the presence of low cardiovascular disease risk profile in middle age: The Coronary Artery Risk Development in (Young) Adults (CARDIA) study. *Circulation* **2012**, *125*, 996–1004. [CrossRef] [PubMed]
60. Chaugai, S.; Meng, W.Y.; Ali Sepehry, A. Effects of RAAS Blockers on Atrial Fibrillation Prophylaxis: An Updated Systematic Review and Meta-Analysis of Randomized Controlled Trials. *J. Cardiovasc. Pharmacol. Ther.* **2016**, *21*, 388–404. [CrossRef] [PubMed]
61. Yamauchi, F.I.; Castro, A. Obesity, adiposopathy, and quantitative imaging biomarkers. *Radiol. Bras.* **2017**, *50*, VII–VIII. [CrossRef] [PubMed]
62. Ogunmoroti, O.; Michos, E.D.; Aronis, K.N.; Salami, J.A.; Blankstein, R.; Virani, S.S.; Spatz, E.S.; Allen, N.B.; Rana, J.S.; Blumenthal, R.S.; et al. Life's Simple 7 and the risk of atrial fibrillation: The Multi-Ethnic Study of Atherosclerosis. *Atherosclerosis* **2018**, *275*, 174–181. [CrossRef]
63. Sagris, M.; Kokkinidis, D.G.; Lempesis, I.G.; Giannopoulos, S.; Rallidis, L.; Mena-Hurtado, C.; Bakoyiannis, C. Nutrition, dietary habits, and weight management to prevent and treat patients with peripheral artery disease. *Rev. Cardiovasc. Med.* **2020**, *21*, 565–575. [CrossRef] [PubMed]
64. Carter, S.; Hartman, Y.; Holder, S.; Thijssen, D.H.; Hopkins, N.D. Sedentary Behavior and Cardiovascular Disease Risk: Mediating Mechanisms. *Exerc. Sport Sci. Rev.* **2017**, *45*, 80–86. [CrossRef] [PubMed]
65. Zhang, N.; Andresen, B.T.; Zhang, C. Inflammation and reactive oxygen species in cardiovascular disease. *World J. Cardiol.* **2010**, *2*, 408–410. [CrossRef]

66. Abed, H.S.; Wittert, G.A.; Leong, D.P.; Shirazi, M.G.; Bahrami, B.; Middeldorp, M.E.; Lorimer, M.F.; Lau, D.H.; Antic, N.A.; Brooks, A.G.; et al. Effect of weight reduction and cardiometabolic risk factor management on symptom burden and severity in patients with atrial fibrillation: A randomized clinical trial. *JAMA* **2013**, *310*, 2050–2060. [CrossRef]
67. Sagris, M.; Giannopoulos, S.; Giannopoulos, S.; Tzoumas, A.; Texakalidis, P.; Charisis, N.; Kokkinidis, D.G.; Malgor, R.D.; Mouawad, N.J.; Bakoyiannis, C. Transcervical carotid artery revascularization: A systematic review and meta-analysis of outcomes. *J. Vasc. Surg.* **2021**, *74*, 657–665.e12. [CrossRef]
68. Lavie, C.J.; Pandey, A.; Lau, D.H.; Alpert, M.A.; Sanders, P. Obesity and Atrial Fibrillation Prevalence, Pathogenesis, and Prognosis: Effects of Weight Loss and Exercise. *J. Am. Coll. Cardiol.* **2017**, *70*, 2022–2035. [CrossRef]
69. Davi, G.; Falco, A. Oxidant stress, inflammation and atherogenesis. *Lupus* **2005**, *14*, 760–764. [CrossRef]
70. Larsson, S.C.; Drca, N.; Wolk, A. Alcohol consumption and risk of atrial fibrillation: A prospective study and dose-response meta-analysis. *J. Am. Coll. Cardiol.* **2014**, *64*, 281–289. [CrossRef]
71. Ariansen, I.; Reims, H.M.; Gjesdal, K.; Olsen, M.H.; Ibsen, H.; Devereux, R.B.; Okin, P.M.; Kjeldsen, S.E.; Dahlof, B.; Wachtell, K. Impact of alcohol habits and smoking on the risk of new-onset atrial fibrillation in hypertensive patients with ECG left ventricular hypertrophy: The LIFE study. *Blood Press* **2012**, *21*, 6–11. [CrossRef]
72. Di Castelnuovo, A.; Costanzo, S.; Bonaccio, M.; Rago, L.; De Curtis, A.; Persichillo, M.; Bracone, F.; Olivieri, M.; Cerletti, C.; Donati, M.B.; et al. Moderate Alcohol Consumption Is Associated With Lower Risk for Heart Failure But Not Atrial Fibrillation. *JACC Heart Fail.* **2017**, *5*, 837–844. [CrossRef] [PubMed]
73. Baczko, I.; Light, P.E. Resveratrol and derivatives for the treatment of atrial fibrillation. *Ann. N. Y. Acad. Sci.* **2015**, *1348*, 68–74. [CrossRef]
74. Stephan, L.S.; Almeida, E.D.; Markoski, M.M.; Garavaglia, J.; Marcadenti, A. Red Wine, Resveratrol and Atrial Fibrillation. *Nutrients* **2017**, *9*, 1190. [CrossRef]
75. Kawada, T. Caffeine Consumption and Atrial Fibrillation: A Risk Assessment. *Cardiology* **2019**, *142*, 194. [CrossRef] [PubMed]
76. Xu, J.; Fan, W.; Budoff, M.J.; Heckbert, S.R.; Amsterdam, E.A.; Alonso, A.; Wong, N.D. Intermittent Nonhabitual Coffee Consumption and Risk of Atrial Fibrillation: The Multi-Ethnic Study of Atherosclerosis. *J. Atr. Fibrillation* **2019**, *12*, 2205. [CrossRef] [PubMed]
77. Cheng, M.; Hu, Z.; Lu, X.; Huang, J.; Gu, D. Caffeine intake and atrial fibrillation incidence: Dose response meta-analysis of prospective cohort studies. *Can. J. Cardiol.* **2014**, *30*, 448–454. [CrossRef] [PubMed]
78. Bodar, V.; Chen, J.; Gaziano, J.M.; Albert, C.; Djousse, L. Coffee Consumption and Risk of Atrial Fibrillation in the Physicians' Health Study. *J. Am. Heart Assoc.* **2019**, *8*, e011346. [CrossRef]
79. Casiglia, E.; Tikhonoff, V.; Albertini, F.; Gasparotti, F.; Mazza, A.; Montagnana, M.; Danese, E.; Benati, M.; Spinella, P.; Palatini, P. Caffeine intake reduces incident atrial fibrillation at a population level. *Eur. J. Prev. Cardiol.* **2018**, *25*, 1055–1062. [CrossRef] [PubMed]
80. Abdelfattah, R.; Kamran, H.; Lazar, J.; Kassotis, J. Does Caffeine Consumption Increase the Risk of New-Onset Atrial Fibrillation? *Cardiology* **2018**, *140*, 106–114. [CrossRef]
81. Pastori, D.; Carnevale, R.; Bartimoccia, S.; Nocella, C.; Tanzilli, G.; Cangemi, R.; Vicario, T.; Catena, M.; Violi, F.; Pignatelli, P. Does Mediterranean Diet Reduce Cardiovascular Events and Oxidative Stress in Atrial Fibrillation? *Antioxid Redox Signal.* **2015**, *23*, 682–687. [CrossRef]
82. Huang, W.L.; Yang, J.; Yang, J.; Wang, H.B.; Yang, C.J.; Yang, Y. Vitamin D and new-onset atrial fibrillation: A meta-analysis of randomized controlled trials. *Hellenic J. Cardiol.* **2018**, *59*, 72–77. [CrossRef] [PubMed]
83. Pastori, D.; Carnevale, R.; Menichelli, D.; Nocella, C.; Bartimoccia, S.; Novo, M.; Leo, I.; Violi, F.; Pignatelli, P. Is There an Interplay Between Adherence to Mediterranean Diet, Antioxidant Status, and Vascular Disease in Atrial Fibrillation Patients? *Antioxid Redox Signal.* **2016**, *25*, 751–755. [CrossRef]
84. Pignatelli, P.; Pastori, D.; Farcomeni, A.; Nocella, C.; Bartimoccia, S.; Vicario, T.; Bucci, T.; Carnevale, R.; Violi, F. Mediterranean diet reduces thromboxane A2 production in atrial fibrillation patients. *Clin. Nutr.* **2015**, *34*, 899–903. [CrossRef]
85. Pastori, D.; Carnevale, R.; Nocella, C.; Novo, M.; Santulli, M.; Cammisotto, V.; Menichelli, D.; Pignatelli, P.; Violi, F. Gut-Derived Serum Lipopolysaccharide is Associated With Enhanced Risk of Major Adverse Cardiovascular Events in Atrial Fibrillation: Effect of Adherence to Mediterranean Diet. *J. Am. Heart Assoc.* **2017**, *6*. [CrossRef] [PubMed]
86. Larsson, S.C.; Drca, N.; Michaelsson, K. Serum Magnesium and Calcium Levels and Risk of Atrial Fibrillation. *Circ. Genom. Precis. Med.* **2019**, *12*, e002349. [CrossRef]
87. Storz, M.A.; Helle, P. Atrial fibrillation risk factor management with a plant-based diet: A review. *J. Arrhythm.* **2019**, *35*, 781–788. [CrossRef]
88. Dinesen, P.T.; Joensen, A.M.; Rix, T.A.; Tjonneland, A.; Schmidt, E.B.; Lundbye-Christensen, S.; Overvad, K. Effect of Dietary Intake of Saturated Fatty Acids on the Development of Atrial Fibrillation and the Effect of Replacement of Saturated With Monounsaturated and Polyunsaturated Fatty Acids. *Am. J. Cardiol.* **2017**, *120*, 1129–1132. [CrossRef] [PubMed]
89. Mortensen, L.M.; Lundbye-Christensen, S.; Schmidt, E.B.; Calder, P.C.; Schierup, M.H.; Tjonneland, A.; Parner, E.T.; Overvad, K. Long-chain n-3 and n-6 polyunsaturated fatty acids and risk of atrial fibrillation: Results from a Danish cohort study. *PLoS ONE* **2017**, *12*, e0190262. [CrossRef]
90. Larsson, S.C.; Wolk, A. Fish, long-chain omega-3 polyunsaturated fatty acid intake and incidence of atrial fibrillation: A pooled analysis of two prospective studies. *Clin. Nutr.* **2017**, *36*, 537–541. [CrossRef]

91. Li, F.R.; Chen, G.C.; Qin, J.; Wu, X. DietaryFish and Long-Chain n-3 Polyunsaturated Fatty Acids Intake and Risk of Atrial Fibrillation: A Meta-Analysis. *Nutrients* **2017**, *9*, 955. [CrossRef]
92. Nattel, S.; Dobrev, D. Electrophysiological and molecular mechanisms of paroxysmal atrial fibrillation. *Nat. Rev. Cardiol.* **2016**, *13*, 575–590. [CrossRef] [PubMed]
93. Levin, M.G.; Judy, R.; Gill, D.; Vujkovic, M.; Verma, S.S.; Bradford, Y.; Regeneron Genetics, C.; Ritchie, M.D.; Hyman, M.C.; Nazarian, S.; et al. Genetics of height and risk of atrial fibrillation: A Mendelian randomization study. *PLoS Med.* **2020**, *17*, e1003288. [CrossRef]
94. Ebana, Y.; Furukawa, T. Networking analysis on superior vena cava arrhythmogenicity in atrial fibrillation. *Int. J. Cardiol. Heart Vasc.* **2019**, *22*, 150–153. [CrossRef]
95. Ebana, Y.; Nitta, J.; Takahashi, Y.; Miyazaki, S.; Suzuki, M.; Liu, L.; Hirao, K.; Kanda, E.; Isobe, M.; Furukawa, T. Association of the Clinical and Genetic Factors With Superior Vena Cava Arrhythmogenicity in Atrial Fibrillation. *Circ. J.* **2017**, *82*, 71–77. [CrossRef] [PubMed]
96. Low, S.K.; Takahashi, A.; Ebana, Y.; Ozaki, K.; Christophersen, I.E.; Ellinor, P.T.; Consortium, A.F.; Ogishima, S.; Yamamoto, M.; Satoh, M.; et al. Identification of six new genetic loci associated with atrial fibrillation in the Japanese population. *Nat. Genet.* **2017**, *49*, 953–958. [CrossRef]
97. Lee, J.Y.; Kim, T.H.; Yang, P.S.; Lim, H.E.; Choi, E.K.; Shim, J.; Shin, E.; Uhm, J.S.; Kim, J.S.; Joung, B.; et al. Korean atrial fibrillation network genome-wide association study for early-onset atrial fibrillation identifies novel susceptibility loci. *Eur. Heart J.* **2017**, *38*, 2586–2594. [CrossRef]
98. Mechakra, A.; Footz, T.; Walter, M.; Aranega, A.; Hernandez-Torres, F.; Morel, E.; Millat, G.; Yang, Y.Q.; Chahine, M.; Chevalier, P.; et al. A Novel PITX2c Gain-of-Function Mutation, p.Met207Val, in Patients With Familial Atrial Fibrillation. *Am. J. Cardiol.* **2019**, *123*, 787–793. [CrossRef] [PubMed]
99. Tao, Y.; Zhang, M.; Li, L.; Bai, Y.; Zhou, Y.; Moon, A.M.; Kaminski, H.J.; Martin, J.F. Pitx2, an atrial fibrillation predisposition gene, directly regulates ion transport and intercalated disc genes. *Circ. Cardiovasc. Genet.* **2014**, *7*, 23–32. [CrossRef]
100. Syeda, F.; Kirchhof, P.; Fabritz, L. PITX2-dependent gene regulation in atrial fibrillation and rhythm control. *J. Physiol.* **2017**, *595*, 4019–4026. [CrossRef]
101. Adam, O.; Lohfelm, B.; Thum, T.; Gupta, S.K.; Puhl, S.L.; Schafers, H.J.; Bohm, M.; Laufs, U. Role of miR-21 in the pathogenesis of atrial fibrosis. *Basic Res. Cardiol.* **2012**, *107*, 278. [CrossRef]
102. Mase, M.; Grasso, M.; Avogaro, L.; Nicolussi Giacomaz, M.; D'Amato, E.; Tessarolo, F.; Graffigna, A.; Denti, M.A.; Ravelli, F. Upregulation of miR-133b and miR-328 in Patients With Atrial Dilatation: Implications for Stretch-Induced Atrial Fibrillation. *Front. Physiol.* **2019**, *10*, 1133. [CrossRef] [PubMed]
103. Shen, N.N.; Zhang, C.; Li, Z.; Kong, L.C.; Wang, X.H.; Gu, Z.C.; Wang, J.L. MicroRNA expression signatures of atrial fibrillation: The critical systematic review and bioinformatics analysis. *Exp. Biol. Med.* **2020**, *245*, 42–53. [CrossRef]
104. Zhelankin, A.V.; Vasiliev, S.V.; Stonogina, D.A.; Babalyan, K.A.; Sharova, E.I.; Doludin, Y.V.; Shchekochikhin, D.Y.; Generozov, E.V.; Akselrod, A.S. Elevated Plasma Levels of Circulating Extracellular miR-320a-3p in Patients with Paroxysmal Atrial Fibrillation. *Int. J. Mol. Sci.* **2020**, *21*, 3485. [CrossRef]
105. Alonso, A.; Krijthe, B.P.; Aspelund, T.; Stepas, K.A.; Pencina, M.J.; Moser, C.B.; Sinner, M.F.; Sotoodehnia, N.; Fontes, J.D.; Janssens, A.C.; et al. Simple risk model predicts incidence of atrial fibrillation in a racially and geographically diverse population: The CHARGE-AF consortium. *J. Am. Heart Assoc.* **2013**, *2*, e000102. [CrossRef] [PubMed]
106. Hindricks, G.; Potpara, T.; Dagres, N.; Arbelo, E.; Bax, J.J.; Blomstrom-Lundqvist, C.; Boriani, G.; Castella, M.; Dan, G.A.; Dilaveris, P.E.; et al. 2020 ESC Guidelines for the diagnosis and management of atrial fibrillation developed in collaboration with the European Association for Cardio-Thoracic Surgery (EACTS): The Task Force for the diagnosis and management of atrial fibrillation of the European Society of Cardiology (ESC) Developed with the special contribution of the European Heart Rhythm Association (EHRA) of the ESC. *Eur. Heart J.* **2021**, *42*, 373–498. [CrossRef] [PubMed]
107. Schnabel, R.B.; Sullivan, L.M.; Levy, D.; Pencina, M.J.; Massaro, J.M.; D'Agostino, R.B., Sr.; Newton-Cheh, C.; Yamamoto, J.F.; Magnani, J.W.; Tadros, T.M.; et al. Development of a risk score for atrial fibrillation (Framingham Heart Study): A community-based cohort study. *Lancet* **2009**, *373*, 739–745. [CrossRef]
108. Khatib, R.; Joseph, P.; Briel, M.; Yusuf, S.; Healey, J. Blockade of the renin-angiotensin-aldosterone system (RAAS) for primary prevention of non-valvular atrial fibrillation: A systematic review and meta analysis of randomized controlled trials. *Int. J. Cardiol.* **2013**, *165*, 17–24. [CrossRef]
109. Kumagai, K.; Nakashima, H.; Urata, H.; Gondo, N.; Arakawa, K.; Saku, K. Effects of angiotensin II type 1 receptor antagonist on electrical and structural remodeling in atrial fibrillation. *J. Am. Coll. Cardiol.* **2003**, *41*, 2197–2204. [CrossRef]
110. Bonora, B.M.; Raschi, E.; Avogaro, A.; Fadini, G.P. SGLT-2 inhibitors and atrial fibrillation in the Food and Drug Administration adverse event reporting system. *Cardiovasc. Diabetol.* **2021**, *20*, 39. [CrossRef] [PubMed]
111. Dobrev, D.; Potpara, T.S. Smart device-based detection of atrial fibrillation: Opportunities and challenges in the emerging world of digital health. *Int. J. Cardiol.* **2020**, *302*, 108–109. [CrossRef] [PubMed]
112. Seshadri, D.R.; Bittel, B.; Browsky, D.; Houghtaling, P.; Drummond, C.K.; Desai, M.Y.; Gillinov, A.M. Accuracy of Apple Watch for Detection of Atrial Fibrillation. *Circulation* **2020**, *141*, 702–703. [CrossRef] [PubMed]
113. Roselli, C.; Rienstra, M.; Ellinor, P.T. Genetics of Atrial Fibrillation in 2020: GWAS, Genome Sequencing, Polygenic Risk, and Beyond. *Circ. Res.* **2020**, *127*, 21–33. [CrossRef] [PubMed]

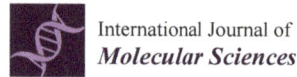 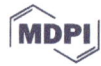

Review

Therapies for the Treatment of Cardiovascular Disease Associated with Type 2 Diabetes and Dyslipidemia

María Aguilar-Ballester [1,†], Gema Hurtado-Genovés [1,†], Alida Taberner-Cortés [1,†], Andrea Herrero-Cervera [1], Sergio Martínez-Hervás [1,2,3,4,*] and Herminia González-Navarro [1,4,*]

1. Health Research Institute Clinic Hospital of Valencia-INCLIVA, 46010 Valencia, Spain; abama4@alumni.uv.es (M.A.-B.); gehurge@alumni.uv.es (G.H.-G.); altacor@doctor.upv.es (A.T.-C.); anhecer@alumni.uv.es (A.H.-C.)
2. Endocrinology and Nutrition Service, Clinic Hospital of Valencia, 46010 Valencia, Spain
3. Department of Medicine, University of Valencia, 46010 Valencia, Spain
4. CIBERDEM (Diabetes and Associated Metabolic Diseases), 28029 Madrid, Spain
* Correspondence: sergio.martinez@uv.es (S.M.-H.); herminia.gonzalez@uv.es (H.G.-N.); Tel.: +34-963864403 (H.G.-N.); Fax: +34-963987860 (H.G.-N.)
† Equal contribution.

Abstract: Cardiovascular disease (CVD) is the leading cause of death worldwide and is the clinical manifestation of the atherosclerosis. Elevated LDL-cholesterol levels are the first line of therapy but the increasing prevalence in type 2 diabetes mellitus (T2DM) has positioned the cardiometabolic risk as the most relevant parameter for treatment. Therefore, the control of this risk, characterized by dyslipidemia, hypertension, obesity, and insulin resistance, has become a major goal in many experimental and clinical studies in the context of CVD. In the present review, we summarized experimental studies and clinical trials of recent anti-diabetic and lipid-lowering therapies targeted to reduce CVD. Specifically, incretin-based therapies, sodium-glucose co-transporter 2 inhibitors, and proprotein convertase subtilisin kexin 9 inactivating therapies are described. Moreover, the novel molecular mechanisms explaining the CVD protection of the drugs reviewed here indicate major effects on vascular cells, inflammatory cells, and cardiomyocytes, beyond their expected anti-diabetic and lipid-lowering control. The revealed key mechanism is a prevention of acute cardiovascular events by restraining atherosclerosis at early stages, with decreased leukocyte adhesion, recruitment, and foam cell formation, and increased plaque stability and diminished necrotic core in advanced plaques. These emergent cardiometabolic therapies have a promising future to reduce CVD burden.

Keywords: cardiometabolic risk; incretin system; dipeptidyl peptidase 4; sodium-glucose-co- transporter 2 inhibitors; proprotein convertase subtilisin kexin 9

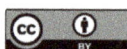

1. Introduction

Despite the existence of different cardiometabolic drugs, cardiovascular disease (CVD) remains the first cause of death worldwide [1]. A main classical risk factor is elevated blood levels of LDL-cholesterol (LDL-C) in the blood which are closely related to atherosclerosis [2], and constitute the first line of therapy [3]. However, the change in lifestyle patterns that promotes sedentarism and an aging of the population have raised the incidence of type 2 diabetes (T2DM), thus becoming a major emergent risk. T2DM features are frequently associated with hypercholesterolemia, dyslipidemia, hypertension, and obesity which altogether represent a cardiometabolic risk whose main complication is the atherosclerotic disease [4].

In recent decades, several mechanisms have been shown to contribute to aggravating atherosclerosis in T2DM patients [5]. Insulin resistance (IR) which plays a pivotal role in the onset of T2DM, increases endothelial cell (EC) dysfunction by diminishing the bioavailability of vasodilators like nitric oxide (NO) [6]. Other mechanisms include IR induced apoptosis in macrophages [4] and reduced survival in vascular smooth muscle cells (VSMC) [7] in lesions. Notably, these seem to be due to inflammatory signaling pathways that promote plaque instability and rupture [4,7,8]. Moreover, hyperglycemia contributes to glucotoxicity and exerts in the vascular bed a proatherogenic synergistic effect alongside dyslipidemia and hypertension. These and other mechanistic studies led to the hypothesis that anti-diabetic drugs might exert atheroprotection by acting directly in vascular cells, prompting many experimental studies and clinical trials to study the expanded use of these drug therapies in additional cardiovascular contexts [9,10].

In the following sections, we will summarize the main current strategies for the management of carbohydrate and lipid metabolism and their relationship with CVD. These include incretin-based therapies, sodium-glucose co-transporter 2 inhibitors (SGLT2i), and proprotein convertase subtilisin kexin 9 (PCSK9) inhibitors. A schematic summary of clinical trials over the years is displayed in Figure 1.

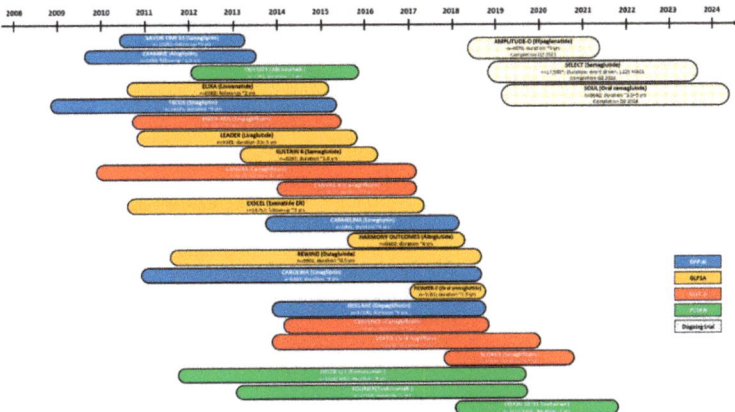

Figure 1. Clinical trials with cardiovascular end-points for T2DM patients in trials for incretin-based and SGLT2i therapies and with LDL-C percentage change from baseline end-points for trials testing PCSK9i. Based on https://clinicaltrials.gov/ct2/home (accessed 10 December 2020).

2. Therapies Based on the Incretin System

2.1. Biology of the Incretins

Incretin hormones are small gut-derived peptides secreted by the endocrine cells of the intestine, mainly in the postprandial state, with potent insulinotropic actions. There are two main incretin hormones, the glucose-dependent insulinotropic polypeptide (GIP), secreted by the enteroendocrine K cells, and the glucagon-like peptide 1 (GLP1), secreted by the gut L cells of the distal small intestine and large bowel [11,12].

GLP1 is produced in response to nutrient intake, mainly sugars and fat, and its two active forms are the GLP1-(7–37) and the GLP1-(7–36)NH(2) generated by selective cleavage of the proglucagon molecule [13]. The GLP1 hormone exerts its effects through the GLP1 receptor (GLP1R) located in the gastrointestinal tract and pancreatic β-cells. However, it is also found in the heart, VSMCs, EC, immune cells, lung, kidney, and nervous system [13]. This protein is a G coupled receptor that mediates GLP1 actions to modulate glucose levels and body weight [13]. In β-cells GLP1 promotes the de novo synthesis and secretion of insulin by increasing cAMP and intracellular calcium levels. GLP1 also enhances β-cell number and mass through β-cell proliferation and neogenesis and decreases glucagon secretion in a glucose-dependent fashion that prevents hypoglycemia. These actions are concomitant to a reduction in food intake, gastric emptying, nutrient absorption and disposal, reduction of appetite by stimulation of the brain satiety center, and enhanced insulin sensitivity in periphery tissues [11]. GLP1 hormone is present at low concentrations in the circulation in fasting and inter-prandial state but, within minutes of food intake, its levels rise up to 2–3 times leading to postprandial insulin secretion [13]. GLP1 in the circulation has a very short half-life and, within 1.5 to 5 min, it is rapidly degraded by the dipeptidyl peptidase 4 (DPP4) into smaller peptides whose functions are not fully understood [14].

GIP production in the enteroendocrine K-cells of the proximal small intestine is mediated by the prohormone convertase (PC) one-third to a full-length peptide form. Alternatively, GIP can be processed by the PC2 to a C-terminal truncated form named GIP(1-30) [11] and it can be secreted under carbohydrate and fat regulation. In β-cells, GIP promotes insulin secretion by increasing cAMP and calcium intracellular levels and by regulating volatage-potassium Kv channel expression. Since its receptor, GIPR, is expressed in multiple tissues—such as the pancreas, gastrointestinal tract, adipose tissue, heart, testis, bone, lung, adrenal cortex, and central nervous system—other effects are under study. In the pancreas, GIP and GLP1 functions overlap, although inactivation of GIP in mice leads to impaired glucose tolerance and insulin release, hence indicating its metabolic relevance [11].

2.2. Degradation of the Incretins by Dipeptidyl Peptidase 4 (DPP4)

GLP1 and GIP incretins are cleaved by DPP4 during the passage across the hepatic bed. They are further processed in peripheral tissues into smaller metabolites to be finally eliminated by the kidney. DPP4, also known as CD26, is a transmembrane cell surface glycoprotein that cleaves N-terminal dipeptides position, mostly from GLP1 and GIP, thus holding an important antihyperglycemic effect. DPP4 is mainly expressed in exocrine glands and absorptive epithelium, hepatocytes, fibroblasts, leukocytes, and epithelial cells of the kidney and intestine [15]. It can be found membrane-bound or soluble.

DPP4 is also an adipokine produced by proteolytic cleavage from fully differentiated adipocytes [16] in some settings. Its production correlates with the degree of IR, inflammation, adipocyte size, and the amount of visceral adipose tissue (VAT) [16,17]. Both insulin and TNFα increase up to 50% the release of soluble DPP4 and it is believed to participate in the crosstalk between adipocytes, macrophages, and the inflamed stroma-vascular fraction [16]. DPP4 levels increase with insulin and leptin and inversely correlate with age and adiponectin levels [16,18].

Consistently, rats with genetic DPP4 deficiency, such as the strain F344/DuCrj or Dark Agouti rats, display improved IR, glucose tolerance, lipid profile, and enhanced GLP1 activity. Likewise, DPP4-deficent mice have enhanced glucose tolerance, glucose-stimulated insulin, and GLP1 release, and improved insulin sensitivity and liver homeostasis [19]. Dendritic cells (DC) and macrophages from VAT, in mice and humans, exhibit elevated DPP4 levels which promote T cell activation, proliferation, and inflammation [20]. In ECs, DPP4 promotes T cell transendothelial migration [21] and in human VSMCs promotes inflammation. Hepatic DPP4 secretion is elevated in obesity and IR while specific hepatic DPP4 deletion through a short hairpin RNA (shRNA) strategy diminished adipose tissue macrophage infiltration and IR [22]. In agreement with these studies, T2DM patients also display reduced levels of GLP1 hormone and enhanced DPP4 in the circulation, and IR correlates with the levels of DPP4 released by adipose tissue depots [23].

Altogether indicates that incretin-based therapies display anti-inflammatory and cardiovascular benefits by mechanisms independently from their glucose-lowering effect. Soluble DDP4 has been shown to induce VSMC proliferation by activating mitogen-activated protein kinases (MAPK)-pathway and the nuclear factor kappa B (NF-κB)-mediated inflammation [24]. Likewise, GLP1 hormone activates thymocytes and T cell proliferation and maintains regulatory T cells [25]. Because of this, they have been tested as therapeutic drugs for the treatment of CVD in T2DM patients. Currently, there are two different strategies to increase the benefits of the incretin system: (1) inhibition of the peptidase DPP4 and (2) the use of GLP1 and GIP incretin analogues [26].

2.3. DPP4 Inhibitors as a Therapeutic Target for T2DM

The gliptins are a family of DPP4 inhibitors developed as glucose-lowering agents that increase the half-life and bioavailability of the GLP1 incretin. These display fewer adverse side effects [27] and a low incidence of hypoglycemia [18]. The gliptins can be peptidomimetics and non-peptidomimetics, and both are extracellular competitive reversible inhibitors of the DPP4 substrate. These two groups differ in their half-lives, the strength of the effect, and therapeutic dose being the most currently prescribed: sitagliptin [28] saxagliptin [29], alogliptin [30], linagliptin [18,31], vildagliptin [32], anagliptin, and teneligliptin [18].

Most of them have shown a low frequency of hypoglycemia, pancreatitis, and pancreatic carcinoma, and no effects on heart failure (HF) rate or major adverse cardiovascular events (MACE) effects [27] except for alogliptin [30] and saxagliptin [29], which increase the rate of HF.

2.4. Effects of DPP4 Inhibitors in CVD

Although the initial rational for DPP4 inhibition is the subsequent increase in GLP1 effects, other independent mechanisms have been reported. Thus, beneficial effects have been reported in adipose tissue, vascular ECs, and monocyte/macrophages during atherosclerosis and myocardial injury in preclinical studies as described below, some of them summarized in [33]. In Table 1, a description of the mechanisms found in the preclinical animal model studies and the effects on atherosclerosis are included for incretin-therapies.

Table 1. Preclinical studies of incretin-based therapies in animal models of atherosclerosis, vascular injury, and myocardial infarction.

Animal Model	Incretin Therapy	Mechanism of Action	Reported Effects	References
Apoe-/- mice	DPP4i Anagliptin	Suppressed VSMCs proliferation and macrophages inflammatory responses	Restrained atherosclerosis	[34]
	DPP4i Linagliptin+HFD	Anti-inflammatory phenotype of macrophages	Improved atherosclerosis	[35]
	GIP active forms	Decreased VSMCs proliferation, monocyte infiltration, foam cell formation and related genes (*Cd36*, *Acat1*), and NF-kB-mediated inflammation in macrophages	Stabilization of atherosclerotic plaque	[36]
	GIP and GLP1	Suppressed foam cell formation	Reduced atheroma plaque	[37]
	Liraglutide	Suppressed *Acat1* expression and foam cell formation	Decreased atherosclerosis	[38]
		Anti-inflammatory macrophage polarization	Reduced atherosclerosis	[39]
	Exenatide+CS	Reduced oxidative stress and inflammation	Reduced plaque	[40]
	Exendin-4	Reduced monocyte adhesion and pro-inflammatory cytokines via cAMP/PKA pathway	Decreased lesion size	[41]
APOE*3-Leiden.CETP mice	Exendin-4	Decreased monocyte recruitment and adhesion and foam cell formation	Reduced atherosclerotic lesions	[42]

Table 1. Cont.

Animal Model	Incretin Therapy	Mechanism of Action	Reported Effects	References
Apoe-/-Irs2+/- mice	Liraglutide Lixisenatide	STAT3-mediated macrophage polarization to an anti-inflammatory phenotype	Decreased atherosclerosis, necrotic core	[43]
Apoe-/- and Ldlr-/- mice	Liraglutide Semaglutide+WD	Changes in inflammatory markers	Reduced lesion size	[44]
Lldr-/- mice	DPP4i	Decreased pro-inflammatory genes expression and macrophage content	Decreased plaque size	[45]
Arterial hypertension Angiotensin II-mouse model	Liraglutide	Reduced leukocyte rolling and neutrophils infiltration	—	[46]
C57Bl6 mice	Liraglutide+45% HFD	Reduced eNOS expression and ER-stress response	Reduced cardiac fibrosis, hypertrophy, and necrosis	[47]
Myocardial injury mouse model	Liraglutide	Enhanced GSK3β, PPARβ-δ, Nrf-2, and HO-1 genes	Reduced mortality, infarct size, and rupture	[48]
Ischemia-reperfusion injury rats	Lixisenatide	—	Reduced infarct-size, improved cardiac function	[49]
Restenosis mouse/rat model	Lixisenatide Exendin-4	Reduced VSMC proliferation	Neointimal hyperplasia	[50]
Diabetic rats	Liraglutide	Decreased macrophage ER-stress-induced secretion of microvesicles	Diminished atherosclerosis and intima thickening	[51]
Diabetic rats	GLP1+adenovirus-mediated delivery	Reduced VSMC and monocyte migration and inflammation	Reduced intima thickening	[52]
Rabbits	DPP4i Anagliptin+CD	Reduced macrophage infiltration	Restrained atherosclerosis	[53]
WHHL rabbits	Lixisenatide	Reduced macrophage, calcium deposition, necrosis	Prevention of plaque growth and instability	[54]

ACAT1: acetyl-CoA acetyltransferase; CD: cholesterol diet; CS: chronic stress; eNOS: endothelial nitric oxide synthase; ER: endoplasmatic reticulum; HFD: high fat diet; VSMCs: vascular smooth muscle cells; WD: western diet; WHHL: Watanabe heritable hyperlipidemic.

2.4.1. Mechanisms of Gliptins in Experimental Atherosclerosis

High levels of soluble DPP4 are found in atherosclerosis and many studies have shown that its inhibition results in restrained atherosclerosis progression (Table 1).

Combination of DPP4 inhibitors with granulocyte-colony-stimulating factor (G-CSF) have shown protection against cardiovascular injury by increasing the number of endothelial stem cell and improving cardiac function [25]. The mechanism was an inhibition of DPP4-mediated degradation of the chemokine stromal cell-derived factor-1α (SDF-1α) which promotes endothelial progenitor cells (EPC) bone marrow mobilization to sites of cellular injury [55,56]. In this sense, SDF engineered to be DPP4-resistant showed improved blood flow in an animal model of peripheral artery disease [25].

In human umbilical vein endothelial cells (HUVECs), alogliptin induces endothelial nitric oxide synthase (eNOS), and AKT phosphorylation leading to enhanced NO production and improved homeostasis [24]. Likewise, alogliptin also promoted vascular relaxation via eNOS production of NO and endothelial-derived hyperpolarizing factor-mediated mechanisms [55]. Ex vivo DPP4 inhibition of human arteries from patients undergoing coronary artery bypass surgery reduced vascular oxidative stress and improved endothelial function [57]. DPP4 inhibitor treatment of HUVECs cultured under hypoxic condition prevented apoptosis in a CXCR4/STAT3-dependent manner [58].

In VSMCs, DPP4 activates MAPK and NF-κB increasing proliferation and production of iNOS proinflammatory cytokines [24]. Consistently, in *Apoe-/-* mice, anagliptin restrained atherosclerosis by suppressing VSMC proliferation [34].

DPP4 inhibition also modulates immune cells and inflammation. In diabetic patients, DPP4 inhibitors treatment resulted in a reduced production of reactive oxygen species and inflammatory mediators TNFα, JNK1, TLR2, TLR4, IL1β, and SOCS3 by monocytes [25]. DPP4 is highly expressed in bone marrow-derived CD11b+ cells. In *Lldr-/-* mice, DPP4 inhibitors downregulated proinflammatory genes and diminished aortic plaque macrophage content and lesion size [45]. In agreement with these results, treatment with linagliptin of high-fat diet-fed *Apoe-/-* mice, ameliorated atherosclerosis by inducing an anti-inflammatory phenotype in macrophages [35]. Likewise, anagliptin treatment restrained atherosclerosis by reducing macrophage plaque infiltration in cholesterol-fed rabbits [53] and suppressed inflammatory responses in macrophages in *Apoe-/-* mice [34].

In T cells, the non-cleaved membrane-bound DPP4 interacts with the T cell receptor (TCR)/CD3, promoting the phosphorylation cascade and antigen-presenting cell interactions engaging NF-κB inflammatory pathway activation [17].

2.4.2. Clinical Studies on DPP4 Inhibitors in T2DM with CVD

Both sitagliptin and anagliptin are being evaluated in clinical trials for their potential in the regulation of lipid metabolism and CVD in T2DM patients (Table 2). Anagliptin has been shown to decrease LDL-C triglycerides, total cholesterol, and non-HDL-C levels in a mechanism independent from its hypoglycemic effects [59]. Other gliptins increase adiponectin levels and reduce intestinal cholesterol absorption [18].

Table 2. Clinical trials of incretin-based therapies.

Incretin-Therapy	Clinical Trial	Patients	Reported Effects	References
DPP4i saxagliptin	SAVOR-TIMI 53 [NCT01107866]	T2DM patients with CV risk	-Unaffected CV risk -Increased HF hospitalization rate	[29]
DPP4i alogliptin	EXAMINE [NCT00968708]	T2DM patients with ACS	-Unaffected CV death and hospital admission for HF	[30]
DPP4i sitagliptin	TECOS [NCT00790205]	T2DM patients with established CVD	-Unaffected MACE or hospitalization for HF risk	[60]
DPP4i Linagliptin	CAROLINA [NCT01243424]	T2DM patients and CV risk	-Unaffected CV risk	[61]
	CARMELINA [NCT01897532]	T2DM patients and CV risk and kidney disease	-Unaffected HF incidence -No influence of kidney disease -Reduced albuminuria	[31,62]
Lixisenatide (exendin-4 based)	ELIXA [NCT01147250]	T2DM patients with a recent ACS	-No effects on MACE, hospitalization for HF -Decreased SBP and heart rate	[63]
Exenatide (exendin-4 synthetic)	EXSCEL [NCT01144338]	T2DM patients with or without CVD	-Unaffected incidence of MACE, retinopathy or renal outcomes -Modest reduction in SBP but increased heart rate	[64]
			-Modest reduction in CV risk	[65]

Table 2. Cont.

Incretin-Therapy	Clinical Trial	Patients	Reported Effects	References
Liraglutide (human GLP1A)	LEADER [NCT01179048]	T2DM patients at high CV risk	-Reduced rates of MACE and death -Reduced SBP and microvascular renal and retinal complications -Enhanced heart rate	[66]
			-Same benefits for polyvascular and single vascular disease	[67]
			-Reduced CV outcomes (MI/stroke) and CVD	[68]
			-Unaffected HF hospitalization and death risk after MI	[69]
			-Decreased rates of diabetic kidney disease	[70]
Semaglutide (human GLP1A)	SUSTAIN-6 [NCT01720446]	T2DM patients at high CV risk	-Reduced rates of CV death and non-fatal MI/stroke -Decreased SBP but enhanced mean pulse rate	[71]
	PIONEER 6 [NCT02692716]	T2DM patients with high CV risk	-Unaffected CV risk -Decreased SBP and LDL-C -Gastrointestinal adverse events	[72]
Albiglutide (modified human GLP1)	Harmony Outcomes [NCT02465515]	T2DM and CVD patients	-Decreased SBP but augmented heart rate -improved glomerular filtration rate -Reduced risk of MACE -Unaffected CV death	[73]
Dulaglutide (modified human GLP1)	REWIND [NCT01394952]	T2DM patients at high CV risk	-Unaffected all-cause mortality rate -Decreased SBP, pulse pressure and arterial pressure but enhanced heart rate -Reduced risk of CV outcomes, total CV, or fatal event burden	[74,75]
Dulaglutide (modified human GLP-1) and tirzepatide (LY3298176)	SURPASS-CVOT [NCT04255433]	T2DM patients with atherosclerotic CVD	Estimated completion date: October 2024	https://clinicaltrials.gov/NCT04255433
Efpeglenatide	AMPLITUDE-O [NCT03496298]	T2DM patients with high CDV risk	Estimated completion date: April 2021	https://clinicaltrials.gov/NCT03496298
NNC0090-2746 (RG7697) [NCT02205528]	Phase 2 trial	T2DM patients	-Improved glycemia control -Diminished body weight, cholesterol, and leptin.	[76]
Tirzepatide (LY3298176) [NCT03131687]	Phase 2 trial	T2DM patients	-Improved glycemic and body weight control -Enhanced pulse rate -Acceptable safety and tolerability profile	[77,78]

ACS: acute coronary syndrome; HF: heart failure; CV: cardiovascular; CVD: cardiovascular disease; DBP: Diastolic blood pressure; LDL-C: low density lipoprotein cholesterol; MACE: major adverse cardiovascular events; MI: myocardial infarction; SBP: systolic blood pressure; T2DM: type 2 diabetes mellitus.

Over the years, the cardiosafety of DPP4 inhibitors in T2DM patients with high cardiovascular risk has been confirmed in several clinical trials (Table 2). The SAVOR-TIMI 53 trial [29], the EXAMINE trial [30], the TECOS trial [60], and the CAROLINA [61] and CARMELINA [31,62] trials, that evaluated saxagliptin, alogliptin, sitagliptin, and linagliptin treatment, respectively, are considered the most important. Nevertheless, no cardiovascular benefits were reported in comparison with the placebo group. In fact, in the SAVOR-TIMI 53 trial, an increase in the rate of HF in patients with no previous history, was detected in the treated groups. The SAVOR-TIMI 53 trial [29], the EXAMINE trial [30] and TECOS trial [60] showed very low frequencies of hypoglycemia, pancreatitis, and pancreatic carcinoma [27]. However, the CARMELINA trial did not detect any effect on kidney disease or cardiovascular and kidney events.

2.5. GLP1 Analogues as Therapeutic Strategies

2.5.1. Development of Drugs Based on GLP1 and Rational Design

Given that GLP1 stimulates insulin secretion, soon after its discovery, this incretin became useful for T2DM treatment [79]. The native peptide has no clinical applicability due to its short plasma life-time of less than 2 min [80]. Therefore, the GLP1 analogues (GLP1A) approved for clinical use [81] are either derivatives of the human native GLP1, with chemical modifications to increase its stability and half-life [82] or peptides based on exendin-4. Exendin-4 is a GLP1A peptide isolated from the saliva of the lizard *Heloderma suspectum* [83], whose an amino acidic identity of 53% to the mammalian GLP1 that allows it to bind to the human GLP1 receptor [11].

Exenatide was the first GLP1A approved in 2005 and it is a synthetic version of the exendin-4. It has a half-life of up to 2.4 h, 10 times longer than endogenous GLP1, because its resistance to human DPP4 degradation [81,82]. Since the first generated GLP1As have a subcutaneous administration twice daily, other compounds have been developed to extend durability [84]. The optimization approach was addressed to keep the human GLP1 backbone to avoid immunogenic problems [84] and to get DPP4 action resistance through GLP1-(7-36) region modifications [26,81]. These modifications consist in the replacement of the penultimate alanine at the N-terminal end of the peptide by a glycine, serine, D-alanine, or by the most optimal chemical group, aminoisobutyric acid (Aib) [80], since it does not interfere with GLP1 receptor binding [85]. Other modifications were a replacement of the histidine residue at the N-terminal end by a glucitol group or by performing a deamination [80]. To increase the GLP1 half-life, the addition of fatty acids to the C-terminal domain was also performed to allow binding to the albumin and protection to renal filtration [26,86].

By combining all of the above-mentioned modifications, the approved GLP1As were designed and generated progressively over time: liraglutide (2009), exenatide (2005) and exenatide once-weekly (2011), lixisenatide (2013), albiglutide (2014) dulaglutide (2014), and semaglutide (2017), whose specific modifications can be found elsewhere [79,81].

These compounds have shown favorable effects in experimental and clinical studies with the limitation of parenteral administration [26,82]. Therefore, current research is focused on developing novel small GLP1As to be administered orally [26,84]. Among these, oral semaglutide stands out, which is a small acetylated peptide [79] whose oral daily administration has recently been approved in combination with sodium N-(8-(2-hydroxybenzoyl) amino) caprylate (SNAC) [84].

2.5.2. Studies in Preclinical Models of T2DM, Atherosclerosis, and CVD

As summarized in Table 1, studies in rodents and rabbits have shown beneficial actions of GLP1As in atherosclerosis, vascular injury, and cardiac function. Liraglutide treatment in diabetic rats led to diminished atherosclerotic lesion formation and intima-media thickening through a decrease of macrophage secretion of ER-stress induced microvesicles [51]. Similarly, the expression of GLP1 by adenovirus-mediated delivery in diabetic rats reduced intima-media thickening, VSMC and monocyte migration, and inflammatory processes [52].

In *Apoe-/-* mice, treatment with both native GIP and GLP1 incretins diminished atherosclerosis by suppressing macrophage foam cell formation [37]. In *Apoe-/-* mice liraglutide suppressed acyl-coenzyme A *cholesterol acyltransferase* 1 (*Acat*1) expression, foam cell formation and decreased atherosclerosis [38], and inhibited progression of early-onset atherosclerosis lesions in a GLP1R-dependent fashion [87]. Liraglutide administration also improved cardiac function through reduced cardiac fibrosis, hypertrophy, and necrosis by ameliorating endothelial NOS expression and ER-stress response in 45% high-fat diet (HFD) fed C57Bl6 mice [47].

Studies conducted by us have shown diminished atherosclerosis by lixisenatide and liraglutide in a mouse model of atherosclerosis and IR, the *Apoe-/-Irs2+/-* mice. Moreover, lixisenatide generated more stable plaques with thicker fibrous caps, smaller necrotic cores, and reduced inflammatory cell infiltration [43]. Lixisenatide also promoted macrophage polarization toward a pro-resolving phenotype in a STAT3-dependent manner [43]. A similar mechanism was found in *Apoe-/-* mice where liraglutide modulated polarization of macrophages toward a pro-resolving phenotype too [39]. Likewise, exenatide exerted protective effects in cultured macrophages via STAT3 activation which promoted adiponectin secretion when co-cultured with 3T3-L1 adipocytes [88]. In another investigation, liraglutide, and semaglutide treatments reduced lesion development in both *Apoe-/-* and *Low density lipoprotein-deficient* (*Ldlr-/-*) mice fed western diet, through major changes in inflammatory markers in aortic tissue [44]. Similarly, exenatide beneficial effects in atherosclerosis in *Apoe-/-* mice were attributed to reduced plaque oxidative stress, inflammation, and proteolysis in mice under chronic stress [40]. In the same line of results, lixisenatide treatment of Watanabe heritable hyperlipidemic (WHHL) rabbits prevented plaque growth and instability by decreasing macrophage infiltration, calcium deposition, and necrosis, as well as increased fibrotic content in VSMC-rich plaques [54]. On the other hand, exendin-4 treatment also decreased lesion size in *Apoe-/-* mice through a reduction of monocyte adhesion and expression of pro-inflammatory cytokines in activated macrophages via cAMP/PKA pathway [41]. Exendin-4 also diminished liver inflammation and atherosclerotic lesions through monocyte/macrophage recruitment and adhesion, and foam cell formation in the atherosclerotic mouse model *APOE*3-Leiden.CETP* [42].

In in vitro studies, treatment of HUVECs with exendin-4 [89] or liraglutide [90] incremented the activity, phosphorylation, and protein levels of eNOS, thus protecting against proatherosclerotic factors [89,90]. Besides, liraglutide in HUVECs diminished high-glucose-induced NF-kB phosphorylation and associated endothelial dysfunction [90]. Liraglutide also alleviated TNFα and LPS-mediated monocyte adhesion in cultured human aortic endothelial cells (HAECs) by increasing Ca^{2+} and CAMKKβ/AMPK activities and diminishing E-selectin and VCAM1 expression [91]. On the other hand, exendin-4 reversed glucolipotoxic gene dysregulation in diabetic human coronary artery endothelial cells (HCAECs) by upregulating eNOS and proangiogenic genes, while downregulating inflammatory, prothrombotic, and apoptosis genes [92].

In ischemia-reperfusion injury rat models (Table 1), prolonged treatment with lixisenatide reduced infarct-size and improved cardiac function [49]. Furthermore, in restenosis mouse and rat models, exendin-4 and lixisenatide reduced VSMC proliferation and neointimal hyperplasia, respectively [50]. In a mouse model of myocardial injury, liraglutide pretreatment reduced mortality and infarct size by enhancing cardioprotective genes such as PPARβ-δ, Nrf-2, and HO-1. Moreover, liraglutide-treated cardiomyocytes displayed diminished caspase-3 activation and increased cAMP production [48]. In another study, which employed an arterial hypertension angiotensin II-mouse model, liraglutide reduced leukocyte rolling and infiltration of myeloid neutrophils into the vascular wall [46].

2.5.3. Clinical Studies on GLP1-Based Strategies in T2DM with CVD

Many clinical trials based on GLP1 analogues have been designed to approve their use in CVD complications in T2DM subjects (Table 2).

In the ELIXA (Evaluation of Lixisenatide in Acute Coronary Syndrome [NCT01147250]) trial, T2DM patients with a recent acute coronary syndrome were enrolled to test a daily injection of lixisenatide, an exendin-4-based analogue, for 25 months. Results showed no effects on MACE or other serious adverse events in T2DM patients who had recently suffered an acute coronary event [63]. The HF hospitalization rates and death remained unchanged but systolic blood pressure (SBP) and heart rate were reduced [63].

The effect on cardiovascular events of weekly injections of exenatide, another exendin-4 based analogue, was evaluated in the EXSCEL [NCT01144338] clinical trial. The study included T2DM patients of which 70% exhibited CVD and 30% did not displayed any CVD. In this study CVD was defined as atherosclerosis peripheral artery disease, coronary artery disease or stroke. The follow-up of patients, which were randomly treated with once-weekly exenatide (2 mg) or placebo for 5 years, did not show differences in MACE. A modest decrease in SBP and LDL-C was seen but treated patients also showed enhanced heart rate. The lack of effect was related to a shorter follow-up period and lower glycated hemoglobin baseline levels in the patients that in the other trials [64]. Once-weekly exenatide did not affect retinopathy or renal outcomes and produced a modest reduction in CV risk in subjects with mild loss of kidney function (estimated glomerular filtration rate, eGFR $\geq$ 60 mL/min/1.73 m^2) [65].

In the LEADER (Liraglutide Effect and Action in Diabetes: Evaluation of Cardiovascular Outcome Results [NCT01179048]) clinical trial, the human GLP1-based analogue liraglutide or placebo were administered once daily as a subcutaneous injections to T2DM patients at high cardiovascular risk with a median follow-up of 3.8 years. In the first analysis, the treated group had lower rates of cardiovascular events and death from any cause but they also suffered more episodes of gallstone disease. The liraglutide group displayed a reduced risk of MACE, defined as cardiovascular death, non-fatal stroke, and non-fatal, first or recurrent MI. Analysis of vascular function showed decreased SBP and microvascular retinal and renal complications but also augmented DBP and heart rate [66]. A second analysis of this trial indicated the same benefits for polyvascular and single vascular disease in T2DM patients, independently of a previous history of MI [67]. In a posthoc analysis which took into account T2DM patients with high cardiovascular risk—due to MI, stroke, or atherosclerosis—liraglutide reduced cariovascular outcomes [68]. In another analysis of the LEADER trial, there was no evidence of decreased cardiovascular outcomes in patients with MI treated with liraglutide [69]. In a third clinical study, liraglutide treatment in T2DM patients resulted in a lower rate of diabetic kidney disease development and progression than placebo [70].

Likewise, semaglutide, whose structure is also based on human GLP1, injected once-weekly at two doses (0.5 mg or 1.0 mg) for 104 weeks in the SUSTAIN-6 trial (NCT01720446) reduced the rate of cardiovascular death and non-fatal MI and stroke in patients with T2DM at high cardiovascular risk. Consistent with the other GLP1A, SBP was reduced but mean pulse rate enhanced [71]. However, in the PIONEER 6 (NCT02692716) trial, once-daily oral semaglutide did not alter the cardiovascular risk profile of T2DM patients at high cardiovascular risk, but decreaed SBP and LDL-C parameters. Moreover, gastrointestinal adverse events were more common in patients receiving oral semaglutide than patients with placebo [72].

Another chemical variant of human GLP1, albiglutide, which consists of two tandem copies of modified human GLP1 bound to human albumin, showed increased effectivity due to its long-acting effect. In the Harmony Outcomes (NCT02465515) clinical trial, albiglutide in subjects of 40 or more years of age with T2DM and CVD, showed reduced MACE, SBP, and improved glomerular filtration rate in a follow up of 1.6 years. However, no effect was observed in death from cardiovascular causes [73].

A long-acting GLP1A, called dulaglutide, has also been generated. This analogue is the human GLP1 peptide covalently linked to a Fc fragment of a human IgG4 that protects against DPP4 degradation. The REWIND (NCT01394952) clinical trial, which tested weekly subcutaneous injection of dulaglutide in T2DM patients with a previous cardiovascular event or cardiovascular risk factors, showed no effect in all-cause mortality rate but reduced the risk of CV outcomes, SBP, pulse and arterial pressure although increased heart rate [74]. A subsequent analysis showed that weekly subcutaneous dulaglutide injections reduced total cardiovascular or fatal event burden [75].

Ongoing clinical trials are the SURPASS-CVOT (NCT04255433) with an estimated enrollment of 12,500 participants and the AMPLITUDE-O (NCT03496298) with 4076 patients. In the first trial, the effect in MACE of two incretins, tirzepatide (LY3298176) and dulaglutide is being compared in T2DM patients and the completion date of the study is in October 2024 (https://clinicaltrials.gov/NCT04255433). The second trial studies the effect of efpeglenatide in T2DM patients at high CVD risk and its estimated completion date is April 2021 (https://clinicaltrials.gov/NCT03496298).

2.6. GIP1 Emergent Therapies

2.6.1. Development of Drugs Based on GIP and Rational Design

Currently, there are no clinical therapies using GIPR agonists [93]. Experimental results of GLP1R/GIPR dual co-agonists derived from intermixed incretin sequence have shown augmented antihyperglycemic and insulinotropic effect compared with specific GLP1 agonist in *db/db* mice, ZDF diabetic rats, monkeys and humans [94,95]. Moreover, these dual agonists have been shown to reduce plasma biomarkers of cardiovascular risk in diet-induced obese mice [95,96].

2.6.2. Investigations of GIP Therapies in Preclinical Models

GIP has been related to different signalling pathways in vascular cells with both anti-atherogenic via NO production, or pro-atherogenic effects through increased endothelin-1 and VSMCs osteopontin expression [93]. In HUVECs cultures GIP/GIPR and GLP1/GLP1R interactions reduce the advanced glycation end products (AGEs) receptor (RAGE) expression, blocking the signalling pathways associated with diabetes-associated vascular damage [97].

On the other hand, as shown in Table 1, GIPR levels are diminished in diabetic experimental models and consequently, administration of GIP in *Apoe-/-* and *db/db* diabetic mice reduced atherosclerotic plaque lesions and foam cell formation [37,98]. Furthermore, the administration of GIP active forms to *Apoe-/-* mice increased atherosclerotic collagen content [36], suppressed VSMCs proliferation and reduced aortic endothelial expression of MCP1, VCAM1, ICAM1, and PAI1 [37,93] and monocyte migration and macrophage activation in a NFkB-dependent manner [36]. Other observed actions are the blocking of proinflammatory monocyte aortic infiltration, the decrease in *Cd36* and *Acat1* expression, foam cell formation, LPS-induced IL-6 secretion, and MMP-9 activity [36,37,93].

2.6.3. Studies in Humans with T2DM and CVD

GIP serum levels are elevated in patients with atherosclerotic vascular disease [36]. In humans, physiological doses of GIP increased heart rate, arterial blood pressure, and blood levels of osteopontin CCL8 and CCL2, accordingly with reduced CCL2/CCR2-mediated migration of cultured human monocytes (THP-1 cells) [93].

GLP1R/GIPR co-agonist NNC0090-2746 tested in T2DM patients in a randomized, placebo-controlled, double-blind phase 2 trial, administered subcutaneously once a day, showed an important effect in glycemia control and diminished body weight, cholesterol levels, and leptin [76] (Table 1). On the other hand, the dual co-agonist LY3298176 (tirzepatide) biased towards GIPR agonism obtained promising results as antidiabetic treatments in T2DM clinical trials as it showed improvements in glycemic and body weight control although is also showed an increased pulse rate [77,78,96]. Further research is needed about their cardioprotective effects, while interest in new GLP1R/GIPR co-agonists development increases [94].

3. Therapies to Inhibit Sodium-Glucose Co-Transporter 2

3.1. Structure of Sodium-Glucose Co-Transporters and Mechanism of Action

Human sodium-glucose co-transporters (SGLTs), encoded by *SLC5*, are a family of 12 secondary active glucose transporters, being the SGLT1 and SGLT2 the most important. The core domain structure of this LeuT-superfamily is a five-helix inverted repeat motif [99,100] with a substrate-binding site in the middle of the protein and with an outer and an inner gate. Glucose adsorption by SGLT1 mostly takes place in the intestine and SGLT2 plays a key role in the renal glucose reabsorption with a highly similar sodium-coupled sugar transport mechanism.

SGLTs transport glucose across the brush-border membrane of the proximal renal tubule segments. SGLT2 mostly located in the S1 segment accounts for up to 90% of glucose reabsorption and SGLT1 in the S3 segment accounts for 10% of reabsorption [100,101]. The transport mechanism consists of Na^+ binding to the transporter in the apical side of the epithelial cells, the opening of the external gate and glucose binding. This is followed by the closing of the external gate, the opening of the inner gate, the release of both substrates to the cytosolic side of the cell and the adoption of the ligand-free conformation [101,102]. Through the basolateral membrane of the epithelial cells, GLUT2 transporters and Na^+/K^+ pump alleviate the intracellular accumulation of sodium and glucose by delivering both molecules in the blood.

3.2. Development of SGLT Inhibitors

The rational for developing SGLT2 inhibitors (SGLT2i) is the existence of up to 50 human mutations of SGLT2 resulting in renal glucosuria and important urinary glucose losses. These suggested that SGLT2i could be of use for hyperglycemic states such as T2DM patients [103].

Phlorizin, a glucoside of phloretin found in the apple tree, was the lead of the SGLT inhibitors as studies on IR diabetic rats showed that its administration subcutaneously normalized plasma glucose profiles and insulin sensitivity [104]. Because of its poor solubility, low bioavailability, and unselective SGLT1/2 inhibition, it was set aside as a therapeutic candidate. Their synthetic derivates, T-1095A and T-1095, had better results though their clinical development did not continue because of the same limitations [103,105].

Novel molecules with a C-glycosylation modification that conferred the phlorizin resistance to hydrolysis by endogenous β-glucosidases, increasing their half-life, were developed [103]. Selective SGLT2i based on this meta-C-glycosylated diarylmethane pharmacophore led to dapagliflozin, canagliflozin, empagliflozin, and ertugliflozin. The gliflozins have a higher selectivity profiles for SGLT2 over SGLT1, except for sotagliflozin with a selectivity for SGLT1 of about 20:1. Sergliflozin is another SGLT2i based on benzylphenol glucoside that did not undergo further development after phase II (https://adisinsight.springer.com/search). Others SGLT2i are ipragliflozin, tofogliflozin, and luseogliflozin, which are approved and available in Japan [106].

Effects of gliflozins also include actions on pancreatic islet cells and modulation of endogenous glucose production in insulin-sensitive tissues. Hence, empagliflozin treatment of T2DM subjects improved β-cell function [107], while dapagliflozin affects glucagon secretion by α-cells [108]. Moreover, T2DM patients treated with dapagliflozin and empagliflozin have shown an endogenous production of glucose and improved insulin sensitivity [107,109].

3.3. Effect of Gliflozins in Preclinical Models of CVD

Tahara et al. [110] studied different gliflozins (dapagliflozin, empagliflozin, canagliflozin, luseogliflozin, ipragliflozin, tofogliflozin) in KK/Ay T2DM mice (Table 3). The treatment with these gliflozins decreased hyperglycemia, lowered plasma levels of inflammatory mediators and improved endothelial dysfunction associated with human atherosclerosis.

Table 3. Summary of the studies about the effect of SGLT2i in preclinical animal models and in clinical trials of T2DM patients.

Drug	Animal Model	Effect on Lipids	Effect on Atherosclerosis	References
Dapagliflozin	KK/A^y mice	Decreased T-Chol, TG, and NEFAs (ipragliflozin and dapagliflozin)	-Decreased ED (CAMs and E-selectin) and plasmatic inflammatory parameters	[110]
Ipragliflozin				
Canagliflozin				
Luseogliflozin				
Empagliflozin				
Tofogliflozin				
Empagliflozin	db/db mice	No change in TG and T-Chol	-Reduced aortic and endothelial cell stiffness	[111]
Empagliflozin	ZDF rats	No change in TG, T-Chol, HDL, and LDL	-Reduced oxidative stress and inflammation -ED partially prevented	[112]
Dapagliflozin	db/db mice	—	-Lower arterial stiffness -Improved ED and VSMC dysfunction	[113]
Ipragliflozin Dapagliflozin	STZ Apoe-/- mice db/db mice	No changes in TG, HDL and T-chol	-Dapagliflozin decreased macrophage infiltration, atherosclerotic lesions and plaque size -Ipragliflozin decreased foam cell formation	[114]
Dapagliflozin	Apoe-/- mice	—	-Attenuated ED and VCAMs expression -Induced vasorelaxation	[115]
Empagliflozin	Apoe-/- mice	Decreased TG and increased HDL	-Decreased atherosclerotic plaque and inflammation	[116]
Canagliflozin	Apoe-/- mice	Decreased TG, T-chol and LDL	-Increased plaque stability -Reduced atherosclerosis and inflammatory parameters	[117]
Dapagliflozin	ob/ob mice	Decreased of TG	-Reduced expression of inflammatory parameters	[118]
Drug	Trial	Structural basis	Effect on vascular and blood parameters, and MACE	References
Empagliflozin	EMPA-REG OUTCOME	C-glycosyl compound	-Decreased CV death (HR = 0.86), SBP and DBP -Increased HDL-C and LDL-C	[119]
Canagliflozin	CANVAS/CANVAS-R		-No effect (HR = 0.86) -Increased HDL-C and LDL-C	[120]
Canagliflozin	CREDENCE		-Decreased nonfatal stroke/MI and CV death (HR = 0.80)	[121]
Dapagliflozin	DECLARE-TIMI 58		-No effect (HR = 0.93) -Decreased SBP and DBP	[122]
Dapagliflozin	DEFINE-HF		-No decrease in HF (HR = 0.84)	[123]
Ertugliflozin	VERTIS-CV		-No effect (HR = 0.97) -Decreased SBP	[124]
Sotagliflozin	SCORED		-Decreased CV death (HR = 0.84)	[125]
Sotagliflozin	SOLOIST-WHF		-Decreased CV death (HR = 0.72)	[126]

CAMs: cellular adhesion molecules; CV: cardiovascular; CVD: cardiovascular disease; DBP: dyastolic blood pressure; ED: endothelial dysfunction; HF: heart failure; HR: hazard ratio for three-component; HDL cholesterol; LDL-C: LDL cholesterol; MACE; MACE: major adverse cardiovascular events; MI: myocardial infarction; SBP: systolic blood pressure; T-chol: total cholesterol; TG: triglycerides; VSM: vascular smooth muscle; VCAMs: vascular cell adhesion molecules.

Studies with empagliflozin in diabetic ZDF rats and *db/db* mice also showed an improvement of vascular stiffness and endothelial function by preventing oxidative stress, AGE-dependent signaling and inflammation [111,112]. Likewise, dapagliflozin treatment of C57BLKS/J-lepr*db*/lepr*db* mice, alleviated arterial stiffness and endothelial and VSMC dysfunction. Interestingly, a decrease in circulating markers of inflammation and alterations in microbial richness and diversity were reported [113].

In vascular disease, dapagliflozin decreased atherosclerosis in streptozotocin-induced diabetic *Apoe-/-* mice, but not in non-diabetic *Apoe-/-* mouse counterparts. Moreover, analysis of peritoneal macrophages from dapagliflozin-treated diabetic *Apoe-/-* mice and ipragliflozin-treated *db/db* mice showed decreased cholesterol-ester accumulation, suggesting less macrophage foam cell formation capacity compared. Both SGLT2i normalized the expression of *lectin-like ox-LDL receptor1* (*Lox1*), *Acat1*, and *ATP-binding cassette transporter A1* (*Abca1*) in peritoneal macrophages from diabetic *Apoe-/-* and *db/db* mice. These results suggested that SGLT2i exert an anti-atherogenic effect in diabetic conditions by modulating genes involved in cholesterol accumulation in macrophages [114].

Studies carried out in *Apoe-/-* mice showed that dapagliflozin improved EC function without variations in plasma glucose concentrations [115] and that empagliflozin reduced plaque formation in the aortic arch and ameliorated insulin sensitivity [116]. A decrease in inflammatory mediators, like VCAM and NFκB [115] and TNFα and IL6 [116] were also observed in these studies. These results point to an atheroprotection through anti-inflammatory mechanisms. Consistently, high-fat diet fed *Apoe-/-* mice, treated with canagliflozin, developed smaller and more stable plaques and displayed decreased *Vcam* and *Mcp1* expression [117].

In the T2DM mouse model, the *ob/ob* mice, dapagliflozin improved left ventricular function, attenuated activation of the Nlrp3 inflammasome and reduced inflammatory mediators by an AMPK-dependent mechanism. These changes were observed also in cardiomyofibroblasts derived from mice and were independent of the glucose-lowering effect [118].

3.4. Clinical Studies of Gliflozins in HF and CVD

In the EMPA-REG OUTCOME (NCT01131676) study, the empagliflozin treatment of patients with T2DM and CVD reduced MACE, death and hospitalization for HF. Both SBP and DBP were reduced while HDL-C and LDL-C levels were increased. However, it did not ameliorate non-fatal MI and stroke, and patients showed an increased rate of genital infection [119] (Table 3).

In the CANVAS (NCT01032629) and CANVAS-R (NCT01989754) program, canagliflozin treatment of patients with T2DM at high CV risk resulted in diminished MACE but it did not alter the occurrence of CV death or overall mortality. Like empaglifliozin, it enhanced the levels of HDL-C and LDL-C and the treated patients displayed a greater risk of fractures and amputations [120].

Differences between EMPA-REG OUTCOME and CANVAS trial might be due to the study design. Thus, in the EMPA-REG all subjects had prior CV disease and additional treatments (i.e., statins, RAS inhibitors, and acetylsalicylic acid), while in the CANVAS study only 65% of patients had prior CV disease [127].

Canagliflozin tested in T2DM and albuminuric chronic kidney disease patients in the CREDENCE (NCT02065791) clinical trial, demonstrated that, besides a lower risk of cardiovascular death, MI or stroke, this drug also diminishes the risk of end-stage kidney disease without changes in the amputation and fracture rates [121].

In the DECLARE-TIMI 58 (NCT01730534) trial with T2DM and CVD patients, dapagliflozin treatment failed to reduce MACE, although the rates of cardiovascular death or hospitalization for HF were lower. In this study reductions in SBP and DBP were described for dapagliflozin-treated patients [122]. Dapagliflozin in the DEFINE-HF (NCT02653482) trial with patients displaying chronic HF, both patients with or without T2DM, did not reduce HF determined as B-type natriuretic peptide levels [123].

Similar to dapagliflozin in the DECLARE-TIMI 58, ertugliflozin in the VERTIS CV (NCT01986881) trial, which included T2DM and CVD patients, did not reduce MACE or neither modify the death rate attributed to CV causes. However, ertugliflozin reduced SBP [124].

Two trials were carried out with sotagliflozin, the SCORED (NCT03315143) clinical trial [125] with TD2M chronic kidney disease and CVD participants, and the SOLOIST-WHF (NCT03521934) trial [126], with TD2M patients with HF. In both trials, a decrease in MACE was observed, but patients in the treatment group of the SCORED trial suffered more genital infections and volume depletion, in addition to diarrhea and hypoglycemia in both trials.

4. Lipid-Lowering Therapies Based on the Proprotein Convertase Subtilisin Kexin 9 Inhibition

As mentioned in the introduction one main mechanism for the regulation of blood LDL-C levels relies on its clearance by LDLR located on the surface of hepatic cells. This receptor binds the apoprotein B-100 (Apo B-100) present in LDL, VLDL, and IDL particles. After LDL binding, the receptor leads to the clathrin-mediated endocytosis of the ligand-receptor complex, which finishes in LDL degradation into amino acids and cholesterol. LDLR undergoes internalization and degradation by the proprotein convertase subtilisin kexin 9 (PCSK9), thus playing a pivotal role in the regulation of lipoprotein clearance [128]. *PCSK9* gene was identified in 2003 in a family with Familial hypercholesterolemia (FH), an autosomal dominant disease with elevated LDL-C in blood [129]. FH was attributed to two missense mutations in the coding region of the *PCSK9* gene with "gain of function—GOF", hence promoting LDLR degradation [129]. Two years later, lower plasmatic levels of LDL-C were associated with the existence of two "loss of function mutations—LOF" in *PCSK9* that resulted in elevated LDLR concentration in hepatic cells [130,131]. All these findings pointed to PCSK9 protein inhibition as a new potential lipid-lowering therapeutic target. To reduce CVD, PSCK9 inhibition has been set as a therapy in patients with FH, in those resistant to statin treatment or in subjects that did not reach the LDL-C goal levels at maximum statin dose [132,133]. By contrary, no recommendations exist today for T2DM patients' treatment.

4.1. Biology of PCSK9 in Lipid Metabolism and Vascular Homeostasis

PCSK9, also known as neural apoptosis-regulated convertase 1, is the ninth member of the secretory serine proteases of the subtilase family. Although it is mainly expressed by hepatocytes, PCSK9 is also present in the small intestine, kidney, pancreas, brain [128,134,135], and ischemic heart [136]. The 25-kb *PCSK9* human gene on chromosome 1p32 has 12 exons and 11 introns and is under the regulation of SREBP-2 (the sterol regulatory element-binding protein) [132,135]. It encodes a 692 amino acid serine protease that is synthesized as an inactive precursor, pre-proPCSK9. The pre-proPCSK9, stored in the ER, is processed to pro-PCSK9 and this last into mature PCSK9 which is bound to a cleaved prodomain that acts as a catalytic inhibitor and chaperone until its secretion into the circulation. The prodomain-mature PCSK9 heterodimer, with a plasma half-life of 5 min, binds to high-affinity specific proteins, leading to their intracellular degradation [135].

PCSK9 function is to regulate the amount of LDLR by forming a PCSK9-LDLR complex in the hepatocyte surface which is internalized by endocytosis and engaged into endosomal-lysosomal degradation [135,137]. PCSK9 can also bind to LDLR intracellularly through a Golgi-lysosome pathway for degradation [135,138].

Recent findings indicate the participation of PCSK9 in other processes beyond lipid homeostasis such as cell cycle, apoptosis, and inflammation with a potential effect on atherosclerosis [139]. Thus, LPS upregulate PCSK9 in liver and kidney in mice, in human EC and VSMCs [140]. Consistently, the injection of LPS into *Pcsk9* deficient mice resulted in less synthesis of pro-inflammatory IL-6 and TNFα cytokines and reduced expression of adhesion molecules in ECs and VSMCs [141].

PCSK9 expression is promoted by TNF in liver and VSMCs and by oxidized LDL in ECs, macrophages, VSMCs, and DC [140,141]. In experimental atherosclerosis, PCSK9 is mostly found in VSMCs, although its expression is LDLR-dependent, as *Ldlr-/-* mice do not display *Pcsk9* expression [142]. Notably, *Pcsk9* expression is localized in the artery branches with low shear stress and mirrors cytokine expression of these sites indicating a proatherogenic effect [142]. On the other hand, *Apoe-/-* mice overexpressing human *PCSK9* specifically in the bone marrow displayed augmented levels of proinflammatory Ly6C^{hi} monocyte infiltration in atheromas. Moreover, human PCSK9-overexpresing macrophages displayed enhanced pro-inflammatory *Tnf* and *Il1b* genes and diminished anti-inflammatory *Il10* and *Arg* genes [143]. In agreement with these, in vivo Pcsk9 gene silencing by lentiviral transduction of Apoe-/- mice decreased lesion size and macrophage infiltration and expression of *Nfkb*, *Tnfa*, *Il1*, and *Tlr4* in atherosclerotic plaques [144]. In macrophages, PCSK9 stimulates proinflammatory cytokine expression and foam cell formation by upregulating *Sra* and *Cd36*. Other actions of PCSK9 include activation of T cells, monocyte migration, and VSMC apoptosis [142]. Altogether indicates a role of PCSK9 in atheroma lesion development by regulating inflammatory pathways. Notwithstanding, the clinical relevance of these anti-inflammatory actions remains to be established, as patients treated with PSCK9 inhibitors (PSCK9i) do not display altered levels of the hs-CRP inflammatory marker [142].

4.2. Rational for PCSK9 Inhibition as a Potential Therapy

The main rational for the development of PCSK9i as CVD therapy were the positive correlation between high PCSK9 levels and increased CVD risk and the association between different *PCSK9* polymorphisms and vascular illness [145,146]. Moreover, the moderately-high prevalence and the lack of harmful effects of *PCSK9* LOF mutations in healthy individuals suggested a high safety of a potential PCSK9 therapeutic inhibition [132,146].

On the other hand, experimental animal data also gave a foundation for the development of PCSK9i. *Pcsk9-/-* mice displayed up to 80% decrease in plasma LDL-C levels due to increased hepatic LDLR and LDL clearance [147], which resulted in dramatic reductions in aortic atherosclerosis [148].

To date, up to nine PCSK9 inhibitory strategies, acting either preventing its binding to the LDLR, or its maturation, secretion, or synthesis, have been or are being developed [149]. These therapies, described below and summarized in Table 4, include the use of monoclonal antibodies (mAb) against PCSK9 [150], antisense oligonucleotides (ASOs), small interfering RNA (siRNAs), vaccines, and small molecules [151].

Table 4. Pre-clinical and clinical trials studying PCSK9 inhibitors in the context of hypercholesterolemia.

Inhibition Strategy	Animal Models	Effects on Lipids	Effects on Atherosclerosis	References
PCSK9 mAb	Cynomolgus monkeys	Decreased LDL-C (80%), T-Chol (48%)	—	[153]
PCSK9 mAb	C57BL/6 mice Cynomolgus monkeys	Decreased LDL-C (40%)	—	[154]
PCSK9 mAb: alirocumab	APOE*3Leiden.CETP mice	Decreased non-HDL-C and TGs	-Decreased inflammation and atherosclerotic lesion -Increased plaque stability	[152]
siRNA PCSK9	Cynomolgus monkeys C57BL/6 mice Sprague–Dawley rats	Decrease of LDL-C and T-Chol (60%)	—	[155]

Table 4. *Cont.*

Inhibition Strategy	Trial Name	Type of Patients	Reported Effects	References
PCSK9 mAb: evolocumab	FOURIER/OSLER [NCT01764633; NCT01439880] Phase III	Patients with atherosclerotic CVD	-Increased LDLR and HDL-C -Decreased LDL-C (61%), Total-C (36.1%), TG (12.6%), and Lp(a) (25.5%). -Increased Apolipoprotein A1 and HDL-C -Reduced CV (12–19%)	[156,157]
PCAK9 mAb: alirocumab	ODYSSEY [NCT01507831] Phase III	ACS patients	-Increased hepatic LDLR and HDL-C (4%) -Decreased LDL-C (58%), Total-C (37.8%), TG (15.6%), and Lp(a) (29.3%) and MACE -Increased ApoA1 and HDL-C -Reduced CV events (48%)	[158,159]
PCSK9 mAb: alirocumab, evolocumab	Meta-analysis	Alirocumab or evolocumab-treated patients	-Decreased nonfatal CV events and mortality. -Improved atherogenic events	[150,160]
PCSK9 siRNA: ALN-PCS	Phase I dose-escalation study [NCT01437059]	Healthy adult volunteers	-Reduced LDL-C (40%)	[161]
PCSK9 siRNA: ALN-60212 (Inclisirian)	ORION 1 Phase II: [NCT02597127] Phase III 10, 11: [NCT03399370; NCT03400800]	Patients at CVD risk with elevated LDL-C and some receiving statins	-Reduced LDL-C (52.6%) relative to base-line, as well as apoB and non-HDL-C.	[162,163]

ACS: Acute coronary syndrome; ApoA1: Apolipoprotein A1; CV: cardiovascular; CVD: cardiovascular disease; HDL-C: HDL cholesterol; LDL-C: LDL cholesterol; LDLR: LDL receptor; Lp(a): lipoprotein (a); MACE: Major adverse cardiovascular events; Total-C: total cholesterol; TG: triglycerides.

4.2.1. PCSK9 Monoclonal Antibodies

The only current clinical therapy to inhibit PCSK9 function in use is the administration of human mAb against soluble PCSK9. A single intravenous injection of the PCSK9 mAb, alirocumab, in hyperlipidemic *APOE*3Leiden.CETP* transgenic mice, decreased non-HDL-C, inflammatory parameters, and atherosclerosis lesion size and improved plaque stability in a dose-dependent manner [152]. Similarly, administration of a PCSK9 mAb reduced about 80% the levels of LDL-C in non-human primates [153]. An improved version of this mAb, with greater antigen affinity and resistance to degradation, achieved a reduction of around 40% in LDL-C levels at lower doses and an efficiency of 2.8 times longer [154].

The two monoclonal antibodies approved as a PCSK9-blocking therapies are alirocumab (SAR236553/REGN727 from Regeneron Pharmaceuticals/Sanofi) and evolocumab (AMG145 from Amgen). These are currently prescribed to reduce the risk of atherosclerotic CVD and lower LDL-C levels in patients with FH and resistance to statin therapy, among others [150,164]. Alirocumab is a human IgG1 mAb that strongly binds PCSK9 with a maximum effect between 8 and 15 days after its subcutaneous administration [165]. Evolocumab is a human mAb of the isotype G2 against PCSK9 with a maximum efficacy between the first and second week after subcutaneous administration [166].

Evolocumab was tested in the FOURIER (Further Cardiovascular Outcomes Research with PCSK9 Inhibition in Subjects with Elevated Risk [NCT01764633]) and OSLER (Open-label Extension Study of Evolocumab [NCT01439880]) trials [156,157], and alirocumab was evaluated in the ODYSSEY trial (Evaluation of Cardiovascular Outcomes After an

Acute Coronary Syndrome With Alirocumab) [158,159]. These showed increased hepatic LDLR and reduced circulating levels of LDL-C by up to 60% as well as VLDL [167]. Both alirocumab and evolocumab slightly increased HDL levels and apolipoprotein A1 and diminished plasmatic lipoprotein(a) [132]. A current meta-analysis have shown that PCSK9 antibodies reduce nonfatal cardiovascular events and all-cause mortality [156,160], improve several atherogenic events [150], and promote plaque regression [168].

Notwithstanding, the use of mAbs as PCSK9 inhibitors for CVD therapy holds several limitations, such as the high cost (about 14,500 USD per patient each year), a limited lifetime, and administration frequency of twice a month [149]. Because of this, novel approaches to pharmacologically inhibit PCSK9 are under development consisting of gene silencing either with siRNAs or by using ASOs.

4.2.2. Small Interfering RNA (siRNA)

The mechanism of action of *PCSK9* gene silencing uses a duplex 20 bp RNA molecule acting as a siRNA. Within the cell, it renders an anti-sense strand that binds to the mRNA gene, generating an incomplete duplex RNA later processed by DICER [151], thus preventing *PCSK9* translation and increasing LDLR protein hepatic content.

Pre-clinical trials have shown that *PCSK9* gene silencing by siRNA reduced cholesterol levels in monkeys by 60% due to a 50–70% decrease in the *PCSK9* mRNA levels [155]. *PCSK9* siRNA suppressed the inflammatory response by diminishing the generation of ROS and LDL oxidation-induced apoptosis in ECs and macrophages, respectively [145]. In clinical trial phase I, this same *PCSK9* siRNA reduced LDL-C levels by 40% [161] but the effects were not lasting and an improved version of the siRNA was developed giving rise to Inclisiran (ALN-60212 from Alnylam) [149,169]. Inclisiran has been designed for hepatic cellular internalization, does not induce immunogenic reactions, and has a greater resistance to degradation by nucleases [169]. In phase I clinical trial, intravenous injection of Inclisiran, a siRNA in a lipid nanoparticle (ALN-60212), reduced the levels of PCSK9 and LDL-C by 74.5% and 50.6% respectively, with lasting effects between 3 to 6 months and decreases in non-HDL-C and apolipoprotein B (apoB) [170]. Phase II trial ORION-1, which evaluated different Inclisiran doses in patients who had a history of atherogenic CVD or high atherosclerotic CVD-risk with elevated LDL-C levels, showed a dose-dependent decrease in PCSK9 and LDL-C levels [162]. Besides, patients who received two doses presented a reduction of 69.1% and 52.6% of PCSK9 and LDL-C [151,162], without adverse reactions [169]. Results of ORION phase III trials (ORION 10 and 11) have shown the effectivity of Inclisiran in patients with CVD, CVD risk or with elevated LDL-C levels despite statin-treatment at the maximum dose, with reductions in LDL-C, non-HDL-C, and apoB [163].

Because its potent and long-lasting effect lowering LDL-C levels, the administration frequency (once/twice per year) [149], low cost and easier long-term storage, Inclisiran holds great promise as an hypolipemiant agent.

4.3. Other Developing Approaches to PCSK9 Inhibition

Other drug strategies to inhibit PCSK9 function include the use of ASOs (antisense oligonucleotides), small-molecules inhibitors, PCSK9 vaccination or the CRISPR/Cas9 system (clustered regularly interspaced short palindromic repeat associated protein 9) to lower PCSK9 concentration [151]. These approaches, in preclinical phase or phase I [150], are expected to offer a number of several additional benefits such as prolonged effects, easier production and lower cost [149]. The administration of an ASO, which is a 15–30 pb single-strand DNA that hybridizes with *PCSK9* mRNA and ensues RNase H degradation route [164], resulted in a high specific decrease of LDL-C and PCSK9 levels of 25–50% and 50–85%, respectively, in a phase I clinical trial [151]. Notably, berberine, a natural product obtained from a plant, and its derivatives have been shown to inhibit the transcription of *PCSK9*, and therefore it could also be useful in the management of patients with CVD risk [149,168].

5. Conclusions

The investigations reviewed here indicate that the new emergent clinical therapies designed to restore metabolic homeostasis have major effects on the cardiovascular system beyond metabolic control. In addition to their expected anti-diabetic and lipid-lowering actions, the main common mechanisms for CVD prevention and atheroprotection of the three class drugs in the studies reviewed here are a direct modulation of vascular and inflammatory cell phenotypes and an improvement of the vascular and cardiomyocyte function. These effects of the incretin-therapies, SGLT2i and PCSK9i in vascular, immune cells and cardiomyocytes have been summarized in Figure 2. These have been shown to prevent early stages of atherosclerosis such as decreased leukocyte adhesion, endothelial dysfunction, immune cell recruitment, and foam cell formation. Moreover, several animal studies also demonstrated that these strategies stabilize atheromas and diminish necrotic cores of advanced plaques. A promising future of incretin-based therapies and SGLT2i for their use in cardiovascular prevention, and possibly, the use of small molecules as PCSK9i for more affordable therapeutics, is anticipated. Notwithstanding, completion of the ongoing clinical trials and further insight about the mechanisms of action of these drugs is needed to reduce the burden of CVD in the future.

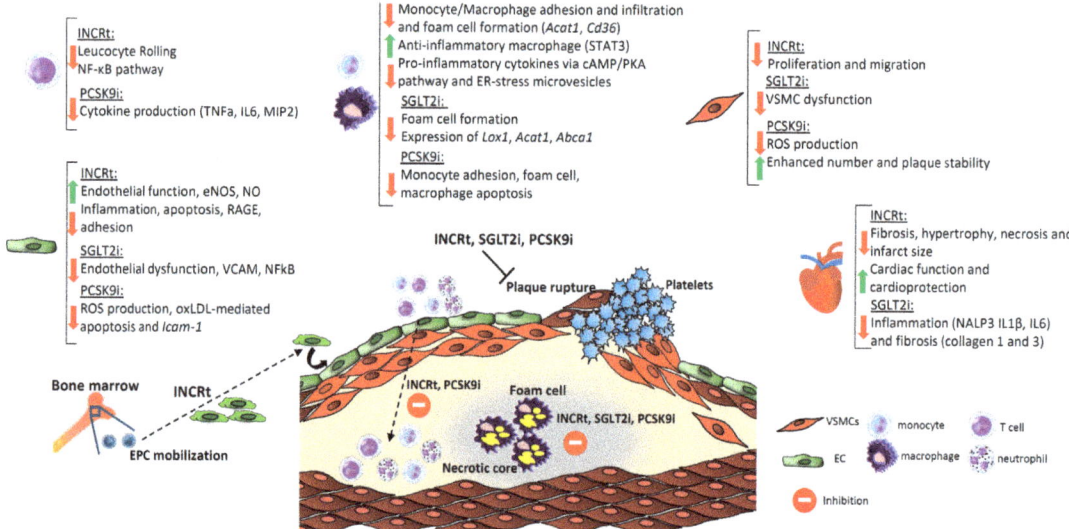

Figure 2. Common mechanism of action of incretin-therapies, SGLT2i and PCSK9i in immune and vascular cells involved in atherosclerosis progression and in cardiomyocyte function. The main protective mechanisms of PCSK9i and INCRt in T cells include the impairment of leukocyte rolling and a decrease in NFkB activation and cytokine secretion. Both PCSK9i and INCRt also reduce monocyte adhesion and recruitment while in macrophages all three class drugs decrease macrophage foam cell formation. INCRt also decreases inflammatory genes in macrophages and PCSK9i impairs restrains proatherogenic apoptosis. Endothelial function is improved by all three class drugs by several mechanisms such as enhanced eNOS, reduced adhesion of leukocytes and inflammatory molecules and diminished ROS production. Notably, INCrt also promote endothelial cell repair by the mobilization of EPC from the bone marrow. In VSMCs' INCRt decrease proliferation and hyperplasia, PCSK9i promotes plaque stability by enhancing VSMC number, and SGLT2i reduce their dysfunction. All these mechanisms lead to a decrease in leukocyte retention in the subendothelial space, less foam cell formation, reduced necrotic core and prevention of plaque rupture that, in patients, ensues the acute cardiovascular events. Lastly, among the actions observed in cardiomyocytes stands out the improved cardiac function by INCRt and SGLT2i by decreasing inflammation and fibrosis and necrosis. EPC: endothelial progenitor cell; INCRt: incretin-therapies; SGLT2i: sodium-glucose co-transporter 2 inhibitor; PCSK9i: proprotein convertase subtilisin kexin 9 inhibitor.

Author Contributions: M.A.-B., G.H.-G., and A.T.-C. reviewed all the literature helped to write the manuscript. A.H.-C. help to write some sections of the manuscript. S.M.-H. and H.G.-N. designed the review, supervised the literature, and wrote the manuscript. All authors have read and agreed to the published version of the manuscript.

Funding: This research was funded by from Carlos III Health Institute and the European Regional Development Fund (FEDER) (CB07/08/0043, PI19/00169 to H.G.-N., S.M.-H.), and JR18/00051 from Generalitat Valenciana, (GenT CDEI-04/20-B to H.G.-N.).

Data Availability Statement: Data sharing not applicable.

Conflicts of Interest: The authors declare no conflict of interest.

References

1. Naghavi, M.; Abajobir, A.A.; Abbafati, C.; Abbas, K.M.; Abd-Allah, F.; Abera, S.F.; Aboyans, V.; Adetokunboh, O.; Ärnlöv, J.; Afshin, A.; et al. Global, regional, and national age-sex specifc mortality for 264 causes of death, 1980–2016: A systematic analysis for the global burden of disease study 2016. *Lancet* **2017**, *390*, 1151–1210. [CrossRef]
2. Ference, B.A.; Ginsberg, H.N.; Graham, I.; Ray, K.K.; Packard, C.J.; Bruckert, E.; Hegele, R.A.; Krauss, R.M.; Raal, F.J.; Schunkert, H.; et al. Low-density lipoproteins cause atherosclerotic cardiovascular disease. 1: Evidence from genetic, epidemiologic, and clinical studies. A consensus statement fromthe European Atherosclerosis Society Consensus Panel. *Eur. Heart J.* **2017**, *38*, 2459–2472. [CrossRef] [PubMed]
3. Stone, N.J.; Robinson, J.G.; Lichtenstein, A.H.; Bairey Merz, C.N.; Blum, C.B.; Eckel, R.H.; Goldberg, A.C.; Gordon, D.; Levy, D.; Lloyd-Jones, D.M.; et al. 2013 ACC/AHA guideline on the treatment of blood cholesterol to reduce atherosclerotic cardiovascular risk in adults: A report of the American college of cardiology/American heart association task force on practice guidelines. *J. Am. Coll. Cardiol.* **2014**, *63*, 2889–2934. [CrossRef] [PubMed]
4. Bornfeldt, K.E. Uncomplicating the macrovascular complications of diabetes: The 2014 edwin bierman award lecture. *Diabetes* **2015**, *64*, 2689–2697. [CrossRef] [PubMed]
5. Adeva-Andany, M.M.; Martínez-Rodríguez, J.; González-Lucán, M.; Fernández-Fernández, C.; Castro-Quintela, E. Insulin resistance is a cardiovascular risk factor in humans. *Diabetes Metab. Syndr. Clin. Res. Rev.* **2019**, *13*, 1449–1455. [CrossRef]
6. Kubota, T.; Kubota, N.; Kumagai, H.; Yamaguchi, S.; Kozono, H.; Takahashi, T.; Inoue, M.; Itoh, S.; Takamoto, I.; Sasako, T.; et al. Impaired insulin signaling in endothelial cells reduces insulin-induced glucose uptake by skeletal muscle. *Cell Metab.* **2011**, *13*, 294–307. [CrossRef]
7. Martínez-Hervás, S.; Vinué, Á.; Núñez, L.; Andrés-Blasco, I.; Piqueras, L.; TomásReal, J.; Ascaso, J.F.; Burks, D.J.; Sanz, M.J.; González-Navarro, H. Insulin resistance aggravates atherosclerosis by reducing vascular smoothmuscle cell survival and increasing CX3CL1/CX3CR1 axis. *Cardiovasc. Res.* **2014**, *103*, 324–336. [CrossRef]
8. Van Dijk, R.A.; Duinisveld, A.J.F.; Schaapherder, A.F.; Mulder-Stapel, A.; Hamming, J.F.; Kuiper, J.; de Boer, O.J.; van der Wal, A.C.; Kolodgie, F.D.; Virmani, R.; et al. A change in inflammatory footprint precedes plaque instability: A systematic evaluation of cellular aspects of the adaptive immune response in human atherosclerosis. *J. Am. Heart Assoc.* **2015**, *4*. [CrossRef]
9. Lytvyn, Y.; Bjornstad, P.; Pun, N.; Cherney, D.Z.I. New and old agents in the management of diabetic nephropathy. *Curr. Opin. Nephrol. Hypertens.* **2016**, *25*, 232–239. [CrossRef]
10. White, W.B.; Baker, W.L. Cardiovascular effects of incretin-based therapies. *Annu. Rev. Med.* **2016**, *67*, 245–260. [CrossRef]
11. Baggio, L.L.; Drucker, D.J. Biology of incretins: GLP-1 and GIP. *Gastroenterology* **2007**, *132*, 2131–2157. [CrossRef] [PubMed]
12. Drucker, D.J. The biology of incretin hormones. *Cell Metab.* **2006**, *3*, 153–165. [CrossRef] [PubMed]
13. Müller, T.D.; Finan, B.; Bloom, S.R.; D'Alessio, D.; Drucker, D.J.; Flatt, P.R.; Fritsche, A.; Gribble, F.; Grill, H.J.; Habener, J.F.; et al. Glucagon-like peptide 1 (GLP-1). *Mol. Metab.* **2019**, *30*, 72–130. [CrossRef] [PubMed]
14. Ussher, J.R.; Drucker, D.J. Cardiovascular actions of incretin-based therapies. *Circ. Res.* **2014**, *114*, 1788–1803. [CrossRef]
15. Lambeir, A.M.; Durinx, C.; Scharpé, S.; De Meester, I. Dipeptidyl-peptidase IV from bench to bedside: An update on structural properties, functions, and clinical aspects of the enzyme DPP IV. *Crit. Rev. Clin. Lab. Sci.* **2003**, *40*, 209–294. [CrossRef]
16. Lamers, D.; Famulla, S.; Wronkowitz, N.; Hartwig, S.; Lehr, S.; Ouwens, D.M.; Eckardt, K.; Kaufman, J.M.; Ryden, M.; Müller, S.; et al. Dipeptidyl peptidase 4 is a novel adipokine potentially linking obesity to the metabolic syndrome. *Diabetes* **2011**, *60*, 1917–1925. [CrossRef]
17. Zhong, J.; Maiseyeu, A.; Davis, S.N.; Rajagopalan, S. DPP4 in cardiometabolic disease: Recent insights from the laboratory and clinical trials of DPP4 inhibition. *Circ. Res.* **2015**, *116*, 1491–1504. [CrossRef]
18. Fisman, E.Z.; Tenenbaum, A. Antidiabetic treatment with gliptins: Focus on cardiovascular effects and outcomes. *Cardiovasc. Diabetol.* **2015**, *14*, 1–13. [CrossRef]
19. Röhrborn, D.; Wronkowitz, N.; Eckel, J. DPP4 in diabetes. *Front. Immunol.* **2015**, *6*, 386. [CrossRef]
20. Zhong, J.; Rao, X.; Deiuliis, J.; Braunstein, Z.; Narula, V.; Hazey, J.; Mikami, D.; Needleman, B.; Satoskar, A.R.; Rajagopalan, S. A potential role for dendritic cell/macrophage-expressing DPP4 in obesity-induced visceral inflammation. *Diabetes* **2013**, *62*, 149–157. [CrossRef]

21. Ikushima, H.; Munakata, Y.; Iwata, S.; Ohnuma, K.; Kobayashi, S.; Dang, N.H.; Morimoto, C. Soluble CD26/dipeptidyl peptidase IV enhances transendothelial migration via its interaction with mannose 6-phosphate/insulin-like growth factor II receptor. *Cell. Immunol.* **2002**, *215*, 106–110. [CrossRef]
22. Ghorpade, D.S.; Ozcan, L.; Zheng, Z.; Nicoloro, S.M.; Shen, Y.; Chen, E.; Blüher, M.; Czech, M.P.; Tabas, I. Hepatocyte-secreted DPP4 in obesity promotes adipose inflammation and insulin resistance HHS Public Access. *Nature* **2018**, *555*, 673–677. [CrossRef] [PubMed]
23. Sell, H.; Blüher, M.; Klöting, N.; Schlich, R.; Willems, M.; Ruppe, F.; Knoefel, W.T.; Dietrich, A.; Fielding, B.A.; Arner, P.; et al. Adipose dipeptidyl peptidase-4 and obesity: Correlation with insulin resistance and depot-specific release from adipose tissue in vivo and in vitro. *Diabetes Care* **2013**, *36*, 4083–4090. [CrossRef] [PubMed]
24. Wronkowitz, N.; Görgens, S.W.; Romacho, T.; Villalobos, L.A.; Sánchez-Ferrer, C.F.; Peiró, C.; Sell, H.; Eckel, J. Soluble DPP4 induces inflammation and proliferation of human smooth muscle cells via protease-activated receptor 2. *Biochim. Biophys. Acta Mol. Basis Dis.* **2014**, *1842*, 1613–1621. [CrossRef] [PubMed]
25. Alonso, N.; Teresa Julián, M.; Puig-Domingo, M.; Vives-Pi, M. Incretin hormones as immunomodulators of atherosclerosis. *Front. Endocrinol.* **2012**, *3*, 112. [CrossRef]
26. Deng, X.; Tavallaie, M.S.; Sun, R.; Wang, J.; Cai, Q.; Shen, J.; Lei, S.; Fu, L.; Jiang, F. Drug discovery approaches targeting the incretin pathway. *Bioorg. Chem.* **2020**, *99*. [CrossRef]
27. Standl, E.; Schnell, O.; McGuire, D.K.; Ceriello, A.; Rydén, L. Integration of recent evidence into management of patients with atherosclerotic cardiovascular disease and type 2 diabetes. *Lancet Diabetes Endocrinol.* **2017**, *5*, 391–402. [CrossRef]
28. McGuire, D.K.; van de Werf, F.; Armstrong, P.W.; Standl, E.; Koglin, J.; Green, J.B.; Bethel, M.A.; Cornel, J.H.; Lopes, R.D.; Halvorsen, S.; et al. Association between sitagliptin use and heart failure hospitalization and related outcomes in type 2 diabetes mellitus: Secondary analysis of a randomized clinical trial. *JAMA Cardiol.* **2016**, *1*, 126–135. [CrossRef]
29. Scirica, B.M.; Bhatt, D.L.; Braunwald, E.; Steg, P.G.; Davidson, J.; Hirshberg, B.; Ohman, P.; Frederich, R.; Wiviott, S.D.; Hoffman, E.B.; et al. Saxagliptin and cardiovascular outcomes in patients with type 2 diabetes mellitus. *N. Engl. J. Med.* **2013**, *369*, 1317–1326. [CrossRef]
30. Zannad, F.; Cannon, C.P.; Cushman, W.C.; Bakris, G.L.; Menon, V.; Perez, A.T.; Fleck, P.R.; Mehta, C.R.; Kupfer, S.; Wilson, C.; et al. Heart failure and mortality outcomes in patients with type 2 diabetes taking alogliptin versus placebo in EXAMINE: A multicentre, randomised, double-blind trial. *Lancet* **2015**, *385*, 2067–2076. [CrossRef]
31. McGuire, D.K.; Alexander, J.H.; Johansen, O.E.; Perkovic, V.; Rosenstock, J.; Cooper, M.E.; Wanner, C.; Kahn, S.E.; Toto, R.D.; Zinman, B.; et al. Linagliptin effects on heart failure and related outcomes in individuals with type 2 diabetes mellitus at high cardiovascular and renal risk in CARMELINA. *Circulation* **2019**, *139*, 351–361. [CrossRef] [PubMed]
32. Mcinnes, G.; Evans, M.; del Prato, S.; Stumvoll, M.; Schweizer, A.; Lukashevich, V.; Shao, Q.; Kothny, W. Cardiovascular and heart failure safety profile of vildagliptin: A meta-analysis of 17,000 patients. *Diabetes Obes. Metab.* **2015**, *17*, 1085–1092. [CrossRef] [PubMed]
33. Remm, F.; Franz, W.M.; Brenner, C. Gliptins and their target dipeptidyl peptidase 4: Implications for the treatment of vascular disease. *Eur. Hear. J. Cardiovasc. Pharm.* **2016**, *2*, 185–193. [CrossRef] [PubMed]
34. Ervinna, N.; Mita, T.; Yasunari, E.; Azuma, K.; Tanaka, R.; Fujimura, S.; Sukmawati, D.; Nomiyama, T.; Kanazawa, A.; Kawamori, R.; et al. Anagliptin, a DPP-4 inhibitor, suppresses proliferation of vascular smooth muscles and monocyte inflammatory reaction and attenuates atherosclerosis in male apo e-deficient mice. *Endocrinology* **2013**, *154*, 1260–1270. [CrossRef]
35. Nishida, S.; Matsumura, T.; Senokuchi, T.; Murakami-Nishida, S.; Ishii, N.; Morita, Y.; Yagi, Y.; Motoshima, H.; Kondo, T.; Araki, E. Inhibition of inflammation-mediated DPP-4 expression by linagliptin increases M2 macrophages in atherosclerotic lesions. *Biochem. Biophys. Res. Commun.* **2020**, *524*, 8–15. [CrossRef]
36. Kahles, F.; Liberman, A.; Halim, C.; Rau, M.; Möllmann, J.; Mertens, R.W.; Rückbeil, M.; Diepolder, I.; Walla, B.; Diebold, S.; et al. The incretin hormone GIP is upregulated in patients with atherosclerosis and stabilizes plaques in ApoE−/− mice by blocking monocyte/macrophage activation. *Mol. Metab.* **2018**, *14*, 150–157. [CrossRef]
37. Nagashima, M.; Watanabe, T.; Terasaki, M.; Tomoyasu, M.; Nohtomi, K.; Kim-Kaneyama, J.; Miyazaki, A.; Hirano, T. Native incretins prevent the development of atherosclerotic lesions in apolipoprotein e knockout mice. *Diabetologia* **2011**, *54*, 2649–2659. [CrossRef]
38. Tashiro, Y.; Sato, K.; Watanabe, T.; Nohtomi, K.; Terasaki, M.; Nagashima, M.; Hirano, T. A glucagon-like peptide-1 analog liraglutide suppresses macrophage foam cell formation and atherosclerosis. *Peptides* **2014**, *54*, 19–26. [CrossRef]
39. Bruen, R.; Curley, S.; Kajani, S.; Crean, D.; O'Reilly, M.E.; Lucitt, M.B.; Godson, C.G.; McGillicuddy, F.C.; Belton, O. Liraglutide dictates macrophage phenotype in apolipoprotein E null mice during early atherosclerosis. *Cardiovasc. Diabetol.* **2017**, *16*. [CrossRef]
40. Yang, G.; Lei, Y.; Inoue, A.; Piao, L.; Hu, L.; Jiang, H.; Sasaki, T.; Wu, H.; Xu, W.; Yu, C.; et al. Exenatide mitigated diet-induced vascular aging and atherosclerotic plaque growth in ApoE-deficient mice under chronic stress. *Atherosclerosis* **2017**, *264*, 1–10. [CrossRef]
41. Arakawa, M.; Mita, T.; Azuma, K.; Ebato, C.; Goto, H.; Nomiyama, T.; Fujitani, Y.; Hirose, T.; Kawamori, R.; Watada, H. Inhibition of monocyte adhesion to endothelial cells and attenuation of atherosclerotic lesion by a glucagon-like peptide-1 receptor agonist, exendin-4. *Diabetes* **2010**, *59*, 1030–1037. [CrossRef] [PubMed]

42. Wang, Y.; Parlevliet, E.T.; Geerling, J.J.; van der Tuin, S.J.L.; Zhang, H.; Bieghs, V.; Jawad, A.H.M.; Shiri-Sverdlov, R.; Bot, I.; de Jager, S.C.A.; et al. Exendin-4 decreases liver inflammation and atherosclerosis development simultaneously by reducing macrophage infiltration. *Br. J. Pharm.* **2014**, *171*, 723–734. [CrossRef]
43. Vinué, Á.; Navarro, J.; Herrero-Cervera, A.; García-Cubas, M.; Andrés-Blasco, I.; Martínez-Hervás, S.; Real, J.T.; Ascaso, J.F.; González-Navarro, H. The GLP-1 analogue lixisenatide decreases atherosclerosis in insulin-resistant mice by modulating macrophage phenotype. *Diabetologia* **2017**, *60*, 1801–1812. [CrossRef] [PubMed]
44. Rakipovski, G.; Rolin, B.; Nøhr, J.; Klewe, I.; Frederiksen, K.S.; Augustin, R.; Hecksher-Sørensen, J.; Ingvorsen, C.; Polex-Wolf, J.; Knudsen, L.B. The GLP-1 analogs liraglutide and semaglutide reduce atherosclerosis in ApoE/− and LDLr/Mice by a mechanism that includes inflammatory pathways. *JACC Basic Transl. Sci.* **2018**, *3*, 844–857. [CrossRef] [PubMed]
45. Shah, Z.; Kampfrath, T.; Deiuliis, J.A.; Zhong, J.; Pineda, C.; Ying, Z.; Xu, X.; Lu, B.; Moffatt-Bruce, S.; Durairaj, R.; et al. Long-term dipeptidyl-peptidase 4 inhibition reduces atherosclerosis and inflammation via effects on monocyte recruitment and chemotaxis. *Circulation* **2011**, *124*, 2338–2349. [CrossRef] [PubMed]
46. Helmstädter, J.; Frenis, K.; Filippou, K.; Grill, A.; Dib, M.; Kalinovic, S.; Pawelke, F.; Kus, K.; Kröller-Schön, S.; Oelze, M.; et al. Endothelial GLP-1 (Glucagon-Like Peptide-1) receptor mediates cardiovascular protection by liraglutide in mice with experimental arterial hypertension. *Arter. Thromb. Vasc. Biol.* **2020**, *40*, 145–158. [CrossRef]
47. Noyan-Ashraf, M.H.; Shikatani, E.A.; Schuiki, I.; Mukovozov, I.; Wu, J.; Li, R.K.; Volchuk, A.; Robinson, L.A.; Billia, F.; Drucker, D.J.; et al. A glucagon-like peptide-1 analog reverses the molecular pathology and cardiac dysfunction of a mouse model of obesity. *Circulation* **2013**, *127*, 74–85. [CrossRef]
48. Noyan-Ashraf, M.H.; Abdul Momen, M.; Ban, K.; Sadi, A.M.; Zhou, Y.Q.; Riazi, A.M.; Baggio, L.L.; Henkelman, R.M.; Husain, M.; Drucker, D.J. GLP-1R agonist liraglutide activates cytoprotective pathways and improves outcomes after experimental myocardial infarction in mice. *Diabetes* **2009**, *58*, 975–983. [CrossRef]
49. Wohlfart, P.; Linz, W.; Hübschle, T.; Linz, D.; Huber, J.; Hess, S.; Crowther, D.; Werner, U.; Ruetten, H. Cardioprotective effects of lixisenatide in rat myocardial ischemia-reperfusion injury studies. *J. Transl. Med.* **2013**, *11*, 84. [CrossRef]
50. Hirano, T.; Mori, Y. Anti-atherogenic and anti-inflammatory properties of glucagon-like peptide-1, glucose-dependent insulinotropic polypepide, and dipeptidyl peptidase-4 inhibitors in experimental animals. *J. Diabetes Investig.* **2016**, *7*, 80–86. [CrossRef]
51. Li, Y.; Liu, X.; Fang, Q.; Ding, M.; Li, C. Liraglutide attenuates atherosclerosis via inhibiting ER-induced macrophage derived microvesicles production in T2DM rats. *Diabetol. Metab. Syndr.* **2017**, *9*. [CrossRef] [PubMed]
52. Lim, S.; Lee, G.Y.; Park, H.S.; Lee, D.H.; Jung, O.T.; Min, K.K.; Kim, Y.B.; Jun, H.S.; Chul, J.H.; Park, K.S. Attenuation of carotid neointimal formation after direct delivery of a recombinant adenovirus expressing glucagon-like peptide-1 in diabetic rats. *Cardiovasc. Res.* **2017**, *113*, 183–194. [CrossRef] [PubMed]
53. Hirano, T.; Yamashita, S.; Takahashi, M.; Hashimoto, H.; Mori, Y.; Goto, M. Anagliptin, a dipeptidyl peptidase-4 inhibitor, decreases macrophage infiltration and suppresses atherosclerosis in aortic and coronary arteries in cholesterol-fed rabbits. *Metabolism* **2016**, *65*, 893–903. [CrossRef] [PubMed]
54. Sudo, M.; Li, Y.; Hiro, T.; Takayama, T.; Mitsumata, M.; Shiomi, M.; Sugitani, M.; Matsumoto, T.; Hao, H.; Hirayama, A. Inhibition of plaque progression and promotion of plaque stability by glucagon-like peptide-1 receptor agonist: Serial In vivo findings from iMap-IVUS in Watanabe heritable hyperlipidemic rabbits. *Atherosclerosis* **2017**, *265*, 283–291. [CrossRef] [PubMed]
55. Oyama, J.I.; Higashi, Y.; Node, K. Do incretins improve endothelial function? *Cardiovasc. Diabetol.* **2014**, *13*, 21. [CrossRef] [PubMed]
56. Huang, C.-Y.; Shih, C.-M.; Tsao, N.-W.; Lin, Y.-W.; Huang, P.-H.; Wu, S.-C.; Lee, A.-W.; Kao, Y.-T.; Chang, N.-C.; Nakagami, H.; et al. Dipeptidyl peptidase-4 inhibitor improves neovascularization by increasing circulating endothelial progenitor cells. *Br. J. Pharm.* **2012**, *167*, 1506–1519. [CrossRef] [PubMed]
57. Akoumianakis, I.; Badi, I.; Douglas, G.; Chuaiphichai, S.; Herdman, L.; Akawi, N.; Margaritis, M.; Antonopoulos, A.S.; Oikonomou, E.K.; Psarros, C.; et al. Insulin-induced vascular redox dysregulation in human atherosclerosis is ameliorated by dipeptidyl peptidase 4 inhibition. *Sci. Transl. Med.* **2020**, *12*. [CrossRef]
58. Nagamine, A.; Hasegawa, H.; Hashimoto, N.; Yamada-Inagawa, T.; Hirose, Y.; Kobara, Y.; Tadokoro, H.; Kobayashi, Y.; Takano, H. The effects of DPP-4 inhibitor on hypoxia-induced apoptosis in human umbilical vein endothelial cells. *J. Pharm. Sci.* **2017**, *133*, 42–48. [CrossRef]
59. Chihara, A.; Tanaka, A.; Morimoto, T.; Sakuma, M.; Shimabukuro, M.; Nomiyama, T.; Arasaki, O.; Ueda, S.; Node, K. Differences in lipid metabolism between anagliptin and sitagliptin in patients with type 2 diabetes on statin therapy: A secondary analysis of the REASON trial. *Cardiovasc. Diabetol.* **2019**, *18*, 158. [CrossRef]
60. Green, J.B.; Bethel, M.A.; Armstrong, P.W.; Buse, J.B.; Engel, S.S.; Garg, J.; Josse, R.; Kaufman, K.D.; Koglin, J.; Korn, S.; et al. Effect of sitagliptin on cardiovascular outcomes in type 2 diabetes. *N. Engl. J. Med.* **2015**, *373*, 232–242. [CrossRef] [PubMed]
61. Rosenstock, J.; Kahn, S.E.; Johansen, O.E.; Zinman, B.; Espeland, M.A.; Woerle, H.J.; Pfarr, E.; Keller, A.; Mattheus, M.; Baanstra, D.; et al. Effect of linagliptin vs. glimepiride on major adverse cardiovascular outcomes in patients with type 2 diabetes: The Carolina randomized clinical trial. *JAMA J. Am. Med. Assoc.* **2019**, *322*, 1155–1166. [CrossRef] [PubMed]
62. Perkovic, V.; Toto, R.; Cooper, M.E.; Mann, J.F.E.; Rosenstock, J.; McGuire, D.K.; Kahn, S.E.; Marx, N.; Alexander, J.H.; Zinman, B.; et al. Effects of linagliptin on cardiovascular and kidney outcomes in people with normal and reduced kidney function: Secondary analysis of the carmelina randomized trial. *Diabetes Care* **2020**, *43*, 1803–1812. [CrossRef] [PubMed]

63. Pfeffer, M.A.; Claggett, B.; Diaz, R.; Dickstein, K.; Gerstein, H.C.; Køber, L.V.; Lawson, F.C.; Ping, L.; Wei, X.; Lewis, E.F.; et al. Lixisenatide in patients with type 2 diabetes and acute coronary syndrome. *N. Engl. J. Med.* **2015**, *373*, 2247–2257. [CrossRef]
64. Holman, R.R.; Bethel, M.A.; Mentz, R.J.; Thompson, V.P.; Lokhnygina, Y.; Buse, J.B.; Chan, J.C.; Choi, J.; Gustavson, S.M.; Iqbal, N.; et al. Effects of once-weekly exenatide on cardiovascular outcomes in type 2 diabetes. *N. Engl. J. Med.* **2017**, *377*, 1228–1239. [CrossRef]
65. Angelyn Bethel, M.; Mentz, R.J.; Merrill, P.; Buse, J.B.; Chan, J.C.; Goodman, S.G.; Iqbal, N.; Jakuboniene, N.; Katona, B.; Lokhnygina, Y.; et al. Microvascular and cardiovascular outcomes according to renal function in patients treated with once-weekly exenatide: Insights from the EXSCEL trial. *Diabetes Care* **2020**, *43*. [CrossRef]
66. Marso, S.P.; Daniels, G.H.; Frandsen, K.B.; Kristensen, P.; Mann, J.F.E.; Nauck, M.A.; Nissen, S.E.; Pocock, S.; Poulter, N.R.; Ravn, L.S.; et al. Liraglutide and cardiovascular outcomes in type 2 diabetes. *N. Engl. J. Med.* **2016**, *375*, 311–322. [CrossRef] [PubMed]
67. Verma, S.; Bhatt, D.L.; Bain, S.C.; Buse, J.B.; Mann, J.F.E.; Marso, S.P.; Nauck, M.A.; Poulter, N.R.; Pratley, R.E.; Zinman, B.; et al. Effect of liraglutide on cardiovascular events in patients with type 2 diabetes mellitus and polyvascular disease results of the LEADER trial. *Circulation* **2018**, *137*, 2179–2183. [CrossRef] [PubMed]
68. Verma, S.; Poulter, N.R.; Bhatt, D.L.; Bain, S.C.; Buse, J.B.; Leiter, L.A.; Nauck, M.A.; Pratley, R.E.; Zinman, B.; Ørsted, D.D.; et al. Effects of liraglutide on cardiovascular outcomes in patients with type 2 diabetes mellitus with or without history of myocardial infarction or stroke: Post hoc analysis from the leader trial. *Circulation* **2018**, *138*, 2884–2894. [CrossRef]
69. Nauck, M.A.; Tornøe, K.; Rasmussen, S.; Treppendahl, M.B.; Marso, S.P. Cardiovascular outcomes in patients who experienced a myocardial infarction while treated with liraglutide versus placebo in the LEADER trial. *Diabetes Vasc. Dis. Res.* **2018**, *15*, 465–468. [CrossRef]
70. Mann, J.F.E.; Ørsted, D.D.; Brown-Frandsen, K.; Marso, S.P.; Poulter, N.R.; Rasmussen, S.; Tornøe, K.; Zinman, B.; Buse, J.B. Liraglutide and renal outcomes in type 2 diabetes. *N. Engl. J. Med.* **2017**, *377*, 839–848. [CrossRef]
71. Marso, S.P.; Bain, S.C.; Consoli, A.; Eliaschewitz, F.G.; Jodar, E.; Leiter, L.A.; Lingvay, I.; Rosenstock, J.; Seufert, J.; Warren, M.L.; et al. Semaglutide and cardiovascular outcomes in patients with type 2 diabetes. *N. Engl. J. Med.* **2016**, *375*, 1834–1844. [CrossRef] [PubMed]
72. Husain, M.; Birkenfeld, A.L.; Donsmark, M.; Dungan, K.; Eliaschewitz, F.G.; Franco, D.R.; Jeppesen, O.K.; Lingvay, I.; Mosenzon, O.; Pedersen, S.D.; et al. Oral semaglutide and cardiovascular outcomes in patients with type 2 diabetes. *N. Engl. J. Med.* **2019**, *381*, 841–851. [CrossRef] [PubMed]
73. Hernandez, A.F.; Green, J.B.; Janmohamed, S.; D'Agostino, R.B.; Granger, C.B.; Jones, N.P.; Leiter, L.A.; Rosenberg, A.E.; Sigmon, K.N.; Somerville, M.C.; et al. Albiglutide and cardiovascular outcomes in patients with type 2 diabetes and cardiovascular disease (Harmony Outcomes): A double-blind, randomised placebo-controlled trial. *Lancet* **2018**, *392*, 1519–1529. [CrossRef]
74. Gerstein, H.C.; Colhoun, H.M.; Dagenais, G.R.; Diaz, R.; Lakshmanan, M.; Pais, P.; Probstfield, J.; Riesmeyer, J.S.; Riddle, M.C.; Rydén, L.; et al. Dulaglutide and cardiovascular outcomes in type 2 diabetes (REWIND): A double-blind, randomised placebo-controlled trial. *Lancet* **2019**, *394*, 121–130. [CrossRef]
75. Dagenais, G.R.; Rydén, L.; Leiter, L.A.; Lakshmanan, M.; Dyal, L.; Probstfield, J.L.; Atisso, C.M.; Shaw, J.E.; Conget, I.; Cushman, W.C.; et al. Total cardiovascular or fatal events in people with type 2 diabetes and cardiovascular risk factors treated with dulaglutide in the REWIND trail: A post hoc analysis. *Cardiovasc. Diabetol.* **2020**, *19*, 199. [CrossRef]
76. Frias, J.P.; Bastyr, E.J.; Vignati, L.; Tschöp, M.H.; Schmitt, C.; Owen, K.; Christensen, R.H.; DiMarchi, R.D. The sustained effects of a dual GIP/GLP-1 receptor agonist, NNC0090-2746, in patients with type 2 diabetes. *Cell Metab.* **2017**, *26*, 343–352. [CrossRef]
77. Frias, J.P.; Nauck, M.A.; Van, J.; Kutner, M.E.; Cui, X.; Benson, C.; Urva, S.; Gimeno, R.E.; Milicevic, Z.; Robins, D.; et al. Efficacy and safety of LY3298176, a novel dual GIP and GLP-1 receptor agonist, in patients with type 2 diabetes: A randomised, placebo-controlled and active comparator-controlled phase 2 trial. *Lancet* **2018**, *392*, 2180–2193. [CrossRef]
78. Coskun, T.; Sloop, K.W.; Loghin, C.; Alsina-Fernandez, J.; Urva, S.; Bokvist, K.B.; Cui, X.; Briere, D.A.; Cabrera, O.; Roell, W.C.; et al. LY3298176, a novel dual GIP and GLP-1 receptor agonist for the treatment of type 2 diabetes mellitus: From discovery to clinical proof of concept. *Mol. Metab.* **2018**, *18*, 3–14. [CrossRef]
79. Drucker, D.J. Mechanisms of Action and Therapeutic Application of Glucagon-Like Peptide-1. *Cell Metab.* **2018**, *27*, 740–756. [CrossRef]
80. Baggio, L.L.; Drucker, D.J. Harnessing the Therapeutic Potential of Glucagon-Like Peptide-1: A Critical Review. *Treat Endocrinol.* **2002**, *1*, 117–125. [CrossRef]
81. Aroda, V.R. A Review of GLP-1 Receptor Agonists: Evolution and Advancement, Through the Lens of Randomised Controlled Trials. *Diabetes Obes. Metab.* **2018**, 22–33. [CrossRef] [PubMed]
82. Knudsen, L.B.; Lau, J. The Discovery and Development of Liraglutide and Semaglutide. *Front. Endocrinol.* **2019**, *10*, 155. [CrossRef]
83. Eng, J.; Kleinman, W.A.; Singh, L.; Singh, G.; Raufman, J.P. Isolation and characterization of exendin-4, an exendin-3 analogue, from Heloderma suspectum venom. Further evidence for an exendin receptor on dispersed acini from guinea pig pancreas. *J. Biol. Chem.* **1992**, *267*, 7402–7405. [CrossRef]
84. Nauck, M.A.; Quast, D.R.; Wefers, J.; Meier, J.J. GLP-1 Receptor Agonists in the Treatment of type 2 Diabetes—State-of-the-Art. *Mol. Metab.* **2020**, 101–102. [CrossRef]
85. Deacon, C.F.; Knudsen, L.B.; Madsen, K.; Wiberg, F.C.; Jacobsen, O.; Holst, J.J. Dipeptidyl peptidase IV resistant analogues of glucagon-like peptide-1 which have extended metabolic stability and improved biological activity. *Diabetologia* **1998**, *41*, 271–278. [CrossRef] [PubMed]

86. Knudsen, J.G.; Hamilton, A.; Ramracheya, R.; Tarasov, A.I.; Brereton, M.; Haythorne, E.; Chibalina, M.V.; Spégel, P.; Mulder, H.; Zhang, Q.; et al. Dysregulation of glucagon secretion by hyperglycemia-induced sodium-dependent reduction of ATP production. *Cell Metab.* **2019**, *29*, 430–442. [CrossRef]
87. Gaspari, T.; Welungoda, I.; Widdop, R.E.; Simpson, R.W.; Dear, A.E. The GLP-1 receptor agonist liraglutide inhibits progression of vascular disease via effects on atherogenesis, plaque stability and endothelial function in an ApoE/mouse model. *Diabetes Vasc. Dis. Res.* **2013**, *10*, 353–360. [CrossRef]
88. Shiraishi, D.; Fujiwara, Y.; Komohara, Y.; Mizuta, H.; Takeya, M. Glucagon-like peptide-1 (GLP-1) induces M2 polarization of human macrophages via STAT3 activation. *Biochem. Biophys. Res. Commun.* **2012**, *425*, 304–308. [CrossRef]
89. Ding, L.; Zhang, J. Glucagon-like peptide-1 activates endothelial nitric oxide synthase in human umbilical vein endothelial cells. *Acta Pharm. Sin.* **2012**, *33*, 75–81. [CrossRef]
90. Dai, Y.; Mehta, J.L.; Chen, M. Glucagon-like peptide-1 receptor agonist liraglutide inhibits endothelin-1 in endothelial cell by repressing nuclear factor-kappa B activation. *Cardiovasc. Drugs Ther.* **2013**, *27*, 371–380. [CrossRef]
91. Krasner, N.M.; Ido, Y.; Ruderman, N.B.; Cacicedo, J.M. Glucagon-Like Peptide-1 (GLP-1) analog liraglutide inhibits endothelial cell inflammation through a calcium and AMPK dependent mechanism. *PLoS ONE* **2014**, *9*. [CrossRef] [PubMed]
92. Erdogdu, Ö.; Eriksson, L.; Nyström, T.; Sjöholm, Å.; Zhang, Q. Exendin-4 restores glucolipotoxicity-induced gene expression in human coronary artery endothelial cells. *Biochem. Biophys. Res. Commun.* **2012**, *419*, 790–795. [CrossRef] [PubMed]
93. Mori, Y.; Matsui, T.; Hirano, T.; Yamagishi, S.I. Gip as a potential therapeutic target for atherosclerotic cardiovascular disease–a systematic review. *Int. J. Mol. Sci.* **2020**, *21*, 1509. [CrossRef] [PubMed]
94. Finan, B.; Ma, T.; Ottaway, N.; Müller, T.D.; Habegger, K.M.; Heppner, K.M.; Kirchner, H.; Holland, J.; Hembree, J.; Raver, C.; et al. Unimolecular dual incretins maximize metabolic benefits in rodents, monkeys, and humans. *Sci. Transl. Med.* **2013**, *5*. [CrossRef]
95. Sachs, S.; Niu, L.; Geyer, P.; Jall, S.; Kleinert, M.; Feuchtinger, A.; Stemmer, K.; Brielmeier, M.; Finan, B.; DiMarchi, R.D.; et al. Plasma proteome profiles treatment efficacy of incretin dual agonism in diet-induced obese female and male mice. *Diabetes Obes. Metab.* **2020**. [CrossRef]
96. Khoo, B.; Tan, T.M.M. Combination gut hormones: Prospects and questions for the future of obesity and diabetes therapy. *J. Endocrinol.* **2020**, *246*, R65–R74. [CrossRef]
97. Yamagishi, S.I.; Fukami, K.; Matsui, T. Crosstalk between advanced glycation end products (AGEs)-receptor RAGE axis and dipeptidyl peptidase-4-incretin system in diabetic vascular complications. *Cardiovasc. Diabetol.* **2015**, *14*, 1–12. [CrossRef]
98. Nogi, Y.; Nagashima, M.; Terasaki, M.; Nohtomi, K.; Watanabe, T.; Hirano, T. Glucose-dependent insulinotropic polypeptide prevents the progression of macrophage-driven atherosclerosis in diabetic apolipoprotein E-null mice. *PLoS ONE* **2012**, *7*. [CrossRef]
99. Watanabe, A.; Choe, S.; Chaptal, V.; Rosenberg, J.M.; Wright, E.M.; Grabe, M.; Abramson, J. The mechanism of sodium and substrate release from the binding pocket of vSGLT. *Nature* **2010**, *468*, 988–991. [CrossRef]
100. Wright, E.M.; Loo, D.D.F.L.; Hirayama, B.A. Biology of human sodium glucose transporters. *Physiol. Rev.* **2011**, *91*, 733–794. [CrossRef]
101. Ghezzi, C.; Loo, D.D.F.; Wright, E.M. Physiology of renal glucose handling via SGLT1, SGLT2 and GLUT2. *Diabetologia* **2018**, *61*, 2087–2097. [CrossRef] [PubMed]
102. Bakris, G.L.; Fonseca, V.A.; Sharma, K.; Wright, E.M. Renal sodium-glucose transport: Role in diabetes mellitus and potential clinical implications. *Kidney Int.* **2009**, *75*, 1272–1277. [CrossRef]
103. Rieg, T.; Vallon, V. Development of SGLT1 and SGLT2 inhibitors. *Diabetologia* **2018**, *61*, 2079–2086. [CrossRef] [PubMed]
104. Rossetti, L.; Smith, D.; Shulman, G.I.; Papachristou, D.; DeFronzo, R.A. Correction of hyperglycemia with phlorizin normalizes tissues sensitivity to insulin in diabetic rats. *J. Clin. Investig.* **1987**, *79*, 1510–1515. [CrossRef]
105. Oku, A.; Ueta, K.; Arakawa, K.; Ishihara, T.; Nawano, M.; Kuronuma, Y.; Matsumoto, M.; Saito, A.; Tsujihara, K.; Anai, M.; et al. T-1095, an inhibitor of renal Na+-glucose cotransporters, may provide a novel approach to treating diabetes. *Diabetes* **1999**, *48*, 1794–1800. [CrossRef] [PubMed]
106. Brown, E.; Rajeev, S.P.; Cuthbertson, D.J.; Wilding, J.P.H. A review of the mechanism of action, metabolic profile and hemodynamic effects of sodium-glucose co-transporter-2 inhibitors. *Diabetes Obes. Metab.* **2019**, *21*, 9–18. [CrossRef] [PubMed]
107. Ferrannini, E.; Muscelli, E.; Frascerra, S.; Baldi, S.; Mari, A.; Heise, T.; Broedl, U.C.; Woerle, H.J. Metabolic response to sodium-glucose cotransporter 2 inhibition in type 2 diabetic patients. *J. Clin. Investig.* **2014**, *124*, 499–508. [CrossRef] [PubMed]
108. Bonner, C.; Kerr-Conte, J.; Gmyr, V.; Queniat, G.; Moerman, E.; Thévenet, J.; Beaucamps, C.; Delalleau, N.; Popescu, I.; Malaisse, W.J.; et al. Inhibition of the glucose transporter SGLT2 with dapagliflozin in pancreatic alpha cells triggers glucagon secretion. *Nat. Med.* **2015**, *21*, 512–517. [CrossRef]
109. Merovci, A.; Solis-Herrera, C.; Daniele, G.; Eldor, R.; Vanessa Fiorentino, T.; Tripathy, D.; Xiong, J.; Perez, Z.; Norton, L.; Abdul-Ghani, M.A.; et al. Dapagliflozin improves muscle insulin sensitivity but enhances endogenous glucose production. *J. Clin. Investig.* **2014**, *124*, 509–514. [CrossRef]
110. Tahara, A.; Takasu, T.; Yokono, M.; Imamura, M.; Kurosaki, E. Characterization and comparison of SGLT2 inhibitors: Part 3. Effects on diabetic complications in type 2 diabetic mice. *Eur. J. Pharm.* **2017**, *809*, 163–171. [CrossRef]
111. Aroor, A.R.; Das, N.A.; Carpenter, A.J.; Habibi, J.; Jia, G.; Ramirez-Perez, F.I.; Martinez-Lemus, L.; Manrique-Acevedo, C.M.; Hayden, M.R.; Duta, C.; et al. Glycemic control by the SGLT2 inhibitor empagliflozin decreases aortic stiffness, renal resistivity index and kidney injury. *Cardiovasc. Diabetol.* **2018**, *17*. [CrossRef] [PubMed]

112. Steven, S.; Oelze, M.; Hanf, A.; Kröller-Schön, S.; Kashani, F.; Roohani, S.; Welschof, P.; Kopp, M.; Gödtel-Armbrust, U.; Xia, N.; et al. The SGLT2 inhibitor empagliflozin improves the primary diabetic complications in ZDF rats. *Redox Biol.* **2017**, *13*, 370–385. [CrossRef] [PubMed]
113. Lee, D.M.; Battson, M.L.; Jarrell, D.K.; Hou, S.; Ecton, K.E.; Weir, T.L.; Gentile, C.L. SGLT2 inhibition via dapagliflozin improves generalized vascular dysfunction and alters the gut microbiota in type 2 diabetic mice. *Cardiovasc. Diabetol.* **2018**, *17*, 62. [CrossRef] [PubMed]
114. Terasaki, M.; Hiromura, M.; Mori, Y.; Kohashi, K.; Nagashima, M.; Kushima, H.; Watanabe, T.; Hirano, T. Amelioration of hyperglycemia with a sodium-glucose cotransporter 2 inhibitor prevents macrophage-driven atherosclerosis through macrophage foam cell formation suppression in type 1 and type 2 diabetic mice. *PLoS ONE* **2015**, *10*, e143396. [CrossRef] [PubMed]
115. Gaspari, T.; Spizzo, I.; Liu, H.; Hu, Y.; Simpson, R.W.; Widdop, R.E.; Dear, A.E. Dapagliflozin attenuates human vascular endothelial cell activation and induces vasorelaxation: A potential mechanism for inhibition of atherogenesis. *Diabetes Vasc. Dis. Res.* **2018**, *15*, 64–73. [CrossRef] [PubMed]
116. Han, J.H.; Oh, T.J.; Lee, G.; Maeng, H.J.; Lee, D.H.; Kim, K.M.; Choi, S.H.; Jang, H.C.; Lee, H.S.; Park, K.S.; et al. The beneficial effects of empagliflozin, an SGLT2 inhibitor, on atherosclerosis in ApoE −/− mice fed a western diet. *Diabetologia* **2017**, *60*, 364–376. [CrossRef]
117. Nasiri-Ansari, N.; Dimitriadis, G.K.; Agrogiannis, G.; Perrea, D.; Kostakis, I.D.; Kaltsas, G.; Papavassiliou, A.G.; Randeva, H.S.; Kassi, E.; Nasiri-Ansari, N.; et al. Canagliflozin attenuates the progression of atherosclerosis and inflammation process in APOE knockout mice. *Cardiovasc. Diabetol.* **2018**, *17*, 106. [CrossRef]
118. Ye, Y.; Bajaj, M.; Yang, H.C.; Perez-Polo, J.R.; Birnbaum, Y. SGLT-2 Inhibition with dapagliflozin reduces the activation of the Nlrp3/ASC Inflammasome and attenuates the development of diabetic cardiomyopathy in mice with type 2 diabetes. Further augmentation of the effects with saxagliptin, a DPP4 inhibitor. *Cardiovasc. Drugs* **2017**, *31*, 119–132. [CrossRef]
119. Zinman, B.; Wanner, C.; Lachin, J.M.; Fitchett, D.; Bluhmki, E.; Hantel, S.; Mattheus, M.; Devins, T.; Johansen, O.E.; Woerle, H.J.; et al. Empagliflozin, cardiovascular outcomes, and mortality in type 2 diabetes. *N. Engl. J. Med.* **2015**, *373*, 2117–2128. [CrossRef]
120. Neal, B.; Perkovic, V.; Mahaffey, K.W.; de Zeeuw, D.; Fulcher, G.; Erondu, N.; Shaw, W.; Law, G.; Desai, M.; Matthews, D.R. Canagliflozin and cardiovascular and renal events in type 2 diabetes. *N. Engl. J. Med.* **2017**, *377*, 644–657. [CrossRef]
121. Perkovic, V.; Jardine, M.J.; Neal, B.; Bompoint, S.; Heerspink, H.J.L.; Charytan, D.M.; Edwards, R.; Agarwal, R.; Bakris, G.; Bull, S.; et al. Canagliflozin and renal outcomes in type 2 diabetes and nephropathy. *N. Engl. J. Med.* **2019**, *380*, 2295–2306. [CrossRef] [PubMed]
122. Wiviott, S.D.; Raz, I.; Bonaca, M.P.; Mosenzon, O.; Kato, E.T.; Cahn, A.; Silverman, M.G.; Zelniker, T.A.; Kuder, J.F.; Murphy, S.A.; et al. Dapagliflozin and cardiovascular outcomes in type 2 diabetes. *N. Engl. J. Med.* **2019**, *380*, 347–357. [CrossRef] [PubMed]
123. Nassif, M.E.; Windsor, S.; Tang, F.; Khariton, Y.; Husain, M.; Inzucchi, S.; McGuire, D.; Pitt, B.; Scirica, B.; Austin, B.; et al. Dapagliflozin effects on biomarkers, symptoms, and functional status in patients with heart failure with reduced ejection fraction. *Circulation* **2019**, *140*, 1463–1476. [CrossRef] [PubMed]
124. Cannon, C.P.; Pratley, R.; Dagogo-Jack, S.; Mancuso, J.; Huyck, S.; Masiukiewicz, U.; Charbonnel, B.; Frederich, R.; Gallo, S.; Cosentino, F.; et al. Cardiovascular outcomes with ertugliflozin in type 2 diabetes. *N. Engl. J. Med.* **2020**, *383*, 1425–1435. [CrossRef] [PubMed]
125. Bhatt, D.L.; Szarek, M.; Pitt, B.; Cannon, C.P.; Leiter, L.A.; McGuire, D.K.; Lewis, J.B.; Riddle, M.C.; Inzucchi, S.E.; Kosiborod, M.N.; et al. Sotagliflozin in patients with diabetes and chronic kidney disease. *N. Engl. J. Med.* **2020**. [CrossRef] [PubMed]
126. Bhatt, D.L.; Szarek, M.; Steg, P.G.; Cannon, C.P.; Leiter, L.A.; McGuire, D.K.; Lewis, J.B.; Riddle, M.C.; Voors, A.A.; Metra, M.; et al. Sotagliflozin in patients with diabetes and recent worsening heart failure. *N. Engl. J. Med.* **2020**. [CrossRef] [PubMed]
127. Bailey, C.J.; Marx, N. Cardiovascular protection in type 2 diabetes: Insights from recent outcome trials. *Diabetes Obes. Metab.* **2019**, *21*, 3–14. [CrossRef]
128. Seidah, N.G.; Awan, Z.; Chrétien, M.; Mbikay, M. PCSK9: A key modulator of cardiovascular health. *Circ. Res.* **2014**, *114*, 1022–1036. [CrossRef]
129. Abifadel, M.; Varret, M.; Rabès, J.P.; Allard, D.; Ouguerram, K.; Devillers, M.; Cruaud, C.; Benjannet, S.; Wickham, L.; Erlich, D.; et al. Mutations in PCSK9 cause autosomal dominant hypercholesterolemia. *Nat. Genet.* **2003**, *34*, 154–156. [CrossRef]
130. Cohen, J.; Pertsemlidis, A.; Kotowski, I.K.; Graham, R.; Garcia, C.K.; Hobbs, H.H. Low LDL cholesterol in individuals of African descent resulting from frequent nonsense mutations in PCSK9. *Nat. Genet.* **2005**, *37*, 161–165. [CrossRef]
131. Cohen, J.C.; Boerwinkle, E.; Mosley, T.H.; Hobbs, H.H. Sequence variations in PCSK9, low LDL, and protection against coronary heart disease. *N. Engl. J. Med.* **2006**, *354*, 1264–1272. [CrossRef] [PubMed]
132. Stoekenbroek, R.M.; Lambert, G.; Cariou, B.; Hovingh, G.K. Inhibiting PCSK9—Biology beyond LDL control. *Nat. Rev. Endocrinol.* **2018**, *15*, 52–62. [CrossRef] [PubMed]
133. Seidah, N.G.; Prat, A.; Pirillo, A.; Catapano, A.L.; Danilo Norata, G. Novel strategies to target proprotein convertase subtilisin kexin 9: Beyond monoclonal antibodies. *Cardiovasc. Pathol.* **2019**, *115*, 510–519. [CrossRef] [PubMed]
134. Seidah, N.G.; Benjannet, S.; Wickham, L.; Marcinkiewicz, J.; Bélanger Jasmin, S.; Stifani, S.; Basak, A.; Prat, A.; Chrétien, M. The secretory proprotein convertase neural apoptosis-regulated convertase 1 (NARC-1): Liver regeneration and neuronal differentiation. *Proc. Natl. Acad. Sci. USA* **2003**, *100*, 928–933. [CrossRef] [PubMed]
135. Shapiro, M.D.; Tavori, H.; Fazio, S. PCSK9 from basic science discoveries to clinical trials. *Circ. Res.* **2018**, *122*, 1420–1438. [CrossRef] [PubMed]

136. Ding, Z.; Wang, X.; Liu, S.; Shahanawaz, J.; Theus, S.; Fan, Y.; Deng, X.; Zhou, S.; Mehta, J.L. PCSK9 expression in the ischemic heart and its relationship to infarct size, cardiac function, and development of autophagy. *Cardiovasc. Res.* **2018**, *114*, 1738–1751. [CrossRef]
137. Seidah, N.G.; Prat, A. The biology and therapeutic targeting of the proprotein convertases. *Nat. Rev. Drug Discov.* **2012**, *11*, 367–383. [CrossRef]
138. Lagace, T.A. PCSK9 and LDLR degradation: Regulatory mechanisms in circulation and in cells. *Curr. Opin. Lipidol.* **2014**, *25*, 387–393. [CrossRef]
139. Lan, H.; Pang, L.; Smith, M.M.; Levitan, D.; Ding, W.; Liu, L.; Shan, L.; Shah, V.V.; Laverty, M.; Arreaza, G.; et al. Proprotein convertase subtilisin/kexin type 9 (PCSK9) affects gene expression pathways beyond cholesterol metabolism in liver cells. *J. Cell. Physiol.* **2010**, *224*, 273–281. [CrossRef]
140. Tang, Z.H.; Li, T.H.; Peng, J.; Zheng, J.; Li, T.T.; Liu, L.S.; Jiang, Z.S.; Zheng, X.L. PCSK9: A novel inflammation modulator in atherosclerosis? *J. Cell. Physiol.* **2019**, *234*, 2345–2355. [CrossRef]
141. Ding, Z.; Liu, S.; Wang, X.; Deng, X.; Fan, Y.; Shahanawaz, J.; Reis, R.J.S.; Varughese, K.I.; Sawamura, T.; Mehta, J.L. Cross-Talk between LOX-1 and PCSK9 in vascular tissues. *Cardiovasc. Res.* **2015**, *107*, 556–567. [CrossRef] [PubMed]
142. Ding, Z.; Pothineni, N.V.K.; Goel, A.; Lüscher, T.F.; Mehta, J.L. PCSK9 and inflammation: Role of shear stress, pro-inflammatory cytokines, and LOX-1. *Cardiovasc. Res.* **2020**, *116*, 908–915. [CrossRef] [PubMed]
143. Giunzioni, I.; Tavori, H.; Covarrubias, R.; Major, A.S.; Ding, L.; Zhang, Y.; Devay, R.M.; Hong, L.; Fan, D.; Predazzi, I.M.; et al. Local effects of human PCSK9 on the atherosclerotic lesion. *J. Pathol.* **2016**, *238*, 52–62. [CrossRef] [PubMed]
144. Tang, Z.H.; Peng, J.; Ren, Z.; Yang, J.; Li, T.T.; Li, T.H.; Wang, Z.; Wei, D.H.; Liu, L.S.; Zheng, X.L.; et al. New role of PCSK9 in atherosclerotic inflammation promotion involving the TLR4/NF-κB pathway. *Atherosclerosis* **2017**, *262*, 113–122. [CrossRef]
145. Guo, Y.; Yan, B.; Gui, Y.; Tang, Z.; Tai, S.; Zhou, S.; Zheng, X.L. Physiology and role of PCSK9 in vascular disease: Potential impact of localized PCSK9 in vascular wall. *J. Cell. Physiol.* **2020**. [CrossRef] [PubMed]
146. Urban, D.; Pöss, J.; Böhm, M.; Laufs, U. Targeting the proprotein convertase subtilisin/kexin type 9 for the treatment of dyslipidemia and atherosclerosis. *J. Am. Coll. Cardiol.* **2013**, *62*, 1401–1408. [CrossRef]
147. Rashid, S.; Curtis, D.E.; Garuti, R.; Anderson, N.H.; Bashmakov, Y.; Ho, Y.K.; Hammer, R.E.; Moon, Y.A.; Horton, J.D. Decreased plasma cholesterol and hypersensitivity to statins in mice lacking Pcsk9. *Proc. Natl. Acad. Sci. USA* **2005**, *102*, 5374–5379. [CrossRef]
148. Denis, M.; Marcinkiewicz, J.; Zaid, A.; Gauthier, D.; Poirier, S.; Lazure, C.; Seidah, N.G.; Prat, A. Gene inactivation of proprotein convertase subtilisin/kexin type 9 reduces atherosclerosis in mice. *Circulation* **2012**, *125*, 894–901. [CrossRef]
149. Xu, S.; Luo, S.; Zhu, Z.; Xu, J. Small Molecules as Inhibitors of PCSK9: Current Status and Future Challenges. *Eur. J. Med. Chem.* **2019**, *162*, 212–233. [CrossRef]
150. Warden, B.A.; Fazio, S.; Shapiro, M.D. The PCSK9 Revolution: Current Status, Controversies and Future Directions: The PCSK9 Revolution. *Trends Cardiovasc. Med.* **2020**, *30*, 179–185. [CrossRef]
151. Nishikido, T.; Ray, K.K. Non-antibody approaches to proprotein convertase subtilisin kexin 9 inhibition: SiRNA, antisense oligonucleotides, adnectins, vaccination, and new attempts at small-molecule inhibitors based on new discoveries. *Front. Cardiovasc. Med.* **2019**, *5*. [CrossRef]
152. Kühnast, S.; van der Hoorn, J.W.A.; Pieterman, E.J.; van den Hoek, A.M.; Sasiela, W.J.; Gusarova, V.; Peyman, A.; Schäfer, H.L.; Schwahn, U.; Jukema, J.W.; et al. Alirocumab inhibits atherosclerosis, improves the plaque morphology, and enhances the effects of a statin. *J. Lipid Res.* **2014**, *55*, 2103–2112. [CrossRef] [PubMed]
153. Chan, J.C.Y.; Piper, D.E.; Cao, Q.; Liu, D.; King, C.; Wang, W.; Tang, J.; Liu, Q.; Higbee, J.; Xia, Z.; et al. A proprotein convertase subtilisin/kexin type 9 neutralizing antibody reduces serum cholesterol in mice and nonhuman primates. *Proc. Natl. Acad. Sci. USA* **2009**, *106*, 9820–9825. [CrossRef] [PubMed]
154. Chaparro-Riggers, J.; Liang, H.; deVay, R.M.; Bai, L.; Sutton, J.E.; Chen, W.; Geng, T.; Lindquist, K.; Casas, M.G.; Boustany, L.M.; et al. Increasing serum half-life and extending cholesterol lowering in vivo by engineering antibody with pH-sensitive binding to PCSK9. *J. Biol. Chem.* **2012**, *287*, 11090–11097. [CrossRef] [PubMed]
155. Frank-Kamenetsky, M.; Grefhorst, A.; Anderson, N.N.; Racie, T.S.; Bramlage, B.; Akinc, A.; Butler, D.; Charisse, K.; Dorkin, R.; Fan, Y.; et al. Therapeutic RNAi targeting PCSK9 acutely lowers plasma cholesterol in rodents and LDL cholesterol in nonhuman primates. *Proc. Natl. Acad. Sci. USA* **2008**, *105*, 11915–11920. [CrossRef] [PubMed]
156. Sabatine, M.S.; Giugliano, R.P.; Wiviott, S.D.; Raal, F.J.; Blom, D.J.; Robinson, J.; Ballantyne, C.M.; Somaratne, R.; Legg, J.; Wasserman, S.M.; et al. Efficacy and safety of evolocumab in reducing lipids and cardiovascular events. *N. Engl. J. Med.* **2015**, *372*, 1500–1509. [CrossRef] [PubMed]
157. Sabatine, M.S.; Giugliano, R.P.; Keech, A.C.; Honarpour, N.; Wiviott, S.D.; Murphy, S.A.; Kuder, J.F.; Wang, H.; Liu, T.; Wasserman, S.M.; et al. Evolocumab and clinical outcomes in patients with cardiovascular disease. *N. Engl. J. Med.* **2017**, *376*, 1713–1722. [CrossRef] [PubMed]
158. Schwartz, G.G.; Steg, P.G.; Szarek, M.; Bhatt, D.L.; Bittner, V.A.; Diaz, R.; Edelberg, J.M.; Goodman, S.G.; Hanotin, C.; Harrington, R.A.; et al. Alirocumab and cardiovascular outcomes after acute coronary syndrome. *N. Engl. J. Med.* **2018**, *379*, 2097–2107. [CrossRef]
159. Robinson, J.G.; Farnier, M.; Krempf, M.; Bergeron, J.; Luc, G.; Averna, M.; Stroes, E.S.; Langslet, G.; Raal, F.J.; el Shahawy, M.; et al. Efficacy and safety of alirocumab in reducing lipids and cardiovascular events. *N. Engl. J. Med.* **2015**, *372*, 1489–1499. [CrossRef]

160. Steg, P.G.; Szarek, M.; Bhatt, D.L.; Bittner, V.A.; Brégeault, M.F.; Dalby, A.J.; Diaz, R.; Edelberg, J.M.; Goodman, S.G.; Hanotin, C.; et al. Effect of alirocumab on mortality after acute coronary syndromes: An analysis of the ODYSSEY OUTCOMES randomized clinical trial. *Circulation* **2019**, *140*, 103–112. [CrossRef]
161. Fitzgerald, K.; Frank-Kamenetsky, M.; Shulga-Morskaya, S.; Liebow, A.; Bettencourt, B.R.; Sutherland, J.E.; Hutabarat, R.M.; Clausen, V.A.; Karsten, V.; Cehelsky, J.; et al. Effect of an RNA interference drug on the synthesis of proprotein convertase subtilisin/kexin type 9 (PCSK9) and the concentration of serum LDL cholesterol in healthy volunteers: A randomised, single-blind, placebo-controlled, phase 1 trial. *Lancet* **2014**, *383*, 60–68. [CrossRef]
162. Ray, K.K.; Landmesser, U.; Leiter, L.A.; Kallend, D.; Dufour, R.; Karakas, M.; Hall, T.; Troquay, R.P.T.; Turner, T.; Visseren, F.L.J.; et al. Inclisiran in patients at high cardiovascular risk with elevated LDL cholesterol. *N. Engl. J. Med.* **2017**, *376*, 1430–1440. [CrossRef] [PubMed]
163. Ray, K.K.; Wright, R.S.; Kallend, D.; Koenig, W.; Leiter, L.A.; Raal, F.J.; Bisch, J.A.; Richardson, T.; Jaros, M.; Wijngaard, P.L.J.; et al. Two Phase 3 Trials of Inclisiran in Patients with Elevated LDL Cholesterol. *N. Engl. J. Med.* **2020**, *382*, 1507–1519. [CrossRef] [PubMed]
164. Blanchard, V.; Khantalin, I.; Ramin-Mangata, S.; Chémello, K.; Nativel, B.; Lambert, G. PCSK9: From biology to clinical applications. *Pathology* **2019**, *51*, 177–183. [CrossRef] [PubMed]
165. Tomlinson, B.; Hu, M.; Zhang, Y.; Chan, P.; Liu, Z.M. Alirocumab for the treatment of hypercholesterolemia. *Expert Opin. Biol.* **2017**, *17*, 633–643. [CrossRef]
166. Kasichayanula, S.; Grover, A.; Emery, M.G.; Gibbs, M.A.; Somaratne, R.; Wasserman, S.M.; Gibbs, J.P. Clinical pharmacokinetics and pharmacodynamics of evolocumab, a PCSK9 inhibitor. *Clin. Pharm.* **2018**, *57*, 769–779. [CrossRef]
167. Reyes-Soffer, G.; Pavlyha, M.; Ngai, C.; Thomas, T.; Holleran, S.; Ramakrishnan, R.; Karmally, W.; Nandakumar, R.; Fontanez, N.; Obunike, J.; et al. Effects of PCSK9 inhibition with alirocumab on lipoprotein metabolism in healthy humans. *Circulation* **2017**, *135*, 352–362. [CrossRef]
168. Ogura, M. PCSK9 inhibition in the management of familial hypercholesterolemia. *J. Cardiol.* **2018**, *71*, 1–7. [CrossRef]
169. Stoekenbroek, R.M.; Kallend, D.; Wijngaard, P.L.; Kastelein, J.J. Inclisiran for the treatment of cardiovascular disease: The ORION clinical development program. *Future Cardiol.* **2018**, *14*, 433–442. [CrossRef]
170. Fitzgerald, K.; White, S.; Borodovsky, A.; Bettencourt, B.R.; Strahs, A.; Clausen, V.; Wijngaard, P.; Horton, J.D.; Taubel, J.; Brooks, A.; et al. A highly durable RNAi therapeutic inhibitor of PCSK9. *N. Engl. J. Med.* **2017**, *376*, 41–51. [CrossRef]

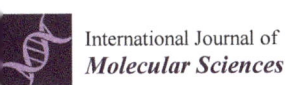

Review

The Protective Role of Sestrin2 in Atherosclerotic and Cardiac Diseases

Yoshimi Kishimoto [1,*], Kazuo Kondo [2] and Yukihiko Momiyama [3]

1. Department of Food Science and Human Nutrition, Faculty of Agriculture, Setsunan University, 45-1 Nagaotouge-cho, Hirakata, Osaka 573-0101, Japan
2. Ochanomizu University, 2-1-1 Otsuka, Bunkyo-ku, Tokyo 112-8610, Japan; k24kondo523@gmail.com
3. Department of Cardiology, National Hospital Organization Tokyo Medical Center, 2-5-1 Higashigaoka, Meguro-ku, Tokyo 152-8902, Japan; ymomiyamajp@gmail.com
* Correspondence: yoshimi.kishimoto@setsunan.ac.jp; Tel.: +81-72-896-6352

Abstract: Atherosclerotic disease, such as coronary artery disease (CAD), is known to be a chronic inflammatory disease, as well as an age-related disease. Excessive oxidative stress produced by reactive oxygen species (ROS) contributes to the pathogenesis of atherosclerosis. Sestrin2 is an anti-oxidant protein that is induced by various stresses such as hypoxia, DNA damage, and oxidative stress. Sestrin2 is also suggested to be associated with aging. Sestrin2 is expressed and secreted mainly by macrophages, endothelial cells, and cardiomyocytes. Sestrin2 plays an important role in suppressing the production and accumulation of ROS, thus protecting cells from oxidative damage. Since sestrin2 is reported to have anti-oxidant and anti-inflammatory properties, it may play a protective role against the progression of atherosclerosis and may be a potential therapeutic target for the amelioration of atherosclerosis. Regarding the association between blood sestrin2 levels and atherosclerotic disease, the blood sestrin2 levels in patients with CAD or carotid atherosclerosis were reported to be high. High blood sestrin2 levels in patients with such atherosclerotic disease may reflect a compensatory response to increased oxidative stress and may help protect against the progression of atherosclerosis. This review describes the protective role of sestrin2 against the progression of atherosclerotic and cardiac diseases.

Keywords: atherosclerosis; carotid plaque; coronary artery disease; inflammation; oxidative stress; sestrin2

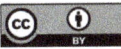

1. Introduction

Cardiovascular diseases, especially atherosclerotic diseases, are known to be associated with oxidative stress produced by excessive reactive oxygen species (ROS) [1,2]. The sestrin family is comprised of antioxidant proteins, and mammals express three sestrins that share nearly 50% identical amino acid sequences: sestrin1, sestrin2, and sestrin3. Sestrins protect against the oxidative stress that is induced by cell or tissue injury by relieving oxidative stress [3–5]. In 1999, sestrin1 was identified as p53-activated gene 26 (PA26), and sestrin2 and sestrin3 were discovered in 2002. Sestrin1 and sestrin2 are recognized to be PA26-related proteins and are regulated mainly by p53 which is induced by oxidative stress, genotoxic stress, and oncogenic stress. Sestrin3 was identified as a PA26 structure-related gene induced by forkhead box O (FOXO) transcription factors, which also contribute to the induction of sestrin1 [3–5]. Among the members of the sestrin family, sestrin2 has been most extensively investigated; it has been demonstrated to be an important stress-induced protein that is responsive to various stresses such as hypoxia, DNA damage, and oxidative stress, and sestrin2 is widely expressed in mammals [3,6]. Sestrin2 has a protective effect on physiological and pathological states, mainly by regulating oxidative stress, endoplasmic reticulum stress, autophagy, metabolism, and inflammation [7]. In addition, sestrin2 regulates cell growth, metabolism and survival in response to various stresses. Its anti-oxidative and anti-aging roles have been the focus of many recent studies [8].

This review describes the protective role of sestrin2 against the progression of atherosclerotic and cardiac diseases.

2. Physiopathological Mechanisms of Sestrin2

2.1. Sestrin2 Signaling Pathways

Sestrin2, a homolog of PA26, is a highly conserved anti-oxidant protein that was originally identified as hypoxia-induced gene 95 (Hi95) [3,4]. Sestrin2 is expressed and secreted mainly by macrophages, T lymphocytes, endothelial cells, and cardiac fibroblasts and cardiomyocytes [6,9,10]. Sestrin2 was shown to accumulate in cells exposed to stress and to play an important role in suppressing the production of ROS, thus protecting cells from oxidative damage [4]. Sestrin2 is recognized to be a negative regulator of mammalian target of rapamycin (mTOR) signaling through its activation of AMP-dependent protein kinase (AMPK) and its phosphorylation of tuberous sclerosis complex 2 (TSC2) [11]. The expression of sestrin2 is regulated by several transcription factors such as p53, activator protein-1 (AP-1), hypoxia inducible factor (HIF)-1α, and nuclear erythroid-related factor 2 (Nrf2), which are activated by stress responses [4,10]. Sestrin2 functions as a stress-inducible metabolic regulator by inhibiting oxidative stress and proinflammatory signaling, mainly via mechanisms that are dependent on AMPK and mTOR complex 1 (mTORC1) [12,13].

Sestrin2 has been recognized to play a protective role against oxidative stress, mainly via the two signaling pathways of Kelch-like ECH-associated protein 1 (Keap1)/Nrf2 and AMPK/mTORC1 as follows:

Keap1 is a cysteine-rich protein that represses Nrf2 activity. Nrf2 localizes in the cytoplasm and binds to Keap1. The Keap1/Nrf2 signaling plays a critical role in maintaining cell homeostasis under oxidative stress. Sestrin2, activated by oxidative stress, increases the expression of sulfiredoxin through the activation of Nrf2. Sestrin2 can also activate Nrf2 by promoting a p62-dependent autophagic degradation of Keap1. Sestrin2 thus decreases the accumulation of ROS and stimulates anti-oxidant defenses via Keap1/Nrf2 signaling activation [8,14].

TOR is a pivotal regulator of cell growth, proliferation, metabolism and autophagy. TOR was first identified as a protein kinase inhibited by rapamycin. mTOR is present in two distinct complexes, mTORC1, which is sensitive to rapamycin, and mTORC2, which is not [15,16]. The regulation of mTORC1 is dependent on tuberous sclerosis complex 1 and 2 (TSC1 and TSC2), of which TSC2 acts as a GTPase-activating protein for the small GTPase Rheb, which negatively controls Rheb and activates mTOR [15,16]. AMPK is an important nutrient-sensing protein kinase that plays a critical role in maintaining metabolic homeostasis [8,17]. The mechanisms of AMPK activation include phosphorylation by its upstream kinases, such as liver kinase B1 (LKB1). Sestrin2 induced by stress inhibits mTORC1 through AMPK activation. Moreover, mTORC1 inhibits autophagy, which plays a critical role in cell viability [18]. As an inhibitor of mTORC1, sestrin2 promotes autophagy. The AMPK/mTORC1 signaling pathway is known to be critical for the role of sestrin2 in controlling cell metabolism and survival under stress conditions [8].

The main signaling pathways and pathophysiological mechanisms of sestrin2 are summarized in Figure 1.

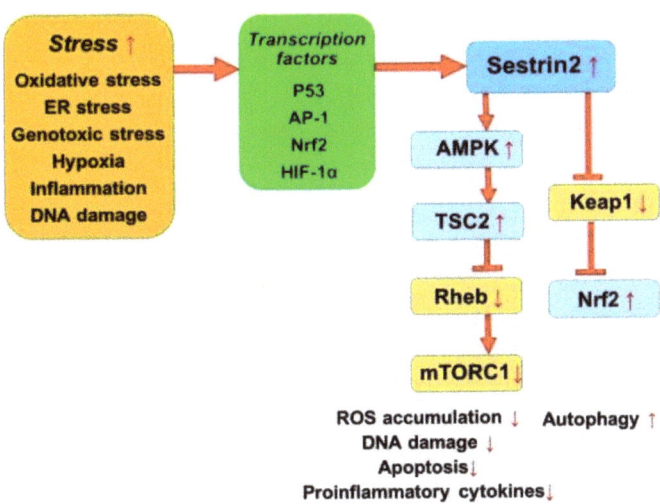

Figure 1. A summary of the main signaling pathways and pathophysiological mechanisms of sestrin2.

2.2. Sestrin2 and Oxidative Stress

Sestrin2 acts as an anti-oxidant protein that diminishes the accumulation of ROS and inhibits mTORC1 signaling. Both the accumulation of ROS and the activation of mTORC1 were shown to be associated with aging and age-related diseases, such as atherosclerotic disease [19].

Hu et al. showed that the expression of sestrin2 was upregulated in macrophages by oxidized low-density lipoprotein (LDL) in a time-dependent and dose-dependent manner, and that the knockdown of sestrin2 with small RNA interference promoted cell apoptosis and the production of ROS induced by oxidized LDL [9]. They suggested that the induction of sestrin2 acts as a compensatory response to oxidized LDL for cell survival.

Yang et al. also reported that the downregulation of sestrin2 increased the production of ROS and elevated blood pressure in mice with dopamine D2 receptor (D2R) silent-induced hypertension [20]. D2R decreased the renal production of ROS and regulated blood pressure, in part via the positive regulation of paraoxonase 2. In D2R-deficient mice, the silencing of D2R in renal proximal tubule cells decreased the expression of sestrin2 and increased hyperoxidized peroxiredoxins. In contrast, D2R stimulation in renal proximal tubule cells increased the sestrin2 expression, decreased hyperoxidized peroxiredoxins, and reduced ROS production. Silencing sestrin2 in renal proximal tubule cells increased hyperoxidized peroxiredoxins and ROS production, abolished a D2R-induced decrease in peroxiredoxin hyperoxidation, and prevented the inhibitory effect of D2R stimulation on ROS production. In mice, renal selective silencing of sestrin2 by small interfering RNA increased renal oxidative stress and blood pressure values. These findings thus suggest that D2R, via paraoxonase 2 and sestrin2, maintains the normal renal redox balance, which contributes to the maintenance of normal blood pressure.

In dendritic cells, sestrin2 knockdown was shown to promote endoplasmic reticulum (ER) stress-related apoptosis and to exacerbate ER disruption and the formation of dilated and aggregated structures [21]. The overexpression of sestrin2 in dendritic cells markedly decreased the apoptotic rate and inhibited ER stress-related protein translation. Moreover, sestrin-deficient mice demonstrated increased apoptosis and an aggravated extent of ER stress. These findings suggest that sestrin2 is a potential regulator to inhibit ER stress signaling that exerts a protective effect on apoptosis in dendritic cells.

The accumulating evidence suggests that sestrin2 acts as an anti-oxidant protein and reduces the production and accumulation of ROS.

2.3. Sestrin2 and Inflammation

Atherosclerotic disease such as coronary artery disease (CAD) is recognized to be a chronic inflammatory disease as well as an age-related disease, and oxidative stress produced by excessive ROS contributes to the pathogenesis of atherosclerosis [1,22]. The excessive production of ROS is implicated in vascular injury. Endogenous anti-oxidants are thought to play a protective role against the progression of atherosclerosis, and the imbalance in oxidant and anti-oxidant mechanisms leads to a state of oxidative stress [1,22]. Atherosclerotic disease is characterized as involving an imbalance between the formation of ROS and the ROS-degrading antioxidant system [23]. Since the progression of atherosclerosis is associated with inflammation with oxidative stress [1,22], sestrin2 would play a protective role against atherosclerotic disease [8,12].

Kim et al. reported that lipopolysaccharide (LPS), a Toll-like receptor 4 (TLR4) ligand, increased the levels of sestrin2 mRNA and protein in macrophages, whereas sestrin1 mRNA and protein were not affected by LPS [10]. The same researchers also showed that sestrin2 almost completely inhibited an LPS-induced release of nitric oxide (NO) and the expression of inducible nitric oxide synthase (iNOS) [24]. Their sestrin2 knockout experiment confirmed the role of sestrin2 in LPS-activated macrophages. The release and expression of proinflammatory cytokines such as tumor necrosis factor (TNF)-α, interleukin (IL)-6 and IL-1β were shown to be inhibited in sestrin2-expressing cells. Sestrin2 prevented LPS-induced apoptosis and ROS production via the inhibition of NADPH oxidase. Those authors suggested that sestrin2 inhibits TLR-induced proinflammatory signaling and protects cells by inhibiting c-Jun N-terminal kinase (JNK)- or p38-mediated c-Jun phosphorylation [24].

Hwang et al. demonstrated that the knockdown of sestrin2 in human umbilical vein endothelial cells (HUVECs) promoted LPS-induced inflammatory responses, apoptosis, and ROS production [25]. In sestrin2-knockdown HUVECs, the LPS-mediated nuclear factor kappa B (NF-κB) phosphorylation, the secretion of pro-inflammatory cytokines such as TNF-α, monocyte chemotactic protein-1 (MCP-1), and IL-6, and the expression of adhesion molecules were significantly increased. LPS-induced ROS production, ER stress, and cell toxicity were also increased after sestrin2 knockdown. All of these effects were fully abrogated by treatment with an AMPK activator. Treatment with an AMPK activator was shown to reduce atherosclerotic lesions in apolipoprotein E-knockout mice [26], and in the aortic tissue samples from the mice, sestrin2 knockdown resulted in the reduction in AMPK phosphorylation and the induction of LPS-mediated NF-κB phosphorylation, thereby leading to the up-regulation of adhesion molecules and ER stress-related signaling [25]. These findings thus suggested that sestrin2 knockdown aggravates atherosclerotic processes by increasing pro-inflammatory reactions and ER stress in the endothelium via an AMPK-dependent mechanism.

These findings therefore indicate that sestrin2 has anti-oxidant and anti-inflammatory properties, thereby protecting against the progression of atherosclerosis. Sestrin2 might be a beneficial target for the amelioration of atherosclerosis, indicating its potential as a therapeutic target in atherosclerotic diseases.

Angiotensin II (AngII) are recognized to induce apoptosis via the activation of AngII receptors, and the activation of AngII signaling triggers proinflammatory effects and the production of ROS in vascular walls by inducing multiple downstream pathways, which consequently causes endothelial dysfunction and cardiovascular diseases [27]. Yi et al. showed that AngII induced the expression of sestrin2 in HUVECs in a time-dependent and dose-dependent manner and that the knockdown of sestrin2 using small RNA interference promoted the cellular toxicity of AngII as well as the reduction in cell viability, the exacerbation of oxidative stress, and the stimulation of apoptosis [28]. They indicated that sestrin2 induction acts as a compensatory response to AngII for survival, implying that the stimulation of sestrin2 expression might be an effective pharmacological target for the treatment of AngII-associated cardiovascular diseases.

In the early phase of atherosclerosis, macrophage-derived foam cells play a major role in atherosclerosis. The AMPK and mTOR signaling pathways were reported to play an essential role in the initiation and progression of atherosclerosis [29,30], and sestrin2 was shown to modulate mTOR activity, thereby regulating glucose and lipid metabolism [31,32]. Sundararajan et al. reported that high-glucose and oxidized LDL treatment mediated the production of proinflammatory cytokine (M1) with a concomitant decrease in anti-inflammatory cytokine (M2) levels in macrophages [33]. M2 macrophages promote the secretion of IL-10, transforming growth factor-β (TGF-β), and extracellular matrix to protect vessels from atherosclerosis, whereas M1 macrophages secrete matrix metalloproteinases (MMPs) and proinflammatory factors such as TNF-α, IL-6, and IL-1β [34]. Glucose and oxidized LDL increased mTOR activation with a marked reduction in AMPK and sestrin2 expression and increased foam cell formation and monocyte adhesion to endothelial cells [33]. In addition, the overexpression of sestrin2 regulated the polarization of macrophages toward anti-inflammatory M2, while the knockdown of sestrin2 directed the polarization toward proinflammatory M1 [33]. These findings suggested that sestrin2 plays a major role in regulating monocyte activation via the AMPK-mTOR signaling pathway under diabetic and dyslipidemic conditions and that sestrin2 has a protective role against atherosclerosis.

3. Sestrin2 and Cardiac Diseases

3.1. Aging and Myocardial Infarction

The hallmarks of aging include accumulated aberrant proteins and oxidative stress, dysfunction of cellular metabolism and organs, and defective homeostasis. It was shown that AMPK activation, mTORC1 suppression, and autophagy stimulation are beneficial for extending lifespan [35]. Sestrin2 is suggested to be associated with aging and age-related diseases [12,36], and blood sestrin2 levels were reported to correlate with age [37,38]. Kishimoto et al. also reported that plasma sestrin2 levels correlated with age (r = 0.29) in 304 patients undergoing coronary angiography [39]. Moreover, sestrin2 was demonstrated to be associated with an aging-related process, and physical exercise can upregulate sestrin2 [40]. Sestrin2 is abundantly expressed in skeletal muscles and is important to the maintenance of muscle homeostasis. Rai et al. reported that the serum sestrin2 levels in 51 frail elderly subjects were low [41]. These findings suggest that sestrin2 is associated with frailty in the elderly.

Damaged myocardium from an ischemia reperfusion (I/R) injury initiates inflammatory responses including those involving macrophages, neutrophils, and inflammatory cytokines [42]. Sestrin2 is suggested to be cardioprotective against inflammation, oxidative stress, and I/R stress. Morrison et al. reported that sestrin2 knockout mice had greater-than-normal myocardial infarct sizes and impaired cardiac function with impaired AMPK activation, and sestrin2 was observed to promote AMPK activation during ischemia and to initiate AMPK phosphorylation via an interaction with LKB1. These findings suggest that sestrin2 plays an important role in cardiac protection against I/R injury, serving as an LKB1-AMPK scaffold to initiate the activation of AMPK during ischemia [43]. The same research group also showed that sestrin2 is an age-related protein that decreases with aging and contributes to the susceptibility of the aged heart toward I/R injury [44]. In mice, ischemic AMPK activation was blunted, and the infarct size was larger in the aged hearts [44]. Moreover, an adeno-associated virus delivery of sestrin2 significantly rescued sestrin2 protein level and ischemic tolerance of aged hearts. These findings suggest that (1) sestrin2 is a scaffold protein that mediates the activation of AMPK in ischemic myocardium, and (2) decreased sestrin2 levels in aging led to blunted ischemic AMPK activation and increased the sensitivity to ischemic insults. In addition, the sestrin2 knockout mice showed an aged-like phenotype in their hearts with excessive oxidative stress, disorganized myocardium, and transcriptomic alterations with I/R stress similar to aged mice [45]. Sestrin2 deficiency increased oxidative stress with up-regulated proinflammatory signaling and greater myocardial damage after I/R stress. These findings indicate that sestrin2 plays critical roles in modulating inflammation and apoptosis in the murine hearts in response to I/R injury.

The inflammatory response plays a crucial role in the progress of myocardial infarction (MI), where it is important in the repair of the myocardium but is also involved in myocardial remodeling and heart failure after an MI. The post-MI inflammatory response includes a substantial recruitment of circulating leukocytes into the infarcted myocardium. Among these infiltrating leukocytes, macrophages are critical players in the modulation of the post-MI inflammatory response [46]. The sestrin2 expression in cardiac macrophages was shown to be upregulated in a mouse model of MI [47]. Sestrin2 overexpression suppressed the inflammatory response of M1 macrophages through the inhibition of mTORC1 signaling both in vitro and in vivo. Together these findings suggest that sestrin2 plays a role in the post-MI inflammatory response, thereby leading to myocardial repair and remodeling.

3.2. Cardiomyopathy

In sestrin2 knockout mice, significantly reduced cardiac function with increased myocardial fibrosis was demonstrated after irradiation [48]. This suggests that sestrin2 is involved in the development of cardiomyopathy after irradiation. Li et al. also reported that the sestrin2 expression was significantly increased after an injection of doxorubicin in mice [49]. In sestrin2 knockout mice, sestrin2 deficiency rendered the mice more vulnerable to doxorubicin and exacerbated doxorubicin-induced cardiomyocyte apoptosis and cardiac dysfunction. Li et al. suggested that sestrin2 is a cardioprotective protein that minimizes cardiac damage in response to doxorubicin insult.

In rat cardiomyocytes, sestrin2 knockdown reduced the AMPK phosphorylation, downregulated antioxidant genes, and increased the ROS production upon LPS treatment [50]. LPS-mediated apoptosis and the expression of MMPs were significantly increased, and these increases were prevented by treatment with 5-aminoimidazole-4-carboxamide ribonucleotide (AICAR), an AMPK activator. Moreover, AMPK phosphorylation was shown to be decreased in the heart tissue from sestrin2 knockdown mice, which was associated with decreased antioxidant gene expression and increased apoptosis. Decreased AMPK phosphorylation by sestrin2 knockdown increased the LPS-mediated expression of cardiac fibrotic factors (e.g., collagen type I and type III). These results suggest that sestrin2 may play a role in the development of cardiomyopathy under inflammatory conditions.

In rats, sestrin2 knockdown was reported to aggravate the cardiomyocyte hypertrophy induced by phenylephrine, and sestrin2 overexpression protected cardiomyocytes from phenylephrine-induced hypertrophy, suggesting a protective effect of sestrin2 against cardiomyocyte hypertrophy [36]. In addition, Quan et al. reported that sestrin2 knockout mice had larger hearts and impaired cardiac function after aortic constriction for pressure overload [51]. Hypertension is the main pathological factor in the development of heart failure, and heart failure caused by hypertension is characterized by cardiac hypertrophy. An adeno-associated virus delivery of sestrin2 rescued the sestrin2 expression, attenuated the activation of mTORC1 and increased the pressure overload tolerance in hearts [51]. These results indicate that sestrin2 inhibits myocardial hypertrophy by inhibiting the mTORC1 pathway, thereby regulating protein synthesis, metabolism, autophagy, and apoptosis.

Wang et al. investigated the plasma sestrin2 levels in 220 patients with heart failure and reported that the patients' plasma sestrin2 levels were high and that their sestrin2 levels gradually increased as the heart failure progressed from New York Heart Association (NYHA) functional class II to IV [6]. High sestrin2 levels were also shown to be associated with major adverse cardiac events in the patients with heart failure. Thus, high plasma levels of sestrin2 in patients with heart failure may reflect a compensatory response to the heart failure and may help protect against the development of adverse cardiac events.

However, the main source and role of high plasma sestrin2 levels in patients with heart failure remain unclear.

The accumulating evidence suggests a role for sestrin2 in the development and progression of cardiomyopathy and heart failure. However, further studies in humans are needed to clarify the roles of sestrin2 in cardiomyopathy and heart failure.

4. Sestrin2 and Atherosclerotic Diseases

4.1. Coronary Artery Disease

Regarding the association between sestrin2 levels and coronary atherosclerosis, Ye et al. measured the plasma sestrin2 levels in 114 patients with CAD (stable angina (SA), $n = 44$; unstable angina (UA), $n = 41$; acute MI (AMI), $n = 29$) and 35 without CAD [37]. They reported that the sestrin2 levels were higher in the patients with CAD than in those without CAD and that the levels were much higher in the patients with UA or AMI compared to the patients with SA. However, a multivariate analysis was not performed in that study despite the involvement of some significant differences in atherosclerotic risk factors between the patients with and without CAD. Ye et al. also showed that the sestrin2 levels correlated with the Gensini score ($r = 0.46$), but this correlation coefficient was analyzed in all patients with CAD including those with AMI.

Kishimoto et al. recently investigated plasma sestrin2 levels in 304 patients undergoing coronary angiography for suspected CAD [39]. Patients with acute coronary syndrome, defined as acute MI and UA, were excluded from the study, and since plasma sestrin2 levels in patients with heart failure were reported to be high [6], patients with heart failure were also excluded. Notably, the plasma sestrin2 levels were significantly higher in the patients with CAD than in those without CAD (Figure 2). A stepwise increase in sestrin2 levels was also observed that depended on the severity of CAD (defined as the number of >50% stenotic vessels), and the sestrin2 levels were highest in the patients with severe CAD (Figure 2). The sestrin2 levels were significantly but weakly correlated with the number of >50% stenotic segments ($r = 0.12$) and age ($r = 0.29$). In a multivariate analysis, the plasma sestrin2 level was a significant factor associated with CAD independent of atherosclerotic risk factors, and the odds ratio for CAD was 1.79 (95%CI: 1.09–2.95) for a high sestrin2 level (>16.0 ng/mL). Thus, high plasma sestrin2 levels were identified in the patients with CAD. However, because sestrin2 is secreted by various types of cells including macrophages, T lymphocytes, endothelial cells, and cardiomyocytes [6,9,10] and because sestrin2 levels were not measured in the coronary sinus in the Kishimoto et al. study [39], the main sources of sestrin2 in patients with CAD remain unclear. Moreover, as shown in Figure 2, there was a substantial overlap in sestrin2 levels between the patients with and without CAD. Therefore, plasma sestrin2 levels in patients with CAD may reflect not only the degree of coronary atherosclerosis but also the degree of atherosclerosis in other vascular beds. Since sestrin2 is considered to have anti-oxidant and anti-inflammatory properties, high plasma levels of sestrin2 in patients with CAD may reflect a compensatory response to increased oxidative stress and may contribute to protection against the progression of CAD. However, further studies are needed to elucidate the main source and role of high plasma sestrin2 levels in patients with CAD.

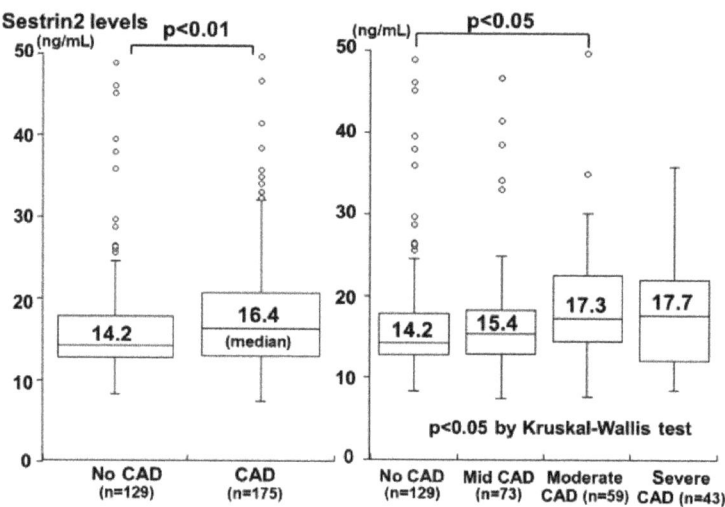

Figure 2. Plasma sestrin2 levels and the presence and severity of CAD. Plasma sestrin2 levels were significantly higher in patients with CAD than in those without CAD (**left**). The sestrin2 levels increased in a stepwise manner depending on the severity of CAD (defined as the number of >50% stenotic vessels) and were highest in the severe CAD group (**right**). The central lines represent the median, and the boxes represent the 25th to 75th percentiles. The whiskers represent the lowest and highest values in the 25th percentile minus 1.5 interquartile range (IQR) and the 75th percentile plus 1.5 IQR, respectively (modified from Kishimoto et al. [39]).

4.2. Carotid Atherosclerosis

Nutritional abundance can lead to chronic mTORC activation, thereby enhancing protein and lipid biosynthesis and inhibiting autophagic catabolism [52]. Chronic mTORC1 stimulation with autophagy inhibition in hepatocytes was reported to lead to insulin resistance and type 2 diabetes mellitus (DM) mainly via the inhibition of phosphorylation of insulin receptor substrates [32]. In obese sestrin2-knockout mice, sestrin2 deficiency was shown to exacerbate obesity-induced mTORC activation, glucose intolerance, insulin resistance, and hepatosteatosis, all of which were reversed by AMPK activation [31]. These findings suggest that sestrin2 may play a role in glucose metabolism. Since DM is a well-known atherosclerotic risk factors, sestrin2 may be associated with an increased risk of atherosclerotic diseases.

Sundararajan et al. reported that the serum sestrin2 levels in 81 patients with type 2 DM were significantly lower compared to those of 46 subjects with normal glucose tolerance [53]. In contrast, Chung et al. investigated the serum sestrin2 levels and the carotid intima-media thickness (IMT) measured by ultrasonography in 46 subjects without DM and 194 with DM [38]; they reported that the sestrin2 levels did not differ among the normal subjects, the DM patients without carotid atherosclerosis, and the DM patients with carotid atherosclerosis. No significant correlation was detected between the sestrin2 levels and carotid IMT, but the sestrin2 levels were correlated with the homeostatic model assessment of insulin resistance (HOMA-IR), waist circumference, percentage body fat, and truncal fat mass.

Kishimoto et al. investigated the plasma sestrin2 levels in 152 subjects (mean age 65 ± 10 years) undergoing carotid ultrasonography for a medical check-up for an evaluation of atherosclerosis [54]. No significant correlation between sestrin2 levels and carotid IMT was identified; however, the plasma sestrin2 levels were significantly higher in the subjects with carotid plaque than in those without plaque (Figure 3). In addition, the sestrin2 levels increased in a stepwise manner depending on the severity of plaque (defined as the plaque score) and were highest in the subjects with severe plaques (Figure 3). Moreover, the plasma sestrin2 levels were significantly correlated with the plaque score (r = 0.24). In a multivariate analysis, age and male gender were significant factors for the presence of plaque, but the sestrin2 level was not. However, the sestrin2 level was a significant factor for severe plaque (plaque score ≥2) independent of atherosclerotic risk factors. The odds ratio for severe plaque was 5.70 (95%CI: 1.99–16.35) for a high sestrin2 level (>13.0 ng/mL). These findings demonstrated that the plasma sestrin2 levels were high in individuals with carotid plaques and were associated with the severity of carotid atherosclerosis, as reported in patients with CAD [39]. High plasma sestrin2 levels may reflect an increased oxidative stress condition and may function to help protect the body against the progression of atherosclerosis.

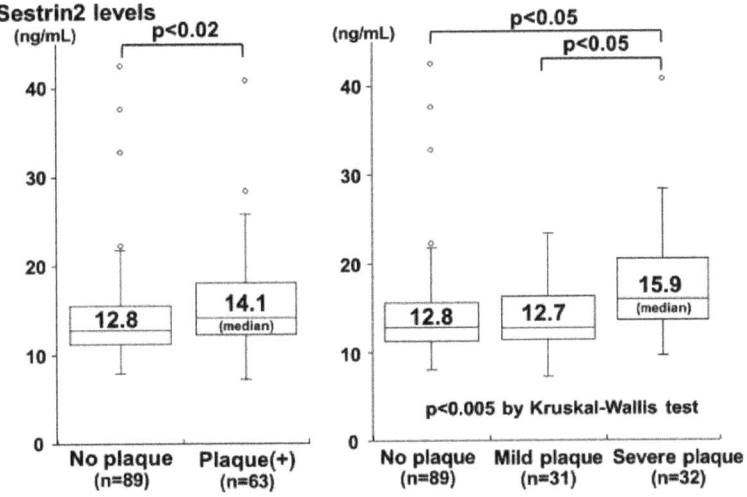

Figure 3. Plasma sestrin2 levels and the presence and severity of carotid plaque. Plasma sestrin2 levels were significantly higher in subjects with plaque than in those without plaque (**left**). Sestrin2 levels increased in a stepwise manner depending on the severity of plaque and were highest in the subjects with severe plaque (score ≥ 2) (**right**) (modified from Kishimoto et al. [54] copyright (2020), with permission from Elsevier).

4.3. Miscellaneous

In addition to CAD and carotid atherosclerosis, Xiao et al. reported that the sestrin2 expression was upregulated in the aortic specimens from 12 patients with aortic dissection, which is recognized to be related to atherosclerosis, and that the plasma sestrin2 levels were high in 120 patients with aortic dissection [55]. They suggested that the upregulation of sestrin2 may help reduce ROS, inflammation, and apoptosis in the aortic tissues of patients with aortic dissection. However, it has not been determined whether or not high plasma sestrin2 levels have a preventative effect on the development of aortic dissection.

Obstructive sleep apnea (OSA) is known to be common among obese individuals. OSA is characterized by repeated apnea during sleep and by intermittent hypoxia, leading to serious complications such as hypertension, DM, and CAD, due to oxidative stress. Intermittent hypoxia increases HIF-1α, thereby leading to an increase in sestrin2 expression. Jiang et al. reported that plasma sestrin2 levels were high in 36 patients with OSA, and that sestrin2 levels decreased after 4-week continuous positive airway pressure (CPAP) treatment [56]. They suggested that high plasma sestrin2 levels may contribute to a reduction in complications such as CAD as well as oxidative stress.

The blood sestrin2 levels in atherosclerotic and cardiometabolic diseases are summarized in Table 1.

Table 1. Summary of blood sestrin2 levels in patients with and without atherosclerotic and cardiometabolic diseases.

Study	Serum/Plasma	Study Subjects	Results
Rai et al. [41]	Serum	51 frail elderly vs. 41 non-frail elderly	Lower in frail elderly than in non-frail elderly.
Wang et al. [6]	Plasma	220 patients with HF vs. 80 controls	Higher in patients with HF than in controls
Xiao et al. [55]	Plasma	120 patients with aortic dissection vs. 40 without dissection	Higher in patients with aortic dissection than in those without dissection
Jiang et al. [56]	Plasma	36 patients with OSA vs. 21 controls	Higher in patients with OSA than in controls
Ye et al. [37]	Plasma	114 patients with CAD (44 SA, 41 UA, 29 AMI) vs. 35 without CAD	Higher in patients with CAD than in those without CAD Higher in patients with UA and AMI than in those with SA
Kishimoto et al. [39]	Plasma	175 patients with CAD vs. 129 without CAD	Higher in patients with CAD than in those without CAD
Sundararajan et al. [53]	Serum	81 patients with DM vs. 46 controls (NGT)	Lower in patients with DM than in controls
Chung et al. [38]	Serum	194 patients with DM vs. 46 without DM	No difference between patients with and without DM
Chung et al. [38]	Serum	80 DM patients with carotid atherosclerosis vs. 114 DM without carotid atherosclerosis	No difference between DM patients with and without carotid atherosclerosis
Kishimoto et al. [54]	Plasma	63 subjects with carotid plaque vs. 89 without carotid plaque	Higher in subjects with carotid plaque than in those without carotid plaque

5. Conclusions

The above results support the notion that sestrin2 has anti-oxidant and anti-inflammatory properties and that sestrin2 may play a protective role against the progression of atherosclerotic diseases such as CAD and carotid atherosclerosis. Sestrin2 may thus be a potential therapeutic target in atherosclerotic diseases. However, since the plasma sestrin2 levels in patients with CAD and those with carotid atherosclerosis were shown to be high, it remains unclear whether or not an exogenous administration of sestrin2 could be beneficial for the prevention of atherosclerotic disease. Further studies are needed to elucidate the roles of high plasma sestrin2 levels in patients with atherosclerotic diseases.

Author Contributions: Investigation and writing—original draft preparation, Y.K.; supervision, K.K.; investigation and writing—review and editing, Y.M. All authors have read and agreed to the published version of the manuscript.

Funding: This work was supported in part by JSPS KAKENHI Grant Number 20K11575.

Conflicts of Interest: The authors declare no conflict of interest. The funders had no role in the design of the study; in the collection, analyses, or interpretation of data; in the writing of the manuscript, or in the decision to publish the results.

References

1. Kattoor, A.J.; Pothineni, N.V.K.; Palagiri, D.; Mehta, J.L. Oxidative stress in atherosclerosis. *Curr. Atheroscler. Rep.* **2017**, *19*, 42. [CrossRef] [PubMed]
2. Cervantes Gracia, K.; Llanas-Cornejo, D.; Husi, H. CVD and oxidative stress. *J. Clin. Med.* **2017**, *6*, 22. [CrossRef] [PubMed]
3. Budanov, A.V.; Shoshani, T.; Faerman, A.; Zelin, E.; Kamer, I.; Kalinski, H.; Gorodin, S.; Fishman, A.; Chajut, A.; Einat, P.; et al. Identification of a novel stress-responsive gene Hi95 involved in regulation of cell viability. *Oncogene* **2002**, *21*, 6017–6031. [CrossRef] [PubMed]

4. Budanov, A.V.; Sablina, A.A.; Feinstein, E.; Koonin, E.V.; Chumakov, P.M. Regeneration of peroxiredoxins by p53-regulated sestrins, homologs of bacterial AhpD. *Science* **2004**, *304*, 596–600. [CrossRef]
5. Budanov, A.V.; Lee, J.H.; Karin, M. Stressin' Sestrins take an aging fight. *EMBO Mol. Med.* **2010**, *2*, 388–400. [CrossRef]
6. Wang, H.; Li, N.; Shao, X.; Li, J.; Guo, L.; Yu, X.; Sun, Y.; Hao, J.; Niu, H.; Xiang, J.; et al. Increased plasma sestrin2 concentrations in patients with chronic heart failure and predicted the occurrence of major adverse cardiac events: A 36-month follow-up cohort study. *Clin. Chim. Acta* **2019**, *495*, 338–344. [CrossRef]
7. Wang, L.X.; Zhu, X.M.; Yao, Y.M. Sestrin2: Its potential role and regulatory mechanism in host immune response in diseases. *Front. Immunol.* **2019**, *10*, 2797. [CrossRef]
8. Sun, W.; Wang, Y.; Zheng, Y.; Quan, N. The emerging role of sestrin2 in cell metabolism, and cardiovascular and age-related diseases. *Aging Dis.* **2020**, *11*, 154–163. [CrossRef]
9. Hu, H.J.; Shi, Z.Y.; Lin, X.L.; Chen, S.M.; Wang, Q.Y.; Tang, S.Y. Upregulation of sestrin2 expression protects against macrophage apoptosis induced by oxidized low-density lipoprotein. *DNA Cell Biol.* **2015**, *34*, 296–302. [CrossRef]
10. Kim, M.G.; Yang, J.H.; Kim, K.M.; Jang, C.H.; Jung, J.Y.; Cho, I.J.; Shin, S.M.; Ki, S.H. Regulation of toll-like receptor-mediated sestrin2 induction by AP-1, Nrf2, and the ubiquitin-proteasome system in macrophages. *Toxicol. Sci.* **2015**, *144*, 425–435. [CrossRef]
11. Budanov, A.V.; Karin, M. p53 target genes sestrin1 and sestrin2 connect genotoxic stress and mTOR signaling. *Cell* **2008**, *134*, 451–460. [CrossRef] [PubMed]
12. Sun, Y.; Wu, Y.; Tang, S.; Liu, H.; Jiang, Y. Sestrin proteins in cardiovascular disease. *Clin. Chim. Acta* **2020**, *508*, 43–46. [CrossRef] [PubMed]
13. Pasha, M.; Eid, A.H.; Eid, A.A.; Gorin, Y.; Munusamy, S. Sestrin2 as a novel biomarker and therapeutic target for various diseases. *Oxid. Med. Cell Longev.* **2017**, *2017*, 3296294. [CrossRef] [PubMed]
14. Bae, S.H.; Sung, S.H.; Oh, S.Y.; Lim, J.M.; Lee, S.K.; Park, Y.N.; Lee, H.E.; Kang, D.; Rhee, S.G. Sestrins activate Nrf2 by promoting p62-dependent autophagic degradation of Keap1 and prevent oxidative liver damage. *Cell Metab.* **2013**, *17*, 73–84. [CrossRef]
15. Alexander, A.; Cai, S.L.; Kim, J.; Nanez, A.; Sahin, M.; MacLean, K.H.; Inoki, K.; Guan, K.L.; Shen, J.; Person, M.D.; et al. ATM signals to TSC2 in the cytoplasm to regulate mTORC1 in response to ROS. *Proc. Natl. Acad. Sci. USA* **2010**, *107*, 4153–4158. [CrossRef]
16. Wullschleger, S.; Loewith, R.; Hall, M.N. TOR signaling in growth and metabolism. *Cell* **2006**, *124*, 471–484. [CrossRef]
17. Kishton, R.J.; Barnes, C.E.; Nichols, A.G.; Cohen, S.; Gerriets, V.A.; Siska, P.J.; Macintyre, A.N.; Goraksha-Hicks, P.; de Cubas, A.A.; Liu, T.; et al. AMPK is essential to balance glycolysis and mitochondrial metabolism to control T-ALL cell stress and survival. *Cell Metab.* **2016**, *23*, 649–662. [CrossRef]
18. Hosokawa, N.; Hara, T.; Kaizuka, T.; Kishi, C.; Takamura, A.; Miura, Y.; Iemura, S.; Natsume, T.; Takehana, K.; Yamada, N.; et al. Nutrient-dependent mTORC1 association with the ULK1-Atg13-FIP200 complex required for autophagy. *Mol. Biol. Cell* **2009**, *20*, 1981–1991. [CrossRef]
19. Finkel, T.; Holbrook, N.J. Oxidants, oxidative stress and the biology of ageing. *Nature* **2000**, *408*, 239–247. [CrossRef]
20. Yang, Y.; Cuevas, S.; Yang, S.; Villar, V.A.; Escano, C.; Asico, L.; Yu, P.; Jiang, X.; Weinman, E.J.; Armando, I.; et al. Sestrin2 decreases renal oxidative stress, lowers blood pressure, and mediates dopamine D2 receptor-induced inhibition of reactive oxygen species production. *Hypertension* **2014**, *64*, 825–832. [CrossRef]
21. Wang, L.X.; Zhu, X.M.; Luo, Y.N.; Wu, Y.; Dong, N.; Tong, Y.L.; Yao, Y.M. Sestrin2 protects dendritic cells against endoplasmic reticulum stress-related apoptosis induced by high mobility group box-1 protein. *Cell Death Dis.* **2020**, *11*, 125. [CrossRef] [PubMed]
22. Steven, S.; Frenis, K.; Oelze, M.; Kalinovic, S.; Kuntic, M.; Bayo Jimenez, M.T.; Vujacic-Mirski, K.; Helmstädter, J.; Kröller-Schön, S.; Münzel, T.; et al. Vascular inflammation and oxidative stress: Major triggers for cardiovascular disease. *Oxid. Med. Cell Longev.* **2019**, *2019*, 7092151. [CrossRef] [PubMed]
23. Griendling, K.K.; FitzGerald, G.A. Oxidative stress and cardiovascular injury: Part I: Basic mechanisms and in vivo monitoring of ROS. *Circulation* **2003**, *108*, 1912–1916. [CrossRef] [PubMed]
24. Yang, J.H.; Kim, K.M.; Kim, M.G.; Seo, K.H.; Han, J.Y.; Ka, S.O.; Park, B.H.; Shin, S.M.; Ku, S.K.; Cho, I.J.; et al. Role of sestrin2 in the regulation of proinflammatory signaling in macrophages. *Free Radic. Biol. Med.* **2015**, *78*, 156–167. [CrossRef]
25. Hwang, H.J.; Jung, T.W.; Choi, J.H.; Lee, H.J.; Chung, H.S.; Seo, J.A.; Kim, S.G.; Kim, N.H.; Choi, K.M.; Choi, D.S.; et al. Knockdown of sestrin2 increases pro-inflammatory reactions and ER stress in the endothelium via an AMPK dependent mechanism. *Biochim. Biophys. Acta Mol. Basis Dis.* **2017**, *1863*, 1436–1444. [CrossRef]
26. Li, D.; Wang, D.; Wang, Y.; Ling, W.; Feng, X.; Xia, M. Adenosine monophosphate-activated protein kinase induces cholesterol efflux from macrophage-derived foam cells and alleviates atherosclerosis in apolipoprotein E-deficient mice. *J. Biol. Chem.* **2010**, *285*, 33499–33509. [CrossRef]
27. Brasier, A.R.; Recinos, A., 3rd; Eledrisi, M.S. Vascular inflammation and the renin-angiotensin system. *Arterioscler. Thromb. Vasc. Biol.* **2002**, *22*, 1257–1266. [CrossRef]
28. Yi, L.; Li, F.; Yong, Y.; Jianting, D.; Liting, Z.; Xuansheng, H.; Fei, L.; Jiewen, L. Upregulation of sestrin-2 expression protects against endothelial toxicity of angiotensin II. *Cell Biol. Toxicol.* **2014**, *30*, 147–156. [CrossRef]
29. Martinet, W.; De Loof, H.; De Meyer, G.R.Y. mTOR inhibition: A promising strategy for stabilization of atherosclerotic plaques. *Atherosclerosis* **2014**, *233*, 601–607. [CrossRef]

30. Kurdi, A.; De Meyer, G.R.; Martinet, W. Potential therapeutic effects of mTOR inhibition in atherosclerosis. *Br. J. Clin. Pharmacol.* **2016**, *82*, 1267–1279. [CrossRef]
31. Lee, J.H.; Budanov, A.V.; Talukdar, S.; Park, E.J.; Park, H.L.; Park, H.W.; Bandyopadhyay, G.; Li, N.; Aghajan, M.; Jang, I.; et al. Maintenance of metabolic homeostasis by Sestrin2 and Sestrin3. *Cell Metab.* **2012**, *16*, 311–321. [CrossRef] [PubMed]
32. Howell, J.J.; Ricoult, S.J.; Ben-Sahra, I.; Manning, B.D. A growing role for mTOR in promoting anabolic metabolism. *Biochem. Soc. Trans.* **2013**, *41*, 906–912. [CrossRef] [PubMed]
33. Sundararajan, S.; Jayachandran, I.; Balasubramanyam, M.; Mohan, V.; Venkatesan, B.; Manickam, N. Sestrin2 regulates monocyte activation through AMPK-mTOR nexus under high-glucose and dyslipidemic conditions. *J. Cell Biochem.* **2018**, *10*, 1002. [CrossRef]
34. Gostner, J.M.; Fuchs, D. Biomarkers for the role of macrophages in the development and progression of atherosclerosis. *Atherosclerosis* **2016**, *255*, 117–118. [CrossRef] [PubMed]
35. Mair, W.; Morantte, I.; Rodrigues, A.P.; Manning, G.; Montminy, M.; Shaw, R.J.; Dillin, A. Lifespan extension induced by AMPK and calcineurin is mediated by CRTC-1 and CREB. *Nature* **2011**, *470*, 404–408. [CrossRef] [PubMed]
36. Dong, B.; Xue, R.; Sun, Y.; Dong, Y.; Liu, C. Sestrin 2 attenuates neonatal rat cardiomyocyte hypertrophy induced by phenylephrine via inhibiting ERK1/2. *Mol. Cell Biochem.* **2017**, *433*, 113–123. [CrossRef] [PubMed]
37. Ye, J.; Wang, M.; Xu, Y.; Liu, J.; Jiang, H.; Wang, Z.; Lin, Y.; Wan, J. Sestrins increase in patients with coronary artery disease and associate with the severity of coronary stenosis. *Clin. Chim. Acta* **2017**, *472*, 51–57. [CrossRef]
38. Chung, H.S.; Hwang, H.J.; Hwang, S.Y.; Kim, N.H.; Seo, J.A.; Kim, S.G.; Kim, N.H.; Baik, S.H.; Choi, K.M.; Yoo, H.J. Association of serum Sestrin2 level with metabolic risk factors in newly diagnosed drug-naive type 2 diabetes. *Diabetes Res. Clin. Pract.* **2018**, *144*, 34–41. [CrossRef]
39. Kishimoto, Y.; Aoyama, M.; Saita, E.; Ikegami, Y.; Ohmori, R.; Kondo, K.; Momiyama, Y. Association between plasma sestrin2 levels and the presence and severity of coronary artery disease. *Dis. Markers* **2020**, *2020*, 7439574. [CrossRef]
40. Sanchis-Gomar, F. Sestrins: Novel antioxidant and AMPK-modulating functions regulated by exercise? *J. Cell Physiol.* **2013**, *228*, 1647–1650. [CrossRef]
41. Rai, N.; Venugopalan, G.; Pradhan, R.; Ambastha, A.; Upadhyay, A.D.; Dwivedi, S.; Dey, A.B.; Dey, S. Exploration of novel anti-oxidant protein sestrin in frailty syndrome in elderly. *Aging Dis.* **2018**, *9*, 220–227. [CrossRef] [PubMed]
42. Buja, L.M. Myocardial ischemia and reperfusion injury. *Cardiovasc. Pathol.* **2005**, *14*, 170–175. [CrossRef] [PubMed]
43. Morrison, A.; Chen, L.; Wang, J.; Zhang, M.; Yang, H.; Ma, Y.; Budanov, A.; Lee, J.H.; Karin, M.; Li, J. Sestrin2 promotes LKB1-mediated AMPK activation in the ischemic heart. *FASEB J.* **2015**, *29*, 408–417. [CrossRef] [PubMed]
44. Quan, N.; Sun, W.; Wang, L.; Chen, X.; Bogan, J.S.; Zhou, X.; Cates, C.; Liu, Q.; Zheng, Y.; Li, J. Sestrin2 prevents age-related intolerance to ischemia and reperfusion injury by modulating substrate metabolism. *FASEB J.* **2017**, *31*, 4153–4167. [CrossRef] [PubMed]
45. Ren, D.; Quan, N.; Fedorova, J.; Zhang, J.; He, Z.; Li, J. Sestrin2 modulates cardiac inflammatory response through maintaining redox homeostasis during ischemia and reperfusion. *Redox Biol.* **2020**, *34*, 101556. [CrossRef]
46. Frangogiannis, N.G.; Smith, C.W.; Entman, M.L. The inflammatory response in myocardial infarction. *Cardiovasc. Res.* **2002**, *53*, 31–47. [CrossRef]
47. Yang, K.; Xu, C.; Zhang, Y.; He, S.; Li, D. Sestrin2 suppresses classically activated macrophages-mediated inflammatory response in myocardial infarction through inhibition of mTORC1 signaling. *Front. Immunol.* **2017**, *8*, 728. [CrossRef]
48. Zeng, Y.C.; Chi, F.; Xing, R.; Zeng, J.; Gao, S.; Chen, J.J.; Wang, H.M.; Duan, Q.Y.; Sun, Y.N.; Niu, N.; et al. Sestrin2 protects the myocardium against radiation-induced damage. *Radiat. Environ. Biophys.* **2016**, *55*, 195–202. [CrossRef]
49. Li, R.; Huang, Y.; Semple, I.; Kim, M.; Zhang, Z.; Lee, J.H. Cardioprotective roles of sestrin 1 and sestrin 2 against doxorubicin cardiotoxicity. *Am. J. Physiol. Heart Circ. Physiol.* **2019**, *317*, H39–H48. [CrossRef]
50. Hwang, H.J.; Kim, J.W.; Chung, H.S.; Seo, J.A.; Kim, S.G.; Kim, N.H.; Choi, K.M.; Baik, S.H.; Yoo, H.J. Knockdown of sestrin2 increases lipopolysaccharide-induced oxidative stress, apoptosis, and fibrotic reactions in H9c2 cells and heart tissues of mice via an AMPK-dependent mechanism. *Mediat. Inflamm.* **2018**, *2018*, 6209140. [CrossRef]
51. Quan, N.; Li, X.; Zhang, J.; Han, Y.; Sun, W.; Ren, D.; Tong, Q.; Li, J. Substrate metabolism regulated by Sestrin2-mTORC1 alleviates pressure overload-induced cardiac hypertrophy in aged heart. *Redox Biol.* **2020**, *36*, 101637. [CrossRef] [PubMed]
52. Zoncu, R.; Efeyan, A.; Sabatini, D.M. mTOR: From growth signal integration to cancer, diabetes and ageing. *Nat. Rev. Mol. Cell Biol.* **2011**, *12*, 21–35. [CrossRef] [PubMed]
53. Sundararajan, S.; Jayachandran, I.; Subramanian, S.C.; Anjana, R.M.; Balasubramanyam, M.; Mohan, V.; Venkatesan, B.; Manickam, N. Decreased sestrin levels in patients with type 2 diabetes and dyslipidemia and their association with the severity of atherogenic index. *J. Endocrinol. Investig.* **2020**. [CrossRef] [PubMed]
54. Kishimoto, Y.; Saita, E.; Ohmori, R.; Kondo, K.; Momiyama, Y. Plasma sestrin2 concentrations and carotid atherosclerosis. *Clin. Chim. Acta* **2020**, *504*, 56–59. [CrossRef]
55. Xiao, T.; Zhang, L.; Huang, Y.; Shi, Y.; Wang, J.; Ji, Q.; Ye, J.; Lin, Y.; Liu, H. Sestrin2 increases in aortas and plasma from aortic dissection patients and alleviates angiotensin II-induced smooth muscle cell apoptosis via the Nrf2 pathway. *Life Sci.* **2019**, *218*, 132–138. [CrossRef]
56. Jiang, R.; Wang, Q.; Zhai, H.; Du, X.; Sun, S.; Wang, H. Exploring the involvement of plasma sestrin2 in obstructive sleep apnea. *Can. Respir. J.* **2019**, *2019*, 2047674. [CrossRef]

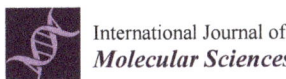

Review

Unraveling the Role of Epicardial Adipose Tissue in Coronary Artery Disease: Partners in Crime?

Glória Conceição, Diana Martins, Isabel M. Miranda, Adelino F. Leite-Moreira, Rui Vitorino and Inês Falcão-Pires *

Cardiovascular R&D Centre (UnIC), Department of Surgery and Physiology, Faculty of Medicine, University of Porto, 4200-319 Porto, Portugal; glorialmeida6100@gmail.com (G.C.); dlfm94@gmail.com (D.M.); imiranda@med.up.pt (I.M.M.); amoreira@med.up.pt (A.F.L.-M.); rvitorino@ua.pt (R.V.)
* Correspondence: ipires@med.up.pt; Tel.: +351-220-426-805; Fax: +351-225-513-646

Received: 23 October 2020; Accepted: 17 November 2020; Published: 23 November 2020

Abstract: The role of epicardial adipose tissue (EAT) in the pathophysiology of coronary artery disease (CAD) remains unclear. The present systematic review aimed at compiling dysregulated proteins/genes from different studies to dissect the potential role of EAT in CAD pathophysiology. Exhaustive literature research was performed using the keywords "epicardial adipose tissue and coronary artery disease", to highlight a group of proteins that were consistently regulated among all studies. Reactome, a pathway analysis database, was used to clarify the function of the selected proteins and their intertwined association. SignalP/SecretomeP was used to clarify the endocrine function of the selected proteins. Overall, 1886 proteins/genes were identified from 44 eligible studies. The proteins were separated according to the control used in each study (EAT non-CAD or subcutaneous adipose tissue (SAT) CAD) and by their regulation (up- or downregulated). Using a Venn diagram, we selected the proteins that were upregulated and downregulated (identified as 27 and 19, respectively) in EAT CAD for both comparisons. The analysis of these proteins revealed the main pathways altered in the EAT and how they could communicate with the heart, potentially contributing to CAD development. In summary, in this study, the identified dysregulated proteins highlight the importance of inflammatory processes to modulate the local environment and the progression of CAD, by cellular and metabolic adaptations of epicardial fat that facilitate the formation and progression of atherogenesis of coronaries.

Keywords: coronary artery disease; epicardial adipose tissue; inflammation; cytokines

1. Introduction

The ever-growing health and socioeconomic burden related to obesity have gathered efforts aimed at revealing the complex association between adipose tissue and cardiovascular disease [1]. Interest in organ-specific adiposity is rapidly increasing as a substantial amount of scientific-based evidence suggests that adipose tissue anatomic specificity is crucial to the pathophysiology of cardiometabolic and endocrine diseases [2]. In this context, epicardial adipose tissue (EAT) has emerged as an exciting fat depot due to its location, peculiar metabolic properties, and clinical measurability [3]. Indeed, several studies have recognized EAT to be an independent predictor of coronary artery disease (CAD) [4,5]; however, the nature of this association remains to be clarified. Thus, this study aims to analyze the current literature focusing on the molecular signature of EAT derived from CAD patients. Our goal is to provide an overview of the potential impact of dysfunctional EAT on CAD pathophysiology.

1.1. Coronary Artery Disease

CAD is one of the most common forms of heart disease and a serious health problem worldwide. CAD can lead to myocardial ischemia, myocardial infarction, heart failure, and ultimately to death. CAD is a severe chronic disease, characterized by progressive atherosclerotic occlusion of the coronary arteries, resulting in a mismatch between myocardial oxygen demand and supply [6]. Atherosclerosis is described as a low-grade inflammatory state of the intima of medium-sized arteries that is accelerated by well-known risk factors such as hypertension, diabetes, obesity, and dyslipidemia [7]. In most observational studies, overweight/obesity has been associated with an increased prevalence of CAD, suggesting that it is the major risk factor associated with the pathophysiology and progression of the disease [8].

Moreover, the risk of developing CAD is not the same for individuals with the same percentage of body fat, which is mainly caused by the different distributions of fat. Patients with visceral obesity develop CAD quickly, demonstrating that this fat pad can predict CAD onset [9]. Figure 1 illustrates an overview of atherosclerosis pathophysiology and progression in CAD. More information can be consulted elsewhere [10,11].

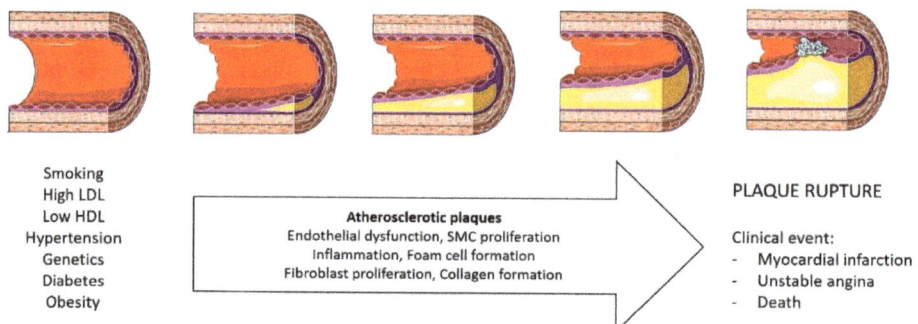

Figure 1. Coronary artery disease progression. LDL, low-density lipoproteins; HDL, high-density lipoproteins; SMC, smooth muscle cells. The figure was produced using Servier Medical Art.

1.2. Obesity as a Risk Factor for Coronary Artery Disease

Obesity is a worldwide epidemic, representing a public health concern. Obesity is determined by a body mass index (BMI) above 30 kg/m^2 [12]. However, is it widely known that BMI is a weak measurement of body fat, being influenced by muscle mass, body water content, and other factors. Furthermore, the relative contribution and burden of central, total, or subcutaneous adiposity to cardiovascular diseases needs further clarification. In lean subjects, subcutaneous adipose tissue (SAT) represents approximately 80% of the total adipose tissue mass, while visceral adipose tissue constitutes 15%. In obese patients, the percentage of visceral adipose tissue increases significantly, representing the most active fat subtype, which secretes adipocytokines that contribute to a systemic proinflammatory state and promote the development of cardiovascular atherosclerosis [13]. Moreover, visceral fat has the highest risk of metabolic dysregulation as a consequence of obesity, type II diabetes mellitus, or insulin resistance [14].

1.3. Epicardial Adipose Tissue

EAT is the fat depot that confers mechanical protection to the heart. It is directly connected to the myocardium, without any separating fascia, and shares the same circulation and blood supply [3]. EAT displays metabolic, thermogenic, and mechanical properties, with the higher rates of lipogenesis and fatty acid metabolism as compared to other fat subtypes. This enrichment and increased metabolism of free fatty acids (FFA) can be functionally important because the heart mostly depends on FFA oxidation as a source of energy [3]. Moreover, as an endocrine organ, EAT is the source of several bioactive adipocytokines that can either protect or adversely affect the myocardium and coronary arteries. Under normal physiological conditions, EAT can trigger cardioprotective actions through paracrine or vasocrine secretion of anti-inflammatory adipocytokines, such as adiponectin. However, upon adipocytes dysfunction, the balance of epicardial fat secretome is disrupted, the production and secretion of protective adipocytokines declines, while the release of proinflammatory adipocytokines through epicardial adipocytes increases [3].

1.4. Epicardial Adipose Tissue and Coronary Artery Disease (CAD)

Currently, several imaging techniques are used to effectively quantify epicardial fat, such as magnetic resonance imaging, transthoracic echocardiography, and cardiac computed tomography [15]. Several populational studies have extensively described the predictive and associative impact of the thickness/volume of epicardial fat on the development and progression of CAD [3,16]. An increasing number of studies has shown that EAT volume was consistently associated with visceral obesity and metabolic syndrome, and potentially represented a marker of CAD in asymptomatic high-risk patients [17,18]. Consequently, the interest in studying EAT volume as a predictor of CAD has increased, demonstrating that it can be a useful marker of CAD in asymptomatic patients with noncalcified plaques and zero calcium scores. Interestingly, EAT significantly correlates with CAD development, independently of the existence of cardiovascular risk factors or the volume of other fat depots [19]. Accordingly, EAT volume correlated with coronary calcification independently of global and visceral abdominal adiposities in a cohort of stable elderly patients [20], supporting the idea that EAT could be involved in all stages of CAD.

Some studies have favored the idea that EAT facilitated coronary atherosclerosis directly through an imbalance between cardioprotective and deleterious adipocytokines secreted. These studies strongly supported adipocytokines paracrine rather than systemic effects [14]. Additionally, EAT from CAD patients have shown more interaction and adherence between cells and cell-to-matrix, an increased inflammatory response through the infiltration of complement factors and platelets, as well as dysfunction of lipid metabolism and mitochondria [21].

2. Methods

2.1. Search Strategy

Records that were published up to December 2019 were retrieved from the PubMed database. The keywords "epicardial adipose tissue" were combined with "coronary artery disease" for the search. Two authors (G.C. and D.M.) independently screened records, compared the results, and discussed discrepancies to obtain consensus at each step based on the criteria of study selection.

2.2. Inclusion and Exclusion Criteria of Study Selection

Studies conducted in CAD patients that performed molecular studies in EAT were included. Case reports, conference/dissertation abstracts, echocardiographic and clinic studies, animal model studies, literature reviews, and in vitro experiments were excluded.

2.3. Data Extraction

Data from the reports were manually curated and organized to extract all genes and proteins that could be identified and whose variation had been assessed between the different conditions. Only studies that reported significant differences ($p < 0.05$) were included. We separated the studies based on the control used (SAT) from CAD patients and EAT from non-CAD patients). The genes/proteins identified were separated by their regulation (up- or downregulated) as compared with a selected control. This resulted in four different lists of proteins/genes, namely: (a) the proteins/genes upregulated in EAT CAD as compared with EAT non-CAD, (b) the proteins downregulated in EAT CAD as compared with EAT non-CAD, (c) the proteins upregulated in EAT CAD as compared with SAT CAD, and (d) the proteins downregulated in EAT CAD as compared with SAT CAD.

2.4. Bioinformatic Analysis

The identified genes and proteins were analyzed using the following bioinformatics tools: (1) PANTHER database (http://www.pantherdb.org) was used to perform gene ontology (GO) analyses, based on the biological process; (2) FunRich tool (http://www.funrich.org) was used to construct Venn diagrams, to perform an integrative analysis of the proteins/genes between the different groups; (3) SignalP and SecretomeP bioinformatics analysis were performed to search for putative secreted proteins [22] to elucidate the endocrine function of EAT in CAD, i.e., SignalP predicts classically secreted proteins based on signal peptide triggered protein secretion and SecretomeP predicts non-classical secreted proteins; and (4) Reactome, an open-source, peer-reviewed pathway analysis database [23], was used to clarify the relevance and to further explore the function of the proteins and their intertwined associations (http://reactome.org.). The set of selected genes from the Venn diagram and SignalP/SecretomeP analysis were placed into the "analysis" section of reactome. The program matches these proteins/genes to pathways and provides a pictogram of significant pathways (see Figure S1). The Reactome analysis program lists entities found in each pathway, along with a ratio of those genes found versus total molecules in the pathway, with a p value signifying "overrepresentation", i.e., a larger number than would be expected if the set were random, with a Benjamin–Hochberg correction. Only the top 10 entities in the upregulated and the downregulated groups were detailed. The list also includes a false discovery rate (FDR) for each entity, indicating the expected proportion of rejected genes that were incorrect rejections.

3. Results

Over 571 abstracts were retrieved and reviewed, taking into account the exclusion and inclusion criteria, achieving 44 valid reports for further analysis (Figure 2). In a total of 44 studies, the average of participants ranged from 45 to 74 years. Mostly, EAT samples were collected adjacent to the right coronary artery to perform molecular studies, such as polymerase chain reaction (PCR), Western blot, and other methods. The characteristics for each paper analyzed and a list of the proteins identified can be found in Table S1.

From these 44 eligible studies, 1886 proteins/genes were identified as dysregulated in EAT and subjected to bioinformatic analysis to filter the most relevant information, as summarized in Figure 3. From these, 1108 were identified from studies with SAT CAD as the control and 778 were recognized from studies EAT CAD versus EAT non-CAD (Table S2). Figure 4A,B illustrates the expression pattern of each one of these comparisons. From all proteins identified in EAT as compared with EAT from non-CAD patients, 301 proteins were described as upregulated and 417 proteins as downregulated. Contrarily, 30 proteins were inconsistently regulated. Relative to EAT proteins with SAT CAD as the control, 635 proteins were upregulated and 393 proteins were downregulated, and 40 proteins were inconsistently regulated.

For further understanding of the different proteins differentially identified, the proteins were queried in the PANTHER database v15.0 and annotated GO terms based on biological processes. The classification results are illustrated in Figure 4C,D. Independent of the group used as the control, the 3 main biological processes in EAT CAD with more proteins were metabolic process (GO:0008152, $p = 6.10 \times 10^{-29}$ vs. EAT non-CAD and $p = 1.83 \times 10^{-12}$ vs. SAT CAD), cellular process (GO:0009987, $p = 2.93 \times 10^{-28}$ vs. EAT non-CAD and $p = 9.99 \times 10^{-16}$ vs. SAT CAD), and biological regulation (GO:0065007, $p = 4.12 \times 10^{-19}$ vs. EAT non-CAD and $p = 6.13 \times 10^{-29}$ vs. SAT CAD). In addition, response to stimulus (GO:0050896, $p = 1.55 \times 10^{-57}$ vs. EAT non-CAD and $p = 4.90 \times 10^{-37}$ vs. SAT CAD), cellular component organization or biogenesis (GO:0071840, $p = 4.56 \times 10^{-8}$ vs. EAT non-CAD and $p = 1.41 \times 10^{-6}$ vs. SAT CAD), localization (GO:0051179, $p = 1.79 \times 10^{-21}$ vs. EAT non-CAD and

$p = 6.71 \times 10^{-21}$ vs. SAT CAD), signaling (GO:0023052, $p = 4.48 \times 10^{-28}$ vs. EAT non-CAD and $p = 3.43 \times 10^{-26}$ vs. SAT CAD), developmental process (GO:0032502, $p = 6.85 \times 10^{-6}$ vs. EAT non-CAD and $p = 4.18 \times 10^{-36}$ vs. SAT CAD), multicellular organismal process (GO:0032501, $p = 2.3 \times 10^{-16}$ vs. EAT non-CAD and $p = 1.46 \times 10^{-38}$ vs. SAT CAD), and immune system process (GO:0002376, $p = 3.73 \times 10^{-29}$ vs. EAT non-CAD and $p = 1.25 \times 10^{-27}$. SAT CAD) were also consistently highlighted.

A Venn diagram representing the differences in protein expression among groups was designed to highlight the most significant proteins underlying the interaction between EAT and CAD (Figure 5 and Table S3). This diagram identifies which proteins were simultaneously upregulated (27 in Figure 5, upregulated subgroup) and simultaneously downregulated (19 in Figure 5, downregulated subgroup) in EAT CAD for both comparisons (Table 1). On the one hand, from the upregulated proteins, one should highlight tumor necrosis factor, C-C motif chemokine 2, C-C motif chemokine 5, and interleukin (IL)-18. On the other hand, from the downregulated proteins, galectin-3, gelsolin, cathepsin K, and macrophage scavenger receptor types I and II should be emphasized.

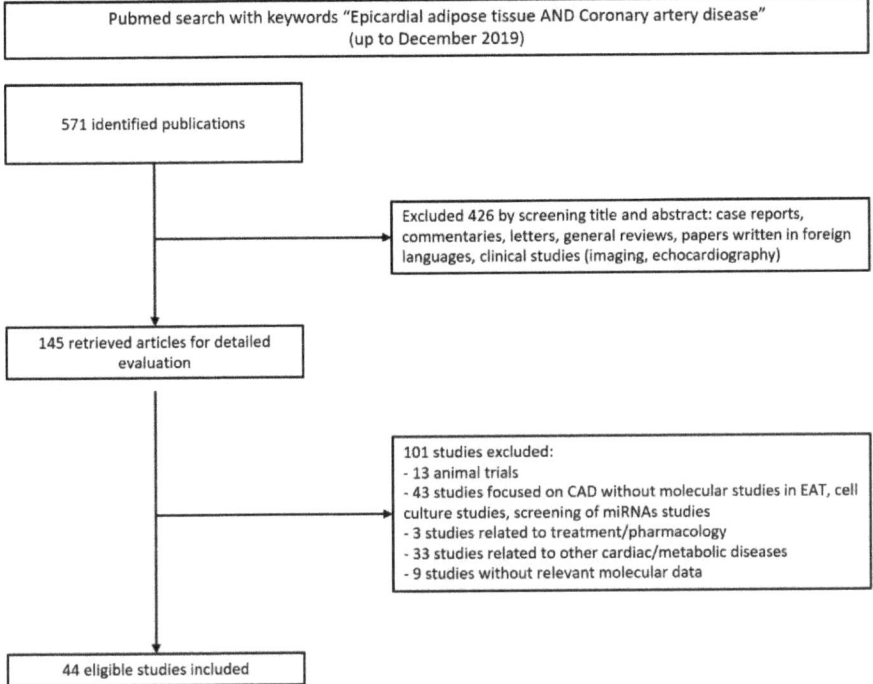

Figure 2. Search strategy flowchart. From the 571 abstracts collected in PubMed, using the keywords "epicardial adipose tissue and coronary artery disease", 44 reports were used for the systematic review and 527 were excluded, according to the criteria above mentioned. CAD, coronary artery disease; EAT, epicardial adipose tissue.

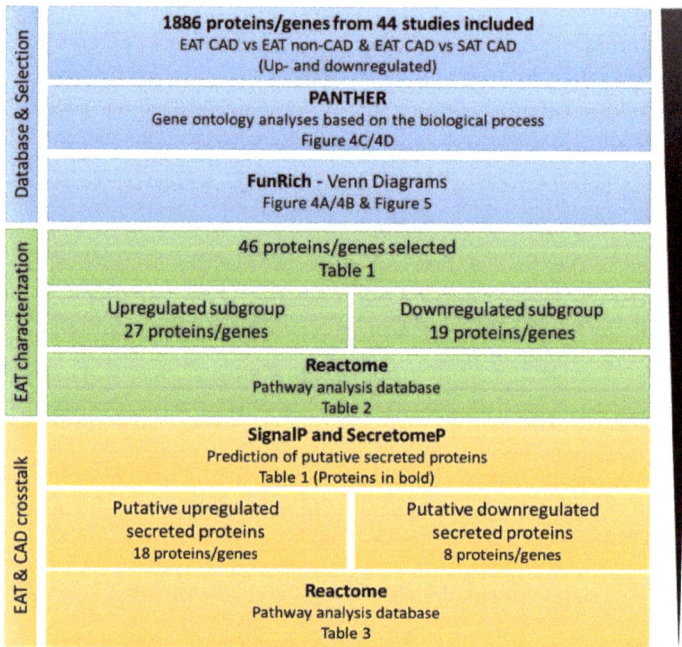

Figure 3. The workflow for proteins/genes analysis using bioinformatic tools. SAT, subcutaneous adipose tissue.

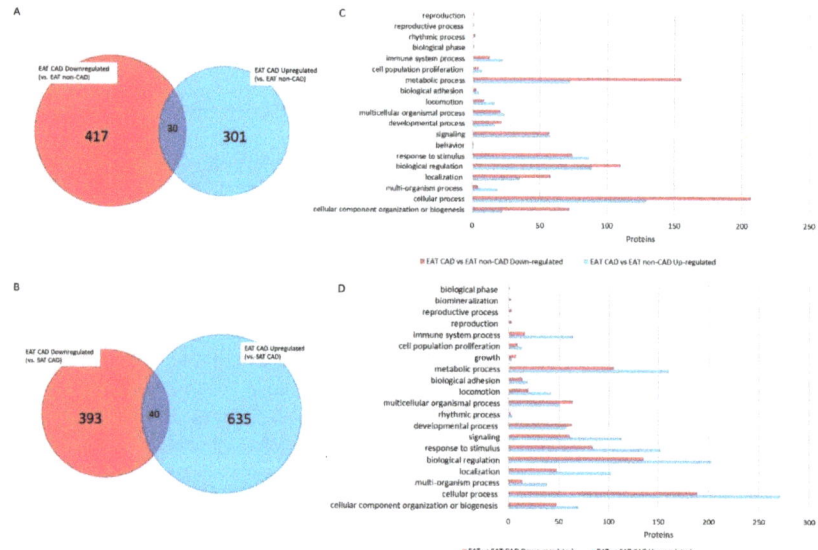

Figure 4. Venn diagram representing the distribution of identified proteins per control evidencing the overlapped and unique proteins. Proteins identified in EAT from studies using EAT non-coronary artery disease (non-CAD) as control (**A**) and corresponding altered biological processes (**C**); Proteins identified in EAT from studies using SAT CAD as control (**B**) and corresponding altered biological processes (**D**).

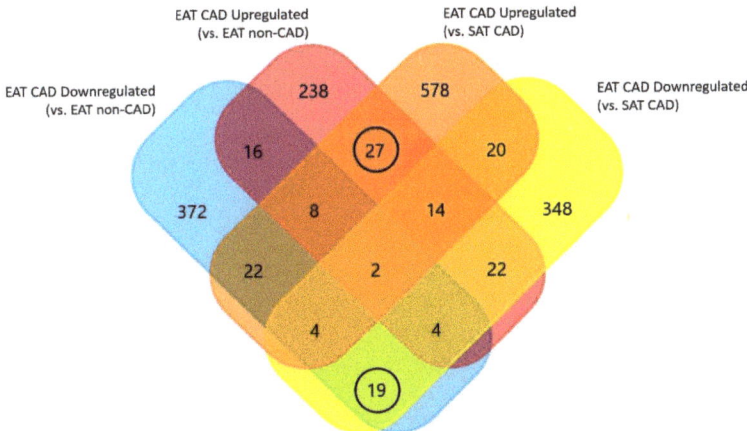

Figure 5. Venn diagram representing the distribution of proteins per control evidencing the overlapped and unique proteins in EAT, using the protein up- and downregulated in EAT CAD as compared with EAT non-CAD and SAT CAD.

Table 1. List of upregulated and downregulated proteins selected to characterize EAT. The putative secreted proteins are identified in bold.

Upregulated Subgroup (27 Proteins, 18 Secreted Proteins)	Downregulated Subgroup (19 Proteins, 8 Secreted Proteins)
Tumor necrosis factor Mitogen-activated protein kinase kinase kinase 8 Scavenger receptor cysteine-rich type 1 protein M130	Tyrosine-protein kinase ABL2 **5-aminolevulinate synthase**
C-C motif chemokine 2 C-C chemokine receptor type 2	erythroid-specific, mitochondrial Amphiphysin
Arachidonate 5-lipoxygenase-activating protein **C-C motif chemokine 5**	Aminopeptidase N
Nitric oxide synthase, endothelial	**Cathepsin K**
Neutrophil cytosol factor 2 Histone-lysine N-methyltransferase PRDM16	Dynamin-1
C-C motif chemokine 18	**Gelsolin**
Cathepsin E Leucine-rich repeat transmembrane protein FLRT3 Interleukin-7 receptor subunit alpha	**Macrophage scavenger receptor types I and II** Ubiquitin carboxyl-terminal hydrolase isozyme L1
C-C motif chemokine 13 T-cell surface glycoprotein CD3 zeta chain	Butyrophilin-like protein 9 Zinc finger and BTB domain-containing protein 16
HLA class I histocompatibility antigen protein P5 Toll-like receptor 2	**Galectin-3**
Interleukin-18	**Secreted frizzled-related protein 2**
E3 SUMO-protein ligase EGR2	**Hormone-sensitive lipase**
Early activation antigen CD69 L-selectin	Prelamin-A/C
Alpha-1-antichymotrypsin	Actin, gamma-enteric smooth muscle
Complement C3	Collagen alpha-1(I) chain
Coronin-1A **Intercellular adhesion molecule 3**	Acyl-CoA-binding protein
Integrin beta-2	Fructose-bisphosphate aldolase C

4. Bioinformatics Analysis Provides a Protein Network Overview from CAD Epicardial Adipose Tissue

4.1. Functional Protein Categorization and Integrative Analysis with REACTOME

To further understand the biological implications of EAT in CAD condition, we performed network enrichment analysis using Reactome. The data revealed that upregulated proteins were integrated into 59 pathways and downregulated proteins were integrated into 47 pathways, with a p value restricted to ≤ 0.05.

The most representative pathways for the upregulated subgroup of proteins were interleukin-10 signaling ($p = 8.66 \times 10^{-8}$), signaling by interleukins ($p = 8.91 \times 10^{-7}$), immune system ($p = 9.07 \times 10^{-7}$), chemokine receptors bind chemokines ($p = 1.15 \times 10^{-5}$), and innate immune system ($p = 6.06 \times 10^{-5}$, Table 2). The most representative pathways for the downregulated subgroup of proteins were depolymerization of the nuclear ($p = 4.05 \times 10^{-4}$), scavenging by class A receptors ($p = 5.7 \times 10^{-4}$), initiation of nuclear envelope reformation ($p = 6.3 \times 10^{-4}$), apoptotic cleavage of cellular proteins ($p = 2.23 \times 10^{-3}$), and apoptotic execution phase ($p = 4.11 \times 10^{-3}$, Table 2).

4.2. Predictions of Putative Secreted Proteins

In order to add new insights regarding EAT and CAD crosstalk, SignalP and SecretomeP bioinformatics analysis of the upregulated and downregulated subgroups of proteins retrieved which proteins were putatively secreted (Table S5). These proteins are highlighted in bold in Table 1 and were reanalyzed with Reactome, showing similar results to those presented in Table 2. Briefly, upregulated secreted proteins were integrated into 47 pathways and downregulated secreted proteins were integrated into 39 pathways, with a p value restricted to ≤ 0.05. The most prevalent pathways associated with upregulated secreted proteins were interleukin-10 signaling ($p = 8.91 \times 10^{-7}$), signaling by interleukins ($p = 5.33 \times 10^{-6}$), immune system ($p = 1.14 \times 10^{-5}$), interleukin-4 and interleukin-13 signaling ($p = 3.08 \times 10^{-5}$), and interleukin-18 signaling ($p = 1.05 \times 10^{-4}$, Table 3). In contrast, the most prevalent pathways associated with downregulated secreted proteins were binding and uptake of ligands by scavenger receptors ($p = 7.75 \times 10^{-5}$), RUNX2 regulates genes involved in differentiation of myeloid cells ($p = 8.6 \times 10^{-4}$), neutrophil degranulation ($p = 3.01 \times 10^{-4}$), degradation of the extracellular matrix (ECM) ($p = 3.41 \times 10^{-3}$), and RUNX1 regulates transcription of genes involved in differentiation of myeloid cells ($p = 3.5 \times 10^{-3}$).

Table 2. The 10 most relevant pathways sorted by p value using the upregulated and downregulated subgroups of proteins. Entities found in each pathway are described in Table S4.

Pathway Name	Entities Found	Entities Total	Entities Ratio	Entities p Value	Entities FDR
Upregulated Proteins					
Interleukin-10 signaling	5	45	0.004	8.66×10^{-8}	1.69×10^{-5}
Signaling by Interleukins	9	456	0.04	8.91×10^{-7}	5.9×10^{-5}
Immune System	18	2398	0.21	9.07×10^{-7}	5.9×10^{-5}
Chemokine receptors bind chemokines	4	57	0.005	1.15×10^{-5}	5.54×10^{-4}
Innate Immune System	11	1187	0.104	6.06×10^{-5}	2.36×10^{-3}
Peptide ligand-binding receptors	5	198	0.017	1.1×10^{-4}	3.53×10^{-3}
Interleukin-4 and Interleukin-13 signaling	4	111	0.01	1.52×10^{-4}	4.09×10^{-3}
Interleukin-18 signaling	2	9	0.001	2.32×10^{-4}	5.56×10^{-3}
Adaptive Immune System	9	944	0.083	2.9×10^{-4}	6.09×10^{-3}
Cytokine Signaling in Immune system	9	981	0.086	3.86×10^{-4}	7.34×10^{-3}
Downregulated Proteins					
Depolymerisation of the Nuclear	2	16	0.001	4.05×10^{-4}	2.65×10^{-2}
Scavenging by Class A Receptors	2	19	0.002	5.7×10^{-4}	2.65×10^{-2}
Initiation of Nuclear Envelope (NE) Reformation	2	20	0.002	6.3×10^{-4}	2.65×10^{-2}
Apoptotic cleavage of cellular proteins	2	38	0.003	2.23×10^{-3}	6.91×10^{-2}
Apoptotic execution phase	2	52	0.005	4.11×10^{-3}	8.17×10^{-2}
Nuclear Envelope Breakdown	2	58	0.005	5.08×10^{-3}	8.17×10^{-2}
Breakdown of the nuclear lamina	1	3	0	5.5×10^{-3}	8.17×10^{-2}
Collagen degration	2	64	0.006	6.14×10^{-3}	8.17×10^{-2}
Nuclear Envelope (NE) Reassembly	2	78	0.007	8.99×10^{-3}	8.17×10^{-2}
RUNX2 regulates genes involved in differentiation of myeloid cells	1	5	0	9.15×10^{-3}	8.17×10^{-2}

Entities reflect proteins, small molecules and genes regarding the pathway. Entities p value indicates that the proteins within this pathway represent more than would be expected if the set were random, corrected for multiple testing (Benjamini-Hochberg) that arises from evaluation of the submitted list of identifiers against every pathway. FDR indicates false discovery rate corrected for the probability of over-representation.

Table 3. The 10 most relevant pathways sorted by p value using upregulated and downregulated proteins predicted to be secreted. Entities found in each pathway are described in Table S6.

Pathway Name	Entities Found	Entities Total	Entities Ratio	Entities p Value	Entities FDR
Upregulated Proteins					
Interleukin-10 signaling	4	45	0.004	8.91×10^{-7}	1.08×10^{-4}
Signaling by Interleukins	7	456	0.04	5.33×10^{-6}	3.2×10^{-4}
Immune System	13	2398	0.21	1.14×10^{-5}	4.58×10^{-4}
Interleukin-4 and Interleukin-13 signaling	4	111	0.01	3.08×10^{-5}	9.23×10^{-4}
Interleukin-18 signaling	2	9	0.001	1.05×10^{-4}	2.27×10^{-3}
Chemokine receptors bind chemokines	3	57	0.005	1.13×10^{-4}	2.27×10^{-3}
Peptide ligand-binding receptors	4	198	0.017	2.84×10^{-4}	4.83×10^{-3}
Cytokine Signaling in Immune system	7	981	0.086	6.86×10^{-4}	9.59×10^{-3}
Purinergic signaling in Leishmaniasis infection	2	25	0.002	8.00×10^{-4}	9.59×10^{-3}
Cell recruitment (proinflammatory response)	2	25	0.002	8.00×10^{-4}	9.59×10^{-3}
Downregulated Proteins					
Binding and Uptake of Ligands by Scavenger Receptors	2	19	0.002	7.7×10^{-5}	4.85×10^{-3}
RUNX2 regulates genes involved in differentiation of myeloid cells	2	64	0.006	8.6×10^{-4}	2.58×10^{-2}
Neutrophil degranulation	2	121	0.011	3.01×10^{-4}	2.58×10^{-2}
Degradation of the extracellular matrix	2	129	0.011	3.41×10^{-3}	2.58×10^{-2}
RUNX1 regulates transcription of genes involved in differentiation of myeloid cells	1	5	0	3.5×10^{-3}	2.58×10^{-2}
RUNX1 regulates transcription of genes involved in differentiation of keratinocytes	3	480	0.042	3.55×10^{-3}	2.58×10^{-2}
Innate Immune System	2	140	0.012	4.01×10^{-3}	2.58×10^{-2}
GP1b-IX-V activation signalling	1	8	0.001	5.59×10^{-3}	2.58×10^{-2}
Caspase-mediated cleavage of cytoskeletal proteins	1	8	0.001	5.59×10^{-3}	2.58×10^{-2}
Transcriptional regulation by RUNX1	4	1187	0.104	5.79×10^{-3}	2.58×10^{-2}

Entities reflect proteins, small molecules and genes regarding the pathway. Entities p value indicates that the proteins within this pathway represent more than would be expected if the set were random, corrected for multiple testing (Benjamini–Hochberg) that arises from evaluation of the submitted list of identifiers against every pathway. FDR indicates false discovery rate corrected for the probability of over-representation.

5. Discussion

This study was the first to compile dysregulated proteins/genes from different studies to scrutinize the potential role of EAT in CAD. Despite the significant amount of research focusing on the impact of EAT on CAD, controversial results still preclude a clear vision of this interaction. This partially results from the fact that some studies have different control groups, while other studies describe different proteins, even if related to the same biological processes. Lastly, some proteins are inconsistently regulated, i.e., being upregulated or downregulated, depending on the study (Figure 5). This inconsistency proves that the same protein can behave differently depending on other comorbidities that cannot be excluded from human studies. With this systematic review, we were able to highlight a group of proteins that were consistently regulated among all studies, accounting for the control used in each study (EAT CAD vs. EAT non-CAD or EAT CAD vs. SAT CAD). The analysis of these proteins revealed the main pathways altered in the EAT and how they could communicate with the heart, potentially contributing to CAD development.

5.1. The Contribution of Epicardial Adipose Tissue to the Proinflammatory Profile of CAD

The bioinformatic analysis, presented in this study, revealed innate and adaptive immunity activation as the most relevant signaling pathways in EAT from CAD patients. Accordingly, it is currently accepted that the adipose tissue represents an important and highly active part of the immune system [24]. Adipose tissue is composed of two distinct entities, i.e., adipocytes and the stromal-vascular fraction formed by ECM with dispersed fibroblasts, preadipocytes, endothelial and immune cells [25]. Adipose tissue-resident immune cells include almost the full spectrum of immune cell types, namely macrophages, B cells, T cells, neutrophils, eosinophils, and mast cells [24]. Cytokines and chemokines are released from a wide range of immune cells, as confirmed by our analysis (Tables 1 and 2). These factors are indispensable for the communication between immune and non-immune cells and for the coordination of inflammatory responses, as well as the crosstalk between innate and adaptive immune system [26]. The chemokines overexpression, such as CCL2, CCL5, CCL13 and CCL18, triggers the recruitment of immune cells and the macrophages migration (Table 1). Macrophages plasticity endows their diverse activities in response to various environmental stimuli [27]. The M1 macrophages stimulate the conversion of unpolarized macrophages to M1 through the release of various proinflammatory and proatherogenic cytokines (IL-6 and TNF-α) and chemokines. For example, TNF-α initiates and amplifies inflammatory cascades through immune cells recruitment, chemokine regulation, and cytokine release, as well as the migration and mitogenesis of vascular smooth muscle and endothelial cells. Indeed, increased levels of TNF-α have been reported in EAT from CAD patients [28] (Table 1). Inversely, M2 macrophages can be activated by cytokines IL-4/IL-13, secreted from various cells in adipose tissue and are crucial to the promotion of preadipocyte survival, wound healing, and control of inflammation via anti-inflammatory cytokines production, such as IL-10, as evident in Table 2. Several studies have reported the influx of macrophages into the epicardial fat and have correlated the ratio of M1/M2 macrophages with the severity of CAD [29]. Indeed, excessive inflammation in CAD results from an imbalance between these two pathways, favoring M1 polarization and proinflammatory environment. Furthermore, other inflammatory pathways have been observed, such as IL-18 signaling, capable of increasing the atherosclerotic lesion size by T-lymphocytes attraction. Activated immune cells secrete several cytokines that influence adipocyte function and its paracrine secretion of cytokines (adipocytokines). Simultaneously, adipocytes produce inflammatory adipocytokines and ECM proteins, supporting infiltration and activation of immune cells. This vicious cycle creates an optimal microenvironment for low-grade inflammation, which underlies adipose tissue dysfunction.

Many studies have reported that CAD progression was closely associated with a higher volume of EAT, independently of obesity. Inflammation promotes adipose tissue expansion either through hypertrophy of existing adipocytes or differentiation of new adipocytes from adipogenic precursor cells (hyperplasia or adipogenesis) [30]. For instance, Sadler et al. showed that low-dose LPS led to adipocyte hyperplasia at the site of administration, associated with a net loss of adipose tissue collagen (Table 2), evidencing that the ability to effectively degrade ECM was essential for adipose tissue expansion [31,32]. In parallel to ECM remodeling, proinflammatory stimuli also promote angiogenesis in adipose tissue. These processes are both essential for adipogenesis in vivo [32] and explain the increased fat volume described in several studies [33]. Moreover, adipocytes hypertrophy is also associated with higher expression of proinflammatory adipocytokines, further perpetuating the vicious cycle of inflammation and fat expansion.

5.2. The Contribution of Epicardial Adipose Tissue to the Atherosclerotic Plaque Formation in CAD

Inflammation is also considered to be a central driver of atherogenesis and of the development of vulnerable atherosclerotic plaques [34,35]. Indeed, the proatherogenic effects of adipose tissue immune cells are carried out in the endocrine and paracrine manner by increased levels of the putative secreted proinflammatory proteins, as described above. Interestingly, we found IL-4, IL-10, and IL-13 signaling to be increased. We trust that the upregulation of these anti-inflammatory pathways might represent a compensatory mechanism to promote M2 polarization and to inhibit many cellular processes underlying plaque progression, rupture, or thrombosis, which include nuclear factor-κB activation, metalloproteinase proteinase production, tissue factor expression, and cell death. Further reinforcing this idea, other studies have shown that these factors were essential to keep the balance of the inflammatory response, to promote tissue repair, and to ensure plaque stability [36,37]. Interestingly, our analysis revealed reduced expression of cathepsin K and galectin-3 proteins, which have both been linked to the progression of atherosclerotic plaque. While cathepsin K has been associated with progression of unstable plaques and closely associated with CAD [38], galectin-3 has been shown to contribute to macrophage differentiation, foam cell formation, endothelial dysfunction, and vascular smooth muscle cells proliferation and migration [39] in the atheroma and its inhibition might reduce plaque progression [40]. Moreover, galectin-3 deficiency, in a mice model of atherosclerosis (ApoE$^{-/-}$), decreased plaque size, its necrotic core, and collagen content [40], which was consistent with our findings (Table 1). The presence of collagen in the fibrous atherosclerotic plaque cape is essential to maintain its stability, avoiding plaque rupture [41]. In addition, we found the macrophage scavenger receptor class A and the transcript factor RUNX2 to be downregulated in EAT. Macrophage scavenger receptor class A is known to be involved in foam cell development, mediating the influx of lipids into the macrophages [42], and therefore knockout mice for this gene have shown lower proinflammatory responses, macrophage apoptosis, and cellular necrosis with better stabilization of atherosclerotic plaques [43].

Similarly, RUNX2 is activated by atherogenic factors such as lipid-derived products from oxidation present in valve lesions that can promote calcification and is increased in advanced calcified lesions, supporting their implication in active osteogenesis and mineralization of human atherosclerotic coronary arteries [44]. Nevertheless, RUNX2 downregulation seems to be crucial to keep EAT expansion in response to inflammation, once RUNX2 upregulation restrains adipogenesis [45]. The proteome of epicardial fat likely acts as a local trigger for coronary plaque growth, calcification and stability in different stages of CAD. Accordingly, an unbalance between calcification promoters and inhibitors in epicardial fat has been reported in advanced stages of CAD [20].

5.3. The Epicardial Adipose Tissue and Atheroma Communication

Notably, the cellular composition of adipose tissue is highly plastic and can be regulated by environmental acute and chronic stimuli [24]. This suggests that the signals arising from the cardiovascular system can modulate the differentiation and function of adipocytes, and consequently adipose tissue quality. This concept supports a bidirectional crosstalk between epicardial fat and the coronary arteries, as represented in Figure 6. Antonopoulos et al., described an increased expression of adiponectin in perivascular adipose tissue in response to the activation of NADPH oxidase in the human arterial wall using an ex vivo model of human internal mammary arteries and perivascular adipose tissue co-cultures [46]. Moreover, inflammation and alteration in adipokines expression were reported in perivascular adipose tissue of rats and pigs as a consequence of balloon-induced vascular injuries and drug-eluting stent-induced coronary vasoconstriction [47,48]. The inflammation present in atherosclerotic coronary arteries may contribute to attracting immune cells to EAT, as observed by the increased number of chemokines upregulated (Tables 1 and 2). By doing so, the atheroma may affect the EAT composition and signaling.

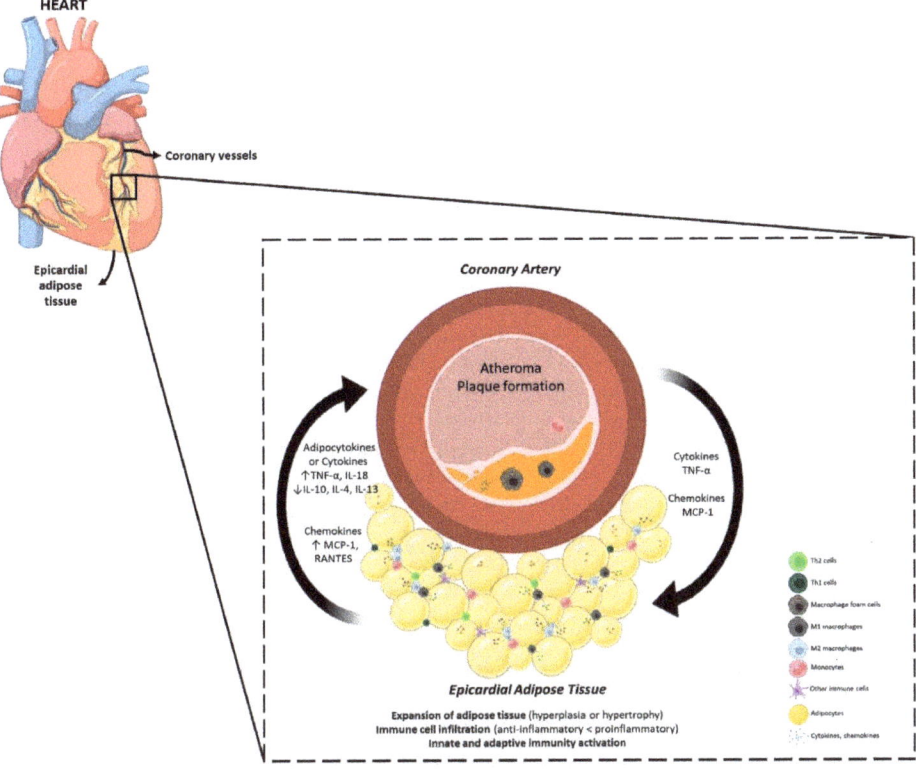

Figure 6. Interactions between EAT and atherosclerotic coronary arteries. In response to inflammatory cytokines released by atheroma, EAT can modulate the differentiation and function of adipocytes. EAT, located in close proximity with heart, can secrete adipocytokines which diffuse directly to the coronary arteries, promoting coronary inflammation. The figure was produced using BioRender and Servier Medical Art.

5.4. Influence of Epicardial Adipose Tissue Proteome on Cardiac Function and Structure

Beyond the influence of EAT on CAD, EAT is also directly connected to the myocardium. Inflammatory mediators have significant repercussions in all myocardial cell types, namely in cardiomyocytes, fibroblasts, and endothelial cells [49,50]. The deleterious effects of the proinflammatory cytokines include myocardial cell death, blunted β-adrenergic signaling, fetal gene reactivation, endothelial dysfunction, and collagen deposition [49], which are major determinants in the pathogenesis of cardiac disorders. There is increasing evidence that proinflammatory adipocytokines trigger cardiomyocyte hypertrophy and apoptosis, fibroblast differentiation into active myofibroblasts, and adhesion of immune cells to the endothelium and trans-endothelial migration [49,51,52]. Moreover, experimental studies have shown that inflammation was responsible for left ventricular (LV) diastolic and endothelial dysfunction and progression towards heart failure with preserved ejection fraction

(HFpEF) [53,54]. Cytokines such as TNF-α (Table 1) promote a direct negative inotropic effect, through downregulation of Ca^{2+}-regulating genes including sarcoplasmic reticulum Ca^{2+} ATPase and Ca^{2+}-release channel [55] and stimulate myofibroblasts activation [56,57]. Transgenic mice with cardiac-specific overexpression of TNF-α developed dilated cardiomyopathy with ventricular hypertrophy, ventricular dilatation, interstitial infiltrates, interstitial fibrosis, and reduced ejection fraction [58]. In contrast, IL-10 signaling suppressed the inflammatory response and contributed to improved LV function and remodeling (Table 2). Treatment approaches with IL-10 seem to be beneficial for preventing hypertrophy, reducing fibrosis, and preserving cardiac function, through the maintenance of cytokine homeostasis [59]. IL-4 and IL-13 signaling also modulate physiological processes, such as tissue repair, ECM remodeling, and metabolism homeostasis [60,61]. Additionally, we have observed a downregulation of RUNX1, that has been identified as a key regulator of adverse cardiac remodeling following myocardial infarction. RUNX1-deficient mice or RUNX1 knockout prevented adverse cardiac remodeling, restrained myocardial scar formation, and assured normal calcium homeostasis in cardiomyocytes [62]. Considering all the identified pathways, we believe that EAT fights to maintain cardiovascular homeostasis, orchestrating the inhibition and promotion of certain pathways.

5.5. Therapeutic Strategies against Inflammation-Related Coronary Artery Disease

Current pharmacological strategies for CAD patients include reducing angina symptoms, exercise-induced ischemia, and preventing cardiovascular events [63]. Taking into account the analysis presented in our study regarding the major impact of inflammation in CAD, therapeutic strategies should target the immune system with anti-inflammatory approaches [52]. Recently, the randomized clinical trial CANTOS assessed the effect of canakinumab, a human monoclonal antibody against IL-1β with anti-inflammatory properties. Canakinumab reduced significantly high-sensitivity C-reactive protein level from baseline in a dose-dependent fashion for three months, which persisted even after the treatment ended [64]. Moreover, the anti-inflammatory therapy targeting the IL-1β reduced the recurrence of cardiovascular events in well-treated CAD patients independent of any lowering effects on low-density lipoproteins (LDL) cholesterol levels [64].

6. Conclusions

The communication between EAT and CAD remains unclear. The dysregulated proteins, identified herein, highlight the importance of inflammatory processes for modulating the local environment and the progression of CAD. Inflammation triggers cellular and metabolic adaptations of epicardial fat that facilitate the formation and progression of atherogenesis of coronaries. Although several authors have supported that EAT thickness was a predictor for CAD, we also trust that the quality of epicardial fat should be assessed. For instance, to evaluate EAT-resident immune cells would ease the comprehension of the dynamic signaling at different time points of CAD progression.

In conclusion, future studies involving immune interventions should envisage clarifying the influence of anti-inflammatory drugs in EAT and how to modulate the paracrine and endocrine communication between epicardial fat and coronary arteries during CAD.

Supplementary Materials: The following are available online at http://www.mdpi.com/1422-0067/21/22/8866/s1, Figure S1: Representative sketch results of enrichment analysis with Reactome, Table S1: Eligible studied included and the proteins identified, Table S2: List of proteins identified in EAT from studies using EAT non-CAD as control or SAT CAD as control, Table S3: Distribution of proteins by Venn diagram, Table S4: Entities found in the 10 most relevant pathways sorted by p value using upregulated and downregulated subgroups of proteins, Table S5: Signal P/SecretomeP report, Table S6: Entities found in the 10 most relevant pathways sorted by p value using the upregulated and downregulated subgroups of potentially secreted proteins.

Funding: This project is supported by Fundo Europeu de Desenvolvimento Regional (FEDER) through Compete 2020, Programa Operacional Competitividade E Internacionalização (POCI); the project DOCNET (norte-01-0145-feder-000003), supported by Norte Portugal regional operational programme (norte 2020), under the

Portugal 2020 partnership agreement, through the European Regional Development Fund (ERDF); the project NETDIAMOND (POCI-01-0145FEDER-016385), supported by European Structural And Investment Funds; Lisbon's regional operational program 2020 and supported by the Cardiovascular R&D Center, financed by national funds through FCT, Fundação para a Ciência e Tecnologia, I.P., under the scope of the project UIDP/00051/2020. Glória Conceição is supported by the PhD grant program (norte-085369-FSE-000024), financed by Norte Portugal Regional Operational Programme (NORTE 2020), through the CCDRN, PORTUGAL 2020 and the European Social Fund (ESF).

Conflicts of Interest: The authors declare no conflict of interest.

References

1. Ng, M.; Fleming, T.; Robinson, M.; Thomson, B.; Graetz, N.; Margono, C.; Mullany, E.C.; Biryukov, S.; Abbafati, C.; Abera, S.F.; et al. Global, regional, and national prevalence of overweight and obesity in children and adults during 1980-2013: A systematic analysis for the Global Burden of Disease Study 2013. *Lancet* **2014**, *384*, 766–781. [CrossRef]
2. Manno, C.; Campobasso, N.; Nardecchia, A.; Triggiani, V.; Zupo, R.; Gesualdo, L.; Silvestris, F.; De Pergola, G. Relationship of para- and perirenal fat and epicardial fat with metabolic parameters in overweight and obese subjects. *Eat. Weight Disord.* **2019**, *24*, 24–67. [CrossRef] [PubMed]
3. Iacobellis, G. Local and systemic effects of the multifaceted epicardial adipose tissue depot. *Nat. Rev. Endocrinol.* **2015**, *11*, 363–371. [CrossRef] [PubMed]
4. Taguchi, R.; Takasu, J.; Itani, Y.; Yamamoto, R.; Yokoyama, K.; Watanabe, S.; Masuda, Y. Pericardial fat accumulation in men as a risk factor for coronary artery disease. *Atherosclerosis* **2001**, *157*, 203–209. [CrossRef]
5. Bettencourt, N.; Toschke, A.M.; Leite, D.; Rocha, J.; Carvalho, M.; Sampaio, F.; Xará, S.; Leite-Moreira, A.; Nagel, E.; Gama, V. Epicardial adipose tissue is an independent predictor of coronary atherosclerotic burden. *Int. J. Cardiol.* **2012**, *158*, 26–32. [CrossRef] [PubMed]
6. Cassar, A.; Holmes, D.R., Jr.; Rihal, C.S.; Gersh, B.J. Chronic coronary artery disease: Diagnosis and management. *Mayo Clin. Proc.* **2009**, *84*, 1130–1146. [CrossRef] [PubMed]
7. Wolf, D.; Ley, K. Immunity and Inflammation in Atherosclerosis. *Circ. Res.* **2019**, *124*, 315–327. [CrossRef] [PubMed]
8. Ades, P.A.; Savage, P.D. Obesity in coronary heart disease: An unaddressed behavioral risk factor. *Prev. Med.* **2017**, *104*, 117–119. [CrossRef] [PubMed]
9. Piche, M.E.; Poirier, P.; Lemieux, I.; Despres, J.P. Overview of Epidemiology and Contribution of Obesity and Body Fat Distribution to Cardiovascular Disease: An Update. *Prog. Cardiovasc. Dis.* **2018**, *61*, 103–113. [CrossRef]
10. Libby, P.; Theroux, P. Pathophysiology of coronary artery disease. *Circulation* **2005**, *111*, 3481–3488. [CrossRef]
11. Libby, P.; Ridker, P.M.; Hansson, G.K. Leducq Transatlantic Network on A. Inflammation in atherosclerosis: From pathophysiology to practice. *J. Am. Coll. Cardiol.* **2009**, *54*, 2129–2138. [CrossRef] [PubMed]
12. Prospective Studies, C.; Whitlock, G.; Lewington, S.; Sherliker, P.; Clarke, R.; Emberson, J.; Halsey, J.; Qizilbash, N.; Collins, R.; Peto, R. Body-mass index and cause-specific mortality in 900 000 adults: Collaborative analyses of 57 prospective studies. *Lancet* **2009**, *373*, 1083–1096. [CrossRef]
13. Fuster, J.J.; Ouchi, N.; Gokce, N.; Walsh, K. Obesity-Induced Changes in Adipose Tissue Microenvironment and Their Impact on Cardiovascular Disease. *Circ. Res.* **2016**, *118*, 1786–1807. [CrossRef] [PubMed]
14. Harada, K.; Shibata, R.; Ouchi, N.; Tokuda, Y.; Funakubo, H.; Suzuki, M.; Kataoka, T.; Nagao, T.; Okumura, S.; Shinoda, N.; et al. Increased expression of the adipocytokine omentin in the epicardial adipose tissue of coronary artery disease patients. *Atherosclerosis* **2016**, *251*, 299–304. [CrossRef] [PubMed]
15. Sicari, R.; Sironi, A.M.; Petz, R.; Frassi, F.; Chubuchny, V.; De Marchi, D.; Positano, V.; Lombardi, M.; Picano, E.; Gastaldelli, A.; et al. Pericardial rather than epicardial fat is a cardiometabolic risk marker: An MRI vs echo study. *J. Am. Soc. Echocardiogr.* **2011**, *24*, 1156–1162. [CrossRef]
16. Iacobellis, G.; Lonn, E.; Lamy, A.; Singh, N.; Sharma, A.M. Epicardial fat thickness and coronary artery disease correlate independently of obesity. *Int. J. Cardiol.* **2011**, *146*, 452–454. [CrossRef]
17. Villasante Fricke, A.C.; Iacobellis, G. Epicardial Adipose Tissue: Clinical Biomarker of Cardio-Metabolic Risk. *Int. J. Mol. Sci.* **2019**, *20*, 5989. [CrossRef]
18. Bachar, G.N.; Dicker, D.; Kornowski, R.; Atar, E. Epicardial adipose tissue as a predictor of coronary artery disease in asymptomatic subjects. *Am. J. Cardiol.* **2012**, *110*, 534–538. [CrossRef]

19. Clauser, M.; Altenberger, J. Obesity and cardiac cachexia in chronic heart failure. *Herz* **2013**, *38*, 610–617. [CrossRef]
20. Mancio, J.; Barros, A.S.; Conceicao, G.; Pessoa-Amorim, G.; Santa, C.; Bartosch, C.; Ferreira, W.; Carvalho, M.; Ferreira, N.; Vouga, L.; et al. Epicardial adipose tissue volume and annexin A2/fetuin-A signalling are linked to coronary calcification in advanced coronary artery disease: Computed tomography and proteomic biomarkers from the EPICHEART study. *Atherosclerosis* **2020**, *292*, 75–83. [CrossRef]
21. Zhao, Y.X.; Zhu, H.J.; Pan, H.; Liu, X.M.; Wang, L.J.; Yang, H.B.; Li, N.; Gong, F.; Sun, W.; Zeng, Y. Comparative Proteome Analysis of Epicardial and Subcutaneous Adipose Tissues from Patients with or without Coronary Artery Disease. *Int. J. Endocrinol.* **2019**, *2019*, 6976712. [CrossRef] [PubMed]
22. Conceicao, G.; Matos, J.; Miranda-Silva, D.; Goncalves, N.; Sousa-Mendes, C.; Goncalves, A.; Ferreira, R.; Leite-Moreira, A.F.; Vitorino, R.; Falcao-Pires, I. Fat Quality Matters: Distinct Proteomic Signatures Between Lean and Obese Cardiac Visceral Adipose Tissue Underlie its Differential Myocardial Impact. *Cell Physiol. Biochem.* **2020**, *54*, 384–400. [PubMed]
23. Jassal, B.; Matthews, L.; Viteri, G.; Gong, C.; Lorente, P.; Fabregat, A.; Sidiropoulos, K.; Cook, J.; Gillespie, M.; Haw, R.; et al. The reactome pathway knowledgebase. *Nucleic Acids Res.* **2020**, *48*, D498–D503. [CrossRef] [PubMed]
24. Grant, R.W.; Dixit, V.D. Adipose tissue as an immunological organ. *Obesity (Silver Spring)* **2015**, *23*, 512–518. [CrossRef] [PubMed]
25. Mraz, M.; Haluzik, M. The role of adipose tissue immune cells in obesity and low-grade inflammation. *J. Endocrinol.* **2014**, *222*, R113–R127. [CrossRef] [PubMed]
26. Lacy, P. Editorial: Secretion of cytokines and chemokines by innate immune cells. *Front. Immunol.* **2015**, *6*, 190. [CrossRef]
27. Wynn, T.A.; Chawla, A.; Pollard, J.W. Macrophage biology in development, homeostasis and disease. *Nature* **2013**, *496*, 445–455. [CrossRef]
28. Mazurek, T.; Zhang, L.; Zalewski, A.; Mannion, J.D.; Diehl, J.T.; Arafat, H.; Sarov-Blat, L.; O'Brien, S.; Keiper, E.A.; Johnson, A.G.; et al. Human epicardial adipose tissue is a source of inflammatory mediators. *Circulation* **2003**, *108*, 2460–2466. [CrossRef]
29. Hirata, Y.; Tabata, M.; Kurobe, H.; Motoki, T.; Akaike, M.; Nishio, C.; Higashida, M.; Mikasa, H.; Nakaya, Y.; Takanashi, S.; et al. Coronary atherosclerosis is associated with macrophage polarization in epicardial adipose tissue. *J. Am. Coll. Cardiol.* **2011**, *58*, 248–255. [CrossRef]
30. Vishvanath, L.; Gupta, R.K. Contribution of adipogenesis to healthy adipose tissue expansion in obesity. *J. Clin. Investig.* **2019**, *129*, 4022–4031. [CrossRef]
31. Sadler, D.; Mattacks, C.A.; Pond, C.M. Changes in adipocytes and dendritic cells in lymph node containing adipose depots during and after many weeks of mild inflammation. *J. Anat.* **2005**, *207*, 769–781. [CrossRef] [PubMed]
32. Wernstedt Asterholm, I.; Tao, C.; Morley, T.S.; Wang, Q.A.; Delgado-Lopez, F.; Wang, Z.V.; Scherer, P.E. Adipocyte inflammation is essential for healthy adipose tissue expansion and remodeling. *Cell Metab.* **2014**, *20*, 103–118. [CrossRef] [PubMed]
33. McClain, J.; Hsu, F.; Brown, E.; Burke, G.; Carr, J.; Harris, T.; Kritchevsky, S.; Szklo, M.; Tracy, R.; Ding, J. Pericardial adipose tissue and coronary artery calcification in the Multi-ethnic Study of Atherosclerosis (MESA). *Obesity (Silver Spring)* **2013**, *21*, 1056–1063. [CrossRef] [PubMed]
34. Raggi, P.; Genest, J.; Giles, J.T.; Rayner, K.J.; Dwivedi, G.; Beanlands, R.S.; Gupta, M. Role of inflammation in the pathogenesis of atherosclerosis and therapeutic interventions. *Atherosclerosis* **2018**, *276*, 98–108. [CrossRef]
35. Antoniades, C.; Kotanidis, C.P.; Berman, D.S. State-of-the-art review article. Atherosclerosis affecting fat: What can we learn by imaging perivascular adipose tissue? *J. Cardiovasc. Comput. Tomogr.* **2019**, *13*, 288–296. [CrossRef]
36. Barrett, T.J. Macrophages in Atherosclerosis Regression. *Arterioscler. Thromb. Vasc. Biol.* **2020**, *40*, 20–33. [CrossRef]
37. Nishihira, K.; Imamura, T.; Yamashita, A.; Hatakeyama, K.; Shibata, Y.; Nagatomo, Y.; Date, H.; Kita, T.; Eto, T.; Asada, Y. Increased expression of interleukin-10 in unstable plaque obtained by directional coronary atherectomy. *Eur. Heart J.* **2006**, *27*, 1685–1689. [CrossRef]
38. Zhao, H.; Qin, X.; Wang, S.; Sun, X.; Dong, B. Decreased cathepsin K levels in human atherosclerotic plaques are associated with plaque instability. *Exp. Ther. Med.* **2017**, *14*, 3471–3476. [CrossRef]

39. Gao, Z.; Liu, Z.; Wang, R.; Zheng, Y.; Li, H.; Yang, L. Galectin-3 Is a Potential Mediator for Atherosclerosis. *J. Immunol. Res.* **2020**, *2020*, 5284728. [CrossRef]
40. MacKinnon, A.C.; Liu, X.; Hadoke, P.W.; Miller, M.R.; Newby, D.E.; Sethi, T. Inhibition of galectin-3 reduces atherosclerosis in apolipoprotein E-deficient mice. *Glycobiology* **2013**, *23*, 654–663. [CrossRef]
41. Hansson, G.K.; Libby, P.; Tabas, I. Inflammation and plaque vulnerability. *J. Intern Med.* **2015**, *278*, 483–493. [CrossRef] [PubMed]
42. de Winther, M.P.; van Dijk, K.W.; Havekes, L.M.; Hofker, M.H. Macrophage scavenger receptor class A: A multifunctional receptor in atherosclerosis. *Arterioscler. Thromb. Vasc. Biol.* **2000**, *20*, 290–297. [CrossRef]
43. Zani, I.A.; Stephen, S.L.; Mughal, N.A.; Russell, D.; Homer-Vanniasinkam, S.; Wheatcroft, S.B.; Ponnambalam, S. Scavenger receptor structure and function in health and disease. *Cells* **2015**, *4*, 178–201. [CrossRef] [PubMed]
44. Alexopoulos, A.; Peroukides, S.; Bravou, V.; Varakis, J.; Pyrgakis, V.; Papadaki, H. Implication of bone regulatory factors in human coronary artery calcification. *Artery Res.* **2011**, *5*, 101–108. [CrossRef]
45. Zhang, Y.Y.; Li, X.; Qian, S.W.; Guo, L.; Huang, H.Y.; He, Q.; Liu, Y.; Ma, C.-G.; Tang, Q.-Q. Down-regulation of type I Runx2 mediated by dexamethasone is required for 3T3-L1 adipogenesis. *Mol. Endocrinol.* **2012**, *26*, 798–808. [CrossRef] [PubMed]
46. Antonopoulos, A.S.; Margaritis, M.; Coutinho, P.; Shirodaria, C.; Psarros, C.; Herdman, L.; Sanna, F.; De Silva, R.; Petrou, M.; Sayeed, R.; et al. Adiponectin as a link between type 2 diabetes and vascular NADPH oxidase activity in the human arterial wall: The regulatory role of perivascular adipose tissue. *Diabetes* **2015**, *64*, 2207–2219. [CrossRef] [PubMed]
47. Takaoka, M.; Suzuki, H.; Shioda, S.; Sekikawa, K.; Saito, Y.; Nagai, R.; Sata, M. Endovascular injury induces rapid phenotypic changes in perivascular adipose tissue. *Arterioscler. Thromb. Vasc. Biol.* **2010**, *30*, 1576–1582. [CrossRef]
48. Ohyama, K.; Matsumoto, Y.; Amamizu, H.; Uzuka, H.; Nishimiya, K.; Morosawa, S.; Hirano, M.; Watabe, H.; Funaki, Y.; Miyata, S.; et al. Association of Coronary Perivascular Adipose Tissue Inflammation and Drug-Eluting Stent-Induced Coronary Hyperconstricting Responses in Pigs: (18)F-Fluorodeoxyglucose Positron Emission Tomography Imaging Study. *Arterioscler. Thromb. Vasc. Biol.* **2017**, *37*, 1757–1764. [CrossRef]
49. Van Linthout, S.; Tschope, C. Inflammation-Cause or Consequence of Heart Failure or Both? *Curr. Heart Fail Rep.* **2017**, *14*, 251–265. [CrossRef]
50. Northcott, J.M.; Yeganeh, A.; Taylor, C.G.; Zahradka, P.; Wigle, J.T. Adipokines and the cardiovascular system: Mechanisms mediating health and disease. *Can. J. Physiol. Pharmacol.* **2012**, *90*, 1029–1059. [CrossRef]
51. Van Linthout, S.; Miteva, K.; Tschope, C. Crosstalk between fibroblasts and inflammatory cells. *Cardiovasc. Res.* **2014**, *102*, 258–269. [CrossRef] [PubMed]
52. Frantz, S.; Falcao-Pires, I.; Balligand, J.L.; Bauersachs, J.; Brutsaert, D.; Ciccarelli, M.; Dawson, D.; De Windt, L.J.; Giacca, M.; Hamdani, N.; et al. The innate immune system in chronic cardiomyopathy: A European Society of Cardiology (ESC) scientific statement from the Working Group on Myocardial Function of the ESC. *Eur. J. Heart Fail* **2018**, *20*, 445–459. [CrossRef] [PubMed]
53. Waddingham, M.T.; Sonobe, T.; Tsuchimochi, H.; Edgley, A.J.; Sukumaran, V.; Chen, Y.C.; Hansra, S.S.; Schwenke, D.O.; Umetani, K.; Aoyama, K.; et al. Diastolic dysfunction is initiated by cardiomyocyte impairment ahead of endothelial dysfunction due to increased oxidative stress and inflammation in an experimental prediabetes model. *J. Mol. Cell. Cardiol.* **2019**, *137*, 119–131. [CrossRef] [PubMed]
54. Franssen, C.; Chen, S.; Unger, A.; Korkmaz, H.I.; De Keulenaer, G.W.; Tschope, C.; Leite-Moreira, A.F.; Musters, R.J.P.; Niessen, H.W.; Linke, W.A.; et al. Myocardial Microvascular Inflammatory Endothelial Activation in Heart Failure With Preserved Ejection Fraction. *JACC Heart Fail* **2016**, *4*, 312–324. [CrossRef] [PubMed]
55. Tsai, C.T.; Wu, C.K.; Lee, J.K.; Chang, S.N.; Kuo, Y.M.; Wang, Y.C.; Lai, L.-P.; Chiang, F.-T.; Hwang, J.-J.; Lin, J.-L.; et al. TNF-alpha down-regulates sarcoplasmic reticulum Ca(2)(+) ATPase expression and leads to left ventricular diastolic dysfunction through binding of NF-kappaB to promoter response element. *Cardiovasc. Res.* **2015**, *105*, 318–329. [CrossRef] [PubMed]
56. Gurantz, D.; Cowling, R.T.; Varki, N.; Frikovsky, E.; Moore, C.D.; Greenberg, B.H. IL-1beta and TNF-alpha upregulate angiotensin II type 1 (AT1) receptors on cardiac fibroblasts and are associated with increased AT1 density in the post-MI heart. *J. Mol. Cell. Cardiol.* **2005**, *38*, 505–515. [CrossRef] [PubMed]

57. Lindner, D.; Zietsch, C.; Tank, J.; Sossalla, S.; Fluschnik, N.; Hinrichs, S.; Maier, L.; Poller, W.; Blankenberg, S.; Schultheiss, H.-P.; et al. Cardiac fibroblasts support cardiac inflammation in heart failure. *Basic Res. Cardiol.* **2014**, *109*, 428. [CrossRef]
58. Kubota, T.; McTiernan, C.F.; Frye, C.S.; Slawson, S.E.; Lemster, B.H.; Koretsky, A.P.; Demetris, A.J.; Feldman, A.M. Dilated cardiomyopathy in transgenic mice with cardiac-specific overexpression of tumor necrosis factor-alpha. *Circ. Res.* **1997**, *81*, 627–635. [CrossRef]
59. Zimmer, A.; Bagchi, A.K.; Vinayak, K.; Bello-Klein, A.; Singal, P.K. Innate immune response in the pathogenesis of heart failure in survivors of myocardial infarction. *Am. J. Physiol. Heart Circ. Physiol.* **2019**, *316*, H435–H45. [CrossRef]
60. Ramos, G.; Frantz, S. Myocardial Metabolism Under Control of a Cytokine Receptor. *J. Am. Heart Assoc.* **2017**, *6*, e006291. [CrossRef]
61. Wodsedalek, D.J.; Paddock, S.J.; Wan, T.C.; Auchampach, J.A.; Kenarsary, A.; Tsaih, S.W.; Flister, M.J.; O'Meara, C.C. IL-13 promotes in vivo neonatal cardiomyocyte cell cycle activity and heart regeneration. *Am. J. Physiol. Heart Circ. Physiol.* **2019**, *316*, H24–H34. [CrossRef] [PubMed]
62. Riddell, A.; McBride, M.; Braun, T.; Nicklin, S.A.; Cameron, E.; Loughrey, C.M.; Martin, T.P. RUNX1: An emerging therapeutic target for cardiovascular disease. *Cardiovasc. Res.* **2020**, *116*, 1410–1423. [CrossRef] [PubMed]
63. Knuuti, J.; Wijns, W.; Saraste, A.; Capodanno, D.; Barbato, E.; Funck-Brentano, C.; Prescott, E.; Storey, R.F.; Deaton, C.; Cuisset, T.; et al. 2019 ESC Guidelines for the diagnosis and management of chronic coronary syndromes. *Eur. Heart J.* **2020**, *41*, 407–477. [CrossRef] [PubMed]
64. Lorenzatti, A.; Servato, M.L. Role of Anti-inflammatory Interventions in Coronary Artery Disease: Understanding the Canakinumab Anti-inflammatory Thrombosis Outcomes Study (CANTOS). *Eur. Cardiol.* **2018**, *13*, 38–41. [CrossRef] [PubMed]

Publisher's Note: MDPI stays neutral with regard to jurisdictional claims in published maps and institutional affiliations.

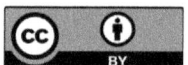

© 2020 by the authors. Licensee MDPI, Basel, Switzerland. This article is an open access article distributed under the terms and conditions of the Creative Commons Attribution (CC BY) license (http://creativecommons.org/licenses/by/4.0/).

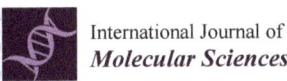

Review

Coronary Artery Ectasia: Review of the Non-Atherosclerotic Molecular and Pathophysiologic Concepts

Gavin H. C. Richards [1], Kathryn L. Hong [1,2], Michael Y. Henein [3], Colm Hanratty [1] and Usama Boles [1,4,*]

[1] Cardiovascular Research Institute (CVRI) Dublin, Mater Private Hospital, D07 WKW8 Dublin, Ireland; gavin.richards@materprivate.ie (G.H.C.R.); kathryn.hong@ucdconnect.ie (K.L.H.); colm.hanratty@materprivate.ie (C.H.)
[2] School of Medicine, University College Dublin, D04 V1W8 Dublin, Ireland
[3] Department of Public Health and Clinical Medicine, Heart Clinic, Umea University, 901 87 Umea, Sweden; michael.henein@umu.se
[4] Cardiology Department, Tipperary University Hospital, E91 VY40 Clonmel, Ireland
* Correspondence: bolesu@tcd.ie

Abstract: Coronary artery ectasia (CAE) is frequently encountered in clinical practice, conjointly with atherosclerotic CAD (CAD). Given the overlapping cardiovascular risk factors for patients with concomitant CAE and atherosclerotic CAD, a common underlying pathophysiology is often postulated. However, coronary artery ectasia may arise independently, as isolated (pure) CAE, thereby raising suspicions of an alternative mechanism. Herein, we review the existing evidence for the pathophysiology of CAE in order to help direct management strategies towards enhanced detection and treatment.

Keywords: coronary artery ectasia; coronary artery aneurysm; CAD; cytokine; lipidome

1. Introduction

Coronary artery ectasia (CAE) is a relatively common coronary angiographic finding, with an incidence of 1.5–5% and geographical variations in prevalence. CAE has been associated with a male predominance (1.7% vs. 0.2%) and more frequently affects the right coronary artery and the proximal vessels. Currently, the pathogenesis of CAE is not fully understood, with some evidence suggesting an atherosclerotic aetiology and other reports describing a distinct pathology [1].

While the terms CAE and coronary artery aneurysm (CAA) are often used interchangeably, they carry distinct phenotypes and definitions. CAE is defined as a diffuse dilatation of the coronary artery of at least 1.5 times the normal artery with a length of over 20 mm or greater than one third of the vessel. It can be further subdivided into diffuse and focal dilations by the length of the dilated vessels. Histologically, it presents with extensive destruction of musculoelastic elements, with marked degradation of collagen and elastic fibres and disruption of the elastic lamina. Conversely, CAA is a dilatation with a focal appearance. It is termed saccular if the transverse diameter is greater than the longitudinal, and fusiform for the opposite [2].

Given that CAE is associated with atherosclerosis in 50% of cases, a common underlying aetiology has been postulated. It is important to note, however, that approximately 30% of cases are associated with vasculitis including Kawasaki disease and Takayasu arteritis, and connective tissue diseases such as Ehlers–Danlos or Marfan's syndrome. The remainder are congenital or idiopathic [3]. In particular, congenital CAE has been documented with other cardiovascular abnormalities including bicuspid aortic valve, aortic aneurysms, pulmonary stenosis, and ventricular septal defects.

2. Acute Myocardial Infarction in CAE

CAE patients with acute myocardial infarction (MI) undergoing percutaneous coronary intervention (PCI) have reported a high thrombus burden and greater use of glycoprotein IIb/IIIa inhibitors (GPI) and post-procedural anticoagulation [4]. Indeed, thrombus formation may be inherently related to abnormal flow within coronary ectatic lesions, resulting in distal embolization. While higher rates of no-reflow and lower Thrombolysis in Myocardial Infarction (TIMI) flow grades have been observed after percutaneous coronary intervention (PCI), long term survival is good [5]. One study reported that no stent was deployed in 44% of patients undergoing coronary angiogram, compared with 7.5% in a comparable group with no CAE [6]. Furthermore, stent deployment conferred a better in-hospital outcome, although long term outcomes were shown to be similar with relatively high rates of non-fatal MI and angina. In a large observational study evaluating the long-term outcomes of 1698 patients with acute MI, the incidence of major adverse cardiac events (MACE) ($p < 0.001$), cardiac death ($p = 0.004$), and non-fatal myocardial infection ($p < 0.001$) was significantly higher in patients with CAE [7]. An increased risk of MACE has also been identified in patients with diffuse CAE as compared to those with focal CAE [8].

3. Clinical Sequelae

While most patients with CAE experience coronary artery disease (CAD), additional clinical manifestations may be related to increased inflammatory markers in the peripheral blood [9] and anomalies present in other blood vessels [10]. Possible aetiologies contributing to the destruction of musculoelastic coronary elements in CAE include vascular endothelial dysfunction, oxidative stress [11], and enzyme destruction [12].

Angina is a frequently reported symptom, resulting from slow coronary flow due to turbulence within ectatic segments. Disturbed blood flow patterns directly affect endothelial cells by promoting the sustained activation of atherogenic genes, such as monocyte chemotactic protein-1 (MCP-1). This subsequently induces monocyte infiltration and platelet-derived growth factors, further increasing endothelial cell turnover and smooth muscle cell migration [13]. Previous reports have even elucidated a higher prevalence in CAE compared with matched patients with severe atherosclerotic CAD [14]. Taken together, patients with CAE may have a higher relative risk for angina and associated risk of adverse cardiac-related outcomes when coupled with obstructive CAD.

The incidence of PCI in CAE with CAD is significantly lower than CAD with no CAE ($p < 0.001$), reflecting the limitations of current technologies to treat ectatic vessels. Coronary embolization in CAE can result from stasis in dilated segments and anticoagulation is frequently prescribed to mitigate this. Rupture of aneurysmal segments is a rare but serious complication [2].

CAE is also associated with ECG markers of arrhythmia including QRS fragmentation [15]. Conlon et al. reported an association between CAE and ECG markers of arrhythmia including prolonged Tp-Te, QTc dispersion, and P wave dispersion. Long Tp-Te interval represents a susceptibility to ventricular arrhythmias and is associated with increased mortality in hypertrophic cardiomyopathy, myocardial infarction, and long QT syndromes [16].

Long term follow-up studies have demonstrated higher incidence of acute coronary syndrome (ACS) in CAE compared to controls, with increasing ACS in higher grade CAE (Markis grades 1 and 2) [17]. Mortality and cardiovascular mortality are also higher in CAE when compared with controls [18], and there is evidence for the role of dilatation extent in predicting these clinical outcomes.

4. Risk Factors

A recent study demonstrated no difference in the incidence of hypertension, diabetes, hyperlipidaemia, family history, or smoking between CAE and CAD. However, higher incidences of hypertension, hyperlipidaemia, triglyceride, and low-density lipoprotein/high-density lipoprotein ratio (LDL/HDL) have been observed in previous studies when CAE patients were compared with matched controls ($p < 0.001$) [19]. This is in accordance with recent evidence describing reduced HDL-C and higher TG/HDL-C monocyte/HDL-C ratios in CAE and CAD groups as compared to controls. The LDL-C/HDL-C ratio was also significantly higher in patients with CAE versus those with CAD [20]. Furthermore, patients with solely (pure) CAE have been found to be younger, have diffuse disease involving the three main epicardial coronary branches, and have less traditional CV risk factors than those with mixed CAE [21].

While coronary angiography is the gold standard diagnostic technique for detecting CAE, intravascular ultrasound is frequently used to confirm CAE morphology and luminal dilatation. To further classify anatomical variations, Markis proposed a classification of CAE based on the extent of ectactic involvement. As described in Table 1, severity type decreases from Type I, diffuse ectasia of two or three vessels, to Type IV, localized or segmental ectasia.

Table 1. Markis classification of coronary artery ectasia.

Type I	Diffuse ectasia of two or three vessels
Type II	Diffuse disease in one vessel only and localised in another vessel
Type III	Diffuse disease in one vessel
Type IV	Localised or segmental ectasia

5. Atherosclerotic vs. Non-Atherosclerotic Inflammatory Response in CAE

Given similar histological characteristics, clinical symptoms, and disease co-existence, an atherosclerotic process has been widely linked to CAE pathogenesis. Indeed, CAE may represent an exaggerated form of extensive vascular remodelling in response to atherosclerotic plaque formation, with extracellular enzymatic degradation playing a major role in ectatic vessel formation. The atherosclerotic process may extend through the intima to the media where hyalinisation and lipid deposition in the intima leads to degradation of the media due to overexpression of matrix metalloproteinases (MMPs). Consequently, MMPs are actively involved in the proteolysis of extracellular matrix proteins, resulting in collagen degradation and pathological dilatation. The overproduction of MMPs may lend itself to the development of ACS and may explain the beneficial role of rosuvastatin in suppressing MMP expression and reducing inflammation in CAE patients [22]. Of note, MMP expression is downregulated in diabetes, which may paradoxically explain the lower incidence of CAE in diabetes.

Local coronary flow disturbances caused by decreased endothelial shear stress has also been proposed as an alternative explanation for the coexistence of CAD and CAE. Intravascular ultrasound (IVUS) evidence suggests that atherosclerotic plaques within ectatic regions of vessels are highly inflamed and meet high-risk plaque criteria [23]. Histopathological evidence of CAE shows intense proteolysis and extracellular matrix destruction within the vascular wall [14].

On the other hand, risk factors for CAD are not a prerequisite for the development of CAE, and many patients are found to have no atherosclerotic plaque. Namely, Kawasaki disease is the second most common aetiology in CAE, presenting with diffuse infiltration of the arterial wall by mononuclear cells, lymphocytes, and macrophages [24]. Moreover, infection-linked CAE is associated with pathogenic invasion of the coronary arteries and immune complex deposition.

6. Immuno-Inflammatory Response in CAE

Mediators of chronic inflammation, such as growth factors and cellular adhesion models, have been widely described in the pathogenesis of CAE. Specifically, the expression of specific inflammatory markers, particularly IL-6 and CRP, is known to be higher in CAE compared with CAD and healthy controls [9]. Most recently, a large meta-analysis elucidated the role of other contributory markers, neutrophil to lymphocyte ratio (NLR) and red cell distribution width (RDW), in the pathogenesis of CAE [25].

A report on immune-inflammatory response in CAE demonstrated significantly higher systemic levels of INF-gamma, TNF-alpha, IL-1ß, and IL-8, and lower levels of IL-2 and IL-4 compared with the control group [26]. In comparison with CAD, CAE patients had significantly higher levels of IL-8 and IL-1ß, and significantly lower levels of IL-2 and IL-4. Analysis of isolated CAE versus mixed CAE did not demonstrate any differences with respect to cytokine levels.

Inflammatory markers, C-reactive protein and albumin are believed to be involved in the progression and severity of CAE. Recently, a significantly higher C-reactive protein-to-albumin ratio has been associated with isolated CAE when compared to obstructive CAD and controls. Notably, C-reactive protein-to-albumin ratio also correlated strongly with the severity of CAE, which provides further evidence for its potential role in detection and management [27].

While the cytokine milieu in CAE shares similarities with CAD, there are some distinct differences. Notably, the higher presence of leukocytes in CAE presents as higher levels of IL-6 and lower levels of IL-2. This cytokine-mediated inflammatory response serves as the basis for impaired coronary circulation.

High levels of TNF-α are known to be present in CAD where stimulation of the Th1 pathway leads to activated M1 macrophages which promote atherogenesis. CAE in the absence of CAD is also associated with high levels of TNF-α, which may imply a common mechanism of macrophage activation. Nevertheless, the low level of IL-2 in CAE may suggest an alternative trigger for the direct activation of the Th1 pathway.

The pro-inflammatory marker, IL-6, has a role in inhibiting macrophage activation by inhibiting macrophage scavenger receptor-A, but is not associated with CAD [28]. Additionally, the non-atherogenic process in CAE may be partially explained by lower levels of IL-4, secreted by Th2. Likewise, the lower levels of IL-2 seen in CAE may also support a non-atherogenic pathway through the absence of Th1 cell response which is associated with CAD and acute coronary syndrome.

Another report [29] found some subtle differences in cytokine levels. Triantafyllis et al. reported high IL-4 and low IL-2 levels in CAE compared with CAD and control subjects, and high IL-6 in CAE and CAD compared with control subjects. They concluded that Th2 activation (in the presence of high IL-4) is a cardinal feature of CAE (Figure 1, Pathway A). The relationship of Th2 with atherogenesis is complex as IL-4 produced by Th2 reduces IFN-y activity and so can be considered antiatherogenic. However, in some circumstances in mouse models, IL-4 was found to be associated with the promotion of atherosclerosis. Other Th2 related cytokines such as IL5 and IL33 are antiatherogenic.

In contrast, Bose et al. reported low IL-4 and IL-2 and high IL-6 in CAE compared with CAD and control groups. They proposed that the activation of smooth muscle cells by IL-6 leads to vascular remodelling and, in the absence of M2 macrophages to limit tissue damage, leads to the development of CAE (Figure 1. Pathway B) [30].

A similar histological examination of CAE and CAD supports the notion that ectasia may be a variant of atherosclerosis. Histology demonstrated extensive destruction of the musculo-elastic element of the vessel wall with degradation of medial collagen and disruption of the internal and external elastic lamina. The expansive remodelling of the external elastic membrane, likely due to the activation of MI macrophages, underlies luminal expansion in CAE. Specifically, elevated TNFa and IFNy from activated M1 macrophages promote macrophage transmigration via ICAM1 and VCAM1 into the intima and induce MMPs that inhibit collagen synthesis.

Further evidence for a common underlying pathogenesis with atherosclerosis emerges from recent reports demonstrating MCP-1 as an independent predictor of CAE. As previously mentioned, MCP-1 is directly responsible for disturbed blood flow and is critical in the development of atherosclerosis, specifically with regard to the recruitment of monocytes into the vascular wall. Additionally, higher levels of MCP-1 have also been associated with higher incidence of acute ischemic events in patients with CAD [13].

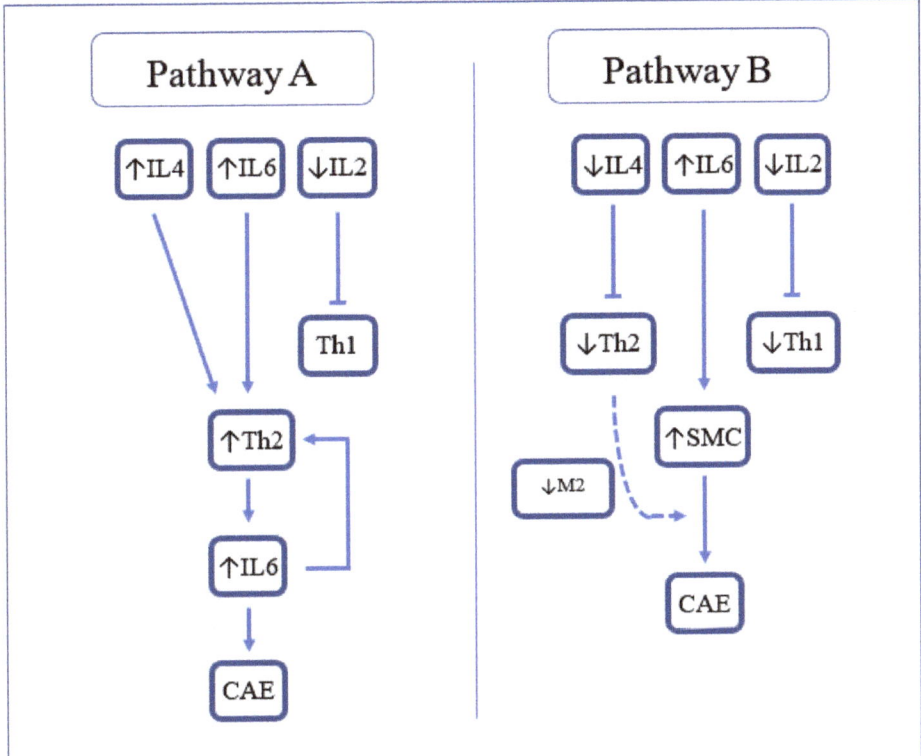

Figure 1. Proposed cytokine-mediated pathways resulting in CAE. IL-2 = Interleukin-2; IL-4 = Interleukin-4; IL-6 = Interleukin-6; Th2 = T-helper 2; CAE = coronary artery ectasia; SMC = smooth muscle cells; and M2 = M2 macrophages.

Of note, significantly elevated mean platelet volume (MPV) has also been observed with CAE and CAD groups compared to controls. Elevated MPV levels result from increased platelet activation and therefore predispose patients to a higher risk of thrombotic events and myocardial infarction [20].

7. Lipid Profiling in CAE

Lipoproteins have been implicated in the remodelling process leading to the development of CAE; however, evidence remains highly elusive. Lipids are known to play an important role in the formation of CAD in the presence of inflammation and oxidative stress. In addition to well-known lipid classes associated with CAD, such as cholesterol and triglycerides, advancements in lipidomic profiling have demonstrated additional lipid classes that are strongly associated with CAD, such as phospholipids [31]. Distinct patterns of individual lipid species within the phospholipid class can potentially differentiate stable from unstable CAD [32].

Previously, a higher prevalence of CAE has been demonstrated in patients with familial hypercholesterolemia alongside higher LDL-C levels, lower HDL-C, and a higher LDL/HDL ratio [19]. Likewise, an elevated LDL-C/HDL-C ratio carries predictive value for CAE development [33]. LDL-C binds to elastin, collagen, and proteoglycans and is subsequently oxidized, hence increasing its affinity to matrix particles. Foam cell formation, and the subsequent extracellular matrix (ECM) breakdown results from the stimulation of macrophages, smooth muscle cells, and ECM-degrading enzymes including MMP-2, MMP-9, and MMP-12 [23]. This is critical in the pathogenesis of dilating vascular diseases, such as CAE, as the ECM provides structural support to the vessel wall, thereby influencing cell behaviour and signalling.

By a similar mechanism, two phospholipid species, specifically sphingomyelin (SM) and phosphatidylcholine (PC), have been found to be significantly downregulated in CAE compared with CAD and healthy controls. In the first lipid profiling study reported for CAE, lipidomic profile in CAE demonstrated distinct patterns of lipid species compared with CAD and healthy controls [34]. SM are carried into the vessel wall on lipoproteins and stimulate foam cell formation [30]. They have also been shown to be incorporated in atherosclerotic plaques in addition to the polyunsaturated cholesteryl esters of long-chain fatty acids. SM levels are independently predictive of the presence of atherosclerotic CAD, a finding that implicates SM in the process of atherosclerotic plaque formation. Notably, low levels of SM in CAE may predispose premature apoptosis within the arterial wall, further promoting ectasia. Lower phosphatidylcholine levels, specifically 16-carbon fatty acyl chain phosphatidylcholines, have also been implicated in the pathogenesis of CAE. PC has a critical role in transporting fatty acids as well as lipid metabolism; thereby providing important knowledge about lipid regulation and disease manifestation. Taken together, downregulated phosphatidylcholine levels and a distinct lipidomic profile in CAE may suggest a non-atherogenic origin of ectasia development.

Similarly, subsequent work in metabolic characterization of fatty acids in patients with CAE can be distinguished from those of controls and CAD. This provides further lipidomic profiling findings that isolated plasma fatty acids profiles with CAE could be seen as biomarkers to distinguish CAE from controls and CAD patients [35].

On the grounds of the aforementioned studies, it may be adequate to conclude that the CAE lipid profile has a clearly distinct pathophysiology from atherosclerosis profile in CAD and hence a distinguished metabolic pathway. The proposed mechanistic pathways underlying the pathogenesis of CAE are depicted in Figure 2.

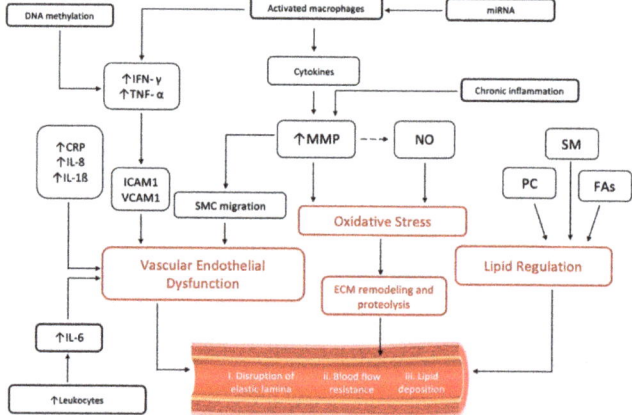

Figure 2. Schematic of proposed pathways underlying vascular remodelling in the pathogenesis of CAE. Proposed triggers such as e.g., viral or Gut microbial metabolites are not included in the figure. IFN-γ = interferon gamma; IFN-α = interferon alfa; IL-6 = interleukin-6; IL-8 = interleukin-8; IL-1β = interleukin 1-beta; CRP = c-reactive protein; ICAM1 = Intercellular Adhesion Molecule 1; VCAM1 = Vascular Cell Adhesion Molecule 1; MMP = Matrix Metalloproteinases; SMC = smooth muscle cells; NO = nitric oxide; ECM = extracellular matrix; SM = sphingomyelin; PC = phosphatidylcholine; FAs = fatty acids; and miRNA = microribonucleic acids.

8. Treatment Options of CAE

Coronary ectasia management is highly dependent on clinical experience and the diagnosis of the disease remains largely incidental, especially for isolated forms of the disease without a preceding history from childhood or adolescence. Adding to this challenge, consensus treatment guidelines have yet to be established, despite increasing evidence of long-term outcomes related to CAE. Available management options include pharmacologic therapy, surgery, and percutaneous intervention.

Given that high grade CAE may predispose to thromboembolic-related ACS, formal anticoagulation has been proposed as a potential treatment strategy. Nevertheless, there still exists a lack of quality data to support this recommendation, and the use of anticoagulation remains controversial.

In the presence of CAD, the prognosis and treatment of CAE are similar to CAD alone. In isolated CAE, however, prognosis is better and antiplatelets are the mainstay treatment option [36]. A rationale for antiplatelet therapy in the absence of atherosclerotic coronary disease may be that platelet activation in isolated CAE is heightened through P-selectin, beta-thromboglobulin and platelet factor 4. Furthermore, given that patients with CAE have been found to have significant elevations of MPV compared to their healthy counterparts, anti-thrombotic therapy may have a beneficial role in management. In general, anticoagulation is recommended with extensive CAE and multi-vessel involvement. In the context of CAE with acute coronary syndrome with obstructive atherosclerotic CAD, the management options should follow the standard guidelines for revascularization.

Nitrates may promote dilatation and potentially exacerbate turbulent flow with a theoretical worsening of ischaemic symptoms, so the use of nitrates is generally avoided.

As statins can inhibit the secretion of MMPs, they may have a therapeutic role in the management of CAE, especially in younger patients. Higher inflammatory marker levels, specifically IL-6 and CRP, have also been observed in younger CAE patients, who have subsequently benefited from rosuvastatin therapy [22].

Overall, standard treatment of co-existent CAD is recommended, including lifestyle modification strategies and cardiovascular risk factor management. For patients with coexisting obstructive lesions and symptoms of significant ischemia despite medical intervention, percutaneous or surgical vascularization may be recommended [37]. Previous reports have described the use of coronary artery bypass grafting for the treatment of significant CAD co-existing with ectatic coronary segments [38].

Most recently, evidence for the prognostic role of serum DAMPs in the pathogenesis of CAE has emerged. The differential regulation of DAMPs S100B, HSP70, DJ-1, and sRAGE in CAE adds to the growing body of literature for novel biomarkers as therapeutic targets in CAE management [39].

9. Epigenetics in CAE Pathogenesis

Emerging evidence has focused on the role of epigenetics and gene regulation in the pathophysiology of cardiovascular disease (CVD) and aging. With regard to CAE, epigenetic modifications have been observed with endothelial cells, vascular smooth muscle cells, and macrophages, in addition to the inflammatory processes governing CAE development [40].

To date, the epigenetic contribution to CAD involves histone modifications, DNA methylation, and RNA-based mechanisms. Interestingly, many of the pro-inflammatory genes involved in CAE pathogenesis, IFN-y and IL-6, appear to be regulated through DNA methylation [41]. In a study investigating the relationship between IL-6 methylation status and CVD risk, lower methylation levels were found in patients with CAD, suggesting an inverse relationship between methylation and CAD risk [42]. Given the tissue heterogeneity of atherosclerosis, the precise mechanisms of DNA methylation in atherosclerosis remain to be elucidated.

Due to the impact of foam cell formation in the pathogenesis of CAE, it is important to note that several cellular microribonucleic acids (miRNAs) have been identified in this process. miRNAs play a role in the inhibition of macrophage cholesterol efflux via ABCA1 [43] as well as regulating the balance between pro-atherosclerotic M1 and anti-atherosclerotic M2 phenotypes specifically via miR-33 [44]. For these reasons, future research should explore circulating miRNAs as potential diagnostic biomarkers in various CAD settings.

As the role of genome sequencing and metabolomics continues to evolve, there is also an increasing need to explore gut microbiome dysbiosis in the progression of CAD. Multiple studies have identified microbial stains associated with CAD [45,46], while alterations in the gut microbiome have been related to the development of several cardiovascular risk factors including diabetes mellitus [47] and obesity [48]. Interestingly, a decrease of *Bacterioidetes* and increase of *Firmicutes, Escherichia-Shigella*, and *Enterococcus* in the gut of CAD patients suggests that a shift in microbiota may underpin the development of CVD [49].

10. Gut Microbial Metabolites in CAE

Metabolites of the gut microbiome, such as trimethylamine (TMA), may promote atheromatous plaque formation through metabolic processes in the systemic circulation. TMA is generated by the gut microbiota from dietary phosphatidylcholine and carnitine and oxidized in the liver to form TMAO, which results in forma cell aggregation [50]. Elevated serum levels of TMAO have been associated with early atherosclerosis, increased risk of CVD mortality, and severity of peripheral artery disease [51]. A larger-scale prospective study established the prognostic value of TMAO in the identification of patients at risk for incident adverse cardiac events at 5 years, including MI and MACE (MI and cardiovascular death) [52].

However, gut microbiome dysregulation decreases the expression of tight junction proteins, thereby increasing the permeability of the intestinal mucosa and allowing Gram-negative bacterial lipopolysaccharide (LPS), or endotoxins, to enter the blood circulation [50]. This triggers the expression of chemokines and cell adhesion molecules, further stimulating the formation of foam cells and the adhesion of monocytes to endothelial cells. Indirectly, bacterial LPS triggers the release of many pro-inflammatory factors involved in CAE pathogenesis, such as TNF-a and IL-1B, while inhibiting the expression of cholesterol transporters [53].

This explanation supports the different metabolite profiling for CAE from both atherosclerotic and normal coronaries [34].

11. Conclusions

While CAE remains an important clinical coronary pathology with associated morbidity and mortality, its exact underlying etiopathogenesis has yet to be fully elucidated. Due to its strong association with coronary atherosclerosis, a heightened immuno-inflammatory response is largely believed to contribute to its pathogenesis. However, CAE can develop in the presence or absence of CAD, suggesting that there may be more than one mechanism involved. Indeed, there are significant differences in the cytokine milieu and the lipidomic profile in CAE compared with CAD and healthy controls, which strongly suggests a distinct pathogenesis is at play, in addition to the development of CAD. Recent evidence has strengthened postulates of an inflammatory mechanism by establishing the role of novel inflammatory markers such as MCP-1 in the pathogenesis of CAE. The mainstay treatment of CAE includes optimal management of coexistent CAD and antiplatelet therapy for the treatment of isolated CAE. Earlier studies confirmed the role of anticoagulant in extensive CAE, however, further studies are warranted to confirm that at larger scale of patients. Novel biomarker targeted therapy in CAE management is considered the ultimate effective approach. CAE has a proven different aetiopathology, metabolites profile, worse clinical prognosis and anatomical appearance than simply atherosclerotic corornaries and hence CAE may represent a different disease.

Author Contributions: Manuscript preparation, review and editing G.H.C.R., K.L.H., M.Y.H., C.H. and U.B. All authors have read and agreed to the published version of the manuscript.

Funding: This research received no external funding.

Conflicts of Interest: The authors declare no conflict of interest.

References

1. Tanner, R.; David, S.; Conlon, R.; Boles, R. Coronary Artery Ectasia; Clinical Updates and Management Options in Acute Presentation. *Med. Res. Arch.* **2017**, *5*. [CrossRef]
2. Kawsara, A.; Gil, I.J.N.; Alqahtani, F.; Moreland, J.; Rihal, C.S.; Alkhouli, M. Management of Coronary Artery Aneurysms. *JACC Cardiovasc. Interv.* **2018**, *11*, 1211–1223. [CrossRef] [PubMed]
3. Boles, U.; Eriksson, P.; Zhao, Y.; Henein, M.Y. Coronary artery ectasia: Remains a clinical dilemma. *Coron. Artery Dis.* **2010**, *21*, 318–320. [CrossRef] [PubMed]
4. Eitan, A.; Roguin, A. Coronary artery ectasia: New insights into pathophysiology, diagnosis, and treatment. *Coron. Artery Dis.* **2016**, *27*, 420–428. [CrossRef] [PubMed]
5. Campanile, A.; Sozzi, F.B.; Consonni, D.; Piscione, F.; Sganzerla, P.; Indolfi, C.; Stabile, A.; Migliorini, A.; Antoniucci, D.; Ferraresi, R.; et al. Primary PCI for the treatment of ectatic infarct-related coronary artery. *Minerva Cardioangiol.* **2014**, *62*, 327–333.
6. Bogana Shanmugam, V.; Psaltis, P.J.; Wong, D.T.L.; Meredith, I.T.; Malaiapan, Y.; Ahmar, W. Outcomes after Primary Percutaneous Coronary Intervention for ST-Elevation Myocardial Infarction Caused by Ectatic Infarct Related Arteries. *Heart Lung Circ.* **2017**, *26*, 1059–1068. [CrossRef]
7. Doi, T.; Kataoka, Y.; Noguchi, T.; Shibata, T.; Nakashima, T.; Kawakami, S.; Nakao, K.; Fujino, M.; Nagai, T.; Kanaya, T.; et al. Coronary Artery Ectasia Predicts Future Cardiac Events in Patients with Acute Myocardial Infarction. *Arterioscler. Thromb. Vasc. Biol.* **2017**, *37*, 2350–2355. [CrossRef]
8. Cai, Z.; Liu, J.; Wang, H.; Yin, D.; Song, W.; Dou, K. Diffuse coronary artery dilation predicted worse long-term outcomes in patients with coronary artery Ectasia. *Int. J. Cardiol.* **2020**, *319*, 20–25. [CrossRef]
9. Li, J.-J.; Nie, S.-P.; Qian, X.-W.; Zeng, H.-S.; Zhang, C.-Y. Chronic inflammatory status in patients with coronary artery ectasia. *Cytokine* **2009**, *46*, 61–64. [CrossRef]
10. Ghetti, G.; Taglieri, N.; Donati, F.; Minnucci, M.; Bruno, A.G.; Palmerini, T.; Saia, F.; Marrozzini, C.; Galié, N. Correlation between aortic root dimension and coronary ectasia. *Coron. Artery Dis.* **2020**, *32*, 335–339. [CrossRef]
11. Antonopoulos, A.S.; Siasos, G.; Oikonomou, E.; Mourouzis, K.; Mavroudeas, S.E.; Papageorgiou, N.; Papaioannou, S.; Tsiamis, E.; Toutouzas, K.; Tousoulis, D. Characterization of vascular phenotype in patients with coronary artery ectasia: The role of endothelial dysfunction. *Int. J. Cardiol.* **2016**, *215*, 138–139. [CrossRef] [PubMed]
12. Liu, R.; Chen, L.; Wu, W.; Chen, H.; Zhang, S. Neutrophil serine proteases and their endogenous inhibitors in coronary artery ectasia patients. *Anatol. J. Cardiol.* **2015**, *16*, 23–28. [CrossRef] [PubMed]
13. Franco-Peláez, J.A.; Martín-Reyes, R.; Pello-Lázaro, A.M.; Aceña, Á.; Lorenzo, Ó.; Martín-Ventura, J.L.; Blanco-Colio, L.; González-Casaus, M.L.; Hernández-González, I.; Carda, R.; et al. Monocyte Chemoattractant Protein-1 Is an Independent Predictor of Coronary Artery Ectasia in Patients with Acute Coronary Syndrome. *J. Clin. Med.* **2020**, *9*, 3037. [CrossRef] [PubMed]
14. Mavrogeni, S. Coronary Artery Ectasia: Diagnosis and Treatment. *E-J. Cardiol. Pract. Hellenic J. Cardiol* **2010**, *51*, 158–163.
15. Şen, F.; Yılmaz, S.; Kuyumcu, M.S.; Ozeke, O.; Balcı, M.M.; Aydogdu, S. The Presence of Fragmented QRS on 12-Lead Electrocardiography in Patients with Coronary Artery Ectasia. *Korean Circ. J.* **2014**, *44*, 307–311. [CrossRef] [PubMed]
16. Conlon, R.; Tanner, R.; David, S.; Szeplaki, G.; Galvin, J.; Keaney, J.; Keelan, E.; Boles, U. Evaluation of the Tp-Te Interval, QTc and P-Wave Dispersion in Patients with Coronary Artery Ectasia. *Cardiol. Res.* **2017**, *8*, 280–285. [CrossRef]
17. Gunasekaran, P.; Stanojevic, D.; Drees, T.; Fritzlen, J.; Haghnegahdar, M.; McCullough, M.; Barua, R.; Mehta, A.; Hockstad, E.; Wiley, M.; et al. Prognostic significance, angiographic characteristics and impact of antithrombotic and anticoagulant therapy on outcomes in high versus low grade coronary artery ectasia: A long-term follow-up study. *Catheter. Cardiovasc. Interv.* **2019**, *93*, 1219–1227. [CrossRef]
18. Boles, U.; Wiklund, U.; David, S.; Ahmed, K.; Henein, M.Y. Coronary artery ectasia carries worse prognosis: A long-term follow-up study. *Pol. Arch. Intern. Med.* **2019**, *129*, 833–835. [CrossRef]
19. Qin, Y.; Tang, C.; Ma, C.; Yan, G. Risk factors for coronary artery ectasia and the relationship between hyperlipidemia and coronary artery ectasia. *Coron. Artery Dis.* **2019**, *30*, 211–215. [CrossRef]
20. Iwańczyk, S.; Borger, M.; Kamiński, M.; Chmara, E.; Cieślewicz, A.; Tykarski, A.; Radziemski, A.; Krasiński, Z.; Lesiak, M.; Araszkiewicz, A. Inflammatory response in patients with coronary artery ectasia and CAD. *Kardiol. Pol.* **2021**, *79*, 773–780. [CrossRef]
21. Boles, U.; Zhao, Y.; David, S.; Eriksson, P.; Henein, M.Y. Pure coronary ectasia differs from atherosclerosis: Morphological and risk factors analysis. *Int. J. Cardiol.* **2012**, *155*, 321–323. [CrossRef] [PubMed]
22. Fan, C.-H.; Hao, Y.; Liu, Y.-H.; Li, X.-L.; Huang, Z.-H.; Luo, Y.; Li, R.-L. Anti-inflammatory effects of rosuvastatin treatment on coronary artery ectasia patients of different age groups. *BMC Cardiovasc. Disord.* **2020**, *20*, 330. [CrossRef] [PubMed]
23. Antoniadis, A.P.; Chatzizisis, Y.S.; Giannoglou, G.D. Pathogenetic mechanisms of coronary ectasia. *Int. J. Cardiol.* **2008**, *130*, 335–343. [CrossRef] [PubMed]

24. Sherif, S.A.; Tok, O.O.; Taşköylü, Ö.; Goktekin, O.; Kilic, I.D. Coronary Artery Aneurysms: A Review of the Epidemiology, Pathophysiology, Diagnosis, and Treatment. *Front. Cardiovasc. Med.* **2017**, *4*, 24. [CrossRef]
25. Vrachatis, D.A.; Papathanasiou, K.A.; Kazantzis, D.; Sanz-Sánchez, J.; Giotaki, S.G.; Raisakis, K.; Kaoukis, A.; Kossyvakis, C.; Deftereos, G.; Reimers, B.; et al. Inflammatory Biomarkers in Coronary Artery Ectasia: A Systematic Review and Meta-Analysis. *Diagnostics* **2022**, *12*, 1026. [CrossRef]
26. Boles, U.; Johansson, A.; Wiklund, U.; Sharif, Z.; David, S.; McGrory, S.; Henein, M.Y. Cytokine Disturbances in Coronary Artery Ectasia Do Not Support Atherosclerosis Pathogenesis. *Int. J. Mol. Sci.* **2018**, *19*, 260. [CrossRef]
27. Dereli, S.; Cerik, I.B.; Kaya, A.; Bektaş, O. Assessment of the Relationship between C-Reactive Protein-to-Albumin Ratio and the Presence and Severity of Isolated Coronary Artery Ectasia. *Angiology* **2020**, *71*, 840–846. [CrossRef]
28. El Bakry, S.A.; Fayez, D.; Morad, C.S.; Abdel-Salam, A.M.; Abdel-Salam, Z.; ElKabarity, R.H.; El Dakrony, A.H.M. Ischemic heart disease and rheumatoid arthritis: Do inflammatory cytokines have a role? *Cytokine* **2017**, *96*, 228–233. [CrossRef]
29. Triantafyllis, A.S.; Kalogeropoulos, A.S.; Rigopoulos, A.G.; Sakadakis, E.A.; Toumpoulis, I.K.; Tsikrikas, S.; Kremastinos, D.T.; Rizos, I. Coronary artery ectasia and inflammatory cytokines: Link with a predominant Th-2 immune response? *Cytokine* **2013**, *64*, 427–432. [CrossRef]
30. Ait-Oufella, H.; Taleb, S.; Mallat, Z.; Tedgui, A. Recent Advances on the Role of Cytokines in Atherosclerosis. *Arterioscler. Thromb. Vasc. Biol.* **2011**, *31*, 969–979. [CrossRef]
31. Kohno, S.; Keenan, A.L.; Ntambi, J.M.; Miyazaki, M. Lipidomic insight into cardiovascular diseases. *Biochem. Biophys. Res. Commun.* **2018**, *504*, 590–595. [CrossRef] [PubMed]
32. Meikle, P.J.; Wong, G.; Tsorotes, D.; Barlow, C.K.; Weir, J.M.; Christopher, M.J.; MacIntosh, G.L.; Goudey, B.; Stern, L.; Kowalczyk, A.; et al. Plasma Lipidomic Analysis of Stable and Unstable Coronary Artery Disease. *Arter. Thromb. Vasc. Biol.* **2011**, *31*, 2723–2732. [CrossRef] [PubMed]
33. Jafari, J.; Daum, A.; Abu Hamed, J.; Osherov, A.; Orlov, Y.; Yosefy, C.; Gallego-Colon, E. Low High-Density Lipoprotein Cholesterol Predisposes to Coronary Artery Ectasia. *Biomedicines* **2019**, *7*, 79. [CrossRef] [PubMed]
34. Boles, U.; Pinto, R.C.; David, S.; Abdullah, A.S.; Henein, M.Y. Dysregulated fatty acid metabolism in coronary ectasia: An extended lipidomic analysis. *Int. J. Cardiol.* **2017**, *228*, 303–308. [CrossRef]
35. Liu, T.; Sun, Y.; Li, H.; Xu, H.; Xiao, N.; Wang, X.; Song, L.; Bai, C.; Wen, H.; Ge, J.; et al. Metabolomic Characterization of Fatty Acids in Patients With Coronary Artery Ectasias. *Front. Physiol.* **2021**, *12*, 770223. [CrossRef]
36. Khedr, A.; Neupane, B.; Proskuriakova, E.; Jada, K.; Kakieu Djossi, S.; Mostafa, J.A. Pharmacologic Management of Coronary Artery Ectasia. *Cureus* **2021**, *13*, e17832. [CrossRef]
37. Mavrogeni, S. Coronary artery ectasia: From diagnosis to treatment. *Hell. J. Cardiol.* **2010**, *51*, 158–163.
38. Hartnell, G.G.; Parnell, B.M.; Pridie, R.B. Coronary artery ectasia, its prevalence and clinical significance in 4993 patients. *Br. Heart J.* **1985**, *54*, 392–395. [CrossRef]
39. Tsoporis, J.N.; Triantafyllis, A.; Gupta, S.; Izhar, S.; Sakadakis, E.; Rigopoulos, A.G.; Parker, T.G.; Rizos, I. Differential Regulation of Circulating Damage-Associated Molecular Patterns in Patients With Coronary Artery Ectasia. *Circulation* **2021**, *144*, A12511. [CrossRef]
40. Rizzacasa, B.; Amati, F.; Romeo, F.; Novelli, G.; Mehta, J.L. Epigenetic Modification in Coronary Atherosclerosis: JACC Review Topic of the Week. *J. Am. Coll. Cardiol.* **2019**, *74*, 1352–1365. [CrossRef]
41. Krishna, S.M.; Dear, A.; Craig, J.M.; Norman, P.E.; Golledge, J. The potential role of homocysteine mediated DNA methylation and associated epigenetic changes in abdominal aortic aneurysm formation. *Atherosclerosis* **2013**, *228*, 295–305. [CrossRef] [PubMed]
42. Zuo, H.P.; Guo, Y.Y.; Che, L.; Wu, X.Z. Hypomethylation of interleukin-6 promoter is associated with the risk of coronary heart disease. *Arq. Bras. Cardiol.* **2016**, *107*, 131–136. [CrossRef] [PubMed]
43. Feinberg, M.W.; Moore, K.J. MicroRNA regulation of atherosclerosis. *Circ. Res.* **2016**, *118*, 703–720. [CrossRef] [PubMed]
44. Ouimet, M.; Ediriweera, H.N.; Gundra, U.M.; Sheedy, F.J.; Ramkhelawon, B.; Hutchison, S.B.; Rinehold, K.; van Solingen, C.; Fullerton, M.D.; Cecchini, K.; et al. MicroRNA-33-dependent regulation of macrophage metabolism directs immune cell polarization in atherosclerosis. *J. Clin. Investig.* **2015**, *125*, 4334–4348. [CrossRef]
45. Tanika, N.K.; Lydia, A.B.; Nadim, J.A.; He, H.; Zhao, J.; Joseph, F.P.; Adolfo, C.; He, J. Gut Microbiome Associates With Lifetime Cardiovascular Disease Risk Profile Among Bogalusa Heart Study Participants. *Circ. Res.* **2016**, *119*, 956–964.
46. Jie, Z.; Xia, H.; Zhong, S.-L.; Feng, Q.; Li, S.; Liang, S.; Zhong, H.; Liu, Z.; Gao, Y.; Zhao, H.; et al. The gut microbiome in atherosclerotic cardiovascular disease. *Nat. Commun.* **2017**, *8*, 845. [CrossRef]
47. Yang, Q.; Lin, S.L.; Kwok, M.K.; Leung, G.M.; Schooling, C.M.; Schooling, C.M. The Roles of 27 Genera of Human Gut Microbiota in Ischemic Heart Disease, Type 2 Diabetes Mellitus, and Their Risk Factors: A Mendelian Randomization Study. *Am. J. Epidemiol.* **2018**, *187*, 1916–1922. [CrossRef]
48. Nakatani, A.; Miyamoto, J.; Inaba, Y.; Sutou, A.; Saito, T.; Sato, T.; Tachibana, N.; Inoue, H.; Kimura, I. Dietary soybean protein ameliorates high-fat diet-induced obesity by modifying the gut microbiota-dependent biotransformation of bile acids. *PLoS ONE* **2018**, *13*, e0202083. [CrossRef]
49. Zhang, B.; Wang, X.; Xia, R.; Li, C. Gut microbiota in coronary artery disease: A friend or foe? *Biosci. Rep.* **2020**, *40*, BSR20200454. [CrossRef]

50. Bennett, B.J.; de Aguiar Vallim, T.Q.; Wang, Z.; Shih, D.M.; Meng, Y.; Gregory, J.; Allayee, H.; Lee, R.; Graham, M.; Crooke, R.; et al. Trimethylamine-N-oxide, a metabolite associated with atherosclerosis, exhibits complex genetic and dietary regulation. *Cell Metab.* **2013**, *17*, 49–60. [CrossRef]
51. Roncal, C.; Martínez-Aguilar, E.; Orbe, J.; Ravassa, S.; Fernandez-Montero, A.; Saenz-Pipaon, G.; Ugarte, A.; de Mendoza, A.E.-H.; Rodriguez, J.A.; Fernández-Alonso, S.; et al. Trimethylamine-N-Oxide (TMAO) Predicts Cardio-vascular Mortality in Peripheral Artery Disease. *Sci. Rep.* **2019**, *9*, 15580. [CrossRef] [PubMed]
52. Amrein, M.; Li, X.S.; Walter, J.; Wang, Z.; Zimmermann, T.; Strebel, I.; Honegger, U.; Leu, K.; Schäfer, I.; Twerenbold, R.; et al. Gut microbiota-dependent metabolite trimethylamine N-oxide (TMAO) and cardiovascular risk in patients with suspected functionally relevant coronary artery disease (fCAD). *Clin. Res. Cardiol.* **2022**. [CrossRef] [PubMed]
53. Chacón, M.R.; Lozano-Bartolomé, J.; Portero-Otín, M.; Rodríguez, M.M.; Xifra, G.; Puig, J.; Blasco, G.; Ricart, W.; Chaves, F.J.; Fernández-Real, J.M.; et al. The gut mycobiome composition is linked to carotid atherosclerosis. *Benef. Microbes* **2018**, *9*, 185–198. [CrossRef] [PubMed]

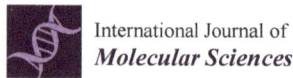
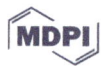

Review

Genetic and Diet-Induced Animal Models for Non-Alcoholic Fatty Liver Disease (NAFLD) Research

Christina-Maria Flessa [1,2], Narjes Nasiri-Ansari [1], Ioannis Kyrou [2,3,4,5,6], Bianca M. Leca [2], Maria Lianou [1], Antonios Chatzigeorgiou [7], Gregory Kaltsas [8], Eva Kassi [1,8,*,†] and Harpal S. Randeva [2,3,*,†]

1. Department of Biological Chemistry, Medical School, National and Kapodistrian University of Athens, 11527 Athens, Greece
2. Warwickshire Institute for the Study of Diabetes, Endocrinology and Metabolism (WISDEM), University Hospitals Coventry and Warwickshire NHS Trust, Coventry CV2 2DX, UK
3. Warwick Medical School, University of Warwick, Coventry CV4 7AL, UK
4. Research Institute for Health and Wellbeing, Coventry University, Coventry CV1 5FB, UK
5. Aston Medical School, College of Health and Life Sciences, Aston University, Birmingham B4 7ET, UK
6. Laboratory of Dietetics and Quality of Life, Department of Food Science and Human Nutrition, School of Food and Nutritional Sciences, Agricultural University of Athens, 11855 Athens, Greece
7. Department of Physiology, Medical School, National and Kapodistrian University of Athens, 11527 Athens, Greece
8. Endocrine Unit, 1st Department of Propaedeutic Internal Medicine, Laiko Hospital, National and Kapodistrian University of Athens, 11527 Athens, Greece
* Correspondence: ekassi@med.uoa.gr (E.K.); harpal.randeva@uhcw.nhs.uk (H.S.R.)
† These authors contributed equally to this work.

Abstract: A rapidly increasing incidence of non-alcoholic fatty liver disease (NAFLD) is noted worldwide due to the adoption of western-type lifestyles and eating habits. This makes the understanding of the molecular mechanisms that drive the pathogenesis of this chronic disease and the development of newly approved treatments of utmost necessity. Animal models are indispensable tools for achieving these ends. Although the ideal mouse model for human NAFLD does not exist yet, several models have arisen with the combination of dietary interventions, genetic manipulations and/or administration of chemical substances. Herein, we present the most common mouse models used in the research of NAFLD, either for the whole disease spectrum or for a particular disease stage (e.g., non-alcoholic steatohepatitis). We also discuss the advantages and disadvantages of each model, along with the challenges facing the researchers who aim to develop and use animal models for translational research in NAFLD. Based on these characteristics and the specific study aims/needs, researchers should select the most appropriate model with caution when translating results from animal to human.

Keywords: non-alcoholic fatty liver disease; NAFLD; non-alcoholic steatohepatitis; NASH; animal models; mouse; cirrhosis

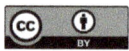

1. Introduction

Non-alcoholic fatty liver disease (NAFLD) is the hepatic manifestation of a cluster of conditions associated with metabolic dysfunction and is characterized by the accumulation of fat in the liver [1]. The global prevalence of NAFLD is constantly increasing and is estimated to be around 25% in the general population [2]. Histopathologically, NAFLD begins with the development of steatosis (accumulation of fat in the form of triglycerides in hepatocytes) with or without mild inflammation (non-alcoholic fatty liver, NAFL) and may progress to non-alcoholic steatohepatitis (NASH) characterized by variable degrees of mainly macrovesicular steatosis, necroinflammation with enlarged and rounded (ballooned) hepatocytes, the development of cytoplasmic inclusions (Mallory-Denk bodies), variable and mixed inflammatory infiltrate and the development of fibrosis with a predominantly perivenular and pericellular distribution [3,4]. Prolonged inflammation with increased oxidative stress, accompanied by DNA damage and consecutive disorganized cell regeneration and apoptosis, can further exacerbate the disease and may lead to advanced fibrosis, cirrhosis and/or the development of hepatocellular carcinoma (HCC) in a minority of patients [3].

The underlying mechanisms leading to NAFLD development and progression are now considered to be complex and multifactorial [5]. Indeed, to describe the consequence of events driving the NAFLD pathophysiology, the "two hits hypothesis" was initially proposed [5]. According to that hypothesis, the rapidly growing consumption of high-fat diets in combination with the adoption of a sedentary lifestyle leads to obesity and insulin resistance, which culminate in hepatic accumulation of lipids, an event that acts as the first hit, further sensitizing the liver to other insults. These insults constitute the "second hit", which in turn activates inflammatory cascades and fibrogenesis [5]. However, this model became outdated since it was viewed as too simplistic to explain the underlying complexity of NAFLD pathogenesis, and, thus, it was replaced by the "multiple-hit hypothesis", according to which the dietary habits and lifestyle, as well as environmental and genetic factors, can cause obesity, insulin resistance, ectopic adipose tissue accumulation and alterations in the intestinal microbiome, all of which are implicated in NAFLD pathogenesis and progression [5]. In this context, insulin resistance through the concomitant upregulated de novo lipogenesis in the liver and the reduced inhibition of lipolysis in the adipose tissue drives the upregulated transport of fatty acids to the liver that leads to steatosis/NASH, while fat accumulation further activates mechanisms related to mitochondrial dysfunction, oxidative stress, endoplasmic reticulum (ER) stress and production of reactive oxygen species (ROS), all of which leads to liver inflammation [5]. On the other hand, the genetic or epigenetic environment can further influence the fat content of liver cells, reinforcing the activation of the aforementioned mechanisms and can also affect several enzymatic procedures and the hepatic inflammatory status [5]. So, in conclusion, the mechanisms of insulin resistance, fat accumulation, mitochondrial dysfunction, oxidative stress, ER stress and ROS production, in association with genetic or epigenetic factors which can alter NAFLD predisposition, affect the fat content of hepatocytes, as well as hepatic pro-inflammatory pathways, culminating in chronic hepatic inflammation which can evolve into hepatocellular death, and activation of hepatic stellate cells that drive fibrogenesis [5].

Although significant efforts have been made over the last 40 years to elucidate the exact natural history and underlying biology of NAFLD, several challenges still exist [1]. The disease is under-recognized to a great extent by healthcare professionals as well as from society as a whole, while the lack of a trustworthy biomarker that would ideally diagnose NAFLD and its possible progression to NASH/HCC, renders invasive techniques, such as liver biopsy, indispensable for diagnosis, thereby inhibiting the early identification of persons in high risk [1]. Another challenge related to the elusive aspects of the underlying NAFLD biology is the significant heterogeneity of the disease and the currently restricted comprehension of its phenotypes [1]. Moreover, while several new drugs are being tested in clinical trials, so far, there are no approved therapies specifically for NAFLD/NASH, with most treatment guidelines focusing on lifestyle modifications with the adoption of a healthier lifestyle with weight loss and regular physical activity, and on the pharmacological treatment of comorbidities, such as anti-obesity and anti-diabetic drugs, and lipid-lowering drugs [1,3].

The need to fully decipher NAFLD pathogenesis and progression, as well as to conduct preclinical testing for potential therapeutic agents, has led to the need for reliable animal models of the disease that ideally display a liver phenotype similar to human NAFLD and can progress to inflammation, fibrosis (NASH), cirrhosis and HCC. Furthermore, these models should also display features of the metabolic syndrome, such as obesity and disturbances in lipid, glucose and insulin metabolism [6]. Towards this direction, several diet- or chemically-induced and genetic animal models have been introduced. Diet-induced models are mainly used in order to recapitulate a situation that mimics metabolic syndrome and to reproduce its main aspects, such as obesity and insulin resistance, that are crucially implicated in NAFLD development [7]. Due to that, the diet-induced models can better mimic the mechanisms, patterns and temporal sequence of events involved in human NAFLD pathogenesis. However, most of them differ from human disease in terms of clinical, morphologic and/or metabolic features [7]. Genetic models have been created to either mimic a human polymorphism implicated in NAFLD occurrence [such as the *patatin-like phospholipase domain-containing 3 (PNPLA3)* polymorphic mice], to recapitulate characteristics of the human metabolic syndrome better than diet induction (such as leptin- or leptin receptor-deficient mice), to better depict or to more rapidly proceed to a particular stage of the NAFLD spectrum. These models can prove to be valuable for the investigation of specific molecular pathways, the mechanisms by which they can alter hepatic homeostasis contributing to NAFLD development and the consequences of their deregulation [8]. However, the genetic induction needed usually makes these mice different from humans who do not have these genes altered [8]. Moreover, many of the genetic murine models are monogenic, while NAFLD and its contributors, such as obesity, are multifactorial situations, and there is more than one route leading to its pathogenesis [9]. Chemically induced NAFLD mouse models are used to better study the progression from one disease stage to another. However, these interventions lead to artificial progression that does not recapitulate human etiology and pathology. Owing to the multifactorial nature of NAFLD, the combination of two or more inductions (diet, genetic or chemical) is a usual approach to better mimic human disease. The choice of the most appropriate model to be used depends on each particular researcher and study question. In this review, we present the key animal models that are currently utilized in each particular stage of NAFLD: (1) non-alcoholic fatty liver (simple steatosis-NAFLD), (2) NASH and (3) NASH-associated HCC.

2. NAFLD Mouse Models

2.1. Diet-Induced Models

2.1.1. High-Fat Diet (HFD)

The increasing incidence of NAFLD in Western countries and its close association with obesity has led to the administration of a high-fat diet (HFD, developed to match Western diets) in order to lead to NAFLD development in animal models [10]. These HFDs range in fat content and source, with fat constituting 45% to 75% of the total calorie intake (kcal) and being derived from saturated fatty acids, polysaturated fatty acids and combinations of them [10–12]. These can lead to the development of metabolic syndrome, hepatic steatosis and NASH in experimental animals [13]. Samuels et al. were the first to implement such an HFD (fat constituted 80% of the total calories) in rats, which led to higher blood glucose levels observed at baseline and during exercise [14]. The most typical of these HFDs consists of 60% kcal as fat, 20% kcal as protein and 20% kcal as carbohydrates [6,15]. However, other such HFDs include a diet that contains 71% total calories (kcal) as fat, 11% as carbohydrate and 18% as protein (first HFD administered to rats inducing NASH) [16,17], or a diet consisting of 45% fat, 35% carbohydrates, and 20% protein [10]. Of note, HFDs fed to wild-type (WT) C57BL/6 mice can have varying effects depending on the time they are administered [6]. More specifically, when WT C57BL/6 mice are fed an HFD for 10–12 weeks, they develop steatosis, as shown by increased lipid accumulation, hyperlipidemia, hypercholesterolemia, hyperinsulinemia and glucose intolerance [10,15], whilst when the HFD is administered for 16 weeks then hepatocyte fat accumulation, ballooning, and Mallory-Denk bodies are observed, as well as decreased serum levels of the anti-inflammatory adipokine adiponectin and higher fasting serum glucose levels [6,17]. After feeding mice an HFD for 19 weeks, further hepatic triglyceride accumulation is observed, accompanied by inflammatory cell infiltration induction [15], while significant increases in circulating liver enzyme levels, i.e., alanine aminotransferase (ALT) and aspartate aminotransferase (AST), are observed after administration of the HFD for 34–36 weeks [6,15]. However, these mice show only minor signs of inflammation and fibrosis even after consuming an HFD for up to 50 weeks [6,15]. Interestingly, an HFD has also been administered as a chronic feeding scheme to C57BL/6 male mice for 80 weeks in order to mimic the lifetime consumption of a diet high in fat by humans [18]. This prolonged HFD feeding led to the development of obesity and insulin resistance, as well as to distinct histopathologic features of NAFLD, such as hepatic steatosis, cell injury, portal and lobular inflammation, fibrosis and hepatic ER stress [18]. Furthermore, this chronic HFD consumption caused changes in gut bacterial composition and led to gut-bacterial dysbiosis, a finding also observed in NAFLD patients [18]. HFD without other ingredients induced only mild steatohepatitis and minimal fibrosis, while the addition of lard enhanced steatosis and fibrosis [7]. In another study, C57BL/6 mice fed an HFD (58% of kcal as fat) supplemented with sucrose for 24–28 weeks displayed microvesicular steatosis and perisinusoidal focal hepatic fibrosis [19]. Overall, in HFD regimes, a higher percentage of cells enriched in fat is observed compared to other types of diets [10].

2.1.2. High-Cholesterol Diet (HCD)

Dietary cholesterol has been recognized by several studies as a key contributor to the development of steatohepatitis in animal models and humans [10,20]. As such, a high-cholesterol diet (HCD) supplemented with 1% cholesterol has been fed to WT C57BL/6 mice [20]. Administration of this HCD leads to the development of simple hepatic steatosis with little inflammation and no fibrosis, as well as a marked increase in serum insulin levels [20]. However, liver weight, plasma triglyceride levels, free fatty acid levels, and serum ALT levels are similar or only slightly elevated compared to the control diet group [10,20]. The addition of cholesterol to this diet reduces bile acid and very low-density lipoprotein (VLDL) synthesis as well as the β-oxidation of fatty acids, mechanisms that could possibly contribute further to the hepatic lipid loading [20].

2.2. Genetic Models

2.2.1. *db/db* Mice

Leptin is the prototype adipokine regulating—among other functions—the feeding behavior by reducing food intake through the promotion of satiety at the level of the hypothalamus [8,10]. *db/db* mice are homozygous for the autosomal recessive diabetic gene (*db*) [21], encoding a point mutation that leads to a lack of the long isoform of the leptin receptor (Ob-Rb), thus resulting in defective leptin signaling [8,10,22]. Consequently, these mice have normal or elevated levels of leptin, but are resistant to its effects [7,8], thus have persistent hyperphagia and are obese and diabetic, exhibiting severe hyperglycemia, hyperinsulinemia, insulin resistance, elevated serum leptin levels and development of macrovesicular hepatic steatosis [7,8,21]. Of note, *db/db* mice do not spontaneously develop inflammation when fed a normal control diet. However, calorie overconsumption for one month or longer could result in more aggravated hepatic inflammation [22]. In the absence of additional interventions, *db/db* mice are good models of NAFLD but not of NASH, since they rarely show NASH features when fed a normal control diet [10]. Despite that, when these mice are challenged with a "second hit" in terms of dietary interventions, they can develop NASH, as will be discussed in the next section [10,22].

2.2.2. *ob/ob* Mice

The *ob/ob* mice were discovered by chance as a mutation arose in a colony at Jackson Laboratory in 1949 [23]. This mutation is recessive, causing sterility in the homozygotes, whilst these mice start becoming phenotypically distinguishable when they reach four to six weeks of age [23]. From that age on, they increase rapidly in weight until they reach a weight three to four times that of normal WT mice [23]. The *ob* gene was identified by positional cloning and was found to encode leptin [24,25]. By carrying this autosomal recessive mutation in the leptin gene, *ob/ob* mice have functional leptin receptors (in contrast to *db/db* mice), but they encode truncated and non-functional leptin [10]. Accordingly, *ob/ob* mice are obese, hyperphagic, inactive, hyperinsulinemic, hyperglycemic, hyperlipidemic, resistant to insulin, and develop intestinal bacterial overgrowth and spontaneous liver steatosis [7,10]. These mice develop fatty liver without fibrosis when fed a normal chow diet, and their resistance to hepatic fibrosis—unlike *db/db* mice—can be attributed to the requirement of leptin for fibrosis development [10,26]. Although *ob/ob* mice do not develop steatohepatitis, the latter can also be induced—like in *db/db* mice—with secondary hits/insults, such as diets other than chow feeding, exposure to low doses of lipopolysaccharide endotoxin [27], ethanol or hepatic ischemia/reperfusion challenge [10,28]

2.2.3. *PNPLA3* Polymorphism

The PNPLA3 (patatin-like phospholipase domain-containing 3) protein is an enzyme with lipase activity towards triglycerides and retinyl esters and with acyltransferase activity on phospholipids [29]. The human *PNPLA3* gene encodes for a protein of 481 amino-acids, whilst the *PNPLA3* rs738409 variant is a cytosine to guanine substitution, which encodes for the isoleucine to methionine substitution at position 148 (I148M) of the protein [29]. The *PNPLA3* I148M variant in humans has been found to increase susceptibility to the whole spectrum of hepatic damage associated with NAFLD while it also promotes hepatic fat accumulation without directly affecting adiposity and insulin resistance to a significant extent [30]. Notably, it has also been associated with a higher risk of liver-related mortality in NAFLD patients and in the general population [30]. In order to mimic PNPLA3-induced fatty liver disease, transgenic mice in a C57BL/6 background were generated that express human PNPLA3 wild-type ($PNPLA3^{WT}$) or the 148M variant ($PNPLA3^{I148M}$) in the liver and adipose tissue [31], or the codon 148 of *Pnpla3* in the mouse genome was changed from ATT to ATG, substituting methionine for isoleucine ($PNPLA3^{I148M}$) [32]. $PNPLA3^{I148M}$ mice with overexpression in the liver mimicked the fatty liver phenotype and other metabolic characteristics caused by this allele in humans and were presented with upregulated amounts of fatty acids and triacylglycerol [31]. Interestingly, when $PNPLA3^{I148M}$ mice were fed a high-sucrose diet (58% sucrose, 0% fat, or 74% sucrose) for 6 or 4 weeks, respectively, the hepatic triacylglycerol levels, as well as the levels of other lipids, increased up to 3-fold leading to steatosis development compared to $PNPLA3^{WT}$ transgenic mice or WT (non-transgenic) animals, while no such effect was observed under an HFD (45% kcal from fat) [31,32]. However, $PNPLA3^{I148M}$ mice display no changes in the expression of genes involved in triglyceride lipolysis, fatty acid oxidation, hepatic inflammation, or fibrosis after high-sucrose diet feeding [32].

2.2.4. *Gankyrin* (*Gank*)-Deficient Mice

Gankyrin (Gank) is a subunit of the 26S proteasome and an oncogene expressed in several types of cancer. Moreover, it also drives liver proliferation and has recently been implicated in NAFLD development [19]. When *Gank* was selectively deleted from the livers of mice, *Gank* liver-specific knockout mice were generated and were administered an HFD (58% of kcal as fat) supplemented with sucrose for 24–28 weeks [19]. The livers of these mice displayed reduced proliferation and no fibrosis with strong macrovesicular steatosis, which was surprisingly associated with health improvement in the animals, while the livers of WT mice under the same diet developed fibrosis but with lower levels of steatosis [19].

3. NASH Mouse Models
3.1. Diet-Induced Models
3.1.1. Methionine and Choline Deficient Diet (MCD)

The typical dietary NASH-inducing model is a diet consisting of high amounts of sucrose (40% of total calorie intake), moderately enriched in fat (10%), which also lacks the essential components of animal and human nutrition methionine and choline [10,11]. Methionine is an essential amino acid necessary for the synthesis of glutathione, an antioxidant protein, which also participates in the regulation of cell proliferation [33]. Choline is the precursor of phosphatidylcholine, which in turn is needed for VLDL secretion [34].

VLDL forms a lipoprotein complex that transports fatty acids from the liver to the adipose tissue [35]. Mice fed an MCD diet develop hepatic steatosis due to the high levels of fatty acid uptake and low levels of VLDL secretion, presenting hepatic inflammation after 2 weeks of feeding, as well as fibrosis after 6 weeks [10,11,36]. Plasma AST and ALT levels are increased, while lobular inflammation and ballooning degeneration of hepatocytes are also observed [10,37]. Furthermore, oxidative stress and an increase in pro-inflammatory cytokines/adipokines and pathways, such as nuclear factor-κB (NF-κB), occur in MCD-fed mice, which exacerbates hepatic damage [11,38,39].

3.1.2. Atherogenic Diet (High Cholesterol and High Cholate)

An atherogenic diet typically contains high cholesterol and high cholate; cholesterol (1–1.25%) and cholate (0.5%) [7,40]. Increased plasma and liver lipid levels are observed in mice fed an atherogenic diet [40], which induces progressive steatosis, fibrosis, and inflammation, in a time-dependent manner ranging from 6 to 24 weeks. Furthermore, hepatocellular ballooning develops after 24 weeks on this diet [40].

3.1.3. High-Fat (HF) Atherogenic Diet

The high cholesterol and high cholate atherogenic diet can be further supplemented with an additional high-fat component, such as 60% fat derived from cocoa butter [40]. Feeding mice this particular diet for 34 weeks leads to steatosis and NASH-like lesions, such as Mallory–Denk bodies and hepatocyte ballooning [7,41]. Furthermore, this diet worsens the histologic severity of NASH and induces insulin resistance and oxidative stress (downregulation of genes encoding antioxidant enzymes) whilst it further enhances the activation of hepatic stellate cells [7,40]. Interestingly, the HF atherogenic diet (60% fat, 20% carbohydrate, 20% protein, 1.25% cholesterol and 0.5% cholic acid) has been compared to the MCD diet (21% fat, 63% carbohydrate, 16% protein), and certain key differences between the two are noteworthy [6,42]. More specifically, while WT C57BL/6 mice fed both diets have high levels of hepatic free fatty acids, the MCD diet-fed mice mainly accumulate triglycerides in their livers, whereas the livers of HF-atherogenic diet-fed mice predominantly accumulate cholesterol [42]. Moreover, the administration of an HF-atherogenic diet does not cause a reduction in the weights of animal livers, while the MCD diet causes such a reduction [42]. Furthermore, compared to the HF-atherogenic diet, the MCD diet exacerbates the hepatic damage (e.g., as indicated by more increased circulating ALT and AST levels) and induces the formation of lipogranulomas (inflammatory nodules composed of macrophages surrounding a lipid droplet), and more pronounced fibrosis [42]. However, both the MCD and the HF-atherogenic diets are considered to induce the classic hepatic histopathological features of NASH, namely steatosis, hepatocyte ballooning and lobular inflammation to the same degree [42]. Additionally, transcriptional analysis has displayed that—although MDC and HF-atherogenic diets lead to the upregulation of hepatic stellate cell activation markers, pro-fibrogenic markers and extracellular matrix proteins—the expression of a subset of genes involved in extracellular matrix remodeling and production, as well as in hepatic stellate cell activation, is more dysregulated in MCD-fed mice than in atherogenic-fed mice [42]. Therefore, a more severe form of NASH is observed in MDC diet-fed mice, where extensive hepatic inflammation and fibrosis are observed quickly after the start of administration (2–10 weeks), probably due to the reduced VLDL synthesis and hepatic-β oxidation [6,42,43]. Notably, liver inflammation, steatohepatitis and elevated serum liver enzyme levels were normalized after switching the diet back to the control within 16 weeks, but fibrosis and CD68-positive macrophages remained present [44].

3.1.4. High-Fat, High-Cholesterol (HFHC) Diets

NASH features are more striking when a high amount of cholesterol is combined with a high amount of fat or cholate in the diet [10]. The administration of a high-fat (33% kcal as fat) and high cholesterol (1% cholesterol) (HFHC) diet to WT C57BL/6 mice leads to greater weight gain, more pronounced hepatic lipid accumulation and steatosis, substantial inflammation, and perisinusoidal fibrosis (namely steatohepatitis) compared to the HCD [20]. This is also associated with adipose tissue inflammation [as indicated by high macrophage gene expression and increased gene expression of monocyte chemotactic factor genes and of the pro-inflammatory cytokine tumor necrosis factor α (TNF-α)], a reduction in circulating adiponectin levels, and a 10-fold elevation of serum ALT levels [20]. In addition, the HFHC diet also induces additional features of human NASH, including hypercholesterolemia and obesity [20].

In another regimen of high fat and cholesterol-enriched diet (containing 45% kcal fat and 0.12% cholesterol), WT C57BL/6 mice become obese and also develop hepatomegaly and hepatic steatosis, with varying degrees of liver fibrosis and steatohepatitis after consuming this diet for a long time (7 months) [45]. Furthermore, about 87% of the mice on this diet for 7 months have elevated plasma ALT [45].

In another study, the long-term consumption (for 20 weeks) of a high-caloric (43%) Western-type diet containing soybean oil with high n-6-polyunsaturated fatty acids (PUFA) (25 g/100 g) and 0.75% cholesterol induces steatosis, ballooning, inflammation and fibrosis, accompanied by hepatic lipid peroxidation, activation of Kupffer cells and oxidative stress in the liver of C57BL/6 mice [46]. Furthermore, the animals under this diet display increased weight gain and insulin resistance compared to those fed either a normal diet or a cholesterol-free HFD, thus showing a phenotype that reflects all clinical features of NASH in patients with metabolic syndrome [46].

In other cholesterol-enriched or choline-deficient high-fat diets, when C57BL/6 mice consumed a high-fat (23%), high-sucrose (424 g/kg) and high-cholesterol (1.9 g/kg) diet or a choline-deficient high-fat diet (CD-HFD) for three months developed marked steatohepatitis [10].

3.1.5. High-Fat, High-Fructose (HFHF) Diets

Modern, western-style diets usually contain significant amounts of food rich in fructose, and this has been associated with a high incidence of obesity and NASH [47]. In order to mimic this pattern of nutrition, male WT C57BL/6 mice were fed a high-fat, high-fructose (HFHF) diet consisting of 58% kcal fat plus drinking water enriched with 42 g/L of carbohydrates at a ratio of 55% fructose and 45% sucrose (w/v) [47]. As a comparison, control animals were administered either a chow diet or an HFD containing 58% kcal fat to assess the effects of fructose consumption. Although weight gain, body fat, insulin resistance, hepatic steatosis, inflammation, and apoptosis were similar between the HFHF diet-fed and HFD-fed mice and increased compared to chow-fed ones, hepatic oxidative stress, pro-inflammatory monocyte populations (probably indicative of stellate cell activation), numbers of CD11b+F4/80+Gr1+ macrophages in the liver, transforming growth factor (TGF)-β1-driven fibrogenesis and collagen deposition were all elevated in the animals consuming the HFHF diet compared to those under the HFD [47]. These data suggest that fructose consumption is necessary for the progression of liver fat deposition to fibrogenesis [47]. In another study, C57BL/6 male mice were fed an HFHF diet (consisting of 60% of kcal as fat and 35% fructose) for 16 weeks, which, apart from the aforementioned increases in hepatic free fatty acid content, serum insulin levels, insulin resistance and oxidative stress, further led to hepatic iron overload, a finding often observed in humans with NAFLD [48].

3.1.6. Amylin Liver NASH (AMLN) Model

Due to the variability in disease onset/progression and the lack of a preclinical mouse model that precisely reproduces the NAFLD-NASH phenotype, the Amylin Liver NASH (AMLN) model was developed [6,49]. The diet administered to these mice consisted of 40% fat (of which nearly 18% was trans-fat), 22% fructose, and 2% cholesterol, with the WT C57BL/6 mice that consumed this diet developing the three stages of NAFLD, namely steatosis, steatohepatitis with fibrosis, and cirrhosis, as assessed histologically and biochemically [49]. In these mice, the development of severe steatosis with necroinflammation and fibrosis, together with the appearance of periportal inflammation and hepatocellular ballooning, which are signs of progression to NASH, occurs after about 30 weeks on the AMLN diet [49]. However, the acceleration of this process and the development of more serious NASH is achieved by the combination of this dietary model with a genetic model. More specifically, when *ob/ob* mice were fed the AMLN diet for at least 8 weeks, key markers and histopathological features of NASH were induced [50,51]. This diet can act as a stimulus leading to NASH development in *ob/ob* mice since they cannot spontaneously proceed from NAFLD to NASH due to leptin absence, given that leptin is necessary for hepatic fibrosis development [26].

3.1.7. Gubra Amylin NASH (GAN) Diet

Following the guidelines of the Food and Drug Administration (FDA) regarding the ban of trans-fats as food additives [52], there was a need for a non-trans-fat Western-type diet that would lead to NASH-like metabolic and hepatic histopathological changes comparable to those caused by the AMLN diet [53]. Thus, the Gubra amylin NASH (GAN) diet was developed with a composition and caloric density similar to the AMLN diet (40% kcal as high-fat, 22% fructose, 10% sucrose, 2% cholesterol) but with the substitution of trans-fat by saturated fat, i.e., palm oil (of the 40% high-fat, 0% was trans-fat and 46% was saturated fatty acids by weight) [53]. Notably, *ob/ob* mice fed the GAN diet for 16 weeks developed steatosis, fibrotic NASH (confirmed with biopsy), lobular inflammation, hepatocyte ballooning, fibrotic liver lesions and hepatic transcriptome changes, features similar to those induced in *ob/ob* mice on the AMLN diet and to those in patients with NASH [53]. The GAN diet induces fibrotic NASH in WT C57BL/6 mice as well, although, within a more prolonged time interval (28 weeks), similar to that needed by the AMLN diet to provoke the same NASH hallmarks [53]. However, the GAN-fed WT C57BL/6 mice displayed significantly higher body weight gain compared to those on the AMLN diet [53]. Moreover, C57BL/6 mice on the GAN diet for 38 weeks or more display morphological characteristics comparable to those in patients with NASH, with similar increases in markers of hepatic lipid accumulation, inflammation and collagen deposition as indicated by histomorphometric analysis. Furthermore, liver biopsies from GAN-fed WT mice and patients with NASH show comparable dynamics in several differentially expressed genes involved in key metabolic and histopathological features of NASH, such as nutrient metabolism, immune function and extracellular matrix organization [54]. Overall, the GAN diet is more obesogenic and impairs glucose tolerance compared to the AMLN diet [53].

3.1.8. Fast-Food-like Diet (High-Fat/High-Fructose/High-Cholesterol Diet)

The administration of a different fast-food-like diet based on a different content of increased fat, fructose and cholesterol concentrations (41% fat, 30% fructose, 2% cholesterol) leads to NASH in different animal models, including the WT C57BL/6, *ob/ob* and KK-A^y mice; the latter being generated when the yellow obese gene (Ay) was transferred into KK-background mice, and exhibiting hyperphagia, obesity and hyperinsulinemia without fully progressing to NASH under normal chow diet [55,56]. Among these models, the *ob/ob* mice developed more marked NAFLD activity scores, fibrosis progression, obesity and hyperinsulinemia [55]. Interestingly, steatohepatitis- and fibrosis-related molecular pathways started displaying alterations after only two weeks of administering this fast-food-like diet in *ob/ob* mice [55]. In another study, C57BL/6 mice were fed an HFHF diet supplemented with high cholesterol as well (providing 40% of energy as fat, with 2% cholesterol and high-fructose corn syrup at 42 g/L final concentration administered in the drinking water of mice) which after six months led to the development of obesity, insulin resistance and steatohepatitis with pronounced ballooning and progressive fibrosis [57]. This was also accompanied by gene expression signature of increased fibrosis, inflammation, ER stress and lipoapoptosis, all key features of the metabolic syndrome and NASH with progressing fibrosis in humans [57].

3.2. Genetic Models

3.2.1. db/db Mice with Iron Supplementation

When genetically obese *db/db* mice are fed a chow diet supplemented with high iron content (20,000 ppm vs. an iron content of 280 ppm in a normal chow diet), they develop a phenotype progressing from NAFLD to NASH [58]. Notably, this was characterized by hepatocellular ballooning, increased hepatic oxidative stress, inflammasome activation, impaired hepatic mitochondrial biogenesis and fatty acid β-oxidation, and activation of other pro-inflammatory/immune mediators [58].

3.2.2. foz/foz Mice

Fat Aussie (*foz/foz*) mice bear a spontaneous deletion of 11bp in the *Alms1* gene, which is mutated in the Alström syndrome in humans, a disorder with distinct metabolic and endocrine features characterized by childhood-onset obesity, metabolic syndrome, and diabetes [59]. The ALMS1 protein localizes at the basal bodies of cilia, playing a role in intracellular trafficking, with the ALMS1-containing cilia in hypothalamic neurons being implicated in the control of satiety [59,60]. Accordingly, *foz/foz* mice fed a chow diet are hyperphagic, obese and glucose intolerant, with insulin resistance, decreased adiponectin levels, and increased total cholesterol, as well as increased hepatic weight, impaired hepatic function and steatosis [61]. Administration of an HFD (21–23% fat, energy content 19.4–20.0 megajoule/kg, 43% energy as fat) to *foz/foz* mice leads to severe NASH progression with significant upregulation of ALT levels, hepatocyte ballooning, inflammation, and fibrosis, as well as further decreased serum adiponectin levels, increased cholesterol levels, and higher hepatic triglyceride levels [59,62]. However, the characteristics and severity of diet-induced NASH are strain-dependent in *foz/foz* mice [63]. More specifically—while both *foz/foz* C57BL/6 and *foz/foz* BALB/c mice were similarly obese-hepatomegaly, hyperinsulinemia, hyperglycemia, and lower adiponectin levels occurred only in *foz/foz* C57BL/6 mice and not in *foz/foz* BALB/c mice after consuming either chow diet or HFD [63]. On the other hand, obese *foz/foz* BALB/c mice had more adipose tissue compared to *foz/foz* C57BL/6 [63]. HFD-fed *foz/foz* C57BL/6 mice present more severe NAFLD, as indicated by serum ALT levels, steatosis, hepatocellular ballooning, liver inflammation and NAFLD activity score, which were all higher compared to *foz/foz* BALB/c mice [63]. Of note, fibrosis after an HFD was severe in *foz/foz* C57BL/6 but absent in *foz/foz* BALB/c mice [63].

3.2.3. MS-NASH Mice

The MS-NASH mouse (formerly known as FATZO/Pco) is a recombinant inbred cross of two strains prone to obesity when fed high-fat, high-calorie diets: C57BL/6J and AKR/J [64,65]. Crossing and selective inbreeding of these two strains lead to obesity, accompanied by significant insulin resistance, hyperlipidemia and hyperglycemia, as well as metabolic syndrome [66]. MS-NASH mice become obese and insulin resistant even when consuming a standard chow diet [64]. When these are fed a high-fat Western-type diet supplemented with 5% fructose in the drinking water for 20 weeks, they become heavier with higher body fat and hypercholesterolemia, with high AST, ALT, hepatic triglyceride levels, and liver over body weight [67]. Additionally, under the aforementioned Western-type, fructose-supplemented diet, markers of liver damage and evidence of NAFLD/NASH progression become more pronounced, particularly in male, and MS-NASH mice develop hepatic steatosis, lobular inflammation, hepatocellular ballooning and fibrosis [64,67].

3.2.4. Ldlr−/− (Low-Density Lipoprotein Receptor Knockout)/Ldlr−/−.Leiden Mice

Deletion of the *low-density lipoprotein receptor* (*ldlr*) gene in mice has highlighted this gene as an important regulator of the transport of lipids and lipoproteins on macrophages and Kuppfer cells, opening a new field for NASH research [6,68]. Hyperlipidemic *ldlr−/−* mice are one of the two best characterized dyslipidemic models [69] and were first used as a model for atherosclerosis research, but when they were fed a high-fat diet with cholesterol (HFC) (21% milk butter, 0.2% cholesterol) for seven days the female mice developed steatosis with severe inflammation characterized by infiltration of macrophages and increased NF-κB signaling, while the male ones developed severe hepatic inflammation in the absence of steatosis [68]. Interestingly, a continuation of this diet for 3 months led to sustained hepatic inflammation in *ldlr−/−* mice, accompanied by increased apoptosis and hepatic fibrosis [70]. Furthermore, *ldlr−/−* mice under this HFC diet display high levels of low-density lipoprotein (LDL) and low levels of high-density lipoprotein (HDL), mimicking the corresponding human lipidemic profile [70]. Analogous to these findings, the administration of a "diabetogenic" high-fat diet supplemented with cholesterol (35.5% carbohydrate, 36.6% fat, 0.15% cholesterol) leads to obesity, insulin resistance, hyperinsulinemia, dyslipidemia, increased hepatic triglycerides and ALT, exacerbated hepatic macrophage infiltration, apoptosis, and oxidative stress, as well as to micro- and macrovesicular steatosis, inflammatory cell foci, and fibrosis in the livers of the *ldlr−/−* mice [71]. Another substrain of the *ldlr−/−* mice have been created with 94% C57BL/6 background and 6% 129S1/SvImJ background, namely the *Ldlr−/−*.Leiden mice (TNO, Metabolic Health Research, Leiden, The Netherlands) [72]. When *ldlr−/−*.Leiden mice are fed an HFD containing 45% kcal fat from lard and 35% kcal from carbohydrates (primarily sucrose) or a fast food diet (FFD) containing 41% kcal fat from milk fat and 44% kcal from carbohydrates (primarily fructose), they develop obesity, hyperlipidemia, hyperinsulinemia, increased ALT and AST levels, progressive macro- and microvesicular steatosis, hepatic inflammation, and fibrosis, along with atherosclerosis [72]. Interestingly, the HFD has been found to cause more severe hyperinsulinemia in these mice, while the FFD induces more severe hepatic inflammation with advanced bridging fibrosis, as well as more severe atherosclerosis [72].

3.2.5. Prostaglandin E2-Deficient Mice

Although prostaglandins, and particularly prostaglandin E2 (PGE2), play a key role during pro-inflammatory processes [73], the role of PGE2 in liver inflammation is not fully elucidated [6,73]. To explore this, mice lacking microsomal PGE synthase 1 (mPGES-1), the key enzyme needed for the production of the majority of PGE2 during inflammation, were fed for 20 weeks a cholesterol-containing HFD with a high content of ω6-polyunsaturated fatty acids (PUFA) (255 g/kg fat, 0.75% cholesterol), which has previously been shown to induce NASH in mice [73]. Of note, these mice presented a strong infiltration of monocyte-derived macrophages and an increase in TNF-α expression in the liver, with the latter causing upregulated interleukin 1β (IL-1β) levels, primarily in hepatocytes and augmented hepatocyte apoptosis [73].

3.2.6. *Apolipoprotein E2* Knock-In (APOE2ki) Mice

The *Apolipoprotein E2* (*APOE2*) knock-in (APOE2ki) mouse model was generated when the murine *Apoe* gene was replaced by a human *Apolipoprotein E2* (*APOE*2*) gene allele via targeted gene replacement in embryonic stem cells and was first used as a model for hyperlipoproteinemia and atherosclerosis [74]. When APOE2ki mice are fed a high-fat/high-cholesterol diet (42% energy as milk butter/fat, 0.2% cholesterol, 46% carbohydrates) from 7/10 days up to three months, they develop early (from the first seven days) increased inflammation indicative of NASH compared to C75BL/6 mice on the same diet which only develop simple steatosis and minor signs of an increase in the infiltrating inflammatory cells [70,75].

3.2.7. *Apolipoprotein E*-deficient (*ApoE−/−*) Mice

Apolipoprotein E (ApoE) acts as a significant component of lipoprotein metabolism in humans and mice [76]. When it is absent, hypercholesterolemia, atherosclerosis and obesity have been reported to occur, thus *Apolipoprotein E*-deficient (*ApoE−/−*) mice display spontaneously increased inflammation and high levels of cholesterol compared to WT mice, and have traditionally served as a metabolic syndrome model used in cardiovascular research [76]. Indeed, *ApoE−/−* mice constitute the other most well-characterized dyslipidemic model [69]. However, when $ApoE-/-$ mice consume a Western-type, cholesterol-enriched diet [42% energy as fat (with coconut oil), 1.25% cholesterol] for seven weeks, they show abnormal glucose tolerance, increased levels of fasting glucose, hepatomegaly, weight gain and develop the full spectrum of NASH spanning from hepatic steatosis and hepatocyte ballooning to inflammation and fibrosis [76]. Recently, $ApoE-/-$ mice on HFD (with compositions ranging from 37–60% of kcal as fat, with a carbohydrate content of 38–44% and supplementation of 0.02–1.5% cholesterol and of 0.5% cholate, administered from seven to 24 weeks [77–91]) have been utilized as NAFLD/NASH models to investigate the pathogenesis and progression of this disease, as well as potential therapeutic treatments.

3.3. Chemically Induced Models

3.3.1. Carbon Tetrachloride (CCl_4) Administration

A way to explore the development of hepatic fibrosis is by inducing it with chemical agents, such as carbon tetrachloride (CCl_4). When male BALB/c mice were given an intraperitoneal injection with CCl_4 (0.4 mL/kg) twice a week for six weeks, their serum levels of aminotransferase and alkaline phosphatase were increased, whilst the anti-oxidative status of the liver was also disturbed [92]. The administration of CCl_4 also caused extensive fibrosis [92]. Moreover, in a more recent model, male C57BL/6 mice were administered CCl_4 and a Liver X receptor (LXR) agonist in combination with HFD feeding, which led to the development of insulin resistance and histopathological characteristics of NASH, such as macrovesicular hepatic steatosis, ballooning hepatocytes, Mallory-Denk bodies, lobular inflammation and fibrosis [93]. In this latter model, the TNF-α and interleukin-6 (IL-6) serum levels were significantly elevated, as well as the expression of mRNAs related to lipogenesis, oxidative stress, fibrosis and steatosis [93].

3.3.2. Thioacetamide (TAA) Administration in Combination to Fast-Food Diet

Thioacetamide (TAA) serves as a hepato-toxin used to induce acute or chronic liver injury in mice and rats [94]. Combined administration of TAA (75 mg/kg, intraperitoneally, three times a week) with a fast food diet [12% saturated fatty acids (SFA) and 2% cholesterol with high fructose corn syrup (42 g/L final concentration)] to C57BL/6 mice for eight weeks leads to the appearance of key histological features of NASH, namely hepatic inflammation, hepatocellular ballooning, collagen deposition and bridging fibrosis [94].

3.4. Thermoneutral Housing

Apart from the genetic and dietary models trying to mimic the human NAFLD spectrum, a novel model focuses on the housing conditions of the animals and their effects on NAFLD development [95]. While mice are usually housed in a temperature range of 20–25 °C, this seems to be based on a human comfort zone and to stress the animals, while the thermoneutral zone or the temperature of metabolic homeostasis, for *Mus musculus* is 30–32 °C [95]. Wild-type C57BL/6 mice housed under thermoneutral conditions display exacerbated pro-inflammatory immune responses that were inhibited under standard housing conditions, and when they simultaneously receive an HFD (60% kcal from fat), they develop signs of deteriorating HFD-induced NASH, including increased steatosis, hepatocyte ballooning, exacerbated hepatic chemokine expression and macrophage infiltration of the liver, as well as more pronounced hepatic damage and elevated expression of genes associated with fibrosis, [95].

4. NASH-HCC Mouse Models

4.1. Diet-Induced Models

4.1.1. Choline-Deficient L-Amino Acid-Defined (CDAA) Diet

The choline-deficient L-amino acid-defined (CDAA) diet is a modification of the MCD diet, in which proteins are substituted by an equimolar mixture of L-amino acids [7,11]. In WT C57BL/6 mice, this causes liver injury that mimics NASH features and can lead to the development of HCC [10]. More specifically, the CDAA diet reduces fatty acid oxidation in hepatocytes of mice, increases lipid deposition (especially after three months of treatment), induces oxidative stress and causes hepatic steatosis and inflammation (after six weeks) [96–98]. However, liver fibrosis develops gradually and takes quite a long time to occur: steatosis and lobular inflammation are induced after six weeks, slight features of fibrosis are displayed after 22 weeks, and finally, HCC is developed after about 36 weeks [96–98]. Although mice under the CDAA diet do not lose weight, they do not gain weight as well at least after 20 weeks on the CDAA diet compared to the control diet (choline-supplemented L-amino acid-defined diet), whilst their insulin sensitivity remains unchanged [99]. However, according to another study by Miura et al., insulin resistance sensitivity can be developed in CDAA-fed mice after 22 weeks, with obesity and increased plasma triglyceride and cholesterol levels, discrepancies probably attributed to the dietary compositions of the diet (e.g., percentage of fat) and the duration of the feeding [11,100].

4.1.2. Choline-Deficient, Ethionine-Supplemented (CDE) Diet

Ethionine is a non-proteinogenic amino acid, the ethyl analog of methionine (an ethyl group instead of a methyl group) [11]. The choline-deficient, ethionine-supplemented (CDE) diet, which is derived from the MCD diet, induces steatohepatitis and inflammation shortly after the start of its administration, which is followed by fibrosis, cirrhosis and HCC in the long-term [11,101]. However, contrary to the NAFLD phenotype in humans, this diet leads to weight loss in CDE-fed animals, whilst it also causes high mortality [11,102,103]. To limit this mortality, some studies alternate the administration of CDE with a normal chow diet or combine a 100% CDE diet with a control diet to reduce the strength of the CDE diet to 75%, 70% or even 67% [101]. This approach minimizes morbidity and mortality while maintaining hepatic steatosis, inflammation and carcinogenesis [11,101].

4.1.3. American Lifestyle-Induced Obesity Syndrome (ALIOS) Diet

In an attempt to recapitulate the western, modern lifestyle and its consequences on liver physiology, a frequently used diet is the American lifestyle-induced obesity syndrome (ALIOS) diet, which is based on the nutritional constitution of commonly consumed fast food, using WT mice kept in conditions that promote sedentary behavior [104]. Mice fed the ALIOS diet were consuming 45% calories in the chow from fat and 30% of the fat as trans-fat in the form of partially hydrogenated vegetable oil [28% saturated, 57% monounsaturated fatty acids (MUFA), 13% PUFA] and were also administered high-fructose corn syrup (HFCS) equivalent (55% fructose, 45% glucose by weight) in drinking water at a concentration of 42 g/L [104]. Furthermore, the cage racks were removed in order to prevent the physical activity of the ALIOS mice and mimic sedentary life [104]. After 16 weeks, the high trans-fat diet without the addition of fructose led to the development of a NASH-like phenotype with associated necroinflammatory changes, obesity, insulin resistance, and high plasma ALT levels accompanied by inflammatory and profibrogenic responses (as shown by the increased liver TNF-α and procollagen mRNA levels), as well as elevated levels of plasma insulin, resistin, and leptin [104,105]. The inclusion of fructose further increased food consumption, obesity, and impaired insulin sensitivity, while it did not alter the plasma ALT levels and the degree of steatosis [104]. The expression of some profibrogenic genes was upregulated, although no histologically detectable fibrosis was found in the mice, at least up to 16 weeks of ALIOS diet consumption [104]. A more prolonged administration of the ALIOS diet led Tetri et al. to the observations that mice display features of early NASH with mild or moderate steatosis at six months and characteristics of more advanced NASH at 12 months, including severe steatosis, liver inflammation, and bridging fibrosis, while Harris et al. reported that the characteristics of more advanced NASH are already present from 6.5 months [105,106]. Furthermore, increased expression of lipid metabolism genes (regulators of lipogenesis and β-oxidation) and insulin signaling genes was observed after six months of the ALIOS diet, which for some continued up to 12 months [106]. Notably, hepatocellular neoplasms were developed in 60% of the ALIOS-fed mice after 12 months, when there was also observed a marked expansion of murine hepatic stem cells, which were closely associated with the neoplastic foci [106]. The ALIOS diet has also been found to change the hepatic transcriptome of mice with the upregulation of genes associated with the reorganization of cellular structures, collagen binding, and inflammatory and immune responses, while genes associated with protein processing and metabolic procedures were downregulated [105].

4.1.4. Diet-Induced Animal Model of Non-Alcoholic Fatty Liver Disease (DIAMOND)

The diet-induced animal model of non-alcoholic fatty liver disease (DIAMOND) was based on an isogenic strain that was derived from a cross between the common WT C57BL/6J strain and the 129S1/SvImJ strain, the latter being a commonly used model to create mice with targeted mutations [6,107]. Almost 60% of this strain's genes come from the C57BL/6 background, while the isogenic nature of mice and the disease phenotype has been followed and confirmed over many generations [8,107]. These mice were fed a Western-type (high fat, high carbohydrate) diet consisting of 42% kcal from fat and 0.1% cholesterol, while they had ad libitum consumption of water with a high fructose and glucose content (23.1 g/L D-fructose plus 18.9 g/L D-glucose) [107]. These rapidly develop obesity, insulin resistance, hypertriglyceridemia, and increased levels of the total- and LDL-cholesterol, AST and ALT [107]. Following administration of this diet for longer periods, these mice gradually develop steatosis (4–8 weeks), steatohepatitis (16–24 weeks), progressive fibrosis (16 weeks onwards), with severe bridging fibrosis (by week 52) and spontaneous HCC (in 89% of mice between 32 and 52 weeks) [107]. Interestingly, DIAMOND mice display a pattern of pathway activation at the transcriptomic level similar to humans with NASH, with lipogenic, inflammatory and apoptotic signaling pathways being activated [107].

4.2. Genetic Models

4.2.1. *Tm6sf2* Hepatic Knockdown or Knockout

Transmembrane 6 superfamily member 2 (TM6SF2) in humans regulates qualitative triglyceride enrichment in VLDL, lipid synthesis and the number of secreted lipoprotein particles [30]. The rs58542926 C > T polymorphism results in an A-to-G substitution in coding nucleotide 499 which replaces glutamate at residue 167 with lysine in the TM6SF2 protein (c.499A > G; p.Glu167Lys/E167K) [30,108]. The E167K variant of the *Tm6sf2* gene is strongly associated with hepatic triglyceride content and favors hepatic fat accumulation in intracellular lipid droplets since it decreases lipid secretion, leading to increased susceptibility to liver damage, including NASH and severe fibrosis, whilst it also predisposes humans to NAFLD with progression to HCC [30,108]. Furthermore, this variant has been associated with an increase in serum ALT, consistent with marked hepatic injury [108]. Selective knockdown of *Tm6sf2* levels in the livers of mice through the introduction of recombinant adeno-associated viral vectors expressing short hairpin RNAs (shRNAs) against *Tm6sf2* leads to 3-fold upregulation of hepatic triglyceride content, a significant decrease of plasma cholesterol levels and a tendency towards lower plasma triglyceride levels, findings consistent with a defect in VLDL secretion in mice consuming a chow diet *ad libitum* [108]. Feeding these mice with a high-sucrose fat-free diet (74% kcal from sucrose) for four weeks exacerbated the effects of *Tm6sf2* knockdown since levels of triglycerides and cholesterol esters were further upregulated in the liver and decreased in plasma [108]. Newberry et al. generated liver-specific *Tm6sf2* knockout mice, which developed spontaneous liver steatosis, with increased numbers of large lipid droplets, triglycerides and diacylglycerol species in the liver, as well as decreased hepatic VLDL triglyceride secretion under normal chow diet [109]. Moreover, *Tm6sf2* liver-specific knockout mice exhibited increased steatosis and fibrosis after the consumption of a high milk-fat diet (60.3% kcal from fat, primary milk fat) for three weeks, with those phenotypes being further exacerbated when mice were fed fibrogenic, high fat/fructose diets for 20 weeks [either a trans-fat, fructose supplemented diet with 45.3% kcal from fat, containing 22% hydrogenated vegetable oil and consuming sugar water containing 55% fructose/45% glucose (4.2g/L) or a palm oil diet (40% kcal fat) supplemented with 20% kcal fructose and 2% cholesterol] [109]. Finally, *Tm6sf2* liver-specific knockout mice are more susceptible to HCC since they display increased steatosis, greater tumor burden, and increased tumor area compared to non-transgenic floxed control mice when tumorigenesis is chemically/dietary induced [109]. Of note, a new rodent model was generated by Luo et al. by inactivating *Tm6sf2* in rats [110]. These *Tm6sf2−/−* rats display a 6-fold higher mean hepatic triglyceride content and lower plasma cholesterol levels than their WT littermates [110].

4.2.2. Fatty Liver Shionogi (FLS) Mice

Inbreeding of dd Shionogi (DS) mice in 1984 resulted in some mice which developed spontaneous fatty liver without obesity, namely the Fatty liver Shionogi (FLS) mice [111]. These also display 5-fold higher hepatic triglyceride concentrations compared to DS mice and higher plasma AST and ALT levels, suggestive of hepatocellular lesions and inflammation [111]. After 2–4 months of age, mononuclear cell infiltration and clusters of foam cells appear in the fatty liver of FLS mice, accompanied by elevated serum ALT levels, suggesting the presence of NASH with inflammatory responses and liver injury [112]. Interestingly, FLS mice over 12 months may develop hepatocellular adenoma and/or HCC, with a frequency of 40% in males at 15–16 months and 9.5% in females at 20–24 months [112]. Interestingly, lipocalin-2 (LCN2), an adipokine, was overexpressed in the liver of FLS mice, particularly in hepatocytes localized around almost all inflammatory cell clusters, while the chemokine C-X-C motif ligand 1 (CXCL1), a pro-inflammatory chemokine exhibited hepatic overexpression localized in steatotic hepatocytes, and CXCL9 (another pro-inflammatory chemokine) was also overexpressed in hepatocytes and the sinusoidal endothelium localized in some areas of inflammatory cell infiltration [113]. When FLS mice were backcrossed to *ob/ob* mice, FLS-Lep^{ob}/Lep^{ob} or FLS-*ob/ob* mice were generated, which display remarkable hyperphagia, obesity, type 2 diabetes, severe hyperinsulinemia and hyperlipidemia, as well as histologically proven severe steatosis, inflammatory changes, increased oxidative stress with advanced fibrosis, and elevated levels of apoptosis later in life with spontaneous hepatic tumors [114,115].

4.2.3. *Phosphatase and Tensin Homolog* (*PTEN*)-Deficient Mice

PTEN is a tumor suppressor gene encoding a multifunctional phosphatase, with both protein and lipid phosphatase activities, whose lipid phosphatase activity is associated with tumor suppression [116,117]. PTEN is mutated in multiple human cancers and is important for maintaining homeostasis and preventing oncogenesis in the liver, where it has been identified as a metabolic regulator of glycose metabolism and insulin signaling [117]. Hepatocyte-specific null mutation of *Pten* in mice has led to *PTEN*-deficient mice that display massive hepatomegaly and steatohepatitis with an accumulation of triglycerides, inflammatory cells and Mallory-Denk bodies, followed by liver fibrosis and HCC, closely mimicking the NASH phenotype/progression in humans [117,118]. These also develop insulin hypersensitivity [117]. Notably, liver tumors appear in 66% of the male and 30% of the female *PTEN*-deficient mice at 40–44 weeks of age and in 100% of PTEN-deficient mice at 74–78 weeks, with 66% of the tumors at 74-78 weeks being HCC (83% in male and 50% in female mice of that genotype) [117].

4.2.4. *Augmenter of Liver Regeneration* (*Alr*) Hepatic Knockout (ALR-H-KO) Mice

Augmenter of liver regeneration (ALR) protein (encoded by the *Gfer* [*growth factor ERV1 homolog of Saccharomyces cerevisiae*]) is pleiotropic and exhibits high expression in the liver (predominantly in hepatocytes), functioning as a hepatic growth factor which is critical for lipid homeostasis and mitochondrial function [119,120]. Global knockout of *Alr* in mice is embryonically lethal, so in order to investigate its role in the liver, mice with hepatocyte-specific deletion of *Alr* [*Alr* hepatic knockout (ALR-H-KO)] have been generated by Gandhi et al. [119]. These mice are normal at birth, but up to the second week of life, present low levels of ALR and ATP in their livers and have diminished mitochondrial respiratory function and increased oxidative stress, compared with livers from control mice, whilst also developing excessive steatosis and hepatocyte apoptosis [119]. Surprisingly, at weeks 2–4 after birth, hepatic lipid accumulation reverses, leading to a reduction in the levels of steatosis and apoptosis, while the numbers of cells that express ALR increase, along with ATP levels [119]. However, at 4–8 weeks after birth, and despite the reversion of steatosis, livers of ALR-H-KO mice develop hepatic inflammation, with hepatocellular necrosis, ductular proliferation, and fibrosis, whilst HCC appears in almost 60% of the mice by 12 months after birth [119]. When ALR-H-KO mice were administered a high-fat/high-carbohydrate (HF/HC) diet (60% kcal fat plus 2.3% fructose and 1.9% sucrose in drinking water) and were compared to WT and hepatocyte-specific ALR-heterozygous (ALR-H-HET) mice consuming the same diet, it was shown that the ALR-H-KO mice gained the least weight and had the least steatosis, whilst also had lower insulin resistance (all these HF/HC-fed mice developed insulin resistance) [120]. In addition, this HF/HC feeding led to severe fibrosis and/or cirrhosis in ALR-H-KO mice, contrary to the ALR-H-HET that only developed modest fibrosis and to WT that did not proceed to fibrosis and cirrhosis [120].

4.2.5. *Melanocortin 4 Receptor* Knockout (*Mc4r*−/−) Mice

Melanocortin 4 receptor (MC4R) is a seven-transmembrane G protein–coupled receptor expressed in the hypothalamic nuclei, which regulates food intake and body weight [121]. In humans, *MC4R* mutations constitute the most common known monogenic cause of obesity [121]. Deletion of this receptor in mice results in the generation of *Melanocortin 4 receptor* knockout (*Mc4r*−/−) mice, which under a normal chow diet develop late-onset obesity, hyperphagia, hyperinsulinemia, and hyperglycemia [122]. *Mc4r*−/− mice consuming an HFD (60% energy as fat) for 20 weeks develop hepatic microvesicular and macrovesicular steatosis, ballooning degeneration, inflammation and pericellular fibrosis, a phenotype compatible with NASH, associated with obesity, insulin resistance, and dyslipidemia [121]. Overall, *Mc4r*−/− mice under HFD for 20 weeks develop both obesity and NASH with moderate fibrosis [123]. Interestingly, these mice when fed a western diet (41% kcal from fat, 43% kcal from carbohydrate, 17% kcal from protein) for 12 weeks, accompanied by intraperitoneal injection of lipopolysaccharide (LPS) twice a week for the last four weeks, develop NASH with rapid accumulation of fibrosis compared to HFD-fed *Mc4r*−/− mice [124]. Of note, *Mc4r*−/− mice further develop well-differentiated HCC after consuming HFD for 12 months [121].

4.2.6. Tsumura-Suzuki Obese Diabetes (TSOD) Mice

Tsumura Suzuki obese diabetes (TSOD) mice spontaneously develop diabetes mellitus, obesity, glucosuria, hyperglycemia, and hyperinsulinemia without any special intervention/treatment, such as gene manipulation or an HFD [125]. The livers of TSOD mice display NASH-like features in the early stage at 3 months of age, which is exacerbated after 4 months of age, with microvesicular steatosis, hepatocellular ballooning, and Mallory-Denk bodies, with all these features worsening over time [125,126]. Interestingly, after 12 months of age, TSOD mice develop hepatic nodules with nuclear and structural atypia, characteristic of human HCC, with increased oxidative stress and elevation of glucose metabolites and L-arginine in the liver [125,127,128]. Although this model is not so common, it has been used over the last years in certain studies that investigated mechanisms implicated in NASH and hepatic carcinogenesis, as well as potential therapeutic agents against these conditions [129,130].

4.2.7. *Keratin 18*-Deficient (*Krt18*−/−) Mice

Keratin 18 deficiency in mice (*Krt18*−/− mice) results in mild to moderate degree of steatosis after 17–20 months from birth, with lobular inflammation and mononuclear cell infiltration, an image that closely resembles NASH in humans [131]. These mice also develop liver tumors resembling human HCC with stemness features, frequently on the basis of chromosomal instability, at a frequency of ~80% and ~35% in male and female mice, respectively [131].

4.2.8. Methionine Adenosyltransferase 1A (*Mat1a*) Knockout Mice

Methionine adenosyltransferases (MATs) are products of two genes, *Mat1a* and *Mat2a*, and catalyze the formation of S-adenosylmethionine (AdoMet), the principal biological methyl donor [132]. *Mat1a* is expressed in the liver, while *Mat2a* is expressed in extrahepatic tissues [132]. Mice with *Mat1a* gene deletion (*Mat1a* knockout mice) have increased hepatic weight compared to WT animals under a normal chow diet, while at eight months of age, they develop spontaneous macrovesicular steatosis and predominantly periportal mononuclear cell infiltration, signs of NASH [132]. Interestingly, these mice spontaneously develop HCC with increasing age (after 18 months of age) at a frequency of around 60% [133]. Notably, it has been now shown that the *Mat1a* gene deficiency impairs VLDL synthesis and dysregulates plasma lipid homeostasis, thereby contributing to the development of the NAFLD spectrum in these mice [134].

4.2.9. Liver-Specific Deletion of *NF-κB Essential Modulator* (*Nemo*) in Mice (NEMO^{LPC-KO} Mice)

NEMO/IKKγ is a subunit of the IkB kinase (IKK), which is essential for the activation of the transcription factor NF-κB, thus regulating cellular responses to inflammation [135]. Deletion of NEMO in hepatic parenchymal cells leads to the development of steatosis and steatohepatitis characterized by immune cell infiltration of the liver parenchyma in 8-week-old NEMO^{LPC-KO} mice [135]. This is followed by inflammatory fibrosis and the appearance of dysplastic nodules at six months of age that culminate in the spontaneous development of HCC in 12-month-old mice [135].

4.2.10. Circadian Rhythm Oscillations

Circadian rhythm has been found to exert multiple effects associated with NAFLD since it drives oscillations in mitochondria dynamics, oxidative stress, hepatic insulin resistance and triglyceride levels [136,137]. Liver-specific *Bmal1* knockout (LBmal1KO) mice accumulate oxidative damage and have been found to develop fatty liver and hepatic insulin resistance [136]. *Bmal1* knockout mice exhibit higher body fat than their WT littermates, impaired glucose metabolism, and high insulin sensitivity [138]. Notably, when these are fed an HFD (60% kcal fat) for 12 weeks, their insulin sensitivity is further increased, and they develop early obesity, to which they rapidly adapt [138]. In *Per1/2−/−* mice that lack a functional clock and consequently feeding rhythms, circadian oscillations in hepatic triglycerides levels persist, although with a completely different phase, pointing towards a role for additional mechanisms that control their circadian accumulation [137]. Interestingly, chronic disruption of the circadian rhythm has been found to disrupt the liver clock and induce NAFLD to NASH progression (high ALT and AST levels, hepatomegaly, chronic liver inflammation and fibrosis), which ultimately leads to HCC [139]. Furthermore, CLOCK mutant mice (*Clk$^{\Delta 19/\Delta 19}$*) display steatosis and steatohepatitis with age when fed a chow diet compared to WT littermates (with differences being evident from 6 up to 12 months). Of note, their hepatic steatosis is accelerated when fed a cholate-containing high-fat diet (37% kcal from fat, 1.25% cholesterol and 0.5% cholate) and a Western diet (42% kcal from fat, 0.2% cholesterol), whilst they develop cirrhosis when challenged with LPS, which induces an inflammatory response, on top of a Western diet [140].

4.3. Chemically Induced Models

4.3.1. Carbon Tetrachloride (CCl$_4$) Administration in Combination with Western Diet

In a further attempt to accelerate the progression of extensive fibrosis and tumor development, a Western-type diet (high-fat, high-fructose and high-cholesterol, 42% kcal from fat, 41% sucrose and 1.25% cholesterol by weight) together with a high sugar solution (23.1 g/L D-fructose and 18.9 g/L D-glucose) was fed to WT C57BL/6 mice, while CCl$_4$

at the dose of 0.2 µL (0.32 µg)/g of body weight was also injected intraperitoneally [141]. This approach resulted in the acceleration of the progression of the disease from simple NAFLD to NASH and tumor development, resulting in rapidly progressive steatosis, stage 3 fibrosis at 12 weeks, and HCC at 24 weeks [141].

4.3.2. STAM Model

Streptozotocin (STZ) is an antibiotic that damages pancreatic islet β-cells and is widely used to generate a model of type 1 diabetes mellitus [142]. Indeed, STZ treatment causes insulin deficiency and hyperglycemia in mice and rats [142]. Accordingly, as an animal model to better understand the progression of NASH to HCC, the STAM mouse model was generated, in which neonatal WT C57BL/6 mice received a single low-dose (200 µg) STZ injection two days after birth followed by administration of an HFD (60% kcal from fat) after four weeks of age [143]. These mice display steatosis with first signs of lobular inflammatory accumulation at six weeks of age, marked inflammation with hepatocyte ballooning and progressive fibrosis at 8–12 weeks of age, and finally, HCC at 16–20 weeks of age [143].

5. Conclusions

The need for better animal models for the whole spectrum of NAFLD becomes even more relevant for translational research, as the NAFLD prevalence is increasing worldwide due to the increasing adoption of Western-type lifestyles and eating habits. Such models would advance our understanding of the molecular mechanisms that drive NAFLD pathogenesis, as well as facilitate the ongoing research for new NAFLD/NASH treatments. HFD feeding in mice is currently a widely used approach that, in comparison to other models, closely mimics the histopathology and pathogenesis of human NAFLD whilst it also presents important features that compose the broader clinical presentation of the disease. However, HFD alone can typically lead only to hepatic steatosis, and further combined interventions are needed to proceed to NASH and HCC in the utilized animal models. Moreover, HFD feeding is a very broad term that exhibits great variations regarding the utilized diet composition and duration of feeding, while it also seems to have different effects on mice of different genetic backgrounds. Similar issues, and especially the lack of a standardized diet regimen, are raised with other dietary interventions that lead to NASH, such as the high fat, high fructose (HFHF) diet or the fast-food-like diet (High-fat/high-fructose/high-cholesterol diet). Moreover, these diets and other NASH-inducing dietary models, such as the methionine and choline-deficient diet (MCD), either display discrepancies from the NASH in humans or require a long time to induce NASH features. Thus, most of the utilized NASH-inducing diets (e.g., the MCD, AMLN, GAN, and fast-food-like-diets) are usually administered to leptin-deficient (*ob/ob*) or leptin receptor-deficient (*db/db*) mice. Overall, the genetic alterations that have been introduced/utilized in mice models for NAFLD are rarely found in humans, or those that predispose to NAFLD in humans and are used to create mouse models (e.g., the $PNPLA3^{I148M}$ and *Tm6sf2* hepatic knockdown or knockout mice) do not seem to induce the same effects in the animal models. Therefore, so far, these models have certain limitations and fail to meet the features of an "ideal" NAFLD animal model. Furthermore, the genetic mouse models for NASH, such as the *Prostaglandin E2*-deficient mice, the APOE2ki and *ApoE*−/− mice, need a dietary stimulus as well to induce key NASH features. Finally, the administration of chemical agents, such as CCl_4, TAA and STZ (in the STAM model), has the additional disadvantage of not reflecting the pathogenesis of NAFLD in humans.

Particularly, for research on NAFLD progression to HCC, the latter can be successfully caused by dietary modifications of the MCD diet (such as the CDAA or CDE diets), as well as by other diet regimes, but these models usually have discrepancies from what is noted in patients. Certain genetic models that have been created (*Krt18*−/−, *Mat1a* knockout and NEMO^{LPC-KO} mice) seem promising for the study of NASH and NASH-HCC since they display several key characteristics of the human disease. However, these have not been used in many studies yet, and thus remain to be further validated as appropriate models. TSOD mice seem another promising model that can develop all stages of NAFLD over time, with hepatic carcinogenesis being developed in a reasonable time range (after 12 months of age), whilst crucially these mice progress from NAFLD to NASH and HCC without the need for the addition of a genetic mutation/manipulation or a specific diet. Although not so common, this model has been used in some recent studies on the NAFLD spectrum [129,130], and its further use will reveal its exact potential as a more holistic NAFLD animal model.

On the other hand, there are also mouse models that can more properly replicate a specific stage of the NALFD but not its entire spectrum. For example, $ldlr-/-$ mice exhibit an inflammatory response developing early within NASH. Thus, this model can serve to study the early onset of NASH [70]. Although not appropriate for mimicking the complete NAFLD human pathophysiology, these animal models provide the opportunity for research into a particular NAFLD stage and/or mechanism.

Given that the ideal animal model for NAFLD does not exist yet, the various animal models that are currently utilized for NAFLD research, with various dietary interventions, genetic manipulations, and administration of chemical substances and their combinations should be critically viewed within the context of their advantages and disadvantages for basic and translational research, as presented in Table 1. Accordingly, taking into consideration the specific research hypothesis/objectives of each study, there are models that can be successfully utilized in order to investigate the NAFLD-related pathophysiologic mechanisms and/or treatments.

Table 1. Key advantages and disadvantages of animal models that are commonly utilized for NAFLD research, according to the stage of the disease they mimic.

	Advantages	Disadvantages
NAFLD Mouse Models		
Diet-Induced Models		
High-fat diet (HFD)	• HFD-fed animals, in contrast to other NAFLD models, closely mimic both the histopathology and pathogenesis of human NAFLD [10]. • Animals on a HFD display the most prominent features of NAFLD observed in humans as well, including obesity and insulin resistance [10].	• HFD does not seem to be the best option to study NAFLD due to extensive variations related to dietary compositions (source, nature and composition of fatty acids in the diet), the age at which HFD feeding starts, duration of HFD feeding, gender and mouse strains (e.g., C57BL/6 mice seem to be susceptible to HFD effects, while BALB/c exhibit reduced hepatic lipid accumulation, maintain normal glucose tolerance and insulin action) [11,144,145]. • Hepatic steatosis in HFD feeding varies in degree and seems to be dependent on various factors other than the diet, including the animal strain [10].
High-cholesterol diet (HCD)	• HCD causes the development of simple hepatic steatosis and a striking increase in serum insulin levels [20].	• HCD-fed mice display similar or only slightly increased liver weight, plasma triglyceride levels, free fatty acid levels, and serum ALT levels compared to the control diet fed animals [10,20].

Table 1. Cont.

	Advantages	Disadvantages
	NAFLD Mouse Models	
	Genetic Models	
db/db and *ob/ob* mice	• *db/db* and *ob/ob* mouse models develop characteristics and simulate many aspects of human metabolic syndrome, in contrast to various diet models [7,10]. • Useful models of NAFLD, since they develop marked hepatic steatosis under the administration of a standard diet without additional hits [10]. • They can develop steatohepatitis and be used to study NASH, as well, when a second hit is added, such as another type of diet [10].	• Congenital leptin deficiency or resistance caused by leptin or leptin receptor mutations are extremely rare in NASH patients and leptin levels poorly correlate with the progression of simple steatosis to steatohepatitis, limiting the ability of *db/db* and *ob/ob* mice to reflect the etiology of human obesity, insulin resistance, and hepatic steatosis [7,10,146]. • Leptin deficiency does not seem to play a role in NAFLD and NASH development in humans; on the contrary, serum leptin levels have been found elevated in NAFLD and NASH patients [147–149]. • *db/db* and *ob/ob* mice consist monogenic animal models and the observations derived from them may not apply to humans in whom obesity is typically multifactorial [11].
PNPLA3^{I148M} mice (PNPLA3 polymorphism)	• *PNPLA3*^{I148M} mice with *PNPLA3*^{I148M} overexpression in the liver develop hepatic steatosis characterized by increased levels of triacylglycerol and other lipids [31]. • *PNPLA3*^{I148M} mice under high-sucrose diet present even higher triacylglycerol and fatty acid levels and more pronounced steatosis [31,32].	• Hepatic fat levels remained unaltered and steatosis was not observed in *PNPLA3*^{I148M} mice under HFD [31]. • *PNPLA3*^{I148M} mice develop diet-dependent hepatic steatosis, pointing towards diet as being the primary cause for PNPLA3-polymorphism-associated steatosis, thus rendering these mice a model that does not cover the full spectrum of NAFLD [6,32].
Gankyrin (*Gank*)-deficient mice	• *Gank* liver-specific knockout mice with reduced liver proliferation develop pronounced macrovesicular hepatic steatosis, but no fibrosis after 6–7 months of HFD-feeding, in contrast to wild type littermates under the same diet that display lower steatosis and fibrosis [19]. • This animal model led to the conclusion that liver proliferation drives fibrosis, while steatosis could probably play a protective role and thus potential NAFLD therapeutic approaches oriented towards inhibition of proliferation rather than inhibition of steatosis should be further investigated [19].	

Table 1. *Cont.*

	Advantages	Disadvantages
	NASH Mouse Models	
	Diet-Induced Models	
Methionine and Choline Deficient diet (MCD)	• MCD diet better emulates the pathological image and mechanisms implicated in the pathogenesis of NASH in humans than other dietary models [10]. • Inflammation, fibrosis and apoptosis of hepatocytes developed more rapidly and severely than in mice fed an HFD or Western diets [10]. • Oxidative stress, endoplasmic reticulum stress, and autophagocytic stress, three important cell stress-related mechanisms implicated in human NASH pathogenesis are significantly more active in MCD than in other dietary models [150]. • Collectively, the MCD diet model is appropriate for studying histologically advanced NASH and the inflammation and fibrosis mechanisms in NASH [10].	• Significant differences from the metabolic profile of human NASH exist in MCD diet: mice fed an MCD diet are not obese, but on the contrary show significant weight loss, cachexia, no insulin resistance, and low serum insulin, fasting glucose, leptin and triglyceride levels [10,151,152]. The main risk factors for the development of NAFLD and NASH in humans, namely increased weight and insulin resistance are lacking in this model [11]. These discrepancies limit the use of MCD diet models. • Due to the aforementioned discrepancies, MCD diets are often fed to *db/db* or *ob/ob* mice to better mimic human NASH [10]. For example, *db/db* mice fed an MCD diet show marked hepatic inflammation and fibrosis [153]. • Mallory-Denk bodies have not been observed in MCD diet-fed mice [7]. • Different mouse strains display variable responsiveness to the MCD diet [10,11,154]. For example, C57BL/6N mice are more susceptible to NASH development when receiving the MCD diet in comparison with C3H/HeN mice [154].
Atherogenic diet	• Atherogenic diet simulates some etiologic aspects of human NASH [7].	• Weight loss, attenuation of insulin resistance and decreased serum triglyceride levels caused by atherogenic diet are not found in human NASH [7,40].
High-fat, high-cholesterol (HFHC) diets	• Supplementation of dietary cholesterol and combination with high fat content triggers experimental hepatic inflammation and fibrosis and closely resembles clinical NASH features [20].	
High-fat, High-fructose (HFHF) diets	• The obesity induced by HFHF diets appears to be a more robust model for human obesity in comparison with HFD [11]. • HFHF diets appear to be a more robust model of NASH compared to HFD as well.	• Lack of a standardized diet regime interferes with reproducibility [11].
Amylin Liver NASH (AMLN) model	• The modifications made to the ALIOS model based on which the AMLN model was developed, namely the higher cholesterol content (2%) and the fact that fructose (22% by weight) was included in the food pellets rather than the drinking water, better mimicked the Western-type diet and the subsequent NASH occurrence [49].	• NASH takes quite a long time to develop in wild type C57BL/6 mice after AMLN diet consumption [49], while acceleration of this process requires the administration of this diet to leptin-deficient *ob/ob* mice [50,51].

Table 1. Cont.

	Advantages	Disadvantages
NASH Mouse Models		
Diet-Induced Models		
Gubra amylin NASH diet (GAN diet)	• GAN diet is highly obesogenic and leads to the development of fibrotic NASH characteristics in *ob/ob* and wild type C57BL/6 mice, rendering it a suitable diet for preclinical therapeutic testing against NASH [53,54]. • This diet induces a NASH image similar to that caused by AMLN diet, but with the substitution of trans-fats with saturated fats, following the latest FDA guidelines and by better replicating the Western type diet consumed by humans [53].	• Fibrotic NASH takes longer to develop in wild type C57BL/6 mice after GAN diet consumption, compared to leptin-deficient *ob/ob* mice [53].
Fast-food-like diet (High-fat/high-fructose/high-cholesterol diet)	• *ob/ob* mice consuming fast-food like diet develop metabolic, histological and transcriptomic characteristics similar to human NASH, and, thus, can serve as a preclinical model for testing drugs against NASH [55].	
Genetic Models		
db/db mice with iron supplementation	• Progression from NAFLD to NASH when genetically obese *db/db* mice are fed a chow diet with high iron content points towards a multifactorial role for iron overload in NASH pathogenesis in the setting of obesity and metabolic syndrome [58].	• NASH development with a chow diet (even in the presence of excess iron) raises concerns about the translatability of this model [8].
foz/foz mice	• *foz/foz* mice fed a chow diet are obese, hyperphagic, develop glucose intolerance, insulin resistance, decreased adiponectin levels, increased total cholesterol, and their livers have increased weight, impaired function and steatosis [61]. • Administration of an HFD leads to severe NASH progression with major upregulation of ALT levels, hepatocyte ballooning, inflammation, and fibrosis, among other manifestations [59,62].	• While both *foz/foz* C57BL/6 and *foz/foz* BALB/c mice become similarly obese after HFD feeding, *foz/foz* C57BL/6 develop more severe NASH, as indicated by higher NAFLD activity scores, fibrosis, hepatocyte ballooning and other necroinflammatory changes, implying that the severity of NASH in *foz/foz* mice is inconsistent and strain-dependent [63]. • The exact role of *Alms1* gene is not fully understood and as a consequence the translational character of *foz/foz* model is rather limited [6].

Table 1. *Cont.*

	Advantages	Disadvantages
	NASH Mouse Models	
	Genetic Models	
MS-NASH mice	• Unlike monogenic leptin deficient *ob/ob* or *db/db* mice, the MS-NASH mice are a polygenic model prone to obesity and type 2 diabetes when fed a standard chow diet, but have an intact leptin pathway, making this model more translatable to the human disease [67]. • Given the metabolic status dysregulation when these mice are fed a Western-type, fructose-supplemented diet, this model can serve as a novel tool for studying NAFLD/NASH with high translational value [6].	• Selective inbreeding can cause significant decrease in the genetic variability that may introduce a bias in preclinical drug testing [11].
Ldlr−/− (low-density lipoprotein receptor knockout)/ Ldlr−/−.Leiden mice	• While most animal models for NASH imitate particularly the late stages of human disease, *ldlr*−/− mice focus on inflammatory response developing early within NASH, thus they can serve as a physiological model to study the early onset of NASH [70]. • Although fibrosis is rather mild, the *ldlr*−/− mice develop more fibrosis compared to C57BL/6 mice consuming a similar high-fat diet supplemented with cholesterol [70]. • *ldlr*−/−.Leiden mice can serve as a translational model of NASH with progressive liver fibrosis and simultaneous atherosclerosis development that can recapitulate human NASH, as indicated by hepatic transcriptome analysis [72]. • Adaptation of the fat content of the HFD or fast food diet (FFD) administered to *ldlr*−/−.Leiden mice, can aggravate either the insulin resistance (HFD), or the hepatic inflammation and fibrosis (FFD) of the animals [72].	• Sex differences are observed between *ldlr*−/−.Leiden mice when fed an HFD (45% kcal fat) for 18 weeks, with female mice being characterized by increased perigonadal fat mass, marked macrovesicular hepatic steatosis and liver inflammation and male mice displaying increased mesenteric fat mass, pronounced adipose tissue inflammation and microvesicular hepatic steatosis [155]. • At young age, male *ldlr*−/−.Leiden mice are more susceptible to the detrimental effects of HFD than female ones [155].
Prostaglandin E2(PGE2)-deficient mice	• Attenuation of PGE2 production by *mPGES-1* ablation in mice enhanced the inflammatory responses caused by TNF-α as well as hepatocyte apoptosis in diet-induced NASH [73].	• The lack of genotype-specific differences in macrophage infiltration or fibrosis in PGE2 deficient mice under a cholesterol-enriched HFD denotes that duration of the feeding intervention (20 weeks) was probably not long enough to allow the development of more advanced stages of the disease [73].
APOE2ki mice	• APOE2ki mice on an HFC (42% energy as milk butter/fat, 0.2% cholesterol, 46% carbohydrates) develop early-onset (from the first seven days) increased inflammation indicative of NASH [70,75].	• The inflammatory response is not sustained in APOE2ki mice, as shown by the gene expression levels of inflammatory genes, and the numbers of infiltrating inflammatory cells that are reduced after three months of HFC diet [70]. • Thus, probably the APOE2 isoform is not directly implicated in inflammation [70].

Table 1. *Cont.*

	Advantages	Disadvantages
NASH Mouse Models		
Genetic Models		
Apolipoprotein E-deficient (ApoE−/−) mice	• ApoE−/− mice rapidly develop NASH within seven weeks of HFD usually—but not always—supplemented with cholesterol. In contrast, other dietary NASH models require a minimum of 15 weeks of diet or even longer induction time [76].	• ApoE−/− mice spontaneously developed atherosclerotic plaques, while displaying some difference from humanized lipoprotein profiles, which suggests that this model is probably less suitable for human NAFLD research [6,76,156]. • ApoE−/− mice show an obesity-resistant phenotype, resulting in remarkable insulin sensitivity, which is in contrast to what is noted for NAFLD in humans [157].
Chemically Induced Models		
Carbon tetrachloride (CCl$_4$) administration	• CCl$_4$ administration is an alternative way to study the development and progression of liver fibrosis [92]. • Combined administration of HFD, CCl$_4$ and a Liver X receptor (LXR) agonist led to the generation of an experimental model with histopathology and pathophysiology similar to human NASH [93].	• The exact pathophysiological mechanism driving fibrinogenesis in the liver, and the role of hepatic stellate cells need further investigation [6].
Thioacetamide (TAA) administration in combination to fast-food diet	• This model develops hepatic inflammation, fibrosis, and collagen deposition, hallmarks of human NASH and NASH-related liver injury [94]. • The rapid development of these features in eight weeks makes this model promising for drug discovery investigation [94].	• The mice of this model do not gain weight compared to control mice on chow diet and with no TAA injection, which is a significant discrepancy from human NAFLD/NASH [94].
Thermoneutral Housing		
Thermoneutral housing	• Thermoneutral housing combined with HFD leads to increased intestinal permeability and intestinal microbiome dysbiosis, features mimicking human NASH [95].	• No signs of liver fibrosis were observed neither in male nor in female mice under HFD and thermoneutral housing, pointing towards the need for an additional dietary stimulus to induce liver fibrosis development [6,95].
NASH-HCC Mouse Models		
Diet-Induced Models		
Choline-deficient L-amino acid-defined (CDAA) diet	• The combination of CDAA diet with HFD (CDAA + 60% kcal fat and 0.1% methionine by weight) can act as an improved CDAA model of rapidly progressive liver fibrosis, capable of reproducing the development of NASH, providing better understanding of human NASH and useful for the development of efficient therapies [6,98].	• Humanized features of metabolic disturbances are missing in this model [6]. • Due to low reproducibility among the different sources of CDAA diet, this model should not be used to study the metabolic profile of the disease [11].

Table 1. Cont.

	Advantages	Disadvantages
	NASH-HCC Mouse Models	
	Diet-Induced Models	
Choline-deficient, ethionine-supplemented (CDE) diet	• CDE diet induces steatohepatitis and inflammation in a relatively short period of time [11,101]. • It recapitulates most of the stages of the spectrum of human NAFLD, progressing from liver damage to fibrosis, and finally HCC [102]. • The fact that ethionine is also hepatocarcinogenic (produces hypomethylated DNA) makes this diet an interesting model for the study of steatohepatitis-related HCC [11,102,158].	• CDE diet leads to weight loss in the animals to which it is administered and brings about high levels of mortality, reaching 60% after 4 months of feeding [11,102,103].
American lifestyle induced obesity syndrome (ALIOS) diet	• The ALIOS diet when administered in mice mimics many of the clinical characteristics of NAFLD and, due to this reason, it serves as a robust and reproducible model for the investigation of NAFLD pathogenesis and progression [105].	• The dietary composition of ALIOS diet differs from that normally consumed by humans, since the amount of trans fat per kilogram is greater than in commonly consumed fast food [6,104].
Diet-induced animal model of non-alcoholic fatty liver disease (DIAMOND)	• DIAMOND mice when fed a Western-type diet (42% kcal fat, 0.1% cholesterol, 23.1 g/L D-fructose and 18.9 g/L D-glucose in drinking water) progressively mimic all key physiological, metabolic, histologic, transcriptomic and cell-signaling features of human NAFLD with progression to NASH and culminating in HCC after four months [107]. • This model can serve as a preclinical model for the development of therapeutic targets of NASH [107].	• A limitation of the DIAMOND model is that HCC develops in a high frequency, while in humans only a small proportion of NAFLD patients finally develops HCC [107]. • DIAMOND mice do not develop neither significant atherosclerosis, nor fully established cirrhosis by week 52, features commonly seen in humans with obesity and NAFLD [107].
	Genetic Models	
Tm6sf2 hepatic knockdown or knockout	• *Tm6sf2* knockdown or knockout in mice livers upregulates hepatic triglyceride content and significantly decreases plasma cholesterol levels, leading to hepatic steatosis pointing towards a defect in VLDL secretion under normal chow diet, with these effects being exacerbated when those mice consume high-sucrose diets, leading to fibrosis development and even HCC after chemical/dietary tumorigenesis induction [108,109]. • Therefore, knockdown of *Tm6sf2* selectively in mouse liver mimics the effects on hepatic triglyceride content and plasma lipids of the Glu167Lys TM6SF2 variant observed in humans [108].	• *Tm6sf2*−/− mice replicate the human phenotype of the disease but are not very suitable for detailed mechanistic studies, a fact that led Luo et al. to the development of *Tm6sf2*−/− rats [110].

Table 1. Cont.

	Advantages	Disadvantages
	NASH-HCC Mouse Models	
	Genetic Models	
Fatty liver Shionogi (FLS) mice and FLS-*ob/ob* mice	• FLS mice spontaneously develop hepatic steatosis, NASH after 2–4 months of age and liver tumors, including HCC after 12 months, although at a frequency less than 50% [111,112]. FLS-*ob/ob* mice are hyperphagic, obese with type 2 diabetes, hyperlipidemic and hyperinsulinemic, with severe steatosis in their livers, inflammatory changes, increased oxidative stress with advanced fibrosis, elevated levels of apoptosis later in life and spontaneous appearance of liver tumors [114,115]. Thus, it seems that these models can mimic the whole spectrum and progression of NAFLD.	• The FLS mice (and not the FLS-*ob/ob*) display a very low rate of HCC incidence and heterogeneity of tumorigenesis; this model needs a long time to be established, and together with the fact that spontaneous HCC models are considered uncontrollable and unpredicted system, this model is rarely used [159].
Phosphatase and tensin homolog (PTEN)-deficient mice	• *PTEN*-deficient mice develop hepatic steatosis, progressing to NASH and HCC development as they grow older up to 74–78 weeks of age, thus this model can prove useful for understanding NASH pathogenesis, progression from NASH to HCC and even for the development of potential NASH treatments [116,118].	• These mice show insulin hypersensitivity and decreased body fat mass, characteristics that contrast with human NASH and limit the translational potential of the model [160].
Augmenter of liver regeneration (Alr) hepatic knockout (ALR-H-KO) mice	• ALR-H-KO mice develop hepatic steatosis early in life, and although this is reversed between 2–4 weeks of age, they proceed to developing NASH, while HCC occurs at a frequency of about 60% after one year of life, thus they can provide a useful model for investigating the pathogenesis of steatohepatitis and its complications and can help in better understanding the progression from hepatic necrosis, inflammation and fibrosis to carcinogenesis [6,119].	
Melanocortin 4 receptor knockout (*Mc4r−/−*) mice	• *Mc4r−/−* mice can serve as a NASH model used to investigate the sequence of events that lead to diet-induced hepatic steatosis, liver fibrosis, and HCC [121]. • HFD-fed *Mc4r−/−* mice closely mimic the liver pathology and function of human NASH and could prove useful for the study of hepatic dysfunction during the fibrotic stage and generally advanced stages of NASH and of the potential effects of drugs on NASH development after HFD feeding [123].	

Table 1. Cont.

	Advantages	Disadvantages
NASH-HCC Mouse Models		
Genetic Models		
Tsumura-Suzuki Obese Diabetes (TSOD) mice	• TSOD mice spontaneously develop NAFLD features, such as obesity, type 2 diabetes, hyperglycemia without any special treatment, diet or genetic manipulation, that quickly (after 3–4 months) proceed to NASH and lead to HCC after 12 months of age [125–127]. • The NASH and HCC that the mice develop display many human-like characteristics, rendering this model a promising one for translational research of the NAFLD/NASH-HCC sequence and for the development of potential therapies [125,127].	
Keratin 18-deficient (Krt18−/−) mice	• Krt-18−/− mice develop steatosis increasing with age, as well as progression to NASH and HCC that share several key characteristics with human disease, suggesting that this model can be used to dissect molecular pathways between NASH and HCC [131]. • Interestingly, the male mice of this animal model display liver tumor formation at a higher frequency than female mice, as also observed in humans [131].	
Methionine adenosyltransferase 1A (Mat1a) knockout mice	• *Methionine adenosyltransferase 1A (Mat1a)* gene deletion in mice impaired VLDL synthesis and plasma lipid homeostasis, thereby contributing to NAFLD development and spontaneous progression to NASH and HCC with increasing age [132–134].	
Liver-specific deletion of NF-κB essential modulator (Nemo) in mice (NEMO^{LPC-KO} mice)	• Liver-specific deletion of *NF-κB essential modulator (Nemo)* leads to the occurrence of steatosis, NASH, inflammatory fibrosis and subsequently HCC with increasing age [135].	
Circadian clock oscillations	• Chronic disruption of circadian rhythm can spontaneously lead to NAFLD progressing to NASH, fibrosis, and cirrhosis, similar to the human situation, pointing towards its translational value [6,139].	
Chemically Induced Models		
Carbon tetrachloride (CCl$_4$) administration in combination with Western diet	• Combination of Western type diet, high-sugar drinking solution and CCl$_4$ results in a mouse model with rapid progression of steatosis, advanced fibrosis and HCC, which also shares many histological, immunological and transcriptomic characteristics with human NASH, rendering it a possible useful experimental tool for preclinical drug testing [141].	• The addition of CCl$_4$ to Western diet results in blunting of weight gain and insulin resistance in those mice, typical features of NAFLD patients [141].

Table 1. *Cont.*

	Advantages	Disadvantages
NASH-HCC Mouse Models		
Chemically Induced Models		
STAM model	• Hepatic lipidemic profile of STAM mice shares many common characteristics with human NASH, despite the chemical intervention and the absence of obesity in this model [161]. • NAFLD progression is an artificial process in this model and cannot accurately mimic the human disease pathology, limiting its preclinical potential [6].	• This model represents NASH with diabetic background [143]. • Weight gain and insulin levels of the STAM model mice are reduced compared to HFD-fed mice [161].

Author Contributions: Writing—original draft preparation, C.-M.F.; writing—review and editing, N.N.-A., I.K., B.M.L., M.L., A.C., G.K., E.K. and H.S.R.; supervision, E.K. and H.S.R. All authors have read and agreed to the published version of the manuscript.

Funding: This research received no external funding.

Institutional Review Board Statement: Not applicable.

Informed Consent Statement: Not applicable.

Data Availability Statement: Not applicable.

Conflicts of Interest: The authors declare no conflict of interest.

References

1. Powell, E.E.; Wong, V.W.; Rinella, M. Non-alcoholic fatty liver disease. *Lancet* **2021**, *397*, 2212–2224. [CrossRef]
2. Younossi, Z.; Anstee, Q.M.; Marietti, M.; Hardy, T.; Henry, L.; Eslam, M.; George, J.; Bugianesi, E. Global burden of NAFLD and NASH: Trends, predictions, risk factors and prevention. *Nat. Rev. Gastroenterol. Hepatol.* **2018**, *15*, 11–20. [CrossRef]
3. Makri, E.; Goulas, A.; Polyzos, S.A. Epidemiology, Pathogenesis, Diagnosis and Emerging Treatment of Nonalcoholic Fatty Liver Disease. *Arch. Med. Res.* **2021**, *52*, 25–37. [CrossRef]
4. Brunt, E.M.; Neuschwander-Tetri, B.A.; Burt, A.D. 6—Fatty liver disease: Alcoholic and non-alcoholic. In *MacSween's Pathology of the Liver*, 6th ed.; Burt, A.D., Portmann, B.C., Ferrell, L.D., Eds.; Churchill Livingstone: Edinburgh, UK, 2012; pp. 293–359. [CrossRef]
5. Buzzetti, E.; Pinzani, M.; Tsochatzis, E.A. The multiple-hit pathogenesis of non-alcoholic fatty liver disease (NAFLD). *Metabolism* **2016**, *65*, 1038–1048. [CrossRef]
6. Oligschlaeger, Y.; Shiri-Sverdlov, R. NAFLD Preclinical Models: More than a Handful, Less of a Concern? *Biomedicines* **2020**, *8*, 28. [CrossRef]
7. Denk, H.; Abuja, P.M.; Zatloukal, K. Animal models of NAFLD from the pathologist's point of view. *Biochim. Biophys. Acta Mol. Basis Dis.* **2019**, *1865*, 929–942. [CrossRef]
8. Santhekadur, P.K.; Kumar, D.P.; Sanyal, A.J. Preclinical models of non-alcoholic fatty liver disease. *J. Hepatol.* **2018**, *68*, 230–237. [CrossRef]
9. Mann, J.P.; Semple, R.K.; Armstrong, M.J. How Useful Are Monogenic Rodent Models for the Study of Human Non-Alcoholic Fatty Liver Disease? *Front. Endocrinol.* **2016**, *7*, 145. [CrossRef]
10. Lau, J.K.; Zhang, X.; Yu, J. Animal models of non-alcoholic fatty liver disease: Current perspectives and recent advances. *J. Pathol.* **2017**, *241*, 36–44. [CrossRef]
11. Soret, P.A.; Magusto, J.; Housset, C.; Gautheron, J. In Vitro and In Vivo Models of Non-Alcoholic Fatty Liver Disease: A Critical Appraisal. *J Clin Med* **2020**, *10*, 36. [CrossRef]
12. Hariri, N.; Thibault, L. High-fat diet-induced obesity in animal models. *Nutr. Res. Rev.* **2010**, *23*, 270–299. [CrossRef]
13. Nevzorova, Y.A.; Boyer-Diaz, Z.; Cubero, F.J.; Gracia-Sancho, J. Animal models for liver disease—A practical approach for translational research. *J. Hepatol.* **2020**, *73*, 423–440. [CrossRef]
14. Samuels, L.T.; Gilmore, R.C.; Reinecke, R.M. The effect of previous diet on the ability of animals to do work during subsequent fasting. *J. Nutr.* **1948**, *36*, 639–651. [CrossRef]
15. Ito, M.; Suzuki, J.; Tsujioka, S.; Sasaki, M.; Gomori, A.; Shirakura, T.; Hirose, H.; Ito, M.; Ishihara, A.; Iwaasa, H.; et al. Longitudinal analysis of murine steatohepatitis model induced by chronic exposure to high-fat diet. *Hepatol. Res.* **2007**, *37*, 50–57. [CrossRef]

16. Lieber, C.S.; Leo, M.A.; Mak, K.M.; Xu, Y.; Cao, Q.; Ren, C.; Ponomarenko, A.; DeCarli, L.M. Model of nonalcoholic steatohepatitis. *Am. J. Clin. Nutr.* **2004**, *79*, 502–509. [CrossRef]
17. Eccleston, H.B.; Andringa, K.K.; Betancourt, A.M.; King, A.L.; Mantena, S.K.; Swain, T.M.; Tinsley, H.N.; Nolte, R.N.; Nagy, T.R.; Abrams, G.A.; et al. Chronic exposure to a high-fat diet induces hepatic steatosis, impairs nitric oxide bioavailability, and modifies the mitochondrial proteome in mice. *Antioxid. Redox Signal.* **2011**, *15*, 447–459. [CrossRef]
18. Velazquez, K.T.; Enos, R.T.; Bader, J.E.; Sougiannis, A.T.; Carson, M.S.; Chatzistamou, I.; Carson, J.A.; Nagarkatti, P.S.; Nagarkatti, M.; Murphy, E.A. Prolonged high-fat-diet feeding promotes non-alcoholic fatty liver disease and alters gut microbiota in mice. *World J. Hepatol.* **2019**, *11*, 619–637. [CrossRef]
19. Cast, A.; Kumbaji, M.; D'Souza, A.; Rodriguez, K.; Gupta, A.; Karns, R.; Timchenko, L.; Timchenko, N. Liver Proliferation Is an Essential Driver of Fibrosis in Mouse Models of Nonalcoholic Fatty Liver Disease. *Hepatol. Commun.* **2019**, *3*, 1036–1049. [CrossRef]
20. Savard, C.; Tartaglione, E.V.; Kuver, R.; Haigh, W.G.; Farrell, G.C.; Subramanian, S.; Chait, A.; Yeh, M.M.; Quinn, L.S.; Ioannou, G.N. Synergistic interaction of dietary cholesterol and dietary fat in inducing experimental steatohepatitis. *Hepatology* **2013**, *57*, 81–92. [CrossRef]
21. Hummel, K.P.; Dickie, M.M.; Coleman, D.L. Diabetes, a new mutation in the mouse. *Science* **1966**, *153*, 1127–1128. [CrossRef]
22. Trak-Smayra, V.; Paradis, V.; Massart, J.; Nasser, S.; Jebara, V.; Fromenty, B. Pathology of the liver in obese and diabetic ob/ob and db/db mice fed a standard or high-calorie diet. *Int. J. Exp. Pathol.* **2011**, *92*, 413–421. [CrossRef]
23. Ingalls, A.M.; Dickie, M.M.; Snell, G.D. Obese, a new mutation in the house mouse. *J. Hered.* **1950**, *41*, 317–318. [CrossRef]
24. Zhang, Y.; Proenca, R.; Maffei, M.; Barone, M.; Leopold, L.; Friedman, J.M. Positional cloning of the mouse obese gene and its human homologue. *Nature* **1994**, *372*, 425–432. [CrossRef]
25. Friedman, J.M.; Halaas, J.L. Leptin and the regulation of body weight in mammals. *Nature* **1998**, *395*, 763–770. [CrossRef]
26. Leclercq, I.A.; Farrell, G.C.; Schriemer, R.; Robertson, G.R. Leptin is essential for the hepatic fibrogenic response to chronic liver injury. *J. Hepatol.* **2002**, *37*, 206–213. [CrossRef]
27. Yang, S.Q.; Lin, H.Z.; Lane, M.D.; Clemens, M.; Diehl, A.M. Obesity increases sensitivity to endotoxin liver injury: Implications for the pathogenesis of steatohepatitis. *Proc. Natl. Acad. Sci. USA* **1997**, *94*, 2557–2562. [CrossRef]
28. Chavin, K.D.; Yang, S.; Lin, H.Z.; Chatham, J.; Chacko, V.P.; Hoek, J.B.; Walajtys-Rode, E.; Rashid, A.; Chen, C.H.; Huang, C.C.; et al. Obesity induces expression of uncoupling protein-2 in hepatocytes and promotes liver ATP depletion. *J. Biol. Chem.* **1999**, *274*, 5692–5700. [CrossRef]
29. Pingitore, P.; Romeo, S. The role of PNPLA3 in health and disease. *Biochim. Biophys. Acta Mol. Cell Biol. Lipids* **2019**, *1864*, 900–906. [CrossRef]
30. Trepo, E.; Valenti, L. Update on NAFLD genetics: From new variants to the clinic. *J. Hepatol.* **2020**, *72*, 1196–1209. [CrossRef]
31. Li, J.Z.; Huang, Y.; Karaman, R.; Ivanova, P.T.; Brown, H.A.; Roddy, T.; Castro-Perez, J.; Cohen, J.C.; Hobbs, H.H. Chronic overexpression of PNPLA3I148M in mouse liver causes hepatic steatosis. *J. Clin. Investig.* **2012**, *122*, 4130–4144. [CrossRef]
32. Smagris, E.; BasuRay, S.; Li, J.; Huang, Y.; Lai, K.M.; Gromada, J.; Cohen, J.C.; Hobbs, H.H. Pnpla3I148M knockin mice accumulate PNPLA3 on lipid droplets and develop hepatic steatosis. *Hepatology* **2015**, *61*, 108–118. [CrossRef] [PubMed]
33. Lu, S.C. Regulation of glutathione synthesis. *Mol. Aspects Med.* **2009**, *30*, 42–59. [CrossRef] [PubMed]
34. Cole, L.K.; Vance, J.E.; Vance, D.E. Phosphatidylcholine biosynthesis and lipoprotein metabolism. *Biochim. Biophys. Acta* **2012**, *1821*, 754–761. [CrossRef] [PubMed]
35. Gibbons, G.F.; Wiggins, D.; Brown, A.M.; Hebbachi, A.M. Synthesis and function of hepatic very-low-density lipoprotein. *Biochem. Soc. Trans.* **2004**, *32*, 59–64. [CrossRef] [PubMed]
36. Yamada, T.; Obata, A.; Kashiwagi, Y.; Rokugawa, T.; Matsushima, S.; Hamada, T.; Watabe, H.; Abe, K. Gd-EOB-DTPA-enhanced-MR imaging in the inflammation stage of nonalcoholic steatohepatitis (NASH) in mice. *Magn. Reson. Imaging* **2016**, *34*, 724–729. [CrossRef]
37. Larter, C.Z.; Yeh, M.M.; Williams, J.; Bell-Anderson, K.S.; Farrell, G.C. MCD-induced steatohepatitis is associated with hepatic adiponectin resistance and adipogenic transformation of hepatocytes. *J. Hepatol.* **2008**, *49*, 407–416. [CrossRef]
38. Greene, M.W.; Burrington, C.M.; Lynch, D.T.; Davenport, S.K.; Johnson, A.K.; Horsman, M.J.; Chowdhry, S.; Zhang, J.; Sparks, J.D.; Tirrell, P.C. Lipid metabolism, oxidative stress and cell death are regulated by PKC delta in a dietary model of nonalcoholic steatohepatitis. *PLoS ONE* **2014**, *9*, e85848. [CrossRef]
39. Dela Pena, A.; Leclercq, I.; Field, J.; George, J.; Jones, B.; Farrell, G. NF-kappaB activation, rather than TNF, mediates hepatic inflammation in a murine dietary model of steatohepatitis. *Gastroenterology* **2005**, *129*, 1663–1674. [CrossRef]
40. Matsuzawa, N.; Takamura, T.; Kurita, S.; Misu, H.; Ota, T.; Ando, H.; Yokoyama, M.; Honda, M.; Zen, Y.; Nakanuma, Y.; et al. Lipid-induced oxidative stress causes steatohepatitis in mice fed an atherogenic diet. *Hepatology* **2007**, *46*, 1392–1403. [CrossRef]
41. Seki, A.; Sakai, Y.; Komura, T.; Nasti, A.; Yoshida, K.; Higashimoto, M.; Honda, M.; Usui, S.; Takamura, M.; Takamura, T.; et al. Adipose tissue-derived stem cells as a regenerative therapy for a mouse steatohepatitis-induced cirrhosis model. *Hepatology* **2013**, *58*, 1133–1142. [CrossRef]
42. Montandon, S.A.; Somm, E.; Loizides-Mangold, U.; de Vito, C.; Dibner, C.; Jornayvaz, F.R. Multi-technique comparison of atherogenic and MCD NASH models highlights changes in sphingolipid metabolism. *Sci. Rep.* **2019**, *9*, 16810. [CrossRef] [PubMed]

43. Chen, K.; Ma, J.; Jia, X.; Ai, W.; Ma, Z.; Pan, Q. Advancing the understanding of NAFLD to hepatocellular carcinoma development: From experimental models to humans. *Biochim. Biophys. Acta Rev. Cancer* **2019**, *1871*, 117–125. [CrossRef] [PubMed]
44. Itagaki, H.; Shimizu, K.; Morikawa, S.; Ogawa, K.; Ezaki, T. Morphological and functional characterization of non-alcoholic fatty liver disease induced by a methionine-choline-deficient diet in C57BL/6 mice. *Int. J. Clin. Exp. Pathol.* **2013**, *6*, 2683–2696. [PubMed]
45. Zheng, S.; Hoos, L.; Cook, J.; Tetzloff, G.; Davis, H., Jr.; van Heek, M.; Hwa, J.J. Ezetimibe improves high fat and cholesterol diet-induced non-alcoholic fatty liver disease in mice. *Eur. J. Pharmacol.* **2008**, *584*, 118–124. [CrossRef] [PubMed]
46. Henkel, J.; Coleman, C.D.; Schraplau, A.; Jhrens, K.; Weber, D.; Castro, J.P.; Hugo, M.; Schulz, T.J.; Kramer, S.; Schurmann, A.; et al. Induction of steatohepatitis (NASH) with insulin resistance in wildtype B6 mice by a western-type diet containing soybean oil and cholesterol. *Mol. Med.* **2017**, *23*, 70–82. [CrossRef] [PubMed]
47. Kohli, R.; Kirby, M.; Xanthakos, S.A.; Softic, S.; Feldstein, A.E.; Saxena, V.; Tang, P.H.; Miles, L.; Miles, M.V.; Balistreri, W.F.; et al. High-fructose, medium chain trans fat diet induces liver fibrosis and elevates plasma coenzyme Q9 in a novel murine model of obesity and nonalcoholic steatohepatitis. *Hepatology* **2010**, *52*, 934–944. [CrossRef]
48. Tsuchiya, H.; Ebata, Y.; Sakabe, T.; Hama, S.; Kogure, K.; Shiota, G. High-fat, high-fructose diet induces hepatic iron overload via a hepcidin-independent mechanism prior to the onset of liver steatosis and insulin resistance in mice. *Metabolism* **2013**, *62*, 62–69. [CrossRef] [PubMed]
49. Clapper, J.R.; Hendricks, M.D.; Gu, G.; Wittmer, C.; Dolman, C.S.; Herich, J.; Athanacio, J.; Villescaz, C.; Ghosh, S.S.; Heilig, J.S.; et al. Diet-induced mouse model of fatty liver disease and nonalcoholic steatohepatitis reflecting clinical disease progression and methods of assessment. *Am. J. Physiol. Gastrointest. Liver Physiol.* **2013**, *305*, G483–G495. [CrossRef] [PubMed]
50. Trevaskis, J.L.; Griffin, P.S.; Wittmer, C.; Neuschwander-Tetri, B.A.; Brunt, E.M.; Dolman, C.S.; Erickson, M.R.; Napora, J.; Parkes, D.G.; Roth, J.D. Glucagon-like peptide-1 receptor agonism improves metabolic, biochemical, and histopathological indices of nonalcoholic steatohepatitis in mice. *Am. J. Physiol. Gastrointest. Liver Physiol.* **2012**, *302*, G762–G772. [CrossRef]
51. Kristiansen, M.N.; Veidal, S.S.; Rigbolt, K.T.; Tolbol, K.S.; Roth, J.D.; Jelsing, J.; Vrang, N.; Feigh, M. Obese diet-induced mouse models of nonalcoholic steatohepatitis-tracking disease by liver biopsy. *World J. Hepatol.* **2016**, *8*, 673–684. [CrossRef]
52. Food and Drug Administration (Ed.) Final Determination Regarding Partially Hydrogenated Oils. *Fed. Regist.* **2018**, *83*, 23358–23359.
53. Boland, M.L.; Oro, D.; Tolbol, K.S.; Thrane, S.T.; Nielsen, J.C.; Cohen, T.S.; Tabor, D.E.; Fernandes, F.; Tovchigrechko, A.; Veidal, S.S.; et al. Towards a standard diet-induced and biopsy-confirmed mouse model of non-alcoholic steatohepatitis: Impact of dietary fat source. *World J. Gastroenterol.* **2019**, *25*, 4904–4920. [CrossRef] [PubMed]
54. Hansen, H.H.; HM, A.E.; Oro, D.; Evers, S.S.; Heeboll, S.; Eriksen, P.L.; Thomsen, K.L.; Bengtsson, A.; Veidal, S.S.; Feigh, M.; et al. Human translatability of the GAN diet-induced obese mouse model of non-alcoholic steatohepatitis. *BMC Gastroenterol.* **2020**, *20*, 210. [CrossRef] [PubMed]
55. Abe, N.; Kato, S.; Tsuchida, T.; Sugimoto, K.; Saito, R.; Verschuren, L.; Kleemann, R.; Oka, K. Longitudinal characterization of diet-induced genetic murine models of non-alcoholic steatohepatitis with metabolic, histological, and transcriptomic hallmarks of human patients. *Biol. Open* **2019**, *8*, bio041251. [CrossRef] [PubMed]
56. Kennedy, A.J.; Ellacott, K.L.; King, V.L.; Hasty, A.H. Mouse models of the metabolic syndrome. *Dis. Models Mech.* **2010**, *3*, 156–166. [CrossRef]
57. Charlton, M.; Krishnan, A.; Viker, K.; Sanderson, S.; Cazanave, S.; McConico, A.; Masuoko, H.; Gores, G. Fast food diet mouse: Novel small animal model of NASH with ballooning, progressive fibrosis, and high physiological fidelity to the human condition. *Am. J. Physiol. Gastrointest. Liver Physiol.* **2011**, *301*, G825–G834. [CrossRef]
58. Handa, P.; Morgan-Stevenson, V.; Maliken, B.D.; Nelson, J.E.; Washington, S.; Westerman, M.; Yeh, M.M.; Kowdley, K.V. Iron overload results in hepatic oxidative stress, immune cell activation, and hepatocellular ballooning injury, leading to nonalcoholic steatohepatitis in genetically obese mice. *Am. J. Physiol. Gastrointest. Liver Physiol.* **2016**, *310*, G117–G127. [CrossRef]
59. Arsov, T.; Silva, D.G.; O'Bryan, M.K.; Sainsbury, A.; Lee, N.J.; Kennedy, C.; Manji, S.S.; Nelms, K.; Liu, C.; Vinuesa, C.G.; et al. Fat aussie—A new Alstrom syndrome mouse showing a critical role for ALMS1 in obesity, diabetes, and spermatogenesis. *Mol. Endocrinol.* **2006**, *20*, 1610–1622. [CrossRef]
60. Heydet, D.; Chen, L.X.; Larter, C.Z.; Inglis, C.; Silverman, M.A.; Farrell, G.C.; Leroux, M.R. A truncating mutation of Alms1 reduces the number of hypothalamic neuronal cilia in obese mice. *Dev. Neurobiol.* **2013**, *73*, 1–13. [CrossRef]
61. Bell-Anderson, K.S.; Aouad, L.; Williams, H.; Sanz, F.R.; Phuyal, J.; Larter, C.Z.; Farrell, G.C.; Caterson, I.D. Coordinated improvement in glucose tolerance, liver steatosis and obesity-associated inflammation by cannabinoid 1 receptor antagonism in fat Aussie mice. *Int. J. Obes.* **2011**, *35*, 1539–1548. [CrossRef]
62. Arsov, T.; Larter, C.Z.; Nolan, C.J.; Petrovsky, N.; Goodnow, C.C.; Teoh, N.C.; Yeh, M.M.; Farrell, G.C. Adaptive failure to high-fat diet characterizes steatohepatitis in Alms1 mutant mice. *Biochem. Biophys. Res. Commun.* **2006**, *342*, 1152–1159. [CrossRef] [PubMed]
63. Farrell, G.C.; Mridha, A.R.; Yeh, M.M.; Arsov, T.; Van Rooyen, D.M.; Brooling, J.; Nguyen, T.; Heydet, D.; Delghingaro-Augusto, V.; Nolan, C.J.; et al. Strain dependence of diet-induced NASH and liver fibrosis in obese mice is linked to diabetes and inflammatory phenotype. *Liver Int.* **2014**, *34*, 1084–1093. [CrossRef] [PubMed]
64. Neff, E.P. Farewell, FATZO: A NASH mouse update. *Lab Anim.* **2019**, *48*, 151. [CrossRef] [PubMed]

65. Alexander, J.; Chang, G.Q.; Dourmashkin, J.T.; Leibowitz, S.F. Distinct phenotypes of obesity-prone AKR/J, DBA2J and C57BL/6J mice compared to control strains. *Int. J. Obes.* **2006**, *30*, 50–59. [CrossRef]
66. Peterson, R.G.; Jackson, C.V.; Zimmerman, K.M.; Alsina-Fernandez, J.; Michael, M.D.; Emmerson, P.J.; Coskun, T. Glucose dysregulation and response to common anti-diabetic agents in the FATZO/Pco mouse. *PLoS ONE* **2017**, *12*, e0179856. [CrossRef]
67. Sun, G.; Jackson, C.V.; Zimmerman, K.; Zhang, L.K.; Finnearty, C.M.; Sandusky, G.E.; Zhang, G.; Peterson, R.G.; Wang, Y.J. The FATZO mouse, a next generation model of type 2 diabetes, develops NAFLD and NASH when fed a Western diet supplemented with fructose. *BMC Gastroenterol.* **2019**, *19*, 41. [CrossRef]
68. Wouters, K.; van Gorp, P.J.; Bieghs, V.; Gijbels, M.J.; Duimel, H.; Lutjohann, D.; Kerksiek, A.; van Kruchten, R.; Maeda, N.; Staels, B.; et al. Dietary cholesterol, rather than liver steatosis, leads to hepatic inflammation in hyperlipidemic mouse models of nonalcoholic steatohepatitis. *Hepatology* **2008**, *48*, 474–486. [CrossRef]
69. Aravani, D.; Kassi, E.; Chatzigeorgiou, A.; Vakrou, S. Cardiometabolic Syndrome: An Update on Available Mouse Models. *Thromb. Haemost.* **2021**, *121*, 703–715. [CrossRef]
70. Bieghs, V.; Van Gorp, P.J.; Wouters, K.; Hendrikx, T.; Gijbels, M.J.; van Bilsen, M.; Bakker, J.; Binder, C.J.; Lutjohann, D.; Staels, B.; et al. LDL receptor knock-out mice are a physiological model particularly vulnerable to study the onset of inflammation in non-alcoholic fatty liver disease. *PLoS ONE* **2012**, *7*, e30668. [CrossRef]
71. Subramanian, S.; Goodspeed, L.; Wang, S.; Kim, J.; Zeng, L.; Ioannou, G.N.; Haigh, W.G.; Yeh, M.M.; Kowdley, K.V.; O'Brien, K.D.; et al. Dietary cholesterol exacerbates hepatic steatosis and inflammation in obese LDL receptor-deficient mice. *J. Lipid Res.* **2011**, *52*, 1626–1635. [CrossRef]
72. van den Hoek, A.M.; Verschuren, L.; Worms, N.; van Nieuwkoop, A.; de Ruiter, C.; Attema, J.; Menke, A.L.; Caspers, M.P.M.; Radhakrishnan, S.; Salic, K.; et al. A Translational Mouse Model for NASH with Advanced Fibrosis and Atherosclerosis Expressing Key Pathways of Human Pathology. *Cells* **2020**, *9*, 2014. [CrossRef]
73. Henkel, J.; Coleman, C.D.; Schraplau, A.; Johrens, K.; Weiss, T.S.; Jonas, W.; Schurmann, A.; Puschel, G.P. Augmented liver inflammation in a microsomal prostaglandin E synthase 1 (mPGES-1)-deficient diet-induced mouse NASH model. *Sci. Rep.* **2018**, *8*, 16127. [CrossRef] [PubMed]
74. Sullivan, P.M.; Mezdour, H.; Quarfordt, S.H.; Maeda, N. Type III hyperlipoproteinemia and spontaneous atherosclerosis in mice resulting from gene replacement of mouse Apoe with human Apoe*2. *J. Clin. Investig.* **1998**, *102*, 130–135. [CrossRef] [PubMed]
75. Baron, M.; Leroyer, A.S.; Majd, Z.; Lalloyer, F.; Vallez, E.; Bantubungi, K.; Chinetti-Gbaguidi, G.; Delerive, P.; Boulanger, C.M.; Staels, B.; et al. PPARalpha activation differently affects microparticle content in atherosclerotic lesions and liver of a mouse model of atherosclerosis and NASH. *Atherosclerosis* **2011**, *218*, 69–76. [CrossRef]
76. Schierwagen, R.; Maybuchen, L.; Zimmer, S.; Hittatiya, K.; Back, C.; Klein, S.; Uschner, F.E.; Reul, W.; Boor, P.; Nickenig, G.; et al. Seven weeks of Western diet in apolipoprotein-E-deficient mice induce metabolic syndrome and non-alcoholic steatohepatitis with liver fibrosis. *Sci. Rep.* **2015**, *5*, 12931. [CrossRef] [PubMed]
77. Zang, S.; Wang, L.; Ma, X.; Zhu, G.; Zhuang, Z.; Xun, Y.; Zhao, F.; Yang, W.; Liu, J.; Luo, Y.; et al. Neutrophils Play a Crucial Role in the Early Stage of Nonalcoholic Steatohepatitis via Neutrophil Elastase in Mice. *Cell Biochem. Biophys.* **2015**, *73*, 479–487. [CrossRef]
78. Allen, J.N.; Dey, A.; Cai, J.; Zhang, J.; Tian, Y.; Kennett, M.; Ma, Y.; Liang, T.J.; Patterson, A.D.; Hankey-Giblin, P.A. Metabolic Profiling Reveals Aggravated Non-Alcoholic Steatohepatitis in High-Fat High-Cholesterol Diet-Fed Apolipoprotein E-Deficient Mice Lacking Ron Receptor Signaling. *Metabolites* **2020**, *10*, 326. [CrossRef]
79. Luo, Y.; Dong, X.; Yu, Y.; Sun, G.; Sun, X. Total aralosides of aralia elata (Miq) seem (TASAES) ameliorate nonalcoholic steatohepatitis by modulating IRE1alpha-mediated JNK and NF-kappaB pathways in ApoE−/− mice. *J. Ethnopharmacol.* **2015**, *163*, 241–250. [CrossRef]
80. Han, H.; Qiu, F.; Zhao, H.; Tang, H.; Li, X.; Shi, D. Dietary Flaxseed Oil Prevents Western-Type Diet-Induced Nonalcoholic Fatty Liver Disease in Apolipoprotein-E Knockout Mice. *Oxid. Med. Cell. Longev.* **2017**, *2017*, 3256241. [CrossRef]
81. Jeon, S.; Park, Y.J.; Kwon, Y.H. Genistein alleviates the development of nonalcoholic steatohepatitis in ApoE(−/−) mice fed a high-fat diet. *Mol. Nutr. Food Res.* **2014**, *58*, 830–841. [CrossRef]
82. Torres, S.; Brol, M.J.; Magdaleno, F.; Schierwagen, R.; Uschner, F.E.; Klein, S.; Ortiz, C.; Tyc, O.; Bachtler, N.; Stunden, J.; et al. The Specific NLRP3 Antagonist IFM-514 Decreases Fibrosis and Inflammation in Experimental Murine Non-Alcoholic Steatohepatitis. *Front. Mol. Biosci.* **2021**, *8*, 715765. [CrossRef] [PubMed]
83. Wang, D.; Cong, H.; Wang, X.; Cao, Y.; Ikuyama, S.; Fan, B.; Gu, J. Pycnogenol protects against diet-induced hepatic steatosis in apolipoprotein-E-deficient mice. *Am. J. Physiol. Endocrinol. Metab.* **2018**, *315*, E218–E228. [CrossRef] [PubMed]
84. Huang, W.C.; Xu, J.W.; Li, S.; Ng, X.E.; Tung, Y.T. Effects of exercise on high-fat diet-induced non-alcoholic fatty liver disease and lipid metabolism in ApoE knockout mice. *Nutr. Metab.* **2022**, *19*, 10. [CrossRef] [PubMed]
85. Nasiri-Ansari, N.; Nikolopoulou, C.; Papoutsi, K.; Kyrou, I.; Mantzoros, C.S.; Kyriakopoulos, G.; Chatzigeorgiou, A.; Kalotychou, V.; Randeva, M.S.; Chatha, K.; et al. Empagliflozin Attenuates Non-Alcoholic Fatty Liver Disease (NAFLD) in High Fat Diet Fed ApoE((−/−)) Mice by Activating Autophagy and Reducing ER Stress and Apoptosis. *Int. J. Mol. Sci.* **2021**, *22*, 818. [CrossRef] [PubMed]
86. Zheng, F.; Cai, Y. Concurrent exercise improves insulin resistance and nonalcoholic fatty liver disease by upregulating PPAR-gamma and genes involved in the beta-oxidation of fatty acids in ApoE-KO mice fed a high-fat diet. *Lipids Health Dis.* **2019**, *18*, 6. [CrossRef]

87. Chen, W.; Zhang, X.; Xu, M.; Jiang, L.; Zhou, M.; Liu, W.; Chen, Z.; Wang, Y.; Zou, Q.; Wang, L. Betaine prevented high-fat diet-induced NAFLD by regulating the FGF10/AMPK signaling pathway in ApoE($-/-$) mice. *Eur. J. Nutr.* **2021**, *60*, 1655–1668. [CrossRef]
88. Wisniewska, A.; Stachowicz, A.; Kus, K.; Ulatowska-Bialas, M.; Toton-Zuranska, J.; Kiepura, A.; Stachyra, K.; Suski, M.; Gajda, M.; Jawien, J.; et al. Inhibition of Atherosclerosis and Liver Steatosis by Agmatine in Western Diet-Fed apoE-Knockout Mice Is Associated with Decrease in Hepatic De Novo Lipogenesis and Reduction in Plasma Triglyceride/High-Density Lipoprotein Cholesterol Ratio. *Int. J. Mol. Sci.* **2021**, *22*, 688. [CrossRef]
89. Santos-Sanchez, G.; Cruz-Chamorro, I.; Alvarez-Rios, A.I.; Fernandez-Santos, J.M.; Vazquez-Roman, M.V.; Rodriguez-Ortiz, B.; Alvarez-Sanchez, N.; Alvarez-Lopez, A.I.; Millan-Linares, M.D.C.; Millan, F.; et al. Lupinus angustifolius Protein Hydrolysates Reduce Abdominal Adiposity and Ameliorate Metabolic Associated Fatty Liver Disease (MAFLD) in Western Diet Fed-ApoE($-/-$) Mice. *Antioxidants* **2021**, *10*, 1222. [CrossRef]
90. Ma, Y.; Chen, K.; Lv, L.; Wu, S.; Guo, Z. Ferulic acid ameliorates nonalcoholic fatty liver disease and modulates the gut microbiota composition in high-fat diet fed ApoE($-/-$) mice. *Biomed. Pharmacother.* **2019**, *113*, 108753. [CrossRef]
91. Joo, H.K.; Lee, Y.R.; Lee, E.O.; Kim, S.; Jin, H.; Kim, S.; Lim, Y.P.; An, C.G.; Jeon, B.H. Protective Role of Dietary Capsanthin in a Mouse Model of Nonalcoholic Fatty Liver Disease. *J. Med. Food* **2021**, *24*, 635–644. [CrossRef]
92. Domitrovic, R.; Jakovac, H.; Tomac, J.; Sain, I. Liver fibrosis in mice induced by carbon tetrachloride and its reversion by luteolin. *Toxicol. Appl. Pharmacol.* **2009**, *241*, 311–321. [CrossRef] [PubMed]
93. Owada, Y.; Tamura, T.; Tanoi, T.; Ozawa, Y.; Shimizu, Y.; Hisakura, K.; Matsuzaka, T.; Shimano, H.; Nakano, N.; Sakashita, S.; et al. Novel non-alcoholic steatohepatitis model with histopathological and insulin-resistant features. *Pathol. Int.* **2018**, *68*, 12–22. [CrossRef] [PubMed]
94. Sharma, L.; Gupta, D.; Abdullah, S.T. Thioacetamide potentiates high cholesterol and high fat diet induced steato-hepatitic changes in livers of C57BL/6J mice: A novel eight weeks model of fibrosing NASH. *Toxicol. Lett.* **2019**, *304*, 21–29. [CrossRef] [PubMed]
95. Giles, D.A.; Moreno-Fernandez, M.E.; Stankiewicz, T.E.; Graspeuntner, S.; Cappelletti, M.; Wu, D.; Mukherjee, R.; Chan, C.C.; Lawson, M.J.; Klarquist, J.; et al. Erratum: Thermoneutral housing exacerbates nonalcoholic fatty liver disease in mice and allows for sex-independent disease modeling. *Nat. Med.* **2017**, *23*, 1241. [CrossRef]
96. Denda, A.; Kitayama, W.; Kishida, H.; Murata, N.; Tsutsumi, M.; Tsujiuchi, T.; Nakae, D.; Konishi, Y. Development of hepatocellular adenomas and carcinomas associated with fibrosis in C57BL/6J male mice given a choline-deficient, L-amino acid-defined diet. *Jpn. J. Cancer Res.* **2002**, *93*, 125–132. [CrossRef]
97. De Minicis, S.; Agostinelli, L.; Rychlicki, C.; Sorice, G.P.; Saccomanno, S.; Candelaresi, C.; Giaccari, A.; Trozzi, L.; Pierantonelli, I.; Mingarelli, E.; et al. HCC development is associated to peripheral insulin resistance in a mouse model of NASH. *PLoS ONE* **2014**, *9*, e97136. [CrossRef]
98. Matsumoto, M.; Hada, N.; Sakamaki, Y.; Uno, A.; Shiga, T.; Tanaka, C.; Ito, T.; Katsume, A.; Sudoh, M. An improved mouse model that rapidly develops fibrosis in non-alcoholic steatohepatitis. *Int. J. Exp. Pathol.* **2013**, *94*, 93–103. [CrossRef]
99. Kodama, Y.; Kisseleva, T.; Iwaisako, K.; Miura, K.; Taura, K.; De Minicis, S.; Osterreicher, C.H.; Schnabl, B.; Seki, E.; Brenner, D.A. c-Jun N-terminal kinase-1 from hematopoietic cells mediates progression from hepatic steatosis to steatohepatitis and fibrosis in mice. *Gastroenterology* **2009**, *137*, 1467–1477 e1465. [CrossRef]
100. Miura, K.; Kodama, Y.; Inokuchi, S.; Schnabl, B.; Aoyama, T.; Ohnishi, H.; Olefsky, J.M.; Brenner, D.A.; Seki, E. Toll-like receptor 9 promotes steatohepatitis by induction of interleukin-1beta in mice. *Gastroenterology* **2010**, *139*, 323–334 e327. [CrossRef]
101. Passman, A.M.; Strauss, R.P.; McSpadden, S.B.; Finch-Edmondson, M.L.; Woo, K.H.; Diepeveen, L.A.; London, R.; Callus, B.A.; Yeoh, G.C. A modified choline-deficient, ethionine-supplemented diet reduces morbidity and retains a liver progenitor cell response in mice. *Dis. Model Mech.* **2015**, *8*, 1635–1641. [CrossRef]
102. Ochoa-Callejero, L.; Perez-Martinez, L.; Rubio-Mediavilla, S.; Oteo, J.A.; Martinez, A.; Blanco, J.R. Maraviroc, a CCR5 antagonist, prevents development of hepatocellular carcinoma in a mouse model. *PLoS ONE* **2013**, *8*, e53992. [CrossRef] [PubMed]
103. Gogoi-Tiwari, J.; Kohn-Gaone, J.; Giles, C.; Schmidt-Arras, D.; Gratte, F.D.; Elsegood, C.L.; McCaughan, G.W.; Ramm, G.A.; Olynyk, J.K.; Tirnitz-Parker, J.E.E. The Murine Choline-Deficient, Ethionine-Supplemented (CDE) Diet Model of Chronic Liver Injury. *J. Vis. Exp.* **2017**, *128*, 56138. [CrossRef] [PubMed]
104. Tetri, L.H.; Basaranoglu, M.; Brunt, E.M.; Yerian, L.M.; Neuschwander-Tetri, B.A. Severe NAFLD with hepatic necroinflammatory changes in mice fed trans fats and a high-fructose corn syrup equivalent. *Am. J. Physiol. Gastrointest. Liver Physiol.* **2008**, *295*, G987–G995. [CrossRef] [PubMed]
105. Harris, S.E.; Poolman, T.M.; Arvaniti, A.; Cox, R.D.; Gathercole, L.L.; Tomlinson, J.W. The American lifestyle-induced obesity syndrome diet in male and female rodents recapitulates the clinical and transcriptomic features of nonalcoholic fatty liver disease and nonalcoholic steatohepatitis. *Am. J. Physiol. Gastrointest. Liver Physiol.* **2020**, *319*, G345–G360. [CrossRef]
106. Dowman, J.K.; Hopkins, L.J.; Reynolds, G.M.; Nikolaou, N.; Armstrong, M.J.; Shaw, J.C.; Houlihan, D.D.; Lalor, P.F.; Tomlinson, J.W.; Hubscher, S.G.; et al. Development of hepatocellular carcinoma in a murine model of nonalcoholic steatohepatitis induced by use of a high-fat/fructose diet and sedentary lifestyle. *Am. J. Pathol.* **2014**, *184*, 1550–1561. [CrossRef] [PubMed]
107. Asgharpour, A.; Cazanave, S.C.; Pacana, T.; Seneshaw, M.; Vincent, R.; Banini, B.A.; Kumar, D.P.; Daita, K.; Min, H.K.; Mirshahi, F.; et al. A diet-induced animal model of non-alcoholic fatty liver disease and hepatocellular cancer. *J. Hepatol.* **2016**, *65*, 579–588. [CrossRef]

108. Kozlitina, J.; Smagris, E.; Stender, S.; Nordestgaard, B.G.; Zhou, H.H.; Tybjaerg-Hansen, A.; Vogt, T.F.; Hobbs, H.H.; Cohen, J.C. Exome-wide association study identifies a TM6SF2 variant that confers susceptibility to nonalcoholic fatty liver disease. *Nat. Genet.* **2014**, *46*, 352–356. [CrossRef]
109. Newberry, E.P.; Hall, Z.; Xie, Y.; Molitor, E.A.; Bayguinov, P.O.; Strout, G.W.; Fitzpatrick, J.A.J.; Brunt, E.M.; Griffin, J.L.; Davidson, N.O. Liver-Specific Deletion of Mouse Tm6sf2 Promotes Steatosis, Fibrosis, and Hepatocellular Cancer. *Hepatology* **2021**, *74*, 1203–1219. [CrossRef]
110. Luo, F.; Smagris, E.; Martin, S.A.; Vale, G.; McDonald, J.G.; Fletcher, J.A.; Burgess, S.C.; Hobbs, H.H.; Cohen, J.C. Hepatic TM6SF2 Is Required for Lipidation of VLDL in a Pre-Golgi Compartment in Mice and Rats. *Cell Mol. Gastroenterol. Hepatol.* **2022**, *13*, 879–899. [CrossRef]
111. Soga, M.; Kishimoto, Y.; Kawaguchi, J.; Nakai, Y.; Kawamura, Y.; Inagaki, S.; Katoh, K.; Oohara, T.; Makino, S.; Oshima, I. The FLS mouse: A new inbred strain with spontaneous fatty liver. *Lab. Anim. Sci.* **1999**, *49*, 269–275.
112. Soga, M.; Kishimoto, Y.; Kawamura, Y.; Inagaki, S.; Makino, S.; Saibara, T. Spontaneous development of hepatocellular carcinomas in the FLS mice with hereditary fatty liver. *Cancer Lett.* **2003**, *196*, 43–48. [CrossRef] [PubMed]
113. Semba, T.; Nishimura, M.; Nishimura, S.; Ohara, O.; Ishige, T.; Ohno, S.; Nonaka, K.; Sogawa, K.; Satoh, M.; Sawai, S.; et al. The FLS (fatty liver Shionogi) mouse reveals local expressions of lipocalin-2, CXCL1 and CXCL9 in the liver with non-alcoholic steatohepatitis. *BMC Gastroenterol.* **2013**, *13*, 120. [CrossRef] [PubMed]
114. Soga, M.; Hashimoto, S.; Kishimoto, Y.; Hirasawa, T.; Makino, S.; Inagaki, S. Insulin resistance, steatohepatitis, and hepatocellular carcinoma in a new congenic strain of Fatty Liver Shionogi (FLS) mice with the Lep(ob) gene. *Exp. Anim.* **2010**, *59*, 407–419. [CrossRef] [PubMed]
115. Sugihara, T.; Koda, M.; Kishina, M.; Kato, J.; Tokunaga, S.; Matono, T.; Ueki, M.; Murawaki, Y. Fatty liver Shionogi-ob/ob mouse: A new candidate for a non-alcoholic steatohepatitis model. *Hepatol. Res.* **2013**, *43*, 547–556. [CrossRef] [PubMed]
116. Horie, Y.; Suzuki, A.; Kataoka, E.; Sasaki, T.; Hamada, K.; Sasaki, J.; Mizuno, K.; Hasegawa, G.; Kishimoto, H.; Iizuka, M.; et al. Hepatocyte-specific Pten deficiency results in steatohepatitis and hepatocellular carcinomas. *J. Clin. Investig.* **2004**, *113*, 1774–1783. [CrossRef] [PubMed]
117. Chen, C.Y.; Chen, J.; He, L.; Stiles, B.L. PTEN: Tumor Suppressor and Metabolic Regulator. *Front. Endocrinol.* **2018**, *9*, 338. [CrossRef]
118. Watanabe, S.; Horie, Y.; Kataoka, E.; Sato, W.; Dohmen, T.; Ohshima, S.; Goto, T.; Suzuki, A. Non-alcoholic steatohepatitis and hepatocellular carcinoma: Lessons from hepatocyte-specific phosphatase and tensin homolog (PTEN)-deficient mice. *J. Gastroenterol. Hepatol.* **2007**, *22* (Suppl. S1), S96–S100. [CrossRef]
119. Gandhi, C.R.; Chaillet, J.R.; Nalesnik, M.A.; Kumar, S.; Dangi, A.; Demetris, A.J.; Ferrell, R.; Wu, T.; Divanovic, S.; Stankeiwicz, T.; et al. Liver-specific deletion of augmenter of liver regeneration accelerates development of steatohepatitis and hepatocellular carcinoma in mice. *Gastroenterology* **2015**, *148*, 379–391 e374. [CrossRef]
120. Kumar, S.; Verma, A.K.; Rani, R.; Sharma, A.; Wang, J.; Shah, S.A.; Behari, J.; Salazar Gonzalez, R.; Kohli, R.; Gandhi, C.R. Hepatic Deficiency of Augmenter of Liver Regeneration Predisposes to Nonalcoholic Steatohepatitis and Fibrosis. *Hepatology* **2020**, *72*, 1586–1604. [CrossRef]
121. Itoh, M.; Suganami, T.; Nakagawa, N.; Tanaka, M.; Yamamoto, Y.; Kamei, Y.; Terai, S.; Sakaida, I.; Ogawa, Y. Melanocortin 4 receptor-deficient mice as a novel mouse model of nonalcoholic steatohepatitis. *Am. J. Pathol.* **2011**, *179*, 2454–2463. [CrossRef]
122. Huszar, D.; Lynch, C.A.; Fairchild-Huntress, V.; Dunmore, J.H.; Fang, Q.; Berkemeier, L.R.; Gu, W.; Kesterson, R.A.; Boston, B.A.; Cone, R.D.; et al. Targeted Disruption of the Melanocortin-4 Receptor Results in Obesity in Mice. *Cell* **1997**, *88*, 131–141. [CrossRef] [PubMed]
123. Yamada, T.; Kashiwagi, Y.; Rokugawa, T.; Kato, H.; Konishi, H.; Hamada, T.; Nagai, R.; Masago, Y.; Itoh, M.; Suganami, T.; et al. Evaluation of hepatic function using dynamic contrast-enhanced magnetic resonance imaging in melanocortin 4 receptor-deficient mice as a model of nonalcoholic steatohepatitis. *Magn. Reson. Imaging* **2019**, *57*, 210–217. [CrossRef]
124. Watanabe, T.; Tsuchiya, A.; Takeuchi, S.; Nojiri, S.; Yoshida, T.; Ogawa, M.; Itoh, M.; Takamura, M.; Suganami, T.; Ogawa, Y.; et al. Development of a non-alcoholic steatohepatitis model with rapid accumulation of fibrosis, and its treatment using mesenchymal stem cells and their small extracellular vesicles. *Regen. Ther.* **2020**, *14*, 252–261. [CrossRef]
125. Nishida, T.; Tsuneyama, K.; Fujimoto, M.; Nomoto, K.; Hayashi, S.; Miwa, S.; Nakajima, T.; Nakanishi, Y.; Sasaki, Y.; Suzuki, W.; et al. Spontaneous onset of nonalcoholic steatohepatitis and hepatocellular carcinoma in a mouse model of metabolic syndrome. *Lab. Investig.* **2013**, *93*, 230–241. [CrossRef] [PubMed]
126. Murotomi, K.; Arai, S.; Uchida, S.; Endo, S.; Mitsuzumi, H.; Tabei, Y.; Yoshida, Y.; Nakajima, Y. Involvement of splenic iron accumulation in the development of nonalcoholic steatohepatitis in Tsumura Suzuki Obese Diabetes mice. *Sci. Rep.* **2016**, *6*, 22476. [CrossRef] [PubMed]
127. Takahashi, T.; Nishida, T.; Baba, H.; Hatta, H.; Imura, J.; Sutoh, M.; Toyohara, S.; Hokao, R.; Watanabe, S.; Ogawa, H.; et al. Histopathological characteristics of glutamine synthetase-positive hepatic tumor lesions in a mouse model of spontaneous metabolic syndrome (TSOD mouse). *Mol. Clin. Oncol.* **2016**, *5*, 267–270. [CrossRef] [PubMed]
128. Kakehashi, A.; Suzuki, S.; Ishii, N.; Okuno, T.; Kuwae, Y.; Fujioka, M.; Gi, M.; Stefanov, V.; Wanibuchi, H. Accumulation of 8-hydroxydeoxyguanosine, L-arginine and Glucose Metabolites by Liver Tumor Cells Are the Important Characteristic Features of Metabolic Syndrome and Non-Alcoholic Steatohepatitis-Associated Hepatocarcinogenesis. *Int. J. Mol. Sci.* **2020**, *21*, 7746. [CrossRef]

129. Ichimura-Shimizu, M.; Kageyama, T.; Oya, T.; Ogawa, H.; Matsumoto, M.; Sumida, S.; Kakimoto, T.; Miyakami, Y.; Nagatomo, R.; Inoue, K.; et al. Verification of the Impact of Blood Glucose Level on Liver Carcinogenesis and the Efficacy of a Dietary Intervention in a Spontaneous Metabolic Syndrome Model. *Int. J. Mol. Sci.* **2021**, *22*, 12844. [CrossRef]
130. Watanabe, S.; Takahashi, T.; Ogawa, H.; Uehara, H.; Tsunematsu, T.; Baba, H.; Morimoto, Y.; Tsuneyama, K. Daily Coffee Intake Inhibits Pancreatic Beta Cell Damage and Nonalcoholic Steatohepatitis in a Mouse Model of Spontaneous Metabolic Syndrome, Tsumura-Suzuki Obese Diabetic Mice. *Metab. Syndr. Relat. Disord.* **2017**, *15*, 170–177. [CrossRef]
131. Bettermann, K.; Mehta, A.K.; Hofer, E.M.; Wohlrab, C.; Golob-Schwarzl, N.; Svendova, V.; Schimek, M.G.; Stumptner, C.; Thuringer, A.; Speicher, M.R.; et al. Keratin 18-deficiency results in steatohepatitis and liver tumors in old mice: A model of steatohepatitis-associated liver carcinogenesis. *Oncotarget* **2016**, *7*, 73309–73322. [CrossRef]
132. Lu, S.C.; Alvarez, L.; Huang, Z.Z.; Chen, L.; An, W.; Corrales, F.J.; Avila, M.A.; Kanel, G.; Mato, J.M. Methionine adenosyltransferase 1A knockout mice are predisposed to liver injury and exhibit increased expression of genes involved in proliferation. *Proc. Natl. Acad. Sci. USA* **2001**, *98*, 5560–5565. [CrossRef] [PubMed]
133. Martinez-Chantar, M.L.; Corrales, F.J.; Martinez-Cruz, L.A.; Garcia-Trevijano, E.R.; Huang, Z.Z.; Chen, L.; Kanel, G.; Avila, M.A.; Mato, J.M.; Lu, S.C. Spontaneous oxidative stress and liver tumors in mice lacking methionine adenosyltransferase 1A. *FASEB J.* **2002**, *16*, 1292–1294. [CrossRef] [PubMed]
134. Cano, A.; Buque, X.; Martinez-Una, M.; Aurrekoetxea, I.; Menor, A.; Garcia-Rodriguez, J.L.; Lu, S.C.; Martinez-Chantar, M.L.; Mato, J.M.; Ochoa, B.; et al. Methionine adenosyltransferase 1A gene deletion disrupts hepatic very low-density lipoprotein assembly in mice. *Hepatology* **2011**, *54*, 1975–1986. [CrossRef] [PubMed]
135. Luedde, T.; Beraza, N.; Kotsikoris, V.; van Loo, G.; Nenci, A.; De Vos, R.; Roskams, T.; Trautwein, C.; Pasparakis, M. Deletion of NEMO/IKKgamma in liver parenchymal cells causes steatohepatitis and hepatocellular carcinoma. *Cancer Cell* **2007**, *11*, 119–132. [CrossRef]
136. Jacobi, D.; Liu, S.; Burkewitz, K.; Kory, N.; Knudsen, N.H.; Alexander, R.K.; Unluturk, U.; Li, X.; Kong, X.; Hyde, A.L.; et al. Hepatic Bmal1 Regulates Rhythmic Mitochondrial Dynamics and Promotes Metabolic Fitness. *Cell Metab.* **2015**, *22*, 709–720. [CrossRef]
137. Adamovich, Y.; Rousso-Noori, L.; Zwighaft, Z.; Neufeld-Cohen, A.; Golik, M.; Kraut-Cohen, J.; Wang, M.; Han, X.; Asher, G. Circadian clocks and feeding time regulate the oscillations and levels of hepatic triglycerides. *Cell Metab.* **2014**, *19*, 319–330. [CrossRef]
138. Jouffe, C.; Weger, B.D.; Martin, E.; Atger, F.; Weger, M.; Gobet, C.; Ramnath, D.; Charpagne, A.; Morin-Rivron, D.; Powell, E.E.; et al. Disruption of the circadian clock component BMAL1 elicits an endocrine adaption impacting on insulin sensitivity and liver disease. *Proc. Natl. Acad. Sci. USA* **2022**, *119*, e2200083119. [CrossRef]
139. Kettner, N.M.; Voicu, H.; Finegold, M.J.; Coarfa, C.; Sreekumar, A.; Putluri, N.; Katchy, C.A.; Lee, C.; Moore, D.D.; Fu, L. Circadian Homeostasis of Liver Metabolism Suppresses Hepatocarcinogenesis. *Cancer Cell* **2016**, *30*, 909–924. [CrossRef]
140. Pan, X.; Queiroz, J.; Hussain, M.M. Nonalcoholic fatty liver disease in CLOCK mutant mice. *J. Clin. Investig.* **2020**, *130*, 4282–4300. [CrossRef]
141. Tsuchida, T.; Lee, Y.A.; Fujiwara, N.; Ybanez, M.; Allen, B.; Martins, S.; Fiel, M.I.; Goossens, N.; Chou, H.I.; Hoshida, Y.; et al. A simple diet- and chemical-induced murine NASH model with rapid progression of steatohepatitis, fibrosis and liver cancer. *J. Hepatol.* **2018**, *69*, 385–395. [CrossRef]
142. Furman, B.L. Streptozotocin-Induced Diabetic Models in Mice and Rats. *Curr. Protoc. Pharmacol.* **2015**, *70*, 5.47.1–5.47.20. [CrossRef] [PubMed]
143. Fujii, M.; Shibazaki, Y.; Wakamatsu, K.; Honda, Y.; Kawauchi, Y.; Suzuki, K.; Arumugam, S.; Watanabe, K.; Ichida, T.; Asakura, H.; et al. A murine model for non-alcoholic steatohepatitis showing evidence of association between diabetes and hepatocellular carcinoma. *Med. Mol. Morphol.* **2013**, *46*, 141–152. [CrossRef] [PubMed]
144. Lai, M.; Chandrasekera, P.C.; Barnard, N.D. You are what you eat, or are you? The challenges of translating high-fat-fed rodents to human obesity and diabetes. *Nutr. Diabetes* **2014**, *4*, e135. [CrossRef] [PubMed]
145. Montgomery, M.K.; Hallahan, N.L.; Brown, S.H.; Liu, M.; Mitchell, T.W.; Cooney, G.J.; Turner, N. Mouse strain-dependent variation in obesity and glucose homeostasis in response to high-fat feeding. *Diabetologia* **2013**, *56*, 1129–1139. [CrossRef]
146. Paz-Filho, G.; Mastronardi, C.; Delibasi, T.; Wong, M.L.; Licinio, J. Congenital leptin deficiency: Diagnosis and effects of leptin replacement therapy. *Arq. Bras. Endocrinol. Metabol.* **2010**, *54*, 690–697. [CrossRef] [PubMed]
147. Uygun, A.; Kadayifci, A.; Yesilova, Z.; Erdil, A.; Yaman, H.; Saka, M.; Deveci, M.S.; Bagci, S.; Gulsen, M.; Karaeren, N.; et al. Serum leptin levels in patients with nonalcoholic steatohepatitis. *Am. J. Gastroenterol.* **2000**, *95*, 3584–3589. [CrossRef]
148. Huang, X.D.; Fan, Y.; Zhang, H.; Wang, P.; Yuan, J.P.; Li, M.J.; Zhan, X.Y. Serum leptin and soluble leptin receptor in non-alcoholic fatty liver disease. *World J. Gastroenterol.* **2008**, *14*, 2888–2893. [CrossRef]
149. Polyzos, S.A.; Kountouras, J.; Mantzoros, C.S. Leptin in nonalcoholic fatty liver disease: A narrative review. *Metabolism* **2015**, *64*, 60–78. [CrossRef]
150. Machado, M.V.; Michelotti, G.A.; Xie, G.; Almeida Pereira, T.; Boursier, J.; Bohnic, B.; Guy, C.D.; Diehl, A.M. Mouse models of diet-induced nonalcoholic steatohepatitis reproduce the heterogeneity of the human disease. *PLoS ONE* **2015**, *10*, e0127991. [CrossRef]
151. Rinella, M.E.; Green, R.M. The methionine-choline deficient dietary model of steatohepatitis does not exhibit insulin resistance. *J. Hepatol.* **2004**, *40*, 47–51. [CrossRef]

152. Rizki, G.; Arnaboldi, L.; Gabrielli, B.; Yan, J.; Lee, G.S.; Ng, R.K.; Turner, S.M.; Badger, T.M.; Pitas, R.E.; Maher, J.J. Mice fed a lipogenic methionine-choline-deficient diet develop hypermetabolism coincident with hepatic suppression of SCD-1. *J. Lipid Res.* **2006**, *47*, 2280–2290. [CrossRef] [PubMed]
153. Sahai, A.; Malladi, P.; Pan, X.; Paul, R.; Melin-Aldana, H.; Green, R.M.; Whitington, P.F. Obese and diabetic db/db mice develop marked liver fibrosis in a model of nonalcoholic steatohepatitis: Role of short-form leptin receptors and osteopontin. *Am. J. Physiol. Gastrointest. Liver Physiol.* **2004**, *287*, G1035–G1043. [CrossRef] [PubMed]
154. Yamazaki, Y.; Kakizaki, S.; Takizawa, D.; Ichikawa, T.; Sato, K.; Takagi, H.; Mori, M. Interstrain differences in susceptibility to non-alcoholic steatohepatitis. *J. Gastroenterol. Hepatol.* **2008**, *23*, 276–282. [CrossRef] [PubMed]
155. Jacobs, S.A.H.; Gart, E.; Vreeken, D.; Franx, B.A.A.; Wekking, L.; Verweij, V.G.M.; Worms, N.; Schoemaker, M.H.; Gross, G.; Morrison, M.C.; et al. Sex-Specific Differences in Fat Storage, Development of Non-Alcoholic Fatty Liver Disease and Brain Structure in Juvenile HFD-Induced Obese Ldlr−/−.Leiden Mice. *Nutrients* **2019**, *11*, 81861. [CrossRef]
156. Mannisto, V.T.; Simonen, M.; Soininen, P.; Tiainen, M.; Kangas, A.J.; Kaminska, D.; Venesmaa, S.; Kakela, P.; Karja, V.; Gylling, H.; et al. Lipoprotein subclass metabolism in nonalcoholic steatohepatitis. *J. Lipid Res.* **2014**, *55*, 2676–2684. [CrossRef]
157. Liu, Z.; Li, P.; Zhao, Z.H.; Zhang, Y.; Ma, Z.M.; Wang, S.X. Vitamin B6 Prevents Endothelial Dysfunction, Insulin Resistance, and Hepatic Lipid Accumulation in Apoe (−/−) Mice Fed with High-Fat Diet. *J. Diabetes Res.* **2016**, *2016*, 1748065. [CrossRef]
158. Shivapurkar, N.; Wilson, M.J.; Poirier, L.A. Hypomethylation of DNA in ethionine-fed rats. *Carcinogenesis* **1984**, *5*, 989–992. [CrossRef]
159. He, L.; Tian, D.A.; Li, P.Y.; He, X.X. Mouse models of liver cancer: Progress and recommendations. *Oncotarget* **2015**, *6*, 23306–23322. [CrossRef]
160. Ibrahim, S.H.; Hirsova, P.; Malhi, H.; Gores, G.J. Animal Models of Nonalcoholic Steatohepatitis: Eat, Delete, and Inflame. *Dig. Dis. Sci.* **2016**, *61*, 1325–1336. [CrossRef]
161. Saito, K.; Uebanso, T.; Maekawa, K.; Ishikawa, M.; Taguchi, R.; Nammo, T.; Nishimaki-Mogami, T.; Udagawa, H.; Fujii, M.; Shibazaki, Y.; et al. Characterization of hepatic lipid profiles in a mouse model with nonalcoholic steatohepatitis and subsequent fibrosis. *Sci. Rep.* **2015**, *5*, 12466. [CrossRef]

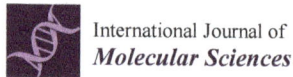

Review

SGLT-2 Inhibitors in NAFLD: Expanding Their Role beyond Diabetes and Cardioprotection

Theodoros Androutsakos [1,†], Narjes Nasiri-Ansari [2,†], Athanasios-Dimitrios Bakasis [1], Ioannis Kyrou [3,4,5,6,7], Efstathios Efstathopoulos [8], Harpal S. Randeva [3,4,*] and Eva Kassi [2,9,*]

1. Department of Pathophysiology, Medical School, National and Kapodistrian University of Athens, 11527 Athens, Greece; t_androutsakos@yahoo.gr (T.A.); th.bacasis@gmail.com (A.-D.B.)
2. Unit of Molecular Endocrinology, Department of Biological Chemistry, Medical School, National and Kapodistrian University of Athens, 11527 Athens, Greece; nnasiri@med.uoa.gr
3. Warwickshire Institute for the Study of Diabetes, Endocrinology and Metabolism (WISDEM), University Hospitals Coventry and Warwickshire NHS Trust, Coventry CV2 2DX, UK; kyrouj@gmail.com
4. Warwick Medical School, University of Warwick, Coventry CV4 7AL, UK
5. Laboratory of Dietetics and Quality of Life, Department of Food Science and Human Nutrition, School of Food and Nutritional Sciences, Agricultural University of Athens, 11855 Athens, Greece
6. Centre for Sport, Exercise and Life Sciences, Research Institute for Health & Wellbeing, Coventry University, Coventry CV1 5FB, UK
7. Aston Medical School, College of Health and Life Sciences, Aston University, Birmingham B4 7ET, UK
8. 2nd Department of Radiology, Medical School, National and Kapodistrian University of Athens, 11527 Athens, Greece; stathise@med.uoa.gr
9. Endocrine Oncology Unit, 1st Department of Propaedeutic Internal Medicine, Laiko Hospital, National and Kapodistrian University of Athens, 11527 Athens, Greece
* Correspondence: harpal.randeva@uhcw.nhs.uk (H.S.R.); ekassi@med.uoa.gr (E.K.)
† These authors contributed equally to this work.

Abstract: Non-alcoholic fatty liver disease (NAFLD) is an 'umbrella' term, comprising a spectrum ranging from benign, liver steatosis to non-alcoholic steatohepatitis, liver fibrosis and eventually cirrhosis and hepatocellular carcinoma. NAFLD has evolved as a major health problem in recent years. Discovering ways to prevent or delay the progression of NAFLD has become a global focus. Lifestyle modifications remain the cornerstone of NAFLD treatment, even though various pharmaceutical interventions are currently under clinical trial. Among them, sodium-glucose co-transporter type-2 inhibitors (SGLT-2i) are emerging as promising agents. Processes regulated by SGLT-2i, such as endoplasmic reticulum (ER) and oxidative stress, low-grade inflammation, autophagy and apoptosis are all implicated in NAFLD pathogenesis. In this review, we summarize the current understanding of the NAFLD pathophysiology, and specifically focus on the potential impact of SGLT-2i in NAFLD development and progression, providing current evidence from in vitro, animal and human studies. Given this evidence, further mechanistic studies would advance our understanding of the exact mechanisms underlying the pathogenesis of NAFLD and the potential beneficial actions of SGLT-2i in the context of NAFLD treatment.

Keywords: non-alcoholic fatty liver disease; NAFLD; MAFLD; SGLT-2; sodium-glucose co-transporter type-2 inhibitors; metabolic syndrome

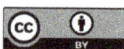

1. Introduction

Non-alcoholic fatty liver disease (NAFLD) has become a major health problem worldwide with an increasing prevalence ranging from 13% in Africa to 42% in South-East Asia [1,2]. The term NAFLD includes a variety of diseases, ranging from liver fat deposition in more than 5% of hepatocytes (steatosis—non-alcoholic fatty liver (NAFL)) to necroinflammation and fibrosis (non-alcoholic steatohepatitis (NASH)), which can progress into NASH-cirrhosis, and eventually to hepatocellular carcinoma [3,4]. Determining ways to delay the progression of NAFLD has become a global focus.

Lifestyle modifications—namely improved diet, weight management and increased physical activity—play a fundamental role in the treatment in NAFLD, since more than half of the patients with NAFLD have a high body mass index (BMI) [5,6]. Of note, drugs for specifically treating NAFLD are now being developed/approved, thus management of co-morbidities such as obesity, dyslipidemia or type 2 diabetes mellitus (T2DM) remains the cornerstone for the treatment of NAFLD patients [7,8].

Interestingly, since the cardiometabolic disorders associated with NAFLD account for the increased morbidity and mortality in these patients, the term metabolic (dysfunction) associated fatty liver disease (MAFLD) has been recently proposed by a panel of international experts as more appropriate, reflecting the underlying pathogenesis of the NAFLD spectrum [9–11]. Masarone et al., revealed that the prevalence of NAFLD was 94.82% among patients with metabolic syndromes (MS) and was presented in all T2DM patients with elevated transaminases when they performed biopsy [12]. Surprisingly, 58.52% of MS and 96.82% of T2DM patients in this study were diagnosed with NASH. As insulin resistance (IR) is crucially linked with both T2DM and NASH pathophysiology [13], they concluded that NASH may be one of the early clinical manifestations of T2DM [12]. Of note, NAFLD, particularly steatohepatitis, has also been associated with an increased risk of cardiovascular-related mortality regardless of age, sex, smoking habit, cholesterolemia and the remaining elements of MS [11]. Several prospective, observational and cross-sectional studies and meta-analyses demonstrated that NAFLD is associated with enhanced preclinical atherosclerotic damage as well as coronary, cerebral and peripheral vascular events with a negative impact on patients' outcome [14]. Furthermore, the severity of liver biopsy-based fibrosis has been independently associated with the worsening of both systolic and diastolic cardiac dysfunction [15,16].

Sodium-glucose co-transporter type-2 (SGLT-2) inhibitors (SGLT-2i) are glucose-lowering agents that improve glucose control, whilst promoting weight loss and lowering serum uric acid levels. These agents have shown great advantages even in patients with no diabetes, gaining approval of use in non-diabetic patients with heart failure and chronic kidney diseases [17,18]. In addition to the anti-hyperglycemic effects and their ability to reduce body weight, SGLT-2i seem to exert potent antioxidant and anti-inflammatory effects making them promising candidates for NAFLD treatment.

Indeed, recent data from animal studies and clinical trials have demonstrated beneficial effects of SGLT-2i on fatty liver accumulation, as judged by improvement of biological markers of NAFLD, as well as by imaging techniques, albeit mainly in T2DM patients.

Herein, we provide current insights into the effects of SGLT-2i on the progression of NAFLD, focusing on the underlying mechanisms of action. Endoplasmic reticulum (ER) stress, oxidative stress, low-grade inflammation, autophagy and apoptosis are among the SGLT-2i-regulated processes that have been shown to mediate the beneficial effects of SGLT-2i on NAFLD. Accordingly, we present the available evidence from in vitro, animal and human studies regarding the potential impact of SGLT-2i on NAFLD development and progression.

2. Overview of NAFLD Pathogenesis

The main theory concerning the pathophysiology of NAFLD has changed over time, reflecting the advances in our understanding of this multi-factorial disease. For years, the "two-hit" theory was the prevailing one. According to this theory, the pathophysiology of NAFLD consisted of a first "hit" representing the stage of simple steatosis alone (NAFL), which involves hepatocytic lipid accumulation and hepatic insulin resistance [19], as well as of a second "hit" from other factors (e.g., oxidative stress, ER stress, other injury), which was required for the development and progression of hepatic inflammation (NASH) and fibrosis. Replacing this initial theory, the "multiple parallel-hit" model [20] has been more recently proposed to better explain the complex pathogenesis and progression of NAFLD. According to this theory, as its name suggests, different amalgamations of numerous (epi)genetic and environmental factors, representing "hits", dynamically interplay with each other, and can drive the development and progression of NAFLD. These factors include specific genetic polymorphisms and epigenetic modifications [21], features of metabolic syndrome [22–25] (western diet, lack of physical activity, central obesity, dysregulation of adipoknes and IR), lipotoxicity [26,27], dysbiosis of the gut microbiota [26], dysregulation of autophagy and mitochondrial function [28–30], ER stress [31], hepatocyte homeostasis and death [32,33], as well as inflammatory and fibrotic responses [34,35]. Notably, when the hepatic capacity to handle the primary metabolic energy substrates is overwhelmed, toxic lipid species accumulate in the liver, leading to hepatocyte dysfunction and apoptosis, along with metabolically triggered inflammation and subsequent fibrosis [36].

The hallmark of NAFLD pathogenesis seems to be an increased adipocyte-like (dys)function of the hepatocytes, when the capacity of adipose tissue to store excess energy from the diet is diminished [37–40]. In conditions of energy surplus, increased metabolic substrates in tissues [27] drive hepatic de novo lipogenesis [41–43], while enhancing IR leading to a vicious cycle. The accumulation of intrahepatic lipid levels are governed by the balance between lipids synthesis, uptake and lysis [44]. Loss of equilibrium between lipogenesis and lipolysis leads to intracellular accumulation of free fatty acids (FFA) and subsequent hepatocellular damage, IR, worsening of liver function, formation of hepatic steatosis and progression to NASH, cirrhosis, and hepatocellular carcinoma [44].

In most individuals with NAFLD, dysregulation of adipokines (e.g., leptin and adiponectin) and metabolic-induced inflammation impair insulin signaling in adipocytes [45,46]. This impairment, in turn, contributes to reduced FA uptake and accelerated lipolysis in subcutaneous adipose tissue, resulting in exces sive delivery to the liver [45–47]. When hepatocytes are overloaded with lipids, physiologically minor pathways of β-oxidation in the peroxisomes and the ER are upregulated, thus increasing the hepatocyte reactive oxygen species (ROS) production [41,48] and generating highly reactive aldehyde by-products [49]. This phenomenon leads to nuclear and mitochondrial DNA damage, phospholipid membrane disruption and cell death. Moreover, due to the mitochondrial dysfunction and the consequent impaired β-oxidation found in patients with NAFLD, FA are alternatively esterified and collected in lipid droplets in the ER [50,51], generating toxic lipid metabolites, such as diacylglycerols [24], ceramides [52,53], and lysophosphatidyl choline species [53], which in turn lead to hepatocyte dysfunction (lipotoxicity) [54,55] and ER stress. The adaptive homeostatic mechanism of ER stress, called the unfolded protein response (UPR) [56], is impaired in NAFLD patients and, thus further cell stress-sensors are activated, whilst inflammatory and apoptotic pathways are upregulated [57,58]. In addition, the gut microbiota seem to also play a critical role in NAFL and NASH pathogenesis. Gut-derived pathogens and damage-associated molecular patterns activate an intrahepatic inflammatory process via Toll-like receptor signaling and NLR family pyrin domain containing-3 (NLRP3) inflammasome activation [35,59,60]. Hepatic innate immune cells, including Kupffer cells and dendritic cells, as well as hepatic stellate cells (HSCs) are then activated and the liver parenchyma is progressively infiltrated by recruited neutrophils, monocytes, T-lymphocytes, and macrophages [34,61]. Subsequently, the secreted cytokines and growth factors intensify the inflammatory process and further contribute to the fibrotic process as an ineffective attempt for tissue regeneration [35]. Overall, NAFLD is characterized by a complex pathogenetic mechanism, where various pathways are implicated, making the discovery of a "wonder drug" a difficult task (Figure 1).

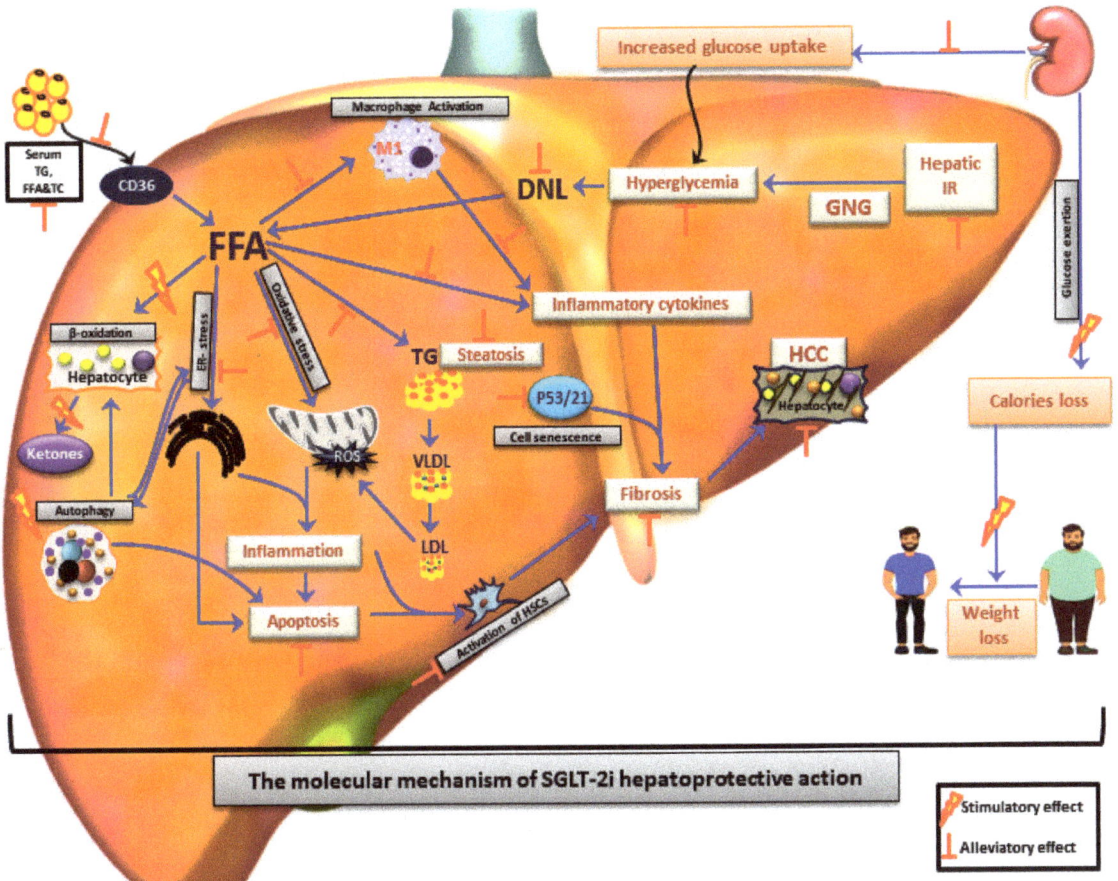

Figure 1. SGLT-2 inhibitors as a promising therapeutic agents for treatment of NAFLD/NASH patients. SGLT-2i treatment contributes to alleviation of NAFLD by reduction of hyperglycaemia, improvement of systematic insulin resistance, elevation of caloric loss and reduction of body weight mostly due to glycosuria. Apart from that, SGLT-2i play a hepatoprotective effect through reduction of hepatic de novo lipogenesis, hepatic inflammation, apoptosis, ER-stress, oxidative stress, and increase of hepatic beta-oxidation. Reduced activation of hepatic satellite cells and p53/p21 pathways by SGLT-2i leads to amelioration of hepatic fibrosis and HCC development. FFA: Free fatty acids; DNL: De novo lipogenesis; HCC: Hepatocellular carcinoma; TC: Total cholesterol; TG: Triglycerides; LDL: Low density lipoprotein; VLDL: Very low density lipoprotein; GNG: Gluconeogenesis; HSC: Hepatic stellate cells; IR: Insulin resistance; ROS: Reactive oxygen species; ER-stress: Endoplasmic reticulum stress.

3. SGLT-2i Overview

Phlorizin, a b-Dglucoside, was the first natural non-selective SGLT-2i isolated from the bark of the apple tree in 1835 and was initially used for fever relief and treatment of infectious diseases [62,63]. Phlorizin contains a glucose moiety and an aglycone in which two aromatic carbocycles are joined by an alkyl spacer. Approximately fifty years later, scientists observed that phlorizin in high dose lowered plasma glucose levels through glucosuria independently of insulin secretion [62–64]. However, the mechanism of phlorizin action through the active glucose transport system of the proximal tubule was revealed in the early 1970s [62,65].

Thereafter, researchers began to discover the exact mechanism of phlorizin action and its potential application in the management of hyperglycaemia. Phlorizin, when delivered orally, undergoes hydrolysis of the O-glycosidic bond by intestinal glucosidases, leading to formation of phloretin, which is capable of GLUT transporter inhibition and uncoupling of oxidative phosphorylation. Due to Phlorizin's low SGLT-2 selectivity, rapid degradation, inhibition of the ubiquitous glucose transporter 1 (GLUT1), poor intestinal absorption and its gastrointestinal side effects (e.g., diarrhea and dehydration), possibly due to its higher potency for SGLT-1, it failed to be developed as an antidiabetic drug [62,66–68].

Nevertheless, in order to overcome the aforementioned side effects of phlorizin, a researcher developed a devphlorizin-based analog with improved bioavailability/stability and more selectivity towards SGLT-2 than SGLT-1. Initially, they focused on the development of O-glucoside analogs such as T-1095, sergliflozin and remogliflozin [69,70]. However, due to their poor stability and incomplete SGLT-2 selectivity, pharmaceutical industries turned to another derivative of phlorizin known as C-glucosides [62].

Since then, there have been numerous attempts to synthesize phlorizin C-glucoside analogs with sufficient potency and selectivity for inhibition of SGLT-2. These attempts led to development of dapagliflozin by Meng et al., in 2008 [71]. Dapagliflozin demonstrated more than 1200-fold higher potency for human SGLT-2 versus SGLT-1. Apart from dapagliflozin, during the next years, several other C-glucoside inhibitors have been developed and approved by United States Food and Drug Administration (FDA). Canagliflozin, characterized by a thiophene derivative of C-glucoside, showed over 400-fold difference in inhibitory activities between human SGLT-2 and SGLT-1 [72]. Thereafter, empagliflozin, which has the highest selectivity for SGLT-2 over SGLT-1 (approximately 2700-fold), was the third agent approved by both the European Medicines Agency (EMA) and the FDA, while other SGLT-2i, namely luseogliflozin and topogliflozin, are approved so far for use only in Japan, and ipragliflozin only in Japan and Russia [73–77].

The structure of phlorizin and currently FDA-approved SGLT-2 inhibitors in the United States, including dapagliflozin, canagliflozin, empagliflozin, and ertugliflozin, along with their chemical formulae and brand names are presented in Figure 2 [78]. Diverse structures of other SGLT-2 inhibitors have been previously disclosed in various articles and in a number of patents [79,80].

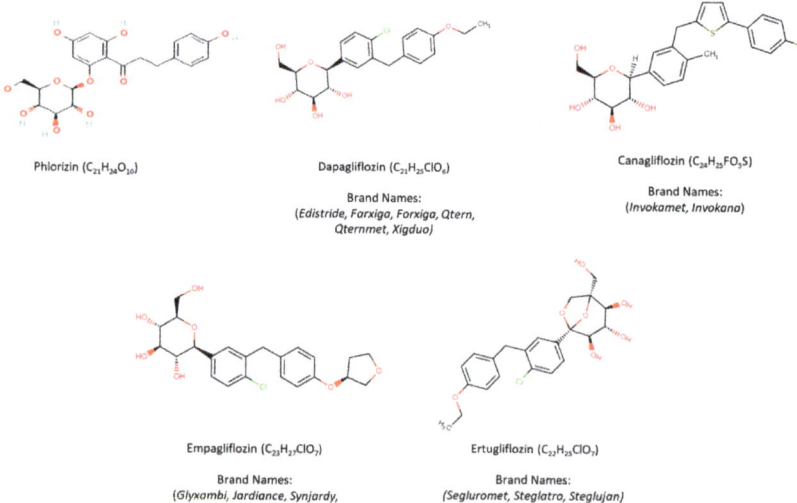

Figure 2. Structure of phlorizin and FDA-approved SGLT-2 inhibitors.

4. SGLT-2 Inhibitors in NAFLD

4.1. Laboratory Experiments

4.1.1. In Vitro Data

The expression of both SGLT-1 and SGLT-2 co-transporters has been reported in human hepatocellular carcinoma cells (HepG2) [81–83], whilst SGLT-2 has also been identified in immortalized human primary hepatocyte cells (HuS-E/2), as well as immortalized normal human hepatocyte-derived liver cells (L02) [84,85].

Studies have indicated that most SGLT-2i exert anti-proliferative activity in several hepatocellular cell lines, through—among other mechanisms—attenuation of glucose uptake [86]. Incubation of both L02 and HepG2 cells with canagliflozin at various concentrations for 24 h resulted in a significant reduction of cell proliferation through an increase in G0/G1 and a decrease in G2/M phase cell population [86]. In addition, an apoptotic effect was exhibited through activation of caspase 3 in HepG2 cells [87]. From a mechanistic point of view, cell growth regulators, cyclins and cyclin-dependent kinases (CDKs) have been indicated as direct targets of SGLT-2i to control proliferation and survival processes. As such, canagliflozin-treated HepG2 cells demonstrated increased expression of the cell growth regulator hepatocyte nuclear factor 4α (HNF4α) [82]. Furthermore, reduced expression of cyclin D1, cyclin D2 and cdk4 leading to cell cycle arrest in a hepatocellular carcinoma (HCC) cell line have been reported after treatment with canagliflozin [82,87]. In another study, incubation of HepG2 cells with canagliflozin resulted in reduced clonogenic cell survival and elevation of anti-carcinogenic potential of γ-irradiation through modulation of ER stress-mediated autophagy and cell apoptosis [88]. On the contrary, trilobatin, a novel SGLT-1/2 inhibitor, increased the HepG2 cell proliferation rate at a dose of 10, 50 and 100 µM, while incubation of human HCC cells with tofogliflozin at various concentrations did not alter the HCC cell proliferation rate [89]. Incubation of HepG2 cells with dapagliflozin, canagliflozin and empagliflozin had no effect on cancer cell survival [81,86] and adhesion capacity [81], while the cell sensitivity to dapagliflozin was induced after UDP Glucuronosyltransferase Family 1 Member A9 (UGT1A9) silencing, indicated by an increased number of floating HepG2 cells; of note, UGT1A9 metabolizes and deactivates dapagliflozin [81].

Dapagliflozin treatment remarkably suppressed oleic acid (OA)-induced lipid accumulation and TG content in L02 cells through increased FA β-oxidation, as indicated by elevated proliferator-activated receptor-gamma coactivator-1 alpha (PGC-1α) levels and activation of the AMP-activated protein kinase (AMPK)/mammalian target of rapamycin (mTOR) signaling pathway [84]. Several in vitro studies have shown that AMPK is a key regulator that mediates the various beneficial effects of SGLT-2i related to cholesterol and glucose metabolism in hepatic cells. AMPK activation by dapagliflozin prevented glucose absorption through reduced SGLT-2 expression in OA-stimulated HuS-E/2 cells [90]. This effect was eliminated after incubation of cells with compound C, a potent AMPK inhibitor [84]. Moreover, treatment of HepG2 cells with canagliflozin facilitated hepatic cholesterol efflux via activation of AMPK. In turn, AMPK activation led to increased expression of the liver X receptor (LXR) and its downstream proteins, resulting in subsequent stimulation of cholesterol reverse transport [91]. LXR activation also accelerates fecal cholesterol disposal through regulation of ATP-binding cassette (ABC) transporters ABCG5 and ABCG8 expression [92]. Canagliflozin treatment resulted in reduced expressions of ABCG5 and ABCG8 and LXR, while this effect was inhibited after treatment of cells with compound C [91]. An increased AMP/ADP ratio leads to AMPK activation. It is known that SGLT-2i reduces cellular ATP levels and indirectly activates the AMPK signaling pathway [83,93]. It has been shown that dapagliflozin alleviates the intracellular ATP levels via regulation of glucose metabolism [84].

Stimulation of hepatic cell lines with palmitic acid (PA) mimics hepatocyte situation in NASH [94,95]. Incubation of PA-stimulated L02 and HepG2 cell lines with dapagliflozin resulted in a significant reduction of intracellular lipid accumulation. This effect was attributed to down-regulation of proteins related to lipid synthesis, up-regulation of genes involved in fatty acid oxidation (e.g., peroxisome proliferator-activated receptor alpha (PPARα) and carnitine palmitoyltransferase 1 (CPT1a)), regulation of AMPK/mTOR pathway and autophagy. Interestingly, incubation of cells with compound C abolished the dapagliflozin beneficial effect on reduction of intracellular lipid accumulation [85]. Collectively, these data suggest that SGLT-2i induced improvement of NAFLD is directly dependent on AMPK signaling activation.

The divergent results of the various relevant studies suggest that the effects of SGLT-2i on cell proliferation, survival and apoptosis—which are important processes in hepatocellular carcinoma development and progression—appear to be drug-, dose- and duration-dependent.

4.1.2. Animal Studies

Overall, the animal models of NAFLD/NASH can be divided into two categories. Of these, one comprises genetically modified animal models, such as leptin deficient (ob/ob), leptin-resistant (db/db), Agouti mutation (KK-Ay), and apolipoprotein E knockout (ApoE$^{-/-}$) mice, as well as the Prague hereditary hypertriglyceridemic (HHTg) rats, Zucker diabetic fatty (ZDF) rats and Otsuka Long-Evans Tokushima Fatty (OLETF) rat. The other category includes dietary/pharmacological manipulation-induced NAFLD/NASH animal models, such as those fed with either a methionine/choline-deficient (MCD) diet, the trans-fat containing AMLN (amylin liver non-alcoholic steatohepatitis, NASH) diet, and the methionine-reduced, choline-deficient and amino acid defined (CDAA) diet, as well as a high-fat diet (HFD), and a HFD + cholesterol diet or a high-fat, high-calorie (HFHC) diet [30,96–100]. Most of the recent data indicate that both SGLT-1 and SGLT-2 genes are expressed in hepatic tissues of mice and rats [30,85,87,101]. High levels of SGLT-2 protein have also been detected in hepatic macrophages and T cells [101]. While the exact underlying molecular mechanisms of SGLT-2i-induced beneficial effects on NAFLD have not yet been fully clarified, most of our knowledge regarding the potential hepato-protective mechanism(s) of SGLT-2i actions comes from animal studies.

Although the SGLT-2i-induced weight loss seems to play an important role in hepatoprotective effects on NAFLD in humans [102–104], data from animal studies suggest that other mechanisms are more likely responsible for the noted SGLT-2i-mediated hepato-protection.

Administration of SGLT-2i leads to net loss of calories and consequent attenuation of body weight gain, while reducing the accumulated white adipose tissue [99,105–107]. In fact, it has been found that SGLT-2i promote weight loss through improvement of systemic IR, increased body temperature and basal metabolism via regulation of the AMP/ATP ratio [19]. Petito da Silva et al., reported that empagliflozin (Table 1) at a dose of 10 mg/kg/day given for five weeks significantly reduces body weight and body mass in HFD-fed male C57Bl/6 mice, despite a slight increase in their appetite [107]. Similar results were observed in HFD-fed C57BL/6J male mice after administration of canagliflozin (Table 2) at 30 mg/kg dose for four weeks in parallel with improvement of liver function, liver TG content and NAS score [108]. Additionally, short term and low dose administration of dapagliflozin (Table 3) reduced both ALT levels and body weight in both HFD and HFD+MCD diet fed C57BL/6J mice [109]. However, it should be noted that not all studies point towards a beneficial effect of SGLT-2i on body weight. Several studies have shown that administration of SGLT-2i does not exert any significant effect on body weight gain, epididymal fat weight or food intake [30,105,110,111]. In addition, although several studies reported strong effects of low dose ipragliflozin (Table 4) on weight loss [100,112,113], supplementation of an AMLN diet with 40 mg ipragliflozin/kg for 8 weeks did not significantly alter the body weight of AMLN diet fed mice, while it improved liver function, hepatic fibrosis and NA score [114]. Empagliflozin at the dose of 10 mg/kg/day improved liver function and NAFLD status, while it had no significant effect on the body weight of

ZDF, HHTg and Wistar rats [115,116], as well as on the body weight and appetite of ApoE knockout mice [30].

Although there are studies showing that administration of SGLT-2i does not exert any significant effect on body weight gain [30,100,110–114], the vast majority of the literature points towards a beneficial effect on weight loss.

However, the protective role of SGLT-2i against NAFLD progression also seems to be mediated by effects beyond those on body weight. Indeed, it has been shown that SGLT-2i treatment improves IR and ameliorates the intracellular FFA, total cholesterol (TC) and TG accumulation through reducing the expression of genes involved in de novo lipogenesis, FA uptake and hepatic TG secretion, whilst it also promotes the expression of key regulatory genes of fatty acid β-oxidation [30,84,100,107,109,112,117]. Specifically, empagliflozin administration has been shown to reduce hepatic triacylglycerol (TAG) levels and improve IR through reduction of lipotoxic intermediates formation, such as diacylglycerols (DAG) [115], which at elevated levels contribute to IR by activating the protein kinase C (PKC)ε pathway [118]. Of note, a recent study by Hüttl et al., demonstrated that reduction of hepatic lipid accumulation following empagliflozin treatment is mediated via increased nuclear factor erythroid 2-related factor 2 (Nrf2), fibroblast growth factor 21 (FGF21) and altered gene expression of the P450 (CYP) enzyme superfamily of cytochrome [115]. Interestingly, Nrf2 and FGF21 regulate lipid metabolism through inhibiting lipogenesis and improving insulin sensitivity, respectively [119,120].

Sterol regulatory element-binding transcription factor 1 (SREBP1) is one of the key regulators of hepatic lipogenesis and plays a crucial role in the regulation of lipogenic genes, such as fatty acid synthase (Fasn), acetyl-CoAcarboxylase 1 (Acc1), and stearoyl-CoA desaturase1 (Scd-1). Increased SREBP1 expression has been linked to the aggravation of hepatic steatosis [121]. While reduced expression of SREBP1 and Scd-1 by both canagliflozin and empagliflozin has been observed in several studies [30,107,108,115], Kern et al., found that empagliflozin treatment for eight weeks does not markedly affect the Scd-1 levels in db/db mice [122]. Dapagliflozin (1 mg/kg/day) treatment for nine weeks resulted in downregulation of Scd-1 gene expression, as well as reduced ACC1 phosphorylation in ZDF rats. Taking into account that SREBP1 activity is directly regulated by mTOR signaling [123], reduced expression of SREBP1 and its downstream lipogenic targets could be due to the reduced mTOR expression/activity observed after SGLT-2i administration [84,123].

Peroxisome proliferator-activated receptor gamma (PPAR-γ) upregulation triggers de novo lipogenesis and consequent deposition of lipid droplets into hepatocytes [124]. Eight weeks of dapagliflozin treatment reduced hepatic weight and prevented progression of hepatic steatosis compared to mice treated with insulin glargine [125]. This effect was found to be mediated through decreased expression of PPAR-γ targeted genes involved in fatty acid synthesis, such as Scd-1, monoacylglycerol O-acyltransferase 1 (Mogat1), Cell death inducing DFFA like effector A (Cidea) and cell death inducing DFFA like effector C (Cidec), without affecting insulin sensitivity, liver TC or oleate content [125].

SGLT-2i have been also shown to reverse the HFD-induced down regulation of genes involved in FA β-oxidation and lipolysis in the liver of various mouse models of NAFLD [30,84,107,108]. Indeed, it has been shown that expression of PPARα is induced by SGLT-2i [84,105,107,114]. PPARα activation is predominant for regulation of genes related to the FA β-oxidation process in mitochondria, such as peroxisomal acyl-CoA oxidase1 (ACOX1) and enoyl-CoA hydratase, CPT1, and cytochrome-mediated (CYP4A1 and CYP4A3) [44]. Ipragliflozin treatment has been shown to result in acceleration of β-oxidation and export of very-low-density lipoprotein (VLDL) through upregulation of PPARα, CPT1A, and Microsomal Triglyceride Transfer Protein (MTTP) gene expression in the liver of AMLN-fed C57BL/6J mice. MTTP plays a crucial role in export of hepatic LDL [114]. Similarly, dapagliflozin attenuated hepatic lipid accumulation in ZDF rats via up-regulation of the FA β-oxidation enzyme ACOX1 [85]. Tofogliflozin administration induced the expression of genes related to FA β-oxidation in non-tumorous liver lesions, while it had no effect on their expression in tumorous liver tissues [126]. However, not all studies show a promotive effect of SGLT-2i on the expression of enzymes and transcription factors involved in the regulation of FA β-oxidation [107,114,126]. Of note, the expression of PPARα remained unaffected in both Wistar and HHTg rats after eight weeks of empagliflozin administration [107,115]. Administration of canagliflozin at doses of 10 and 20 mg/kg/day ameliorated the HFD-induced down-regulation of the expression of the key regulatory molecule of hepatic lipolysis, known as zinc alpha 2 glycoprotein (ZAG). When the same SGLT-2i was given in KK-Ay mice, it reduced the accumulation of lipid droplets in the liver by increasing hepatic prostaglandin E2 (PGE2) protein levels [111]. Furthermore, the combined therapy with canagliflozin and exercise exerted an additive effect on hepatic PPARγ Coactivator 1 Beta (PGC1b) elevation, and reduced expression of hepatic lipogenic genes, such as Scd1 [108]. Notably, PGC1 plays a central role in the control of hepatic gluconeogenesis, while its overexpression has been associated with stimulation of hepatic FA oxidation [127].

The inhibition of de novo lipogenesis, and enhanced lipolysis and β-oxidation by SGLT-2-i lead to a consequent reduction in oxidative stress, hepatic inflammation and apoptosis [128]. Administration of canagliflozin to HFD-fed diabetic Wistar adult male rats resulted in reduced hepatic steatosis through amelioration of oxidative stress, inflammation and apoptosis, as indicated by reduced plasma malondialdehyde (MDA) levels, serum tumor necrosis factor (TNF) and caspase-3 levels, as well as hepatic expression of interleukin-6 (IL-6) [128,129]. Moreover, dapagliflozin treatment reduced the expression of hepatic inflammatory cytokine (TNF-α, IL-1β, IL-18) content and improved hepatic steatosis in HCHF fed male Wistar rats [130]. Tahara et al., have also shown anti-oxidative stress and anti-inflammatory effects of ipragliflozin on HFD-fed and streptozotocin–nicotinamide-induced type 2 diabetic mice [131]. Similarly, dapagliflozin treatment at a dose of 1 mg/kg/day decreased hepatic ROS production of myeloperoxidase (MPO) and F4/80, thus ameliorating serum ALT levels and hepatic fibrosis [132]. MPO is a chlorinating oxidant-generating enzyme that regulates the initiation of an acute inflammatory response and promotes the development of chronic inflammation through oxidant production [133]. Furthermore, canagliflozin treatment of F344 rats for 16 weeks resulted in reduced hepatic ROS production and MDA and 8-hydroxy-2'-deoxyguanosine (8-OHdG) levels [110]. MDA and 8-OHdG are known biomarkers of lipid peroxidation and oxidative DNA damage, respectively. Of note, canagliflozin and teneligliptin combination therapy showed a stronger effect on reduction of hepatic oxidative stress and amelioration of hepatic inflammation [110]. Treatment with both remogliflozin and ipragliflozin also reduced oxidative stress levels, as evaluated by decreased thiobarbituric acid reactive substances (TBARS) levels [100,134]. Instead, administration of dapagliflozin at 1 mg/kg/twice/day for four weeks had no significant effect either on hepatic TBARS and TG levels or on plasma ALT levels [135]. In addition, reduction of oxidative stress by empagliflozin treatment resulted in amelioration of hepatic inflammation [30,107,116] and steatosis, as judged by down-regulation of inflammatory markers [30,107,115]. Of interest, decreased macrophage infiltration expression [107,117,134] as well as elevation of autophagy markers [30,117] have also been linked to the anti-inflammatory actions of SGLT-2-i in the liver. Specifically, oxidative stress was reduced after empagliflozin treatment via up regulation of Nrf2, which led to increased antioxidant enzyme activity (SOD) and reduced hepatic inflammation [115]. Empagliflozin exerted anti-inflammatory actions in diet-induced obese mice and NASH mouse models through, at least in part, suppression of hepatic nuclear factor kappa-light-chain-enhancer of activated B cells (NFκB), monocyte chemoattractant protein-1 (MCP-1) and TNF-α expression, as well as inhibition of the IL17/IL23 axis [115,117,136]. Reduced hepatic inflammation has also been reported in mice and rats after treatment with low dose (1 mg/kg/day) dapagliflozin and ipragliflozin. Indeed, ipragliflozin administration for 12 weeks alleviated hepatic fibrosis through reduced expression of pro-inflammatory markers Emr1 and Itgax in non-tumoric lesions [126]. On the contrary, a recent study in mice by Hupa-Breier et al., demonstrated that four weeks treatment of diet-induced NASH with empagliflozin alone at a dose of 10 mg/kg/day did not exert any beneficial effect on NASH, while it significantly increased expression of pro-inflammatory and pro-fibrotic genes. In the same study, the combination of dulaglutide (a GLP-1 agonist) and empagliflozin exhibited a hepato-protective effect on diabetic background mice through modulation of the pro-inflammatory immune response and microbiome dysbiosis [137].

Meng et al., demonstrated that induction of AMPK/mTOR activity is dominant pathway in empagliflozin-induced beneficial effects on liver inflammation and ALT levels [117]. Dapagliflozin treatment also induced AMPK/mTOR pathway activation through phosphorylation of liver kinase B1 (LKB1; a ubiquitously expressed master serine/threonine kinase that activates downstream kinases of the AMPK pathway) [105,138]. Previous studies have demonstrated that AMPK activation is required for SGLT-2i induced autophagy-dependent lipid catabolism [30,117]. Both dapagliflozin and empagliflozin promote hepatic autophagy through increased AMPK phosphorylation and BECLIN gene expression, as well as reduced P62 levels and mTOR levels and activity [30,85].

Apart from impaired autophagy, ER stress is also implicated in the development of steatosis and the progression of NAFLD/NASH [30,107]. Consistent with the regulatory role of ER stress in the autophagy process, Nasiri-Ansari et al., demonstrated that stimulation of autophagy by empagliflozin leads to amelioration of ER stress and reduced hepatic cell apoptosis [30]. In particular, empagliflozin administration protects against HFD-induced NAFLD through inhibiting all three branches of ER stress, namely inositol-requiring enzyme 1 (IRE1a), X-box binding protein 1 (Xbp1), activating transcription factor 4 (ATF4), C/EBP homologous protein (CHOP) and activating transcription factor 6 (ATF6) [30,107]. A recent study by Chen et al., also showed that down-regulation of the ATF6 signaling diminished ER stress-induced inflammation and apoptosis of hepatic cells [139]. The synergistic ER stress response and autophagy process regulated hepatic cell apoptosis in HFD-fed ApoE$^{-/-}$ mice with NASH, by reducing cleaved caspase 3 levels and elevation of B-cell lymphoma-2 (Bcl-2)/BCL2 Associated X (Bax) ratio [30]. Of note, canagliflozin was previously found to exert an anti-apoptotic effect on HFD-fed mice as revealed by robust Bcl-2 hepatic expression [129].

Chronic liver inflammation leads to transformation of hepatic stellate cells to myofibroblasts, thus contributing to liver fibrosis and progression of NAFLD to NASH [140]. Transforming growth factor beta (TGF-β) is known as the most potent inducer of liver fibrosis. Administration of canagliflozin for 16 and 20 weeks reduced the expression of hepatic TGF-β in both F344 rats and MC4R-KO mice, respectively [101,110]. Interestingly, TGF-β activation leads to increased fibronectin and collagen types I, II, and IV production [141]. Treatment of mice with both empagliflozin and canagliflozin resulted in reduced expression of different types of collagen, implying synergistic action(s) [87,137]. Luseogliflozin also exerts anti-fibrotic effects through reduction of collagen1a1, collagen1a2, TGF-β and smooth muscle actin (SMA) expression [142]. Extensive data exist regarding the crucial role of tissue inhibitors of metalloproteinases (TIMPs) in the progression of hepatic fibrosis. Reduced expression of TIMPs and amelioration of hepatic fibrosis have been observed after luseogliflozin and canagliflozin administration [101,126,142]. On the contrary, empagliflozin treatment did not affect the expression of stellate cell functionality markers, such as galectin-3, a-SMA, and collagen1a1 [99].

NASH has been associated with an increased risk of cirrhosis and HCC development. Hepatic tumorogenesis is the result of DNA instability caused by several factors, such as hepatic lipotoxicity, aberrant metabolism and inflammation [141,143]. As a protective effect of SGLT-2i on NAFLD/NASH progression has been shown in the vast majority of the studies, further research aimed to evaluate the effect of SGLT-2i on development and progression of HCC [87,101,142]. Activation of the hepatic P53/P21 signaling pathway is positively correlated with induced fibrosis and hepatocellular carcinogenesis. A 14-week treatment with tofogliflozin has been shown to effectively reduce the P21 expression, alleviating the progression of NASH through, at least in part, mitigating genes related to the hepatocyte cellular senescence-associated secretory phenotype [89]. Daily administration of canagliflozin prevented the occurrence of HCC in both STAM mice—a NASH model—(11 weeks) and HFD-fed MC4R-KO mice (52 weeks), as indicated by a significantly reduced number of hepatic tumorous lesions [87,101]. Moreover, 66 weeks administration of canagliflozin to CDAA-fed F344 rats exerted an anti-carcinogenic effect, as indicated by a reduced number of cells positively stained for placental glutathione S-transferase (a prominent marker of hepatocarcinogenesis) [110]. Finally, canagliflozin administration reduced the development of hepatic preoplastic lesions in CDAA-fed rats through suppression of hepatic neovascularization markers, namely cluster of differentiation 31 (CD31) and vascular endothelial growth factor (VEGF) [110]. Overall, the key animal studies regarding the impact of SGLT-2i on NAFLD/NASH/HCC are summarized in Tables 1–4.

Table 1. Key animal studies regarding the impact of empagliflozin on NAFLD/NASH.

Study/Reference	Animal Model, Dose, & Duration	Effect on Body Weight and Liver Weight	Effect on Laboratory Values	Mechanism of Action	Effect on Insulin Sensitivity & Glucose Homeostasis	NAFLD Activity Score (NAS) & Fibrosis/Steatosis
Perakakis, N., et al., 2021 [99]	Male C57BL/6JRj on AMLN diet (HFD, fructose + cholesterol) 10 mg/kg/day 12 (w)	No effect	-	↓ Hepatic lactosylceramides	↓ Blood glucose levels No effect on Insulin sensitivity	↓ Lobular inflammation ↓ NAS No effect on the hepatic steatosis and fibrosis
Meng, Z., et al., 2021 [117]	Male C57BL/6J on HFD + streptozotocin injection (T2DM with NAFLD) 10 mg/kg/day 8 (w)	↓ Body weight ↓ Liver/Bw	↓ ALT ↓ TG & TC ↑ HDL	↓ Lipogenesis markers and lipid uptake genes (SREBP1, ChREBP, FASN, ACCα, SCDα, CD36) ↑ Autophagy activation (AMPK/mTOR & BECLIN1, LC3BII) ↓ IL-17/IL-23 axis inhibition (IL-23p19, IL-23, IL-1β, IL-17A, RORγt, p-STAT3/t-STAT3, IL-17) ↓ M1 macrophage marker (CD11C, CD86, NOS2) ↓ Th17-related chemokines and chemokine receptors (CCL20, CCR6, CCR4, CXCL1/CXCL2, CXCL1, CXCR2)	↓ Blood glucose levels	↓ Hepatic steatosis ↓ NAS
Nasiri-Ansari, N., et al., 2021 [30]	Male ApoE knockout mice on HFD 10 mg/kg/day 10 (w)	No effects	↓ ALT, TG, TC levels ↓ Serum TG/HDL levels	↓ Lipogenesis markers (SREBP1, Pck1, FASN) ↓ Inflammatory markers (MCP-1, F4/80) ↓ ER stress markers (GRP78, IRE1α, XBP1, ELF2α, ATF4, CHOP, GRP94) Autophagy markers (↓ mTOR and P62 & ↑ pAMPK/AMPK, BECLIN) ↓ Apoptosis markers (Bax/Bcl-2 Ratio, cleaved Caspase-3)	↓ Blood glucose levels	↓ Lobular inflammation ↓ Hepatic steatosis ↓ NAS No effect on hepatic fibrosis

Table 1. Cont.

Study/Reference	Animal Model, Dose, & Duration	Effect on Body Weight and Liver Weight	Effect on Laboratory Values	Mechanism of Action	Effect on Insulin Sensitivity & Glucose Homeostasis	NAFLD Activity Score (NAS) & Fibrosis/Steatosis
Petito-da-Silva, et al., 2019 [107]	Male C57Bl/6 mice on HFD 10 mg/kg/day 5 (w)	↓BW ↓Liver/Bw	No effect on ALT	↓Lipogenic genes (Fas, SREBP1c, PPARγ) ↓ER- stress markers (CHOP, ATF4, GADD45) Fatty acid β-oxidation (↑PPAR-α, ↓Acox1) ↓lipid droplet-associated protein (Fsp27/cidec) ↓Inflammatory markers (Nfκb, TNF-α)	Improved Glucose intolerence Improved Insulin sensitivity	↓Hepatic TC ↓Hepatic steatosis
Jojima, T., et al., 2016 [136]	Male C57BL/6J on HFD + early STZ injection 10 mg/kg/day 3 (w)	↓Liver/BW	↓GA ↓ALT	↓Inflammatory markers (IL6, TNF-α, MCP-1, SOCS3) ↓Plasma DPP-4 activity (CD26/DPP-4)	↓Plasma glucose Levels	↓Hepatic TG ↓NAS ↓Hepatic fibrosis
Hüttl, M., et al., 2021 [115]	HHTg & Wistar rats 10 mg/kg/day 8 (w)	No effect on BW	↓TAG No effect on serum ALT	↓Lipogenicgenes (Fas, Scd-1, SREBP1c, PPARγ) Improvement of hepatic lipid metabolism (↑Nrf, Cyp2e1, ↓FGF21, Cyp4a1, Cyp1a1, Cyp2b1) ↓Inflammatory markers (MCP-1) ↓Oxidative stress markers (↓Hepatic GSH/GSSG, SOD) ↓Hepatokines (Fetuin-A)	Improved Glucose intolerance Improved Insulin sensitivity	↓Hepatic TG ↓lipotoxic diacylglycerols ↓Fibrosis

Table 2. Key animal studies regarding the impact of canagliflozin on NAFLD/NASH/HCC.

Study/Reference	Animal Model Dose & Duration	Effect on Body & Liver Weight	Effect on Laboratory Values	Mechanism of Action	Effect on Insulin Sensitivity & Glucose Homeostasis	NAFLD Activity Score (NAS) & Fibrosis/Steatosis
Yoshino, K., et al., 2021 [111]	obese diabetic KK-Ay mice putative dose of ~17 mg/kg/day 3 (w)	No effect on body weight No effect epididymal fat weigh ↓Liver/Bw	↓TG No effect on serum ALT	↑Prostaglandin E2 (PGE2) and resolvin E3	↓Plasma glucose levels	↓Hepatic TG
Tanaka K., et al., 2020 [108]	Male C57BL/6J mice on HFD 30 mg/kg/day 4 (w)	↓BW	↓ALT ↑TG, ketone bodies	↑lipid-dependent energy expenditure ↓Respiratory Qquotients ↓Lipogenesis markers (PPAR, FAS, Scd1) ↑Fatty acid β-oxidation markers (CPT1a, PGC1a, PGC1b) ↓Inflammatory markers (IL-1b)	Improved glucose intolerance Improved insulin sensitivity ↓lasma glucose & insulin levels	↓Hepatic TG ↓NAS
Jojima, T., et al., 2019 [87]	STAM mice 30 mg/kg/day 4 & 11 (w)	↓Liver/Bw (11 w)	↓TG (11 w) ↓ALT (11 w)	↓Inflammatory marker and fibrosis marker [SOCS-3, collagen 3 (4 w)] ↓Lipogenesis markers [FAS (11 w)] ↑Inhibits progression of NASH to Hepatocarcinogenesis GS & AFP	↓Plasma glucose levels	↓NAS (11 w) ↓Hepatic fibrosis (4 w) ↓Tumor number (11 w)
Shiba, K., et al., 2018 [101]	MC4R-KO mice on HFD 20–30 mg/kg/day 8, 20 & 52 (w)	↓Liver weight (8 w) ↑Body weight (8 and 52 w)	↑TG (8 and 20 w) ↓ALT (8 and 20 w)	↓Lipogenic markers genes [Acc1 and Scd1 (8 and 20 w), Fasn (8 w)] ↓Gluconeogenic markers (G6pc, Pck1) ↓Inflammatory markers [F4/80 gene (20 w), TNFa (20 w), Cd11c (8 and 20 w)] ↓Fibrosis markers [Col1a1, TIMP-1 (8 and 20w), Acta2, Tgf1b (20 w)]	Improved insulin sensitivity and hyperglycemia (8 and 20 w)	↓Hepatic steatosis (8 w) ↓Hepatic fibrosis (20 w) ↓NAS (20 w) ↓Tumor number (52 w) ↓Hepatic TG content (8 and 20 w)

Table 2. Cont.

Study/Reference	Animal Model Dose & Duration	Effect on Body & Liver Weight	Effect on Laboratory Values	Mechanism of Action	Effect on Insulin Sensitivity & Glucose Homeostasis	NAFLD Activity Score (NAS) & Fibrosis/Steatosis
Ozutsumi, T., et al., 2020 [110]	F344 rats on CDAA diet 10 mg/kg/day 16 (w)	No effect on body weight No effect on Liver/BW	↓ALT	↓Fibrosis markers (αSMA, TGF-β1, α1(I)-procollagen) ↓Inflammatory markers (CCL2, TNF-α, IL-6) ↓Hepatocarcinogenesis markers (GST-P, VEGF, CD31) ↓Oxidative stress markers (MDA, 8-OHdG)	No effect on insulin sensitivity No effect on plasma glucose levels	↓Hepatic fibrosis & Steatosis ↓Hepatic Cirrhosis ↓Hepatic inflammation ↓Hepatic ballooning ↓NAS
Kabil, SI, et al., 2018 [129]	Male Wister rats injected with STZ on HFD 10 and 20 mg/kg/day 8 (w)	↓Liver weight ↓BW (20 mg)	↓ALT ↑TC, TG & NEFA	↑Hepatic lipolytic factor ZAG ↓Inflammatory markers (serum TNF-α, hepatic IL-6) Serum apoptotic markers (↓Caspase3, ↑Bcl-2) Hepatic oxidative stress (↓MDA, ↑SOD and GPx activity) Serum antioxidant enzyme activity (↓TOS and ↑TAS)	No effect on fasting insulin levels Fasting blood glucose	↓Hepatic inflammation ↓Hepatic TC, TG, NEFA ↓Hepatic inflammation Hepatic Steatosis ↓NAS

Table 3. Key animal studies regarding the impact of dapagliflozin on NAFLD/NASH.

Study/Reference	Animal Model Dose & Duration	Effect on Body and Liver Weight	Effect on Laboratory Values	Mechanism of Action	Effect on Insulin Sensitivity & Glucose Homeostasis	NAFLD Activity Score (NAS) & Fibrosis/Steatosis
Han, T., et al., 2021 [105]	Male C57BL/6 J and ob/ob mice on HFD 1 mg/kg/day 4 (w)	No effect on BW	↓TC	↑β-oxidation (PPAR-α, CPT1, PGC1α) ↓Inflammatory markers (MCP1)	↓Fasting blood glucose	↓Hepatic oxidative stress ↓Hepatic lipid accumulation ↓Hepatic steatosis

Table 3. Cont.

Study/Reference	Animal Model Dose & Duration	Effect on Body and Liver Weight	Effect on Laboratory Values	Mechanism of Action	Effect on Insulin Sensitivity & Glucose Homeostasis	NAFLD Activity Score (NAS) & Fibrosis/Steatosis
Luo, J., et al., 2021 [84]	Male NIH mice on HFD 25 mg/kg/day 4 (w)	No effect on BW ↑Food intake	↓ALT	↓Lipogenic markers (SREBP1, ACC, FASN) ↑β-oxidation markers (PPARα, CPT1a) Regulation of lipid metabolism ↑pAMPK and ↓pmTOR	-	↓Hepatic steatosis ↓Hepatic ballooning ↓HepaticTC, TG
Tang, L., et al., 2017 [132]	db/db mice 1.0 mg/kg/day via diet gel 4 (w)	No effect on BW	↓ALT ↓TG	↓Inflammatory markers (MPO, F4/80) ↓Oxidative stress markers (ROS) ↓Fibrosis markers (FN, Col I, Col III, LM)	↓Plasma glucose levels	↓Hepatic injury ↓Hepatic fibrosis ↓Hepatic inflammation
Yabiku, K., et al., 2020 [109]	Male C57BL/6J mice on HFD or HFD + MCDD 0.1 or 1.0 mg/kg/day 2 (w)	↓BW (0.1 and 1 mg) in both diets	↓ALT (0.1 and 1 mg) Mice on HFD	-	Improved glucose tolerance and insulin sensitivity	-
Omori, K., et al., 2019 [125]	db/db mice on ND 1.0 mg/kg/day 8 (w)	No effect on BW ↓Liver weight	↓TG ↓Plasma C-peptide	No significant differences in the expression of fatty acid oxidation markers No significant differences in the expression of inflammatory markers Fatty acid uptake and storage markers (PPARγ targeted genes as compared to Gla group)	Improved glucose tolerance	No significant changes in hepatic TG, Palmitate, Oleate, and Stearate content
Li, L., et al., 2021 [85]	ZDF rats 1 mg/kg/day 9 (w)	↓BW ↓Liver weight ↓Liver weight/BW	↓TG, TC, LDL, HDL	↓Lipogenic markers (SREBP1, ACC1, p-ACC) ↑Fatty acid oxidation markers (ACOX1, CPT1, pACOX) Autophagy-related markers (↑LC3B, Beclin1, activation of AMPK/mTOR pathway and ↓P62)	↓Plasma glucose and insulin levels	↓Hepatic lipid accumulation ↓Hepatic steatosis
ElMahdy, M.K., et al., 2020 [130]	Male Wistar rats on HCHF diet 1 mg/kg/day 5 (w)	No significant effects on liver weight	↓ALT, AST ↓TC, TG, LDL ↑HDL	↓Inflammatory markers (TNF-α, IL-1β, IL-18)	-	↓Hepatic steatosis

Table 4. Key animal studies regarding the impact of ipragliflozin, remogliflozin, tofogliflozin and luseogliflozin on NAFLD/NASH/HCC.

Study/Reference	Animal Model Dose & Duration	Effect on Body Weight & Body Composition	Effect on Laboratory Values	Mechanism of Action	Effect on Insulin Sensitivity & Glucose Homeostasis	NAFLD Activity Score (NAS) & Fibrosis/Steatosis
Ipragliflozin						
Tahara, A. & Takasu, T., 2020 [100]	KK-Ay mice on HFD 0.1, 0.3, 1 and 3 mg/kg/day Alone or with Metformin 4 (w)	↓BW weight (1 & 3 mg) ↓Liver weight (0.3, 1 & 3 mg)	↓TG (0.3, 1 & 3 mg) ↓TC (1 & 3 mg) ↓AST (1 & 3 mg) ↓ALT (0.3, 1 & 3 mg)	↓Inflammatory Markers [serum TNF-α, IL-6, MCP-1 and CRP (1 and 3mg); Liver TNF-α (3 mg) and IL-6, MCP-1 and CRP (1 & 3 mg)] Serum and hepatic oxidative stress markers [TBARS and protein carbonyl (1 & 3 mg)]	Improve glucose intolerance Improved Insulin resistance Improved hyperlipidemia	↓Hepatic TG, TC (1 & 3 mg) ↓Hepatic Hypertrophy (1 & 3 mg) ↓Hepatic Inflammation (1 & 3 mg) ↓Hepatic fibrosis & steatosis (3 mg)
Tahara, A., et al., 2019 [113]	KK-Ay mice on HFD 0.1, 0.3, 1 and 3 mg/kg/day Alone or with Pioglitazone 4 (w)	↓BW weight (1 & 3 mg) ↓Liver weight (0.3, 1 & 3 mg)	↓TC (0.3, 1 & 3 mg) ↓TG (1 & 3 mg) ↓AST (1 & 3 mg) ↓ALT (1 & 3 mg)	↓Genes involved in regulation of insulin sensitivity (Plasma adipocytokines, Leptin & FGF-21) ↓Inflammatory Markers [serum TNF-α, IL-6, MCP-1 and CRP (1 and 3 mg); Liver TNF-α (3 mg) and IL-6, MCP-1 and CRP (1 and 3 mg)] Serum and hepatic oxidative stress markers [TBARS and protein carbonyl (1 & 3 mg)]	↓Plasma glucose and insulin levels (0.3, 1 and 3 mg)	↓Hepatic TG (0.3, 1 & 3 mg) ↓Hepatic TC (1 & 3 mg) ↓Hepatic Hypertrophy (1 & 3 mg) ↓Hepatic Inflammation (3 mg) ↓Hepatic fibrosis (3 mg)
Komiya, Ch., et al., 2016 [112]	ob/ob and WT mice on HFD 11 mg/kg/day 4 (w)	↓Hyperphagia ↓BW weight ↓Liver weight	↓ALT ↓TG ↓Plasma glucagon	↓Lipogenic markers genes (SREBP1, Fasn, Acc1, Scd1) ↓Gluconeogenic markers (Pck1) ↓Inflammatory markers (F4/80, Cd11c)	Improved Insulin resistance Improved fasting glucose levels	↓Hepatic TG ↓Hepatic lipid ↓Hepatic steatosis
Honda, Y., et al., 2016 [114]	C57BL/6J male mice on AMLN diet 40 mg/kg/day 8 (w)	No effect on BW ↓Liver weight	↓ALT, AST ↓FFA	↑β-oxidation (PPAR-α, CPT1, MTTP) ↓Hepatocytes apoptosis (TUNEL) ↓Lipogenic markers genes (SREBP1 & Acc1)	Improved Insulin resistance	↓Hepatic TG & FFA ↓Hepatic fibrosis ↓Hepatocyte ballooning ↓Lobular inflammation ↓NAS

Table 4. Cont.

Study/Reference	Animal Model Dose & Duration	Effect on Body Weight & Body Composition	Effect on Laboratory Values	Mechanism of Action	Effect on Insulin Sensitivity & Glucose Homeostasis	NAFLD Activity Score (NAS) & Fibrosis/Steatosis
Hayashizaki-Someya, Y., et al., 2015 [144]	Male Wistar rats on CDAA diet 0.3 and 3 mg/kg/day 5 (w)	↓ BW weight (3 mg)	No effect on ALT, AST	-	No effect on fasting blood glucose levels	↓ Hepatic TG (3 mg) ↓ Hepatic lipid droplet size ↓ Hepatic fibrosis (0.3 & 3 mg) ↓ Hepatic HP
Yoshioka, N., et al., 2021 [126]	Mc4r KO mice on HFD and injected with single dose of diethylnitrosamine 5 mg/kg/day 12 (w)	↓ BW weight ↓ Liver weight	↓ ALT, AST ↓ LDH	↓ Lipogenic markers genes (Fasn in non-tumor) ↓ Fibrosis markers (Emr1, Itgax in non-tumor) ↓ Cell senescence markers (Cxcl1 in tumor lesion; p21, Cxcl1, MMp12, mmp13 in non-tumor) ↓ β-oxidation (PPAR-α in tumor lesion; PPAR-α, CPT1, PGC1 in non-tumor) ↓ Cell apoptosis (Bax and Pcna)	↓ Plasma glucose & insulin levels	↓ Hepatic TG ↓ Lobular inflammation ↓ Hepatocyte ballooning ↓ NAS ↓ Hepatic steatosis & fibrosis ↓ Hepatic tumor number & size
(Remogliflozin)						
Nakano, S., et al., 2015 [134]	C57BL/6J mice on HFD32 13.2 ± 2.2 and 33.9 ± 2.0 mg/kg/day 4 (w)	↓ Liver weight ↓ Liver/BW	↓ ALT & AST	↓ Inflammatory markers [Hepatic TNF-α (13.2 mg), hepatic MCP-1 (13.2 and 33.9 mg)] ↓ Oxidative stress (serum and hepatic TBARS)	Improved non fasting glucose levels	↓ Hepatic TG ↓ Hepatic fibrosis
Tofogliflozin						
Obara, K., et al., 2017 [89]	db/db mice on HFD and injected with single dose of diethylnitrosamine 1 and 10 mg/kg/day 14 (w)	↓ Liver weight (10 mg)	↓ ALT (10 mg) ↓ FFA (1 & 10 mg)	↓ Inflammatory markers (10 mg) (F4/80)	↓ Plasma glucose levels Improved insulin insensitivity	↓ Foci of cellular alteration (10 mg) ↓ Hepatic pre-neoplastic lesions (10 mg) ↓ Hepatocyte ballooning (10 mg) ↓ Hepatic steatosis (10 mg) ↓ NAS (1 & 10 mg)

Table 4. Cont.

Study/Reference	Animal Model Dose & Duration	Effect on Body Weight & Body Composition	Effect on Laboratory Values	Mechanism of Action	Effect on Insulin Sensitivity & Glucose Homeostasis	NAFLD Activity Score (NAS) & Fibrosis/Steatosis
				Luseoglifozin		
Qiang, Sh, et al., 2015 [142]	C57BL/6 mice injected with STZ on HFDT Mixing in food at 0.1%. w/w food 8 (w)	↓ Liver weight	↓ ALT ↑ TG, NEFA	↓ Hepatic fibrosis markers (collagen1a1, collagen1a2, TGF, SMA, TIMP1) ↓ Inflammatory markers (MCP-1, IL1, IL-12, IL-6, f4/80)	↓ Plasma glucose levels	↓ Hepatic TC, TG & NEFA

Abbreviations: W: week, BW: Body Weight, STZ: streptozotocin, WT: Wild Type, Gla:insulin glargine, ALT: Alanine aminotransferase, TG: Triglycerides, TC: Total cholesterol, FFA: Free fatty acids, GA: glycated albumin, STAT3: Signal Transducer And Activator Of Transcription 3, ROR: RAR Related Orphan Receptor, Bax: BCL2 Associated X, IRE: Inositol-requiring enzyme 1, -Xbp1: X-box binding protein 1, ATF4: Activating transcription factor 4, CHOP: C/EBP homologous protein, ATF-6:Activating transcription factor 6, ChREBP: Carbohydrate response element binding protein, SREBP1: Sterol regulatory element-binding transcription factor 1, Scd1: Stearoyl-CoA desaturase1, ACC1: Acetyl-CoAcarboxylase 1, ACOX: Peroxisomal acyl-CoA oxidase1 Fasn: Fatty acid synthase, IL: Interleukin, TNF-α: Tumor necrosis factor, NFκB: Nuclear factor kappa-light-chain-enhancer of activated B cells, MCP-1:Monocyte chemoattractant protein-1, CRP:C-reactive protein, PPAR-α: Peroxisome proliferator activated receptor alpha, CPT1: Carnitine palmitoyltransferase 1, PGC1: PPARγ coactivator 1, TOS: Total Oxidant Status, TAS: Total antioxidant status, p21: cyclin-dependent kinase inhibitor, Cxcl: Chemokine (C-X-C motif) ligand, MMP: Matrix metalloproteinases, TIMP: Tissue inhibitors of matrix metalloproteinases, CYP: Cytochromes P450, MDA: Malondialdehyde.

4.2. Human Trials

A number of clinical studies have highlighted the benefit of SGLT-2i in patients with T2DM and NAFLD (Table 5) [145–169]. In the majority of them, the administration of SGLT-2i has resulted in improvement of serum levels of liver enzymes and hepatic steatosis, as evaluated by magnetic resonance imaging (MRI), ultrasound (U/S), non-invasive biomarkers, such as AST to platelet ratio (APRI) index, NAFLD fibrosis score (NFS) and Fibrosis-4 (FIB-4) score, or even by liver biopsy (LB). In some of these studies, improvement in hepatic fibrosis was found, using transient elastography (TE) or LB, even though this finding was not univocal [146,153,158,159,164,165,168].

Of note, the overall improvement in hepatic steatosis is also found in patients treated with other classes of anti-diabetic drugs, like thiazolidinediones and dipeptidyl peptidase-4 (DPP-4) inhibitors, raising the question of steatosis improvement due to glycemic control [148,160,162,170]. Moreover, the vast majority of the aforementioned studies are limited by the small sample size, heterogenous inclusion criteria, especially regarding the presence of NAFLD, as well as the duration of follow up, thus meta-analyses have been conducted to better assess the true benefit of SGLT-2i in patients with DM and NAFLD [171–173]. In the largest one, comprising 9 randomized trials, with 7281 and 4088 patients in the SGLT-2i and control arm, (standard of care (SOC) or placebo), respectively, the use of SGLT-2i resulted in improvement of serum transaminases, body weight, and liver fat as measured by proton density fat fraction. Accordingly, the authors discuss that this improvement derives mainly from the achievement of glycemic control and weight loss. However, in a 2020 study by Kahl et al., including 84 patients with DM and excellent glycemic control, randomly assigned to empagliflozin or placebo, patients on empagliflozin had improved liver fat content, as assessed by MRI [161], strongly suggesting that the good glycemic control and weight loss are not the only mechanisms associated with the beneficial effects of SGLT-2i treatment on hepatic steatosis.

In non-DM patients, only a small single center study exists which studied 12 patients under dapagliflozin and 10 patients under teneligliptin, a DPP4 inhibitor, for a total of 12 weeks, showing that after this intervention period, serum transaminases were decreased in both groups, while in the dapagliflozin group, total body water and body fat decreased, leading to decreased total body weight [174].

Regarding the pathophysiology of NAFLD improvement under SGLT-2i treatment, various mechanisms have been suggested. Treatment with SGLT-2i results in decreases in both glucose and insulin levels (especially in patients with DM), which lead to a large reduction of hepatic de novo lipid synthesis [175]. Moreover, glucagon-secreting alpha pancreatic cells also express SGLT-2, thus the administration of SGLT-2i stimulates glucagon secretion [175–177]. In turn, the subsequently elevated plasma glucagon levels stimulate β-oxidation, and this shift from carbohydrate to fatty acid metabolism leads to reduced liver triglyceride content and consequently hepatic steatosis [175,178,179]. Another potential mechanism is mediated by the antioxidant effects of SGLT-2i. Apart from their ability to reduce high glucose-induced oxidative stress, SGLT-2i reduce free radical generation, suppress pro-oxidants, and upregulate antioxidant systems, such as superoxide dismutases (SODs) and glutathione (GSH) peroxidases (Figure 1) [116,180–184].

Table 5. Studies on the impact of SGLT-2i on NAFLD in patients with T2DM.

Study	Study Design	No of Pts	SGLT-2i/Drug Used (No of Pts)	Control Group	Treatment Duration (Weeks)	NAFLD Diagnosis **	Key Results
Eriksson, J., et al., 2018 [150]	Randomised, double-blind, prospective	84	Dapagliflozin (42)	OM-3CA or placebo	12	MRI	Reduction of serum transaminases, CK-18, FGF-21 in Dapagliflozin group and liver fat in Dapagliflozin + OM-3CA group
Kahl, S., et al., 2020, [161]	Randomised, double-blind, prospective	84 *	Empagliflozin (42)	Placebo	24	MRI	LFC improvement only in empagliflozin
Chehrehgosha, H., et al., 2021 [165]	Randomised, double-blind, prospective	78	Empagliflozin (21)	Pioglitazone or placebo	24	TE	Better CAP, LS, no difference vs. pioglitazone for serum transaminases or FIB-4
Gaborit, B., et al., 2021 [167]	Randomised, double-blind, prospective	34	Empagliflozin (18)	Placebo	12	MRI	Reduction in liver fat vs. placebo
Bando, Y., et al., 2017 [145]	Randomised, open label, prospective	62	Ipragliflozin (40)	SOC	12	C/T	Improvement in serum transaminases. VFA, L/S ratio compared to SOC
Ito, D., et al., 2017 [147]	Randomised, open label, prospective	66	Ipragliflozin (32)	Pioglitazone	24	C/T or U/S	Improvement of L/S ratio, ALT, ferritin not statistically significant between 2 groups; ipragliflozin more weight and VFA reduction
Kuchay, M.S., et al., 2018 [152]	Randomised, open label, prospective	42	Empagliflozin (22)	SOC	20	MRI	Reduction of liver fat and ALT
Shibuya, T., et al., 2018 [154]	Randomised, open label, prospective	32	Luseogliflozin (16)	Metformin	26 (6 months)	C/T or U/S	Improvement in L/S ratio compared to baseline
Shimizu, M., et al., 2019 [155]	Randomised, open label, prospective	57	Dapagliflozin (33)	SOC	24	U/S	Improvement of CAP and LS, especially for high LS at the trial beginning
Han, E., et al., 2020 [160]	Randomized, open label, prospective	44	Ipragliflozin (+metformin +pioglitazone) (29)	Metformin + pioglitazone	24	U/S	Better FLI, CAP, NAFLD liver fat score

Table 5. Cont.

Study	Study Design	No of Pts	SGLT-2i/Drug Used (No of Pts)	Control Group	Treatment Duration (Weeks)	NAFLD Diagnosis **	Key Results
Kinoshita, T., et al., 2020 [162]	Randomized, open label, prospective	98	Dapagliflozin (32)	Pioglitazone (33) Glimepiride (33)	28	C/T	Improvement of L/S ratio and ALT with pioglitazone and dapagliflozin
Takahashi, H., et al., 2021 [168]	Randomized, open label, prospective	55	Ipragliflozin (27)	SOC, except pioglitazone, GLP1	72	LB	Statistically significant improvement in NASH resolution and fibrosis improvement in SGLT-2i vs. SOC
Yoneda, M., et al., 2021 [169]	Randomized, open label, prospective	40	Topogliflozin (21)	Pioglitzone	24	MRI	Decrease of liver steatosis in both groups, body weight decrease in topogliflozin
Arai, T., et al., 2021 [164]	Open label, Prospective	100	Canagliflozin (29) Ipragliflozin (12) Tofogliflozin (6) Dapagliflozin (4) Luseogliflozin (4) Empagliflozin (1)	SOC	48	U/S	Decrease in LS and CAP in SGLT-2i during treatment, statistically significant decrease in SGLT-2i vs SOC in ALT, FIB-4
Akuta, N., et al. 2017 [146]	Single-arm, Prospective	5	Canagliflozin (5)	N/A	24	LB	Improvement of NAS score, liver steatosis; fibrosis improvement in 2 pts
Itani, T., et al., 2018 [151]	Single arm, Prospective	35	Canagliflozin (35)	N/A	26 (6 months)	U/S	Improvement in ALT, ferritin, FIB-4 at 3 and 6 months
Miyake, T., et al., 2018 [153]	Single arm, Prospective	43	Ipragliflozin (43)	N/A	24	12 LB, 41 U/S	Reduction in serum transaminases, CAP, not statistically significant reduction in fibrosis
Sumida, Y., et al. 2019 [156]	Single-arm, Prospective	40	Luseogliflozin (40)	N/A	24	U/S	Reduction in transaminases, serum ferritin and liver fat in MRI
Akuta, N., et al. 2019 [157]	Single arm, Prospective	9	Canagliflozin (9)	N/A	24	LB	Histological improvement in all patients

Table 5. Cont.

Study	Study Design	No of Pts	SGLT-2i/Drug Used (No of Pts)	Control Group	Treatment Duration (Weeks)	NAFLD Diagnosis **	Key Results
Akuta, N., et al., 2020 [159]	Single arm, Prospective	7	Canagliflozin (7)	N/A	24	LB	Histopathological improvement at 24 weeks sustained to >1 year, transaminases and ferritin better at 24 weeks
Seko, Y., et al., 2017 [148]	Retrospective	45	Canagliflozin (18) Ipragliflozin (6)	Sitagliptin	24	LB	Significant decrease in serum transaminases with both drugs, not statistically significant between SGLT-2i and sitagliptin
Choi, D.H., et al., 2018 [149]	Retrospective	102 (all abnormal ALT)	Dapagliflozin + Metformin (50)	DPP4 + Metformin	44.4 ± 18.4 for dapagliflozin and 50.4 ± 21.6 for DPP4	U/S	Statistically significant decrease in dapagliflozin vs. DPP4
Yamashima, M., et al., 2019 [158]	Retrospective	22	Ipragliflozin (18) Dapagliflozin (2) Tofogliflozin (1) Empagliflozin (1)	N/A	52 (22 pts) and 104 (15 pts)	12 LB, 10 U/S	Lower serum transaminases levels at 12 and 24 months, better CAR and shear wave velocity at 12 months
Yano, K., et al., 2020 [163]	Retrospective	69	Dapagliflozin (10) Canagliflozin (7) Ipragliflozin (3) Empagliflozin (2)	SOC	162	LB	Improvement of serum transaminases in both groups (No head to head comparison)
Euh, W., et al., 2021 [166]	Retrospective	283	Dapagliflozin (58) Empagliflozin (34) Ipragliflozin (3)	SOC, except GLP-1 and Insulin	39	U/S	Statistically significant reduction in ALT and body weight in SLT2i vs. SOC

* All patients with excellent glycemic control. ** Test used to diagnose/assess NAFLD. Abbreviations: RCT: Randomised controlled trial, L/S ratio: Liver to spleen ratio, VFA: Visceral fat area, C/T: Computed tomography, MRI: Magnetic Resonance Imaging, OM-3CA: omega-3 carboxylic acids, LFC: Liver fat content, FIB-4: Fibrosis-4 index, ALT: Alanine aminotransferase, FLI: Fatty liver index, CAP: Controlled attenuation parameter, SGLT-2i: Sodium-glucose co-transporter type-2 inhibitors, NAS score: NAFLD Activity Score, LB: Liver biopsy, GLP-1: Glucagon-like peptide-1, pts: patients.

5. Conclusions

There is increasing interest regarding the promising effect(s) of SGLT-2i for the treatment of NAFLD, regardless of the co-existence of T2DM. In addition to weight loss, the beneficial effect(s) of SGLT-2i on NAFLD development and progression appear to be mediated directly through regulation of multiple processes, including ER stress, oxidative stress, low-grade inflammation, autophagy and apoptosis, as revealed by in vitro, animal and clinical studies. Moreover, the observed different effects between members of the SGLT-2i class suggest that there are features specific to individual drugs of this class regarding the underlying mechanism(s) of action and their corresponding effects on NAFLD.

Funding: This review article received no external funding.

Institutional Review Board Statement: Not applicable.

Informed Consent Statement: Not applicable.

Data Availability Statement: Not applicable.

Acknowledgments: Not applicable.

Conflicts of Interest: The authors declare no conflict of interest.

References

1. Younossi, Z.M.; Koenig, A.B.; Abdelatif, D.; Fazel, Y.; Henry, L.; Wymer, M. Global epidemiology of nonalcoholic fatty liver disease-Meta-analytic assessment of prevalence, incidence, and outcomes. *Hepatology* **2016**, *64*, 73–84. [CrossRef] [PubMed]
2. Li, J.; Zou, B.; Yeo, Y.H.; Feng, Y.; Xie, X.; Lee, D.H.; Fujii, H.; Wu, Y.; Kam, L.Y.; Ji, F.; et al. Prevalence, incidence, and outcome of non-alcoholic fatty liver disease in Asia, 1999–2019: A systematic review and meta-analysis. *Lancet Gastroenterol. Hepatol.* **2019**, *4*, 389–398. [CrossRef]
3. Hui, J.M.; Kench, J.G.; Chitturi, S.; Sud, A.; Farrell, G.C.; Byth, K.; Hall, P.; Khan, M.; George, J. Long-term outcomes of cirrhosis in nonalcoholic steatohepatitis compared with hepatitis C. *Hepatology* **2003**, *38*, 420–427. [CrossRef] [PubMed]
4. Bugianesi, E.; Leone, N.; Vanni, E.; Marchesini, G.; Brunello, F.; Carucci, P.; Musso, A.; De Paolis, P.; Capussotti, L.; Salizzoni, M.; et al. Expanding the natural history of nonalcoholic steatohepatitis: From cryptogenic cirrhosis to hepatocellular carcinoma. *Gastroenterology* **2002**, *123*, 134–140. [CrossRef] [PubMed]
5. Yki-Jarvinen, H. Non-alcoholic fatty liver disease as a cause and a consequence of metabolic syndrome. *Lancet Diabetes Endocrinol.* **2014**, *2*, 901–910. [CrossRef]
6. Petroni, M.L.; Brodosi, L.; Bugianesi, E.; Marchesini, G. Management of non-alcoholic fatty liver disease. *BMJ* **2021**, *372*, m4747. [CrossRef]
7. European Association for the Study of the Liver (EASL); European Association for the Study of Diabetes (EASD); European Association for the Study of Obesity (EASO). EASL-EASD-EASO Clinical Practice Guidelines for the management of non-alcoholic fatty liver disease. *J. Hepatol.* **2016**, *64*, 1388–1402. [CrossRef]
8. Chalasani, N.; Younossi, Z.; Lavine, J.E.; Charlton, M.; Cusi, K.; Rinella, M.; Harrison, S.A.; Brunt, E.M.; Sanyal, A.J. The diagnosis and management of nonalcoholic fatty liver disease: Practice guidance from the American Association for the Study of Liver Diseases. *Hepatology* **2018**, *67*, 328–357. [CrossRef]
9. Eslam, M.; Sanyal, A.J.; George, J. MAFLD: A Consensus-Driven Proposed Nomenclature for Metabolic Associated Fatty Liver Disease. *Gastroenterology* **2020**, *158*, 1999–2014.e1. [CrossRef]
10. Fouad, Y.; Waked, I.; Bollipo, S.; Gomaa, A.; Ajlouni, Y.; Attia, D. What's in a name? Renaming 'NAFLD' to 'MAFLD'. *Liver Int.* **2020**, *40*, 1254–1261. [CrossRef]
11. Rinaldi, L.; Pafundi, P.C.; Galiero, R.; Caturano, A.; Morone, M.V.; Silvestri, C.; Giordano, M.; Salvatore, T.; Sasso, F.C. Mechanisms of Non-Alcoholic Fatty Liver Disease in the Metabolic Syndrome. A Narrative Review. *Antioxidants* **2021**, *10*, 270. [CrossRef]
12. Masarone, M.; Rosato, V.; Aglitti, A.; Bucci, T.; Caruso, R.; Salvatore, T.; Sasso, F.C.; Tripodi, M.F.; Persico, M. Liver biopsy in type 2 diabetes mellitus: Steatohepatitis represents the sole feature of liver damage. *PLoS ONE* **2017**, *12*, e0178473. [CrossRef]
13. Tanase, D.M.; Gosav, E.M.; Costea, C.F.; Ciocoiu, M.; Lacatusu, C.M.; Maranduca, M.A.; Ouatu, A.; Floria, M. The Intricate Relationship between Type 2 Diabetes Mellitus (T2DM), Insulin Resistance (IR), and Nonalcoholic Fatty Liver Disease (NAFLD). *J. Diabetes Res.* **2020**, *2020*, 3920196. [CrossRef]
14. Fargion, S.; Porzio, M.; Fracanzani, A.L. Nonalcoholic fatty liver disease and vascular disease: State-of-the-art. *World J. Gastroenterol.* **2014**, *20*, 13306–13324. [CrossRef]
15. Galiero, R.; Caturano, A.; Vetrano, E.; Cesaro, A.; Rinaldi, L.; Salvatore, T.; Marfella, R.; Sardu, C.; Moscarella, E.; Gragnano, F.; et al. Pathophysiological mechanisms and clinical evidence of relationship between Nonalcoholic fatty liver disease (NAFLD) and cardiovascular disease. *Rev. Cardiovasc. Med.* **2021**, *22*, 755–768. [CrossRef]

16. Petta, S.; Argano, C.; Colomba, D.; Camma, C.; Di Marco, V.; Cabibi, D.; Tuttolomondo, A.; Marchesini, G.; Pinto, A.; Licata, G.; et al. Epicardial fat, cardiac geometry and cardiac function in patients with non-alcoholic fatty liver disease: Association with the severity of liver disease. *J. Hepatol.* **2015**, *62*, 928–933. [CrossRef]
17. U.S. Food and Drug Administration (FDA). FDA Approves New Treatment for a Type of Heart Failure. Available online: https://www.fda.gov/news-events/press-announcements/fda-approves-new-treatment-type-heart-failure (accessed on 10 December 2021).
18. U.S. Food and Drug Administration (FDA). FDA Approves Treatment for Chronic Kidney Disease. Available online: https://www.fda.gov/news-events/press-announcements/fda-approves-treatment-chronic-kidney-disease (accessed on 15 December 2021).
19. Kim, J.W.; Lee, Y.J.; You, Y.H.; Moon, M.K.; Yoon, K.H.; Ahn, Y.B.; Ko, S.H. Effect of sodium-glucose cotransporter 2 inhibitor, empagliflozin, and alpha-glucosidase inhibitor, voglibose, on hepatic steatosis in an animal model of type 2 diabetes. *J. Cell Biochem.* **2018**, *20*, 8534–8546. [CrossRef]
20. Buzzetti, E.; Pinzani, M.; Tsochatzis, E.A. The multiple-hit pathogenesis of non-alcoholic fatty liver disease (NAFLD). *Metabolism* **2016**, *65*, 1038–1048. [CrossRef]
21. Eslam, M.; Valenti, L.; Romeo, S. Genetics and epigenetics of NAFLD and NASH: Clinical impact. *J. Hepatol.* **2018**, *68*, 268–279. [CrossRef]
22. Mahady, S.E.; George, J. Exercise and diet in the management of nonalcoholic fatty liver disease. *Metabolism* **2016**, *65*, 1172–1182. [CrossRef]
23. Polyzos, S.A.; Kountouras, J.; Mantzoros, C.S. Obesity and nonalcoholic fatty liver disease: From pathophysiology to therapeutics. *Metabolism* **2019**, *92*, 82–97. [CrossRef]
24. Perry, R.J.; Samuel, V.T.; Petersen, K.F.; Shulman, G.I. The role of hepatic lipids in hepatic insulin resistance and type 2 diabetes. *Nature* **2014**, *510*, 84–91. [CrossRef]
25. Marra, F.; Bertolani, C. Adipokines in liver diseases. *Hepatology* **2009**, *50*, 957–969. [CrossRef]
26. Marra, F.; Svegliati-Baroni, G. Lipotoxicity and the gut-liver axis in NASH pathogenesis. *J. Hepatol.* **2018**, *68*, 280–295. [CrossRef]
27. Gluchowski, N.L.; Becuwe, M.; Walther, T.C.; Farese, R.V., Jr. Lipid droplets and liver disease: From basic biology to clinical implications. *Nat. Rev. Gastroenterol. Hepatol.* **2017**, *14*, 343–355. [CrossRef]
28. Mansouri, A.; Gattolliat, C.H.; Asselah, T. Mitochondrial Dysfunction and Signaling in Chronic Liver Diseases. *Gastroenterology* **2018**, *155*, 629–647. [CrossRef]
29. Zhang, Y.; Li, K.; Kong, A.; Zhou, Y.; Chen, D.; Gu, J.; Shi, H. Dysregulation of autophagy acts as a pathogenic mechanism of non-alcoholic fatty liver disease (NAFLD) induced by common environmental pollutants. *Ecotoxicol. Environ. Saf.* **2021**, *217*, 112256. [CrossRef]
30. Nasiri-Ansari, N.; Nikolopoulou, C.; Papoutsi, K.; Kyrou, I.; Mantzoros, C.S.; Kyriakopoulos, G.; Chatzigeorgiou, A.; Kalotychou, V.; Randeva, M.S.; Chatha, K.; et al. Empagliflozin Attenuates Non-Alcoholic Fatty Liver Disease (NAFLD) in High Fat Diet Fed ApoE$^{-/-}$ Mice by Activating Autophagy and Reducing ER Stress and Apoptosis. *Int. J. Mol. Sci.* **2021**, *22*, 818. [CrossRef]
31. Xiong, X.; Wang, X.; Lu, Y.; Wang, E.; Zhang, Z.; Yang, J.; Zhang, H.; Li, X. Hepatic steatosis exacerbated by endoplasmic reticulum stress-mediated downregulation of FXR in aging mice. *J. Hepatol.* **2014**, *60*, 847–854. [CrossRef]
32. Zhang, X.; Han, J.; Man, K.; Li, X.; Du, J.; Chu, E.S.; Go, M.Y.; Sung, J.J.; Yu, J. CXC chemokine receptor 3 promotes steatohepatitis in mice through mediating inflammatory cytokines, macrophages and autophagy. *J. Hepatol.* **2016**, *64*, 160–170. [CrossRef]
33. Alkhouri, N.; Carter-Kent, C.; Feldstein, A.E. Apoptosis in nonalcoholic fatty liver disease: Diagnostic and therapeutic implications. *Expert Rev. Gastroenterol. Hepatol.* **2011**, *5*, 201–212. [CrossRef]
34. Cai, J.; Zhang, X.J.; Li, H. The Role of Innate Immune Cells in Nonalcoholic Steatohepatitis. *Hepatology* **2019**, *70*, 1026–1037. [CrossRef] [PubMed]
35. Lee, Y.A.; Friedman, S.L. Inflammatory and fibrotic mechanisms in NAFLD-Implications for new treatment strategies. *J. Intern. Med.* **2021**, *291*, 11–31. [CrossRef] [PubMed]
36. Ertunc, M.E.; Hotamisligil, G.S. Lipid signaling and lipotoxicity in metaflammation: Indications for metabolic disease pathogenesis and treatment. *J. Lipid Res.* **2016**, *57*, 2099–2114. [CrossRef] [PubMed]
37. Greco, D.; Kotronen, A.; Westerbacka, J.; Puig, O.; Arkkila, P.; Kiviluoto, T.; Laitinen, S.; Kolak, M.; Fisher, R.M.; Hamsten, A.; et al. Gene expression in human NAFLD. *Am. J. Physiol. Gastrointest. Liver Physiol.* **2008**, *294*, G1281–G1287. [CrossRef] [PubMed]
38. Magkos, F.; Fraterrigo, G.; Yoshino, J.; Luecking, C.; Kirbach, K.; Kelly, S.C.; de Las Fuentes, L.; He, S.; Okunade, A.L.; Patterson, B.W.; et al. Effects of Moderate and Subsequent Progressive Weight Loss on Metabolic Function and Adipose Tissue Biology in Humans with Obesity. *Cell Metab.* **2016**, *23*, 591–601. [CrossRef]
39. Vilar-Gomez, E.; Martinez-Perez, Y.; Calzadilla-Bertot, L.; Torres-Gonzalez, A.; Gra-Oramas, B.; Gonzalez-Fabian, L.; Friedman, S.L.; Diago, M.; Romero-Gomez, M. Weight Loss through Lifestyle Modification Significantly Reduces Features of Nonalcoholic Steatohepatitis. *Gastroenterology* **2015**, *149*, 367–378.e5; quiz e14–e15. [CrossRef]
40. Schwarz, J.M.; Noworolski, S.M.; Erkin-Cakmak, A.; Korn, N.J.; Wen, M.J.; Tai, V.W.; Jones, G.M.; Palii, S.P.; Velasco-Alin, M.; Pan, K.; et al. Effects of Dietary Fructose Restriction on Liver Fat, De Novo Lipogenesis, and Insulin Kinetics in Children with Obesity. *Gastroenterology* **2017**, *153*, 743–752. [CrossRef]
41. Donnelly, K.L.; Smith, C.I.; Schwarzenberg, S.J.; Jessurun, J.; Boldt, M.D.; Parks, E.J. Sources of fatty acids stored in liver and secreted via lipoproteins in patients with nonalcoholic fatty liver disease. *J. Clin. Invest.* **2005**, *115*, 1343–1351. [CrossRef]

42. Wang, Y.; Viscarra, J.; Kim, S.J.; Sul, H.S. Transcriptional regulation of hepatic lipogenesis. *Nat. Rev. Mol. Cell Biol.* **2015**, *16*, 678–689. [CrossRef]
43. Abdelmalek, M.F.; Lazo, M.; Horska, A.; Bonekamp, S.; Lipkin, E.W.; Balasubramanyam, A.; Bantle, J.P.; Johnson, R.J.; Diehl, A.M.; Clark, J.M. Higher dietary fructose is associated with impaired hepatic adenosine triphosphate homeostasis in obese individuals with type 2 diabetes. *Hepatology* **2012**, *56*, 952–960. [CrossRef]
44. Ipsen, D.H.; Lykkesfeldt, J.; Tveden-Nyborg, P. Molecular mechanisms of hepatic lipid accumulation in non-alcoholic fatty liver disease. *Cell Mol. Life Sci.* **2018**, *75*, 3313–3327. [CrossRef]
45. Xu, A.; Wang, Y.; Keshaw, H.; Xu, L.Y.; Lam, K.S.; Cooper, G.J. The fat-derived hormone adiponectin alleviates alcoholic and nonalcoholic fatty liver diseases in mice. *J. Clin. Invest.* **2003**, *112*, 91–100. [CrossRef]
46. Myers, M.G.; Cowley, M.A.; Münzberg, H. Mechanisms of leptin action and leptin resistance. *Annu. Rev. Physiol.* **2008**, *70*, 537–556. [CrossRef]
47. Sabio, G.; Das, M.; Mora, A.; Zhang, Z.; Jun, J.Y.; Ko, H.J.; Barrett, T.; Kim, J.K.; Davis, R.J. A stress signaling pathway in adipose tissue regulates hepatic insulin resistance. *Science* **2008**, *322*, 1539–1543. [CrossRef]
48. Aubert, J.; Begriche, K.; Knockaert, L.; Robin, M.A.; Fromenty, B. Increased expression of cytochrome P450 2E1 in nonalcoholic fatty liver disease: Mechanisms and pathophysiological role. *Clin. Res. Hepatol. Gastroenterol.* **2011**, *35*, 630–637. [CrossRef]
49. Delli Bovi, A.P.; Marciano, F.; Mandato, C.; Siano, M.A.; Savoia, M.; Vajro, P. Oxidative Stress in Non-alcoholic Fatty Liver Disease. An Updated Mini Review. *Front. Med.* **2021**, *8*, 595371. [CrossRef]
50. Cases, S.; Smith, S.J.; Zheng, Y.W.; Myers, H.M.; Lear, S.R.; Sande, E.; Novak, S.; Collins, C.; Welch, C.B.; Lusis, A.J.; et al. Identification of a gene encoding an acyl CoA:diacylglycerol acyltransferase, a key enzyme in triacylglycerol synthesis. *Proc. Natl. Acad. Sci. USA* **1998**, *95*, 13018–13023. [CrossRef]
51. Cases, S.; Stone, S.J.; Zhou, P.; Yen, E.; Tow, B.; Lardizabal, K.D.; Voelker, T.; Farese, R.V., Jr. Cloning of DGAT2, a second mammalian diacylglycerol acyltransferase, and related family members. *J. Biol. Chem.* **2001**, *276*, 38870–38876. [CrossRef]
52. Luukkonen, P.K.; Zhou, Y.; Sädevirta, S.; Leivonen, M.; Arola, J.; Orešič, M.; Hyötyläinen, T.; Yki-Järvinen, H. Hepatic ceramides dissociate steatosis and insulin resistance in patients with non-alcoholic fatty liver disease. *J. Hepatol.* **2016**, *64*, 1167–1175. [CrossRef]
53. Han, M.S.; Park, S.Y.; Shinzawa, K.; Kim, S.; Chung, K.W.; Lee, J.H.; Kwon, C.H.; Lee, K.W.; Lee, J.H.; Park, C.K.; et al. Lysophosphatidylcholine as a death effector in the lipoapoptosis of hepatocytes. *J. Lipid Res.* **2008**, *49*, 84–97. [CrossRef] [PubMed]
54. Fassnacht, M.; Kreissl, M.C.; Weismann, D.; Allolio, B. New targets and therapeutic approaches for endocrine malignancies. *Pharmacol. Ther.* **2009**, *123*, 117–141. [CrossRef] [PubMed]
55. Yamaguchi, K.; Yang, L.; McCall, S.; Huang, J.; Yu, X.X.; Pandey, S.K.; Bhanot, S.; Monia, B.P.; Li, Y.X.; Diehl, A.M. Inhibiting triglyceride synthesis improves hepatic steatosis but exacerbates liver damage and fibrosis in obese mice with nonalcoholic steatohepatitis. *Hepatology* **2007**, *45*, 1366–1374. [CrossRef] [PubMed]
56. Puri, P.; Mirshahi, F.; Cheung, O.; Natarajan, R.; Maher, J.W.; Kellum, J.M.; Sanyal, A.J. Activation and dysregulation of the unfolded protein response in nonalcoholic fatty liver disease. *Gastroenterology* **2008**, *134*, 568–576. [CrossRef]
57. Wei, Y.; Wang, D.; Pagliassotti, M.J. Saturated fatty acid-mediated endoplasmic reticulum stress and apoptosis are augmented by trans-10, cis-12-conjugated linoleic acid in liver cells. *Mol. Cell Biochem.* **2007**, *303*, 105–113. [CrossRef]
58. Wei, Y.; Wang, D.; Topczewski, F.; Pagliassotti, M.J. Saturated fatty acids induce endoplasmic reticulum stress and apoptosis independently of ceramide in liver cells. *Am. J. Physiol. Endocrinol. Metab.* **2006**, *291*, E275–E281. [CrossRef]
59. Li, C.; Xu, M.M.; Wang, K.; Adler, A.J.; Vella, A.T.; Zhou, B. Macrophage polarization and meta-inflammation. *Transl. Res.* **2018**, *191*, 29–44. [CrossRef]
60. Tilg, H.; Moschen, A.R.; Szabo, G. Interleukin-1 and inflammasomes in alcoholic liver disease/acute alcoholic hepatitis and nonalcoholic fatty liver disease/nonalcoholic steatohepatitis. *Hepatology* **2016**, *64*, 955–965. [CrossRef]
61. Gomes, A.L.; Teijeiro, A.; Burén, S.; Tummala, K.S.; Yilmaz, M.; Waisman, A.; Theurillat, J.P.; Perna, C.; Djouder, N. Metabolic Inflammation-Associated IL-17A Causes Non-alcoholic Steatohepatitis and Hepatocellular Carcinoma. *Cancer Cell* **2016**, *30*, 161–175. [CrossRef]
62. Choi, C.I. Sodium-Glucose Cotransporter 2 (SGLT2) Inhibitors from Natural Products: Discovery of Next-Generation Antihyperglycemic Agents. *Molecules* **2016**, *21*, 1136. [CrossRef]
63. Hardman, T.C.; Rutherford, P.; Duprey, S.W.; Wierzbicki, A.S. Sodium-glucose co-transporter 2 inhibitors: From apple tree to 'Sweet Pee'. *Curr. Pharm. Des.* **2010**, *16*, 3830–3838. [CrossRef]
64. Blaschek, W. Natural Products as Lead Compounds for Sodium Glucose Cotransporter (SGLT) Inhibitors. *Planta Med.* **2017**, *83*, 985–993. [CrossRef]
65. Vick, H.; Diedrich, D.F.; Baumann, K. Reevaluation of renal tubular glucose transport inhibition by phlorizin analogs. *Am. J. Physiol.* **1973**, *224*, 552–557. [CrossRef]
66. Ehrenkranz, J.R.; Lewis, N.G.; Kahn, C.R.; Roth, J. Phlorizin: A review. *Diabetes Metab. Res. Rev.* **2005**, *21*, 31–38. [CrossRef]
67. Tian, L.; Cao, J.; Zhao, T.; Liu, Y.; Khan, A.; Cheng, G. The Bioavailability, Extraction, Biosynthesis and Distribution of Natural Dihydrochalcone: Phloridzin. *Int. J. Mol. Sci.* **2021**, *22*, 962. [CrossRef]
68. Lehmann, A.; Hornby, P.J. Intestinal SGLT1 in metabolic health and disease. *Am. J. Physiol. Gastrointest. Liver Physiol.* **2016**, *310*, G887–G898. [CrossRef]

69. Katsuno, K.; Fujimori, Y.; Takemura, Y.; Hiratochi, M.; Itoh, F.; Komatsu, Y.; Fujikura, H.; Isaji, M. Sergliflozin, a novel selective inhibitor of low-affinity sodium glucose cotransporter (SGLT2), validates the critical role of SGLT2 in renal glucose reabsorption and modulates plasma glucose level. *J. Pharmacol. Exp. Ther.* **2007**, *320*, 323–330. [CrossRef]
70. Oku, A.; Ueta, K.; Arakawa, K.; Ishihara, T.; Nawano, M.; Kuronuma, Y.; Matsumoto, M.; Saito, A.; Tsujihara, K.; Anai, M.; et al. T-1095, an inhibitor of renal Na^+-glucose cotransporters, may provide a novel approach to treating diabetes. *Diabetes* **1999**, *48*, 1794–1800. [CrossRef]
71. Meng, W.; Ellsworth, B.A.; Nirschl, A.A.; McCann, P.J.; Patel, M.; Girotra, R.N.; Wu, G.; Sher, P.M.; Morrison, E.P.; Biller, S.A.; et al. Discovery of dapagliflozin: A potent, selective renal sodium-dependent glucose cotransporter 2 (SGLT2) inhibitor for the treatment of type 2 diabetes. *J. Med. Chem.* **2008**, *51*, 1145–1149. [CrossRef]
72. Nomura, S.; Sakamaki, S.; Hongu, M.; Kawanishi, E.; Koga, Y.; Sakamoto, T.; Yamamoto, Y.; Ueta, K.; Kimata, H.; Nakayama, K.; et al. Discovery of canagliflozin, a novel C-glucoside with thiophene ring, as sodium-dependent glucose cotransporter 2 inhibitor for the treatment of type 2 diabetes mellitus. *J. Med. Chem.* **2010**, *53*, 6355–6360. [CrossRef]
73. Hsia, D.S.; Grove, O.; Cefalu, W.T. An update on sodium-glucose co-transporter-2 inhibitors for the treatment of diabetes mellitus. *Curr. Opin. Endocrinol. Diabetes Obes.* **2017**, *24*, 73–79. [CrossRef]
74. Markham, A.; Elkinson, S. Luseogliflozin: First global approval. *Drugs* **2014**, *74*, 945–950. [CrossRef]
75. Poole, R.M.; Dungo, R.T. Ipragliflozin: First global approval. *Drugs* **2014**, *74*, 611–617. [CrossRef]
76. Poole, R.M.; Prossler, J.E. Tofogliflozin: First global approval. *Drugs* **2014**, *74*, 939–944. [CrossRef]
77. Xu, J.; Hirai, T.; Koya, D.; Kitada, M. Effects of SGLT2 Inhibitors on Atherosclerosis: Lessons from Cardiovascular Clinical Outcomes in Type 2 Diabetic Patients and Basic Researches. *J. Clin. Med.* **2021**, *11*, 137. [CrossRef]
78. Wishart, D.S.; Feunang, Y.D.; Guo, A.C.; Lo, E.J.; Marcu, A.; Grant, J.R.; Sajed, T.; Johnson, D.; Li, C.; Sayeeda, Z.; et al. DrugBank 5.0: A major update to the DrugBank database for 2018. *Nucleic Acids Res.* **2018**, *46*, D1074–D1082. [CrossRef]
79. Isaji, M. Sodium-glucose cotransporter inhibitors for diabetes. *Curr. Opin. Investig. Drugs* **2007**, *8*, 285–292.
80. Isaji, M. SGLT2 inhibitors: Molecular design and potential differences in effect. *Kidney Int. Suppl.* **2011**, *79* (Suppl. S20), S14–S19. [CrossRef]
81. Okada, J.; Yamada, E.; Saito, T.; Yokoo, H.; Osaki, A.; Shimoda, Y.; Ozawa, A.; Nakajima, Y.; Pessin, J.E.; Okada, S.; et al. Dapagliflozin Inhibits Cell Adhesion to Collagen I and IV and Increases Ectodomain Proteolytic Cleavage of DDR1 by Increasing ADAM10 Activity. *Molecules* **2020**, *25*, 495. [CrossRef]
82. Kaji, K.; Nishimura, N.; Seki, K.; Sato, S.; Saikawa, S.; Nakanishi, K.; Furukawa, M.; Kawaratani, H.; Kitade, M.; Moriya, K.; et al. Sodium glucose cotransporter 2 inhibitor canagliflozin attenuates liver cancer cell growth and angiogenic activity by inhibiting glucose uptake. *Int. J. Cancer* **2018**, *142*, 1712–1722. [CrossRef]
83. Hawley, S.A.; Ford, R.J.; Smith, B.K.; Gowans, G.J.; Mancini, S.J.; Pitt, R.D.; Day, E.A.; Salt, I.P.; Steinberg, G.R.; Hardie, D.G. The Na^+/Glucose Cotransporter Inhibitor Canagliflozin Activates AMPK by Inhibiting Mitochondrial Function and Increasing Cellular AMP Levels. *Diabetes* **2016**, *65*, 2784–2794. [CrossRef]
84. Luo, J.; Sun, P.; Wang, Y.; Chen, Y.; Niu, Y.; Ding, Y.; Xu, N.; Zhang, Y.; Xie, W. Dapagliflozin attenuates steatosis in livers of high-fat diet-induced mice and oleic acid-treated L02 cells via regulating AMPK/mTOR pathway. *Eur. J. Pharmacol.* **2021**, *907*, 174304. [CrossRef] [PubMed]
85. Li, L.; Li, Q.; Huang, W.; Han, Y.; Tan, H.; An, M.; Xiang, Q.; Zhou, R.; Yang, L.; Cheng, Y. Dapagliflozin Alleviates Hepatic Steatosis by Restoring Autophagy via the AMPK-mTOR Pathway. *Front. Pharmacol.* **2021**, *12*, 589273. [CrossRef] [PubMed]
86. Wang, L.; Liu, M.; Yin, F.; Wang, Y.; Li, X.; Wu, Y.; Ye, C.; Liu, J. Trilobatin, a Novel SGLT1/2 Inhibitor, Selectively Induces the Proliferation of Human Hepatoblastoma Cells. *Molecules* **2019**, *24*, 3390. [CrossRef] [PubMed]
87. Jojima, T.; Wakamatsu, S.; Kase, M.; Iijima, T.; Maejima, Y.; Shimomura, K.; Kogai, T.; Tomaru, T.; Usui, I.; Aso, Y. The SGLT2 Inhibitor Canagliflozin Prevents Carcinogenesis in a Mouse Model of Diabetes and Non-Alcoholic Steatohepatitis-Related Hepatocarcinogenesis: Association with SGLT2 Expression in Hepatocellular Carcinoma. *Int. J. Mol. Sci.* **2019**, *20*, 5237. [CrossRef]
88. Abdel-Rafei, M.K.; Thabet, N.M.; Rashed, L.A.; Moustafa, E.M. Canagliflozin, a SGLT-2 inhibitor, relieves ER stress, modulates autophagy and induces apoptosis in irradiated HepG2 cells: Signal transduction between PI3K/AKT/GSK-3beta/mTOR and Wnt/beta-catenin pathways; in vitro. *J. Cancer Res. Ther.* **2021**, *17*, 1404–1418. [CrossRef] [PubMed]
89. Obara, K.; Shirakami, Y.; Maruta, A.; Ideta, T.; Miyazaki, T.; Kochi, T.; Sakai, H.; Tanaka, T.; Seishima, M.; Shimizu, M. Preventive effects of the sodium glucose cotransporter 2 inhibitor tofogliflozin on diethylnitrosamine-induced liver tumorigenesis in obese and diabetic mice. *Oncotarget* **2017**, *8*, 58353–58363. [CrossRef] [PubMed]
90. Chiang, H.; Lee, J.C.; Huang, H.C.; Huang, H.; Liu, H.K.; Huang, C. Delayed intervention with a novel SGLT2 inhibitor NGI001 suppresses diet-induced metabolic dysfunction and non-alcoholic fatty liver disease in mice. *Br. J. Pharmacol.* **2020**, *177*, 239–253. [CrossRef]
91. Zhao, Y.; Li, Y.; Liu, Q.; Tang, Q.; Zhang, Z.; Zhang, J.; Huang, C.; Huang, H.; Zhang, G.; Zhou, J.; et al. Canagliflozin Facilitates Reverse Cholesterol Transport through Activation of AMPK/ABC Transporter Pathway. *Drug Des. Devel. Ther.* **2021**, *15*, 2117–2128. [CrossRef]
92. Wang, B.; Tontonoz, P. Liver X receptors in lipid signalling and membrane homeostasis. *Nat. Rev. Endocrinol.* **2018**, *14*, 452–463. [CrossRef]

93. Zhou, J.; Zhu, J.; Yu, S.J.; Ma, H.L.; Chen, J.; Ding, X.F.; Chen, G.; Liang, Y.; Zhang, Q. Sodium-glucose co-transporter-2 (SGLT-2) inhibition reduces glucose uptake to induce breast cancer cell growth arrest through AMPK/mTOR pathway. *Biomed. Pharmacother.* **2020**, *132*, 110821. [CrossRef]
94. Xiao, Q.; Zhang, S.; Yang, C.; Du, R.; Zhao, J.; Li, J.; Xu, Y.; Qin, Y.; Gao, Y.; Huang, W. Ginsenoside Rg1 Ameliorates Palmitic Acid-Induced Hepatic Steatosis and Inflammation in HepG2 Cells via the AMPK/NF-kappaB Pathway. *Int. J. Endocrinol.* **2019**, *2019*, 7514802. [CrossRef]
95. Soret, P.A.; Magusto, J.; Housset, C.; Gautheron, J. In Vitro and In Vivo Models of Non-Alcoholic Fatty Liver Disease: A Critical Appraisal. *J. Clin. Med.* **2020**, *10*, 36. [CrossRef]
96. Anstee, Q.M.; Goldin, R.D. Mouse models in non-alcoholic fatty liver disease and steatohepatitis research. *Int. J. Exp. Pathol.* **2006**, *87*, 1–16. [CrossRef]
97. Ibrahim, S.H.; Hirsova, P.; Malhi, H.; Gores, G.J. Animal Models of Nonalcoholic Steatohepatitis: Eat, Delete, and Inflame. *Dig. Dis. Sci.* **2016**, *61*, 1325–1336. [CrossRef]
98. Nakamura, A.; Terauchi, Y. Lessons from mouse models of high-fat diet-induced NAFLD. *Int. J. Mol. Sci.* **2013**, *14*, 21240–21257. [CrossRef]
99. Perakakis, N.; Chrysafi, P.; Feigh, M.; Veidal, S.S.; Mantzoros, C.S. Empagliflozin Improves Metabolic and Hepatic Outcomes in a Non-Diabetic Obese Biopsy-Proven Mouse Model of Advanced NASH. *Int. J. Mol. Sci.* **2021**, *22*, 6332. [CrossRef]
100. Tahara, A.; Takasu, T. Therapeutic Effects of SGLT2 Inhibitor Ipragliflozin and Metformin on NASH in Type 2 Diabetic Mice. *Endocr. Res.* **2020**, *45*, 147–161. [CrossRef]
101. Shiba, K.; Tsuchiya, K.; Komiya, C.; Miyachi, Y.; Mori, K.; Shimazu, N.; Yamaguchi, S.; Ogasawara, N.; Katoh, M.; Itoh, M.; et al. Canagliflozin, an SGLT2 inhibitor, attenuates the development of hepatocellular carcinoma in a mouse model of human NASH. *Sci. Rep.* **2018**, *8*, 2362. [CrossRef]
102. Brown, E.; Wilding, J.P.H.; Barber, T.M.; Alam, U.; Cuthbertson, D.J. Weight loss variability with SGLT2 inhibitors and GLP-1 receptor agonists in type 2 diabetes mellitus and obesity: Mechanistic possibilities. *Obes. Rev.* **2019**, *20*, 816–828. [CrossRef]
103. Cai, X.; Yang, W.; Gao, X.; Chen, Y.; Zhou, L.; Zhang, S.; Han, X.; Ji, L. The Association between the Dosage of SGLT2 Inhibitor and Weight Reduction in Type 2 Diabetes Patients: A Meta-Analysis. *Obesity* **2018**, *26*, 70–80. [CrossRef] [PubMed]
104. Cherney, D.Z.I.; Dekkers, C.C.J.; Barbour, S.J.; Cattran, D.; Abdul Gafor, A.H.; Greasley, P.J.; Laverman, G.D.; Lim, S.K.; Di Tanna, G.L.; Reich, H.N.; et al. Effects of the SGLT2 inhibitor dapagliflozin on proteinuria in non-diabetic patients with chronic kidney disease (DIAMOND): A randomised, double-blind, crossover trial. *Lancet Diabetes Endocrinol.* **2020**, *8*, 582–593. [CrossRef]
105. Han, T.; Fan, Y.J.; Gao, J.; Fatima, M.R.; Zhang, Y.L.; Ding, Y.M.; Bai, L.A.; Wang, C.X. Sodium glucose cotransporter 2 inhibitor dapagliflozin depressed adiposity and ameliorated hepatic steatosis in high-fat diet induced obese mice. *Adipocyte* **2021**, *10*, 446–455. [CrossRef] [PubMed]
106. Obata, A.; Kubota, N.; Kubota, T.; Iwamoto, M.; Sato, H.; Sakurai, Y.; Takamoto, I.; Katsuyama, H.; Suzuki, Y.; Fukazawa, M.; et al. Tofogliflozin Improves Insulin Resistance in Skeletal Muscle and Accelerates Lipolysis in Adipose Tissue in Male Mice. *Endocrinology* **2016**, *157*, 1029–1042. [CrossRef]
107. Petito-da-Silva, T.I.; Souza-Mello, V.; Barbosa-da-Silva, S. Empaglifozin mitigates NAFLD in high-fat-fed mice by alleviating insulin resistance, lipogenesis and ER stress. *Mol. Cell Endocrinol.* **2019**, *498*, 110539. [CrossRef]
108. Tanaka, K.; Takahashi, H.; Katagiri, S.; Sasaki, K.; Ohsugi, Y.; Watanabe, K.; Rasadul, I.M.D.; Mine, K.; Nagafuchi, S.; Iwata, T.; et al. Combined effect of canagliflozin and exercise training on high-fat diet-fed mice. *Am. J. Physiol. Endocrinol. Metab.* **2020**, *318*, E492–E503. [CrossRef]
109. Yabiku, K.; Nakamoto, K.; Tsubakimoto, M. Effects of Sodium-Glucose Cotransporter 2 Inhibition on Glucose Metabolism, Liver Function, Ascites, and Hemodynamics in a Mouse Model of Nonalcoholic Steatohepatitis and Type 2 Diabetes. *J. Diabetes Res.* **2020**, *2020*, 1682904. [CrossRef]
110. Ozutsumi, T.; Namisaki, T.; Shimozato, N.; Kaji, K.; Tsuji, Y.; Kaya, D.; Fujinaga, Y.; Furukawa, M.; Nakanishi, K.; Sato, S.; et al. Combined Treatment with Sodium-Glucose Cotransporter-2 Inhibitor (Canagliflozin) and Dipeptidyl Peptidase-4 Inhibitor (Teneligliptin) Alleviates NASH Progression in A Non-Diabetic Rat Model of Steatohepatitis. *Int. J. Mol. Sci.* **2020**, *21*, 2164. [CrossRef]
111. Yoshino, K.; Hosooka, T.; Shinohara, M.; Aoki, C.; Hosokawa, Y.; Imamori, M.; Ogawa, W. Canagliflozin ameliorates hepatic fat deposition in obese diabetic mice: Role of prostaglandin E2. *Biochem. Biophys. Res. Commun.* **2021**, *557*, 62–68. [CrossRef]
112. Komiya, C.; Tsuchiya, K.; Shiba, K.; Miyachi, Y.; Furuke, S.; Shimazu, N.; Yamaguchi, S.; Kanno, K.; Ogawa, Y. Ipragliflozin Improves Hepatic Steatosis in Obese Mice and Liver Dysfunction in Type 2 Diabetic Patients Irrespective of Body Weight Reduction. *PLoS ONE* **2016**, *11*, e0151511. [CrossRef]
113. Tahara, A.; Takasu, T. SGLT2 inhibitor ipragliflozin alone and combined with pioglitazone prevents progression of nonalcoholic steatohepatitis in a type 2 diabetes rodent model. *Physiol. Rep.* **2019**, *7*, e14286. [CrossRef]
114. Honda, Y.; Imajo, K.; Kato, T.; Kessoku, T.; Ogawa, Y.; Tomeno, W.; Kato, S.; Mawatari, H.; Fujita, K.; Yoneda, M.; et al. The Selective SGLT2 Inhibitor Ipragliflozin Has a Therapeutic Effect on Nonalcoholic Steatohepatitis in Mice. *PLoS ONE* **2016**, *11*, e0146337. [CrossRef]
115. Huttl, M.; Markova, I.; Miklankova, D.; Zapletalova, I.; Poruba, M.; Haluzik, M.; Vaneckova, I.; Malinska, H. In a Prediabetic Model, Empagliflozin Improves Hepatic Lipid Metabolism Independently of Obesity and before Onset of Hyperglycemia. *Int. J. Mol. Sci.* **2021**, *22*, 11513. [CrossRef]

116. Steven, S.; Oelze, M.; Hanf, A.; Kroller-Schon, S.; Kashani, F.; Roohani, S.; Welschof, P.; Kopp, M.; Godtel-Armbrust, U.; Xia, N.; et al. The SGLT2 inhibitor empagliflozin improves the primary diabetic complications in ZDF rats. *Redox Biol.* **2017**, *13*, 370–385. [CrossRef]
117. Meng, Z.; Liu, X.; Li, T.; Fang, T.; Cheng, Y.; Han, L.; Sun, B.; Chen, L. The SGLT2 inhibitor empagliflozin negatively regulates IL-17/IL-23 axis-mediated inflammatory responses in T2DM with NAFLD via the AMPK/mTOR/autophagy pathway. *Int. Immunopharmacol.* **2021**, *94*, 107492. [CrossRef]
118. Petersen, M.C.; Shulman, G.I. Roles of Diacylglycerols and Ceramides in Hepatic Insulin Resistance. *Trends Pharmacol. Sci.* **2017**, *38*, 649–665. [CrossRef]
119. Chambel, S.S.; Santos-Goncalves, A.; Duarte, T.L. The Dual Role of Nrf2 in Nonalcoholic Fatty Liver Disease: Regulation of Antioxidant Defenses and Hepatic Lipid Metabolism. *Biomed. Res. Int.* **2015**, *2015*, 597134. [CrossRef]
120. Su, X.; Kong, Y.; Peng, D. Fibroblast growth factor 21 in lipid metabolism and non-alcoholic fatty liver disease. *Clin. Chim. Acta* **2019**, *498*, 30–37. [CrossRef]
121. Eberle, D.; Hegarty, B.; Bossard, P.; Ferre, P.; Foufelle, F. SREBP transcription factors: Master regulators of lipid homeostasis. *Biochimie* **2004**, *86*, 839–848. [CrossRef]
122. Kern, M.; Kloting, N.; Mark, M.; Mayoux, E.; Klein, T.; Bluher, M. The SGLT2 inhibitor empagliflozin improves insulin sensitivity in db/db mice both as monotherapy and in combination with linagliptin. *Metabolism* **2016**, *65*, 114–123. [CrossRef]
123. Bakan, I.; Laplante, M. Connecting mTORC1 signaling to SREBP-1 activation. *Curr. Opin. Lipidol.* **2012**, *23*, 226–234. [CrossRef] [PubMed]
124. Souza-Mello, V. Peroxisome proliferator-activated receptors as targets to treat non-alcoholic fatty liver disease. *World J. Hepatol.* **2015**, *7*, 1012–1019. [CrossRef]
125. Omori, K.; Nakamura, A.; Miyoshi, H.; Takahashi, K.; Kitao, N.; Nomoto, H.; Kameda, H.; Cho, K.Y.; Takagi, R.; Hatanaka, K.C.; et al. Effects of dapagliflozin and/or insulin glargine on beta cell mass and hepatic steatosis in db/db mice. *Metabolism* **2019**, *98*, 27–36. [CrossRef] [PubMed]
126. Yoshioka, N.; Tanaka, M.; Ochi, K.; Watanabe, A.; Ono, K.; Sawada, M.; Ogi, T.; Itoh, M.; Ito, A.; Shiraki, Y.; et al. The sodium-glucose cotransporter-2 inhibitor Tofogliflozin prevents the progression of nonalcoholic steatohepatitis-associated liver tumors in a novel murine model. *Biomed. Pharmacother.* **2021**, *140*, 111738. [CrossRef] [PubMed]
127. Morris, E.M.; Meers, G.M.; Booth, F.W.; Fritsche, K.L.; Hardin, C.D.; Thyfault, J.P.; Ibdah, J.A. PGC-1alpha overexpression results in increased hepatic fatty acid oxidation with reduced triacylglycerol accumulation and secretion. *Am. J. Physiol. Gastrointest. Liver Physiol.* **2012**, *303*, G979–G992. [CrossRef] [PubMed]
128. Chrysavgis, L.; Papatheodoridi, A.M.; Chatzigeorgiou, A.; Cholongitas, E. The impact of sodium glucose co-transporter 2 inhibitors on non-alcoholic fatty liver disease. *J. Gastroenterol. Hepatol.* **2021**, *36*, 893–909. [CrossRef] [PubMed]
129. Kabil, S.L.; Mahmoud, N.M. Canagliflozin protects against non-alcoholic steatohepatitis in type-2 diabetic rats through zinc alpha-2 glycoprotein up-regulation. *Eur. J. Pharmacol.* **2018**, *828*, 135–145. [CrossRef] [PubMed]
130. ElMahdy, M.K.; Helal, M.G.; Ebrahim, T.M. Potential anti-inflammatory effect of dapagliflozin in HCHF diet- induced fatty liver degeneration through inhibition of TNF-alpha, IL-1beta, and IL-18 in rat liver. *Int. Immunopharmacol.* **2020**, *86*, 106730. [CrossRef] [PubMed]
131. Tahara, A.; Kurosaki, E.; Yokono, M.; Yamajuku, D.; Kihara, R.; Hayashizaki, Y.; Takasu, T.; Imamura, M.; Li, Q.; Tomiyama, H.; et al. Effects of SGLT2 selective inhibitor ipragliflozin on hyperglycemia, hyperlipidemia, hepatic steatosis, oxidative stress, inflammation, and obesity in type 2 diabetic mice. *Eur. J. Pharmacol.* **2013**, *715*, 246–255. [CrossRef]
132. Tang, L.; Wu, Y.; Tian, M.; Sjostrom, C.D.; Johansson, U.; Peng, X.R.; Smith, D.M.; Huang, Y. Dapagliflozin slows the progression of the renal and liver fibrosis associated with type 2 diabetes. *Am. J. Physiol. Endocrinol. Metab.* **2017**, *313*, E563–E576. [CrossRef]
133. Klebanoff, S.J. Myeloperoxidase: Friend and foe. *J. Leukoc. Biol.* **2005**, *77*, 598–625. [CrossRef]
134. Nakano, S.; Katsuno, K.; Isaji, M.; Nagasawa, T.; Buehrer, B.; Walker, S.; Wilkison, W.O.; Cheatham, B. Remogliflozin Etabonate Improves Fatty Liver Disease in Diet-Induced Obese Male Mice. *J. Clin. Exp. Hepatol.* **2015**, *5*, 190–198. [CrossRef]
135. Ookawara, M.; Matsuda, K.; Watanabe, M.; Moritoh, Y. The GPR40 Full Agonist SCO-267 Improves Liver Parameters in a Mouse Model of Nonalcoholic Fatty Liver Disease without Affecting Glucose or Body Weight. *J. Pharmacol. Exp. Ther.* **2020**, *375*, 21–27. [CrossRef]
136. Jojima, T.; Tomotsune, T.; Iijima, T.; Akimoto, K.; Suzuki, K.; Aso, Y. Empagliflozin (an SGLT2 inhibitor), alone or in combination with linagliptin (a DPP-4 inhibitor), prevents steatohepatitis in a novel mouse model of non-alcoholic steatohepatitis and diabetes. *Diabetol. Metab. Syndr.* **2016**, *8*, 45. [CrossRef]
137. Hupa-Breier, K.L.; Dywicki, J.; Hartleben, B.; Wellhoner, F.; Heidrich, B.; Taubert, R.; Mederacke, Y.E.; Lieber, M.; Iordanidis, K.; Manns, M.P.; et al. Dulaglutide Alone and in Combination with Empagliflozin Attenuate Inflammatory Pathways and Microbiome Dysbiosis in a Non-Diabetic Mouse Model of NASH. *Biomedicines* **2021**, *9*, 353. [CrossRef]
138. Kuwako, K.I.; Okano, H. Versatile Roles of LKB1 Kinase Signaling in Neural Development and Homeostasis. *Front. Mol. Neurosci.* **2018**, *11*, 354. [CrossRef]
139. Chen, Z.; Liu, Y.; Yang, L.; Liu, P.; Zhang, Y.; Wang, X. MiR-149 attenuates endoplasmic reticulum stress-induced inflammation and apoptosis in nonalcoholic fatty liver disease by negatively targeting ATF6 pathway. *Immunol. Lett.* **2020**, *222*, 40–48. [CrossRef]
140. Heyens, L.J.M.; Busschots, D.; Koek, G.H.; Robaeys, G.; Francque, S. Liver Fibrosis in Non-alcoholic Fatty Liver Disease: From Liver Biopsy to Non-invasive Biomarkers in Diagnosis and Treatment. *Front. Med.* **2021**, *8*, 615978. [CrossRef]

141. Zisser, A.; Ipsen, D.H.; Tveden-Nyborg, P. Hepatic Stellate Cell Activation and Inactivation in NASH-Fibrosis-Roles as Putative Treatment Targets? *Biomedicines* **2021**, *9*, 365. [CrossRef]
142. Qiang, S.; Nakatsu, Y.; Seno, Y.; Fujishiro, M.; Sakoda, H.; Kushiyama, A.; Mori, K.; Matsunaga, Y.; Yamamotoya, T.; Kamata, H.; et al. Treatment with the SGLT2 inhibitor luseogliflozin improves nonalcoholic steatohepatitis in a rodent model with diabetes mellitus. *Diabetol. Metab. Syndr.* **2015**, *7*, 104. [CrossRef]
143. Anstee, Q.M.; Reeves, H.L.; Kotsiliti, E.; Govaere, O.; Heikenwalder, M. From NASH to HCC: Current concepts and future challenges. *Nat. Rev. Gastro Hepat.* **2019**, *16*, 411–428. [CrossRef] [PubMed]
144. Hayashizaki-Someya, Y.; Kurosaki, E.; Takasu, T.; Mitori, H.; Yamazaki, S.; Koide, K.; Takakura, S. Ipragliflozin, an SGLT2 inhibitor, exhibits a prophylactic effect on hepatic steatosis and fibrosis induced by choline-deficient l-amino acid-defined diet in rats. *Eur. J. Pharmacol.* **2015**, *754*, 19–24. [CrossRef] [PubMed]
145. Bando, Y.; Ogawa, A.; Ishikura, K.; Kanehara, H.; Hisada, A.; Notumata, K.; Okafuji, K.; Toya, D. The effects of ipragliflozin on the liver-to-spleen attenuation ratio as assessed by computed tomography and on alanine transaminase levels in Japanese patients with type 2 diabetes mellitus. *Diabetol. Int.* **2017**, *8*, 218–227. [CrossRef] [PubMed]
146. Akuta, N.; Watanabe, C.; Kawamura, Y.; Arase, Y.; Saitoh, S.; Fujiyama, S.; Sezaki, H.; Hosaka, T.; Kobayashi, M.; Kobayashi, M.; et al. Effects of a sodium-glucose cotransporter 2 inhibitor in nonalcoholic fatty liver disease complicated by diabetes mellitus: Preliminary prospective study based on serial liver biopsies. *Hepatol. Commun.* **2017**, *1*, 46–52. [CrossRef] [PubMed]
147. Ito, D.; Shimizu, S.; Inoue, K.; Saito, D.; Yanagisawa, M.; Inukai, K.; Akiyama, Y.; Morimoto, Y.; Noda, M.; Shimada, A. Comparison of Ipragliflozin and Pioglitazone Effects on Nonalcoholic Fatty Liver Disease in Patients with Type 2 Diabetes: A Randomized, 24-Week, Open-Label, Active-Controlled Trial. *Diabetes Care* **2017**, *40*, 1364–1372. [CrossRef]
148. Seko, Y.; Sumida, Y.; Tanaka, S.; Mori, K.; Taketani, H.; Ishiba, H.; Hara, T.; Okajima, A.; Umemura, A.; Nishikawa, T.; et al. Effect of sodium glucose cotransporter 2 inhibitor on liver function tests in Japanese patients with non-alcoholic fatty liver disease and type 2 diabetes mellitus. *Hepatol. Res.* **2017**, *47*, 1072–1078. [CrossRef]
149. Choi, D.H.; Jung, C.H.; Mok, J.O.; Kim, C.H.; Kang, S.K.; Kim, B.Y. Effect of Dapagliflozin on Alanine Aminotransferase Improvement in Type 2 Diabetes Mellitus with Non-alcoholic Fatty Liver Disease. *Endocrinol. Metab.* **2018**, *33*, 387–394. [CrossRef]
150. Eriksson, J.W.; Lundkvist, P.; Jansson, P.A.; Johansson, L.; Kvarnström, M.; Moris, L.; Miliotis, T.; Forsberg, G.B.; Risérus, U.; Lind, L.; et al. Effects of dapagliflozin and n-3 carboxylic acids on non-alcoholic fatty liver disease in people with type 2 diabetes: A double-blind randomised placebo-controlled study. *Diabetologia* **2018**, *61*, 1923–1934. [CrossRef]
151. Itani, T.; Ishihara, T. Efficacy of canagliflozin against nonalcoholic fatty liver disease: A prospective cohort study. *Obes. Sci. Pract.* **2018**, *4*, 477–482. [CrossRef]
152. Kuchay, M.S.; Krishan, S.; Mishra, S.K.; Farooqui, K.J.; Singh, M.K.; Wasir, J.S.; Bansal, B.; Kaur, P.; Jevalikar, G.; Gill, H.K.; et al. Effect of Empagliflozin on Liver Fat in Patients with Type 2 Diabetes and Nonalcoholic Fatty Liver Disease: A Randomized Controlled Trial (E-LIFT Trial). *Diabetes Care* **2018**, *41*, 1801–1808. [CrossRef]
153. Miyake, T.; Yoshida, S.; Furukawa, S.; Sakai, T.; Tada, F.; Senba, H.; Yamamoto, S.; Koizumi, Y.; Yoshida, O.; Hirooka, M.; et al. Ipragliflozin Ameliorates Liver Damage in Non-alcoholic Fatty Liver Disease. *Open Med.* **2018**, *13*, 402–409. [CrossRef] [PubMed]
154. Shibuya, T.; Fushimi, N.; Kawai, M.; Yoshida, Y.; Hachiya, H.; Ito, S.; Kawai, H.; Ohashi, N.; Mori, A. Luseogliflozin improves liver fat deposition compared to metformin in type 2 diabetes patients with non-alcoholic fatty liver disease: A prospective randomized controlled pilot study. *Diabetes Obes. Metab.* **2018**, *20*, 438–442. [CrossRef]
155. Shimizu, M.; Suzuki, K.; Kato, K.; Jojima, T.; Iijima, T.; Murohisa, T.; Iijima, M.; Takekawa, H.; Usui, I.; Hiraishi, H.; et al. Evaluation of the effects of dapagliflozin, a sodium-glucose co-transporter-2 inhibitor, on hepatic steatosis and fibrosis using transient elastography in patients with type 2 diabetes and non-alcoholic fatty liver disease. *Diabetes Obes. Metab.* **2019**, *21*, 285–292. [CrossRef] [PubMed]
156. Sumida, Y.; Murotani, K.; Saito, M.; Tamasawa, A.; Osonoi, Y.; Yoneda, M.; Osonoi, T. Effect of luseogliflozin on hepatic fat content in type 2 diabetes patients with non-alcoholic fatty liver disease: A prospective, single-arm trial (LEAD trial). *Hepatol. Res.* **2019**, *49*, 64–71. [CrossRef] [PubMed]
157. Akuta, N.; Kawamura, Y.; Watanabe, C.; Nishimura, A.; Okubo, M.; Mori, Y.; Fujiyama, S.; Sezaki, H.; Hosaka, T.; Kobayashi, M.; et al. Impact of sodium glucose cotransporter 2 inhibitor on histological features and glucose metabolism of non-alcoholic fatty liver disease complicated by diabetes mellitus. *Hepatol. Res.* **2019**, *49*, 531–539. [CrossRef] [PubMed]
158. Yamashima, M.; Miyaaki, H.; Miuma, S.; Shibata, H.; Sasaki, R.; Haraguchi, M.; Fukushima, M.; Nakao, K. The Long-term Efficacy of Sodium Glucose Co-transporter 2 Inhibitor in Patients with Non-alcoholic Fatty Liver Disease. *Intern. Med.* **2019**, *58*, 1987–1992. [CrossRef]
159. Akuta, N.; Kawamura, Y.; Fujiyama, S.; Sezaki, H.; Hosaka, T.; Kobayashi, M.; Kobayashi, M.; Saitoh, S.; Suzuki, F.; Suzuki, Y.; et al. SGLT2 Inhibitor Treatment Outcome in Nonalcoholic Fatty Liver Disease Complicated with Diabetes Mellitus: The Long-term Effects on Clinical Features and Liver Histopathology. *Intern. Med.* **2020**, *59*, 1931–1937. [CrossRef]
160. Han, E.; Lee, Y.H.; Lee, B.W.; Kang, E.S.; Cha, B.S. Ipragliflozin Additively Ameliorates Non-Alcoholic Fatty Liver Disease in Patients with Type 2 Diabetes Controlled with Metformin and Pioglitazone: A 24-Week Randomized Controlled Trial. *J. Clin. Med.* **2020**, *9*, 259. [CrossRef]
161. Kahl, S.; Gancheva, S.; Straßburger, K.; Herder, C.; Machann, J.; Katsuyama, H.; Kabisch, S.; Henkel, E.; Kopf, S.; Lagerpusch, M.; et al. Empagliflozin Effectively Lowers Liver Fat Content in Well-Controlled Type 2 Diabetes: A Randomized, Double-Blind, Phase 4, Placebo-Controlled Trial. *Diabetes Care* **2020**, *43*, 298–305. [CrossRef]

162. Kinoshita, T.; Shimoda, M.; Nakashima, K.; Fushimi, Y.; Hirata, Y.; Tanabe, A.; Tatsumi, F.; Hirukawa, H.; Sanada, J.; Kohara, K.; et al. Comparison of the effects of three kinds of glucose-lowering drugs on non-alcoholic fatty liver disease in patients with type 2 diabetes: A randomized, open-label, three-arm, active control study. *J. Diabetes Investig.* **2020**, *11*, 1612–1622. [CrossRef]
163. Yano, K.; Seko, Y.; Takahashi, A.; Okishio, S.; Kataoka, S.; Takemura, M.; Okuda, K.; Mizuno, N.; Taketani, H.; Umemura, A.; et al. Effect of Sodium Glucose Cotransporter 2 Inhibitors on Renal Function in Patients with Nonalcoholic Fatty Liver Disease and Type 2 Diabetes in Japan. *Diagnostics* **2020**, *10*, 86. [CrossRef]
164. Arai, T.; Atsukawa, M.; Tsubota, A.; Mikami, S.; Ono, H.; Kawano, T.; Yoshida, Y.; Tanabe, T.; Okubo, T.; Hayama, K.; et al. Effect of sodium-glucose cotransporter 2 inhibitor in patients with non-alcoholic fatty liver disease and type 2 diabetes mellitus: A propensity score-matched analysis of real-world data. *Ther. Adv. Endocrinol. Metab.* **2021**, *12*, 1–13. [CrossRef]
165. Chehrehgosha, H.; Sohrabi, M.R.; Ismail-Beigi, F.; Malek, M.; Reza Babaei, M.; Zamani, F.; Ajdarkosh, H.; Khoonsari, M.; Fallah, A.E.; Khamseh, M.E. Empagliflozin Improves Liver Steatosis and Fibrosis in Patients with Non-Alcoholic Fatty Liver Disease and Type 2 Diabetes: A Randomized, Double-Blind, Placebo-Controlled Clinical Trial. *Diabetes Ther.* **2021**, *12*, 843–861. [CrossRef]
166. Euh, W.; Lim, S.; Kim, J.W. Sodium-Glucose Cotransporter-2 Inhibitors Ameliorate Liver Enzyme Abnormalities in Korean Patients with Type 2 Diabetes Mellitus and Nonalcoholic Fatty Liver Disease. *Front. Endocrinol.* **2021**, *12*, 613389. [CrossRef]
167. Gaborit, B.; Ancel, P.; Abdullah, A.E.; Maurice, F.; Abdesselam, I.; Calen, A.; Soghomonian, A.; Houssays, M.; Varlet, I.; Eisinger, M.; et al. Effect of empagliflozin on ectopic fat stores and myocardial energetics in type 2 diabetes: The EMPACEF study. *Cardiovasc. Diabetol.* **2021**, *20*, 57. [CrossRef]
168. Takahashi, H.; Kessoku, T.; Kawanaka, M.; Nonaka, M.; Hyogo, H.; Fujii, H.; Nakajima, T.; Imajo, K.; Tanaka, K.; Kubotsu, Y.; et al. Ipragliflozin Improves the Hepatic Outcomes of Patients with Diabetes with NAFLD. *Hepatol. Commun.* **2021**, *6*, 120–132. [CrossRef]
169. Yoneda, M.; Honda, Y.; Ogawa, Y.; Kessoku, T.; Kobayashi, T.; Imajo, K.; Ozaki, A.; Nogami, A.; Taguri, M.; Yamanaka, T.; et al. Comparing the effects of tofogliflozin and pioglitazone in non-alcoholic fatty liver disease patients with type 2 diabetes mellitus (ToPiND study): A randomized prospective open-label controlled trial. *BMJ Open Diabetes Res. Care* **2021**, *9*, e001990. [CrossRef]
170. Pradhan, R.; Yin, H.; Yu, O.; Azoulay, L. Glucagon-Like Peptide 1 Receptor Agonists and Sodium-Glucose Cotransporter 2 Inhibitors and Risk of Nonalcoholic Fatty Liver Disease Among Patients with Type 2 Diabetes. *Diabetes Care* **2022**. Online ahead of print. [CrossRef]
171. Sinha, B.; Datta, D.; Ghosal, S. Meta-analysis of the effects of sodium glucose cotransporter 2 inhibitors in non-alcoholic fatty liver disease patients with type 2 diabetes. *JGH Open* **2021**, *5*, 219–227. [CrossRef]
172. Mo, M.; Huang, Z.; Liang, Y.; Liao, Y.; Xia, N. The safety and efficacy evaluation of Sodium-Glucose co-transporter 2 inhibitors for patients with non-alcoholic fatty Liver disease: An updated meta-analysis. *Dig. Liver Dis.* **2021**, in press. [CrossRef]
173. Wong, C.; Yaow, C.Y.L.; Ng, C.H.; Chin, Y.H.; Low, Y.F.; Lim, A.Y.L.; Muthiah, M.D.; Khoo, C.M. Sodium-Glucose Co-Transporter 2 Inhibitors for Non-Alcoholic Fatty Liver Disease in Asian Patients with Type 2 Diabetes: A Meta-Analysis. *Front. Endocrinol.* **2020**, *11*, 609135. [CrossRef] [PubMed]
174. Tobita, H.; Yazaki, T.; Kataoka, M.; Kotani, S.; Oka, A.; Mishiro, T.; Oshima, N.; Kawashima, K.; Ishimura, N.; Naora, K.; et al. Comparison of dapagliflozin and teneligliptin in nonalcoholic fatty liver disease patients without type 2 diabetes mellitus: A prospective randomized study. *J. Clin. Biochem. Nutr.* **2021**, *68*, 173–180. [CrossRef] [PubMed]
175. Daniele, G.; Xiong, J.; Solis-Herrera, C.; Merovci, A.; Eldor, R.; Tripathy, D.; DeFronzo, R.A.; Norton, L.; Abdul-Ghani, M. Dapagliflozin Enhances Fat Oxidation and Ketone Production in Patients with Type 2 Diabetes. *Diabetes Care* **2016**, *39*, 2036–2041. [CrossRef] [PubMed]
176. Wang, D.; Luo, Y.; Wang, X.; Orlicky, D.J.; Myakala, K.; Yang, P.; Levi, M. The Sodium-Glucose Cotransporter 2 Inhibitor Dapagliflozin Prevents Renal and Liver Disease in Western Diet Induced Obesity Mice. *Int. J. Mol. Sci.* **2018**, *19*, 137. [CrossRef]
177. Bonner, C.; Kerr-Conte, J.; Gmyr, V.; Queniat, G.; Moerman, E.; Thévenet, J.; Beaucamps, C.; Delalleau, N.; Popescu, I.; Malaisse, W.J.; et al. Inhibition of the glucose transporter SGLT2 with dapagliflozin in pancreatic alpha cells triggers glucagon secretion. *Nat. Med.* **2015**, *21*, 512–517. [CrossRef]
178. Ferrannini, E.; Baldi, S.; Frascerra, S.; Astiarraga, B.; Heise, T.; Bizzotto, R.; Mari, A.; Pieber, T.R.; Muscelli, E. Shift to Fatty Substrate Utilization in Response to Sodium-Glucose Cotransporter 2 Inhibition in Subjects without Diabetes and Patients with Type 2 Diabetes. *Diabetes* **2016**, *65*, 1190–1195. [CrossRef]
179. Yokono, M.; Takasu, T.; Hayashizaki, Y.; Mitsuoka, K.; Kihara, R.; Muramatsu, Y.; Miyoshi, S.; Tahara, A.; Kurosaki, E.; Li, Q.; et al. SGLT2 selective inhibitor ipragliflozin reduces body fat mass by increasing fatty acid oxidation in high-fat diet-induced obese rats. *Eur. J. Pharmacol.* **2014**, *727*, 66–74. [CrossRef]
180. Terami, N.; Ogawa, D.; Tachibana, H.; Hatanaka, T.; Wada, J.; Nakatsuka, A.; Eguchi, J.; Horiguchi, C.S.; Nishii, N.; Yamada, H.; et al. Long-term treatment with the sodium glucose cotransporter 2 inhibitor, dapagliflozin, ameliorates glucose homeostasis and diabetic nephropathy in db/db mice. *PLoS ONE* **2014**, *9*, e100777. [CrossRef]
181. Tahara, A.; Kurosaki, E.; Yokono, M.; Yamajuku, D.; Kihara, R.; Hayashizaki, Y.; Takasu, T.; Imamura, M.; Li, Q.; Tomiyama, H.; et al. Effects of sodium-glucose cotransporter 2 selective inhibitor ipragliflozin on hyperglycaemia, oxidative stress, inflammation and liver injury in streptozotocin-induced type 1 diabetic rats. *J. Pharm. Pharmacol.* **2014**, *66*, 975–987. [CrossRef]
182. Yaribeygi, H.; Atkin, S.L.; Butler, A.E.; Sahebkar, A. Sodium-glucose cotransporter inhibitors and oxidative stress: An update. *J. Cell Physiol.* **2019**, *234*, 3231–3237. [CrossRef]

183. Oshima, H.; Miki, T.; Kuno, A.; Mizuno, M.; Sato, T.; Tanno, M.; Yano, T.; Nakata, K.; Kimura, Y.; Abe, K.; et al. Empagliflozin, an SGLT2 Inhibitor, Reduced the Mortality Rate after Acute Myocardial Infarction with Modification of Cardiac Metabolomes and Antioxidants in Diabetic Rats. *J. Pharmacol. Exp. Ther.* **2019**, *368*, 524–534. [CrossRef]
184. Osorio, H.; Coronel, I.; Arellano, A.; Pacheco, U.; Bautista, R.; Franco, M.; Escalante, B. Sodium-glucose cotransporter inhibition prevents oxidative stress in the kidney of diabetic rats. *Oxid Med. Cell Longev.* **2012**, *2012*, 542042. [CrossRef]

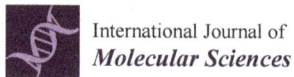

Article

Empagliflozin Attenuates Non-Alcoholic Fatty Liver Disease (NAFLD) in High Fat Diet Fed ApoE$^{(-/-)}$ Mice by Activating Autophagy and Reducing ER Stress and Apoptosis

Narjes Nasiri-Ansari [1,†], Chrysa Nikolopoulou [1,†], Katerina Papoutsi [1,†], Ioannis Kyrou [2,3,4], Christos S. Mantzoros [5,6], Georgios Kyriakopoulos [1,7], Antonios Chatzigeorgiou [8], Vassiliki Kalotychou [9], Manpal S. Randeva [10], Kamaljit Chatha [11], Konstantinos Kontzoglou [12], Gregory Kaltsas [13], Athanasios G. Papavassiliou [1], Harpal S. Randeva [2,10,14,*,‡] and Eva Kassi [1,13,*,‡]

1. Department of Biological Chemistry, Medical School, National and Kapodistrian University of Athens, 11527 Athens, Greece; nnasiri@med.uoa.gr (N.N.-A.); chrysa_nikolopoulou@hotmail.com (C.N.); pap.katerina@hotmail.com (K.P.); geokyr11@hotmail.gr (G.K.); papavas@med.uoa.gr (A.G.P.)
2. Warwickshire Institute for the Study of Diabetes, Endocrinology and Metabolism (WISDEM), University Hospitals Coventry and Warwickshire NHS Trust, Coventry CV2 2DX, UK; kyrouj@gmail.com
3. Aston Medical Research Institute, Aston Medical School, Aston University, Birmingham B4 7ET, UK
4. Division of Biomedical Sciences, Warwick Medical School, University of Warwick, Coventry CV4 7AL, UK
5. Division of Endocrinology, Diabetes and Metabolism, Beth Israel Deaconess Medical Center, Harvard Medical School, Boston, MA 02215, USA; cmantzor@bidmc.harvard.edu
6. Section of Endocrinology, Boston VA Healthcare System, Harvard Medical School, Boston, MA 02215, USA
7. Department of Pathology, Evangelismos Hospital, 10676 Athens, Greece
8. Department of Physiology, Medical School, National and Kapodistrian University of Athens, 11527 Athens, Greece; achatzig@med.uoa.gr
9. 1st Department of Internal Medicine, Laiko Hospital, Medical School, National and Kapodistrian University of Athens, 11527 Athens, Greece; vkalotyc@med.uoa.gr
10. Human Metabolism Research Unit, WISDEM Centre, NHS Trust, Coventry CV2 2DX, UK; manpalrandeva@hotmail.com
11. Department of Biochemistry & Immunology, University Hospitals Coventry and Warwickshire NHS Trust, Coventry CV2 2DX, UK; kamaljit.chatha@uhcw.nhs.uk
12. Laboratory of Experimental Surgery and Surgical Research N.S. Christeas, Athens University Medical School, National and Kapodistrian University of Athens, 11527 Athens, Greece; kckont@med.uoa.gr
13. Endocrine Oncology Unit, 1st Department of Propaupedic Internal Medicine, Laiko Hospital, National and Kapodistrian University of Athens, 11527 Athens, Greece; gkaltsas@endo.gr
14. Division of Translational and Experimental Medicine-Metabolic and Vascular Health, Warwick Medical School, University of Warwick, Coventry CV4 7AL, UK
* Correspondence: harpal.randeva@uhcw.nhs.uk (H.S.R.); ekassi@med.uoa.gr (E.K.)
† Joint first authors.
‡ Joint last authors and corresponding authors.

Citation: Nasiri-Ansari, N.; Nikolopoulou, C.; Papoutsi, K.; Kyrou, I.; Mantzoros, C.S.; Kyriakopoulos, G.; Chatzigeorgiou, A.; Kalotychou, V.; Randeva, M.S.; Chatha, K.; et al. Empagliflozin Attenuates Non-Alcoholic Fatty Liver Disease (NAFLD) in High Fat Diet Fed ApoE$^{(-/-)}$ Mice by Activating Autophagy and Reducing ER Stress and Apoptosis. *Int. J. Mol. Sci.* **2021**, *22*, 818. https://doi.org/10.3390/ijms22020818

Received: 4 December 2020
Accepted: 12 January 2021
Published: 15 January 2021

Publisher's Note: MDPI stays neutral with regard to jurisdictional claims in published maps and institutional affiliations.

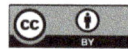

Copyright: © 2021 by the authors. Licensee MDPI, Basel, Switzerland. This article is an open access article distributed under the terms and conditions of the Creative Commons Attribution (CC BY) license (https://creativecommons.org/licenses/by/4.0/).

Abstract: Aims/hypothesis: SGLT-2 inhibitors (SGLT-2i) have been studied as potential treatments against NAFLD, showing varying beneficial effects. The molecular mechanisms mediating these effects have not been fully clarified. Herein, we investigated the impact of empagliflozin on NAFLD, focusing particularly on ER stress, autophagy and apoptosis. Methods: Five-week old ApoE$^{(-/-)}$ mice were switched from normal to a high-fat diet (HFD). After five weeks, mice were randomly allocated into a control group (HFD + vehicle) and Empa group (HFD + empagliflozin 10 mg/kg/day) for five weeks. At the end of treatment, histomorphometric analysis was performed in liver, mRNA levels of *Fasn, Screbp-1, Scd-1, Ppar-γ, Pck-1, Mcp-1, Tnf-α, Il-6, F4/80, Atf4, Elf2α, Chop, Grp78, Grp94, Xbp1, Ire1α, Atf6, mTor, Lc3b, Beclin-1, P62, Bcl-2* and *Bax* were measured by qRT-PCR, and protein levels of p-EIF2α, EIF2a, CHOP, LC3II, P62, BECLIN-1 and cleaved CASPASE-8 were assessed by immunoblotting. Results: Empagliflozin-treated mice exhibited reduced fasting glucose, total cholesterol and triglyceride serum levels, as well as decreased NAFLD activity score, decreased expression of lipogenic enzymes (*Fasn, Screbp-1c* and *Pck-1*) and inflammatory molecules (*Mcp-1* and *F4/80*), compared to the Control group. Empagliflozin significantly decreased the expression of ER stress molecules *Grp78, Ire1α, Xbp1, Elf2α, Atf4, Atf6, Chop, P62(Sqstm1)* and *Grp94*; whilst activating autophagy via increased AMPK phosphorylation, decreased *mTOR* and increased *LC3B* expression. Finally, empagliflozin increased the *Bcl2/Bax* ratio and inhibited CASPASE-8 cleavage, reducing liver cell apoptosis. Immunoblotting analysis confirmed the qPCR results. Conclusion: These novel findings indicate that empagliflozin treatment for five weeks attenuates NAFLD progression in ApoE$^{(-/-)}$ mice by promoting autophagy, reducing ER stress and inhibiting hepatic apoptosis.

Keywords: NAFLD; SGLT-2 inhibitors; autophagy; ER stress; apoptosis; inflammation

1. Introduction

Non-alcoholic fatty liver disease (NAFLD) is one of the most common causes of chronic liver disease worldwide [1,2]. NAFLD ranges from simple steatosis without inflammation to non-alcoholic steatohepatitis (NASH), which, in some cases, can lead to cirrhosis and even hepatocellular carcinoma [1,2]. Despite its high prevalence and morbidity, there is currently no approved therapy for NAFLD/NASH.

Higher prevalence of type 2 diabetes (DMT2) has been documented among NAFLD and NASH patients, while NAFLD also markedly increases the risk of developing DMT2 [3]. NAFLD and DMT2 share common pathophysiologic features, with insulin resistance playing a key pathogenic role [4]. As such, anti-diabetic drugs (e.g., metformin, thiazolidinediones and GLP-1 analogues) have been studied as potential treatments against NAFLD/NASH development and progression [5,6]. Sodium-glucose co-transporter-2 inhibitors (SGLT-2i) represent a new class of anti-diabetic drugs which act mainly through increasing urinary glucose excretion and, thus, improve glucose control independently of insulin secretion [7]. In addition to glucose reduction, SGLT-2i has also been shown to exert certain beneficial cardio-metabolic effects, including weight reduction and cardiovascular disease (CVD) protection [8–10].

Recently, a number of randomized and non-randomized clinical trials have reported beneficial effects of SGLT-2i on NAFLD, as assessed either by surrogate biomarkers/indices (e.g., alanine aminotransferase (ALT), aspartate aminotransferase (AST), gamma-glutamyl transferase (γ-GT), triglycerides, hepatic insulin sensitivity indices), or by intrahepatic fat content on CT, MRI and proton-magnetic resonance spectroscopy imaging [6,11]. Of note, a recent large, placebo-controlled randomized clinical trial, i.e., the EMPA-REG OUTCOME trial, further supported these results, showing that empagliflozin treatment for 24 weeks in patients with DMT2 significantly reduced glutamic-pyruvic transaminase (SGPT) levels (a surrogate biomarker of liver fat) independently of changes in haemoglobin A1c (HbA1c) and body weight [12]. Interestingly, this improvement was more pronounced in the empagliflozin-treated arm compared to glimepiride, suggesting direct empagliflozin-induced effects on NAFLD progression, irrespective of glycemic control [12]. The E-LIFT trial also showed that treatment with empagliflozin (10 mg daily) for 20 weeks significantly reduced liver enzymes and liver fat in in 50 patients with DMT2 and NAFLD [13]. Although such data indicate that SGLT-2i may constitute a promising treatment option against NAFLD/NASH, the molecular mechanisms mediating the beneficial effects of SGLT-2i on biochemical and/or histological NAFLD features remain incompletely explored.

Recently, endoplasmic reticulum (ER) stress and autophagy have emerged as important underlying mechanisms in NAFLD/NASH development and progression, both regulating hepatic cell apoptosis [14,15]. Indeed, it is now well-known that both hyperglycaemia and lipid accumulation can cause proteostasis and trigger ER stress in hepatocytes [16]. In turn, an adaptive signalling pathway, i.e., the unfolded protein response (UPR), is activated to restore it [16]. To that effect, UPR enhances ER protein folding and induces clearance of aggregate-prone proteins by promoting autophagy. Subsequently, autophagy stimulates the degradation of intracellular lipid droplets (lipophagy). However, under chronic ER stress the UPR turns from adaptive to terminal, leading to hepatocyte death by increasing inflammation, reducing autophagic processes and activating pro-apoptotic pathways [17].

Although a number of studies have investigated SGLT-2i effects on ER stress in renal tubular cells, cardiomyocytes and pancreatic β-cells [18–20] data on their role in ER stress related pathways in NAFLD are sparse [21], and even completely lacking regarding the potential impact of SGLT-2i in NAFLD-related autophagy processes. As such, the aim of the present study was to investigate the effect of empagliflozin in NAFLD progression, focusing specifically on ER stress, autophagy and apoptosis.

2. Results

2.1. Empagliflozin Administration for Five Weeks Improves Fasting Blood Glucose and Lipid Profiles

No significant difference in daily food intake was observed between the two groups ($p = 0.5$). Empagliflozin administration had no significant effect on body weight as both HFD-fed ApoE$^{(-/-)}$ mice groups significantly increased their body weight at the end of the five-week intervention compared to baseline (18.7% and 17.9% increase in body weight in the Empa and the control group, respectively). Empagliflozin treatment resulted in significantly reduced fasting glucose, total cholesterol, and triglyceride serum levels at the end of the five-week intervention compared to baseline (all p-values < 0.01). Additionally, fasting glucose, total cholesterol, and triglyceride serum levels were significantly lower in the Empa group compared to the control group at the end of the five-week intervention ($p < 0.01$, $p < 0.01$, and $p < 0.001$, respectively) (Figure 1a).

Recent data indicate that the triglyceride/HDL cholesterol ratio can be used as a new marker for prediction of endothelial dysfunction and as an indicator of increased risk of developing metabolic and cardiovascular complications in human [22]. To this end, we next measured the TG/HDL ratio in mice, and our result showed that at the end of Empagliflozin/placebo oral treatment, there was a significant difference from baseline in TG/HDL ($p < 0.05$) between groups (Figure 1b).

After completion of the five-week empagliflozin treatment, oxaloacetic transaminase (SGOT) levels were marginally decreased ($p = 0.07$), while a significant reduction in SGPT levels ($p = 0.048$) was observed in the Empa group as compared to the control group (Figure 1c).

2.2. Empagliflozin Administration for Five Weeks Improves Hepatic Lipid Accumulation

ApoE mice in the control group had higher liver weights than the Empa group ($p = 0.047$); however, the liver weight to body weight ratio was not different ($p = 0.2$) between the two groups (Figure 2B).

The effect of empagliflozin/vehicle treatment on hepatic lipid accumulation and injury was evaluated in H&E staining. In the Empa group an overall beneficial effect was noted on steatohepatitis-related parameters, including decreased steatosis percentage, intrahepatic ballooning and lobular inflammation, thus leading to significantly improved liver histology (Figure 2A). As such, NAS was significantly lower in the Empa group compared to control ($p = 0.04$), attributed mainly to the significantly reduced lobular inflammation ($p = 0.04$) and steatosis ($p = 0.04$) (Figure 2C).

Of note, no liver fibrosis was detected at the end of intervention neither in the control nor Empa group (data not shown).

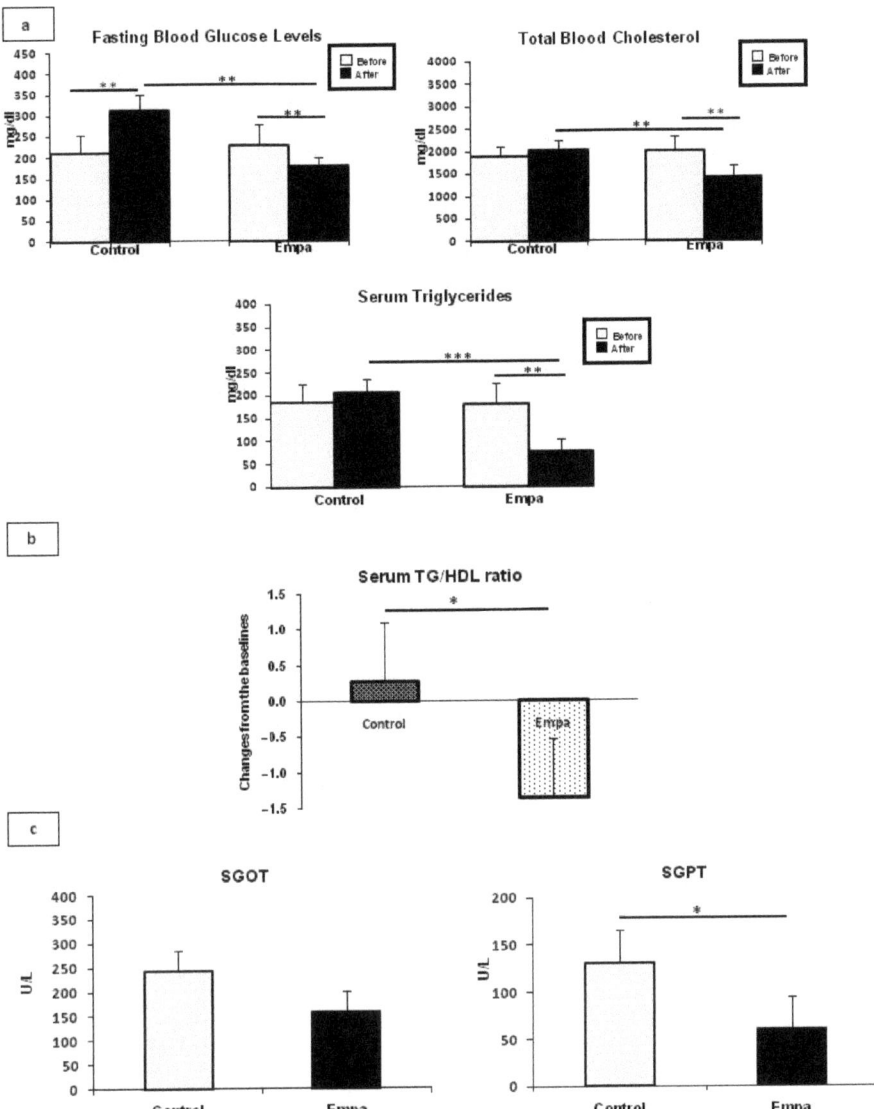

Figure 1. Serum fasting glucose, lipid, SGOT and SGPT concentrations in the Empa and control groups after five weeks of empagliflozin/vehicle oral administration. (**a**). A significant reduction in fasting blood glucose, total cholesterol, triglyceride levels was observed in the Empa group at the end of the treatment period compared to baseline. Fasting glucose was the only significantly increased parameter in the control group at the end of intervention as compared to baseline values. (**b**). Significant changes were detected from baseline in triglyceride/HDL ratio between two groups. (**c**). Serum SGOT and SGPT levels were reduced in Empa group as compared to Control group ($p = 0.07$ and $p = 0.048$, respectively) ($n = 8$ per group). Data are shown as the mean ± SD (***: $p < 0.001$; **: $p < 0.01$, *: $p < 0.05$).

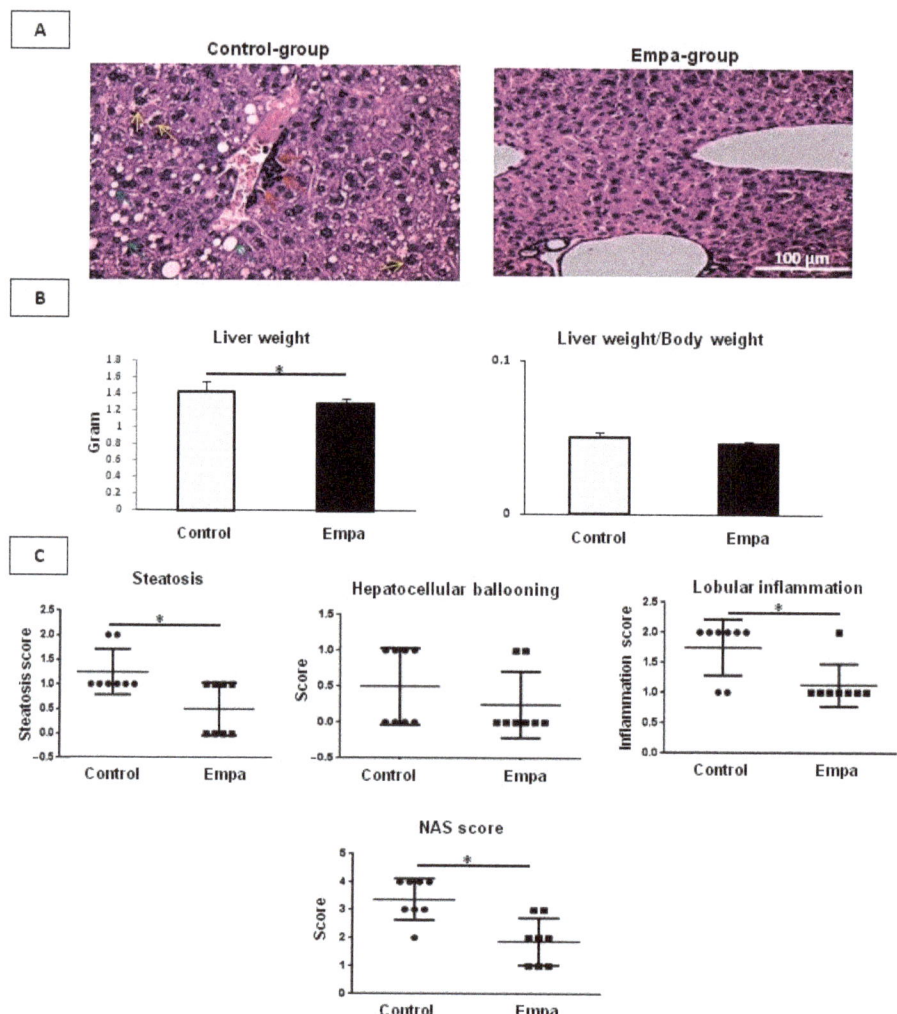

Figure 2. Histological assessment of NAFLD/NASH severity. (**A**) Representative images of H&E-stained slides of ApoE[(-/-)] mice after five weeks of empagliflozin/vehicle oral administration. Lobular inflammation, ballooning cells and cytoplasmic lipid droplets are shown by red, yellow and green arrows, respectively. (**B**) The liver weight and the ratio of liver weight to body weight. (**C**) Histological evaluation of steatosis, hepatocellular ballooning, lobular inflammation and NAS score. Data are shown as the mean ± SD (*: $p < 0.05$).

2.3. Empagliflozin Administration for Five Weeks Reduces the Expression of Lipogenic Enzymes and Inflammatory Markers

Peroxisome proliferator-activated receptor-gamma (*Ppar-γ*) is a known regulator of de novo lipogenesis (DNL) and its upregulation leads to the consequent lipid droplets deposition within hepatocytes. The *Srebp1c* plays a central role in controlling expression of genes involved in DNL such as *Acaca*, *Fasn* and *Scd-1*. *Pck1* is a regulator of re-esterification of free fatty acid into triacylglycerol [16,21]. As such, we evaluated whether empagliflozin had an impact on the hepatic lipogenesis pathway by measuring the expression of these lipogenic genes. The *Fasn*, *Srebp-1c* and *Pck-1* gene expression was significantly lower in Empa group as compared to the Control group ($p = 0.03$, $p = 0.02$, $p = 0.02$, respectively). A marginal reduction in the expression of *Acaca* and *Scd-1* was also observed in Empa group when compared to the Control group ($p < 0.1$) (Figure 3A). No difference was observed in *Ppar-γ* expression between the two groups ($p = 0.2$).

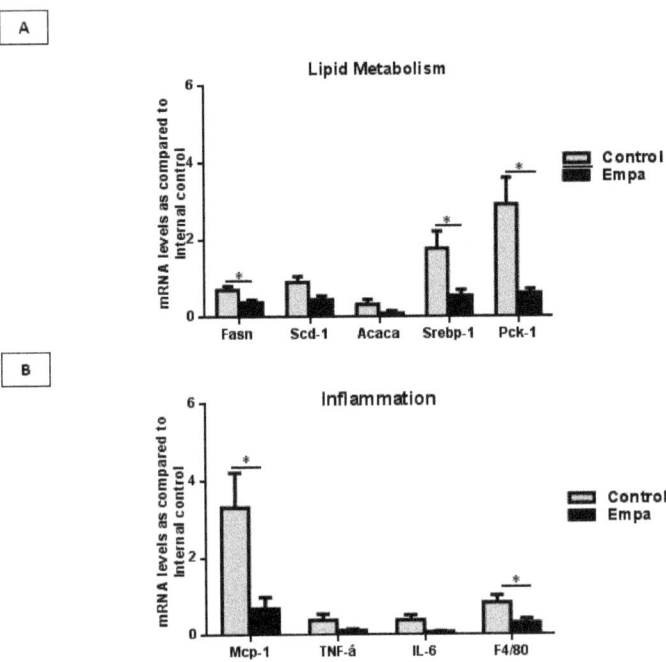

Figure 3. The hepatic expression of lipogenic enzymes and inflammatory markers in ApoE$^{(-/-)}$ mice after five weeks of empagliflozin/vehicle oral administration. (**A**). The mRNA levels of *Fasn*, *Screbp-1* and *Pck-1* were significantly reduced in the Empa group as compared to the Control group. (**B**) Empagliflozin oral administration for five weeks resulted in significant reduction in *Mcp-1* and *F4/80* mRNA levels. Data are shown as the mean ± SEM (*: $p < 0.05$).

Mcp-1 recruits and activates monocytes/macrophages to the site of tissue injury, and regulates the expression of pro-inflammatory cytokines, such as TNF-α and IL-6. F4/80 is a known marker of resident macrophages. Thus, we assessed the effect of empagliflozin on the expression of the aforementioned pro-inflammatory genes. Our results showed that the expression of *Mcp-1* and *F4/80* was significantly reduced by five weeks of empagliflozin administration ($p = 0.02$ in both cases). A borderline decrease in the expression of *TNF-α* and *IL-6* in the Empa group was observed, compared to the control group ($p < 0.1$) (Figure 3B).

Of note, the liver in all mice expressed *SGLT-1* mRNA levels without any significant difference between two groups, while *SGLT-2* mRNA was faintly detected in almost half of the animals in each groups.

2.4. Empagliflozin Administration for Five Weeks Reduces the Expression of ER Stress Markers

The mRNA levels of factors involved in the regulation of the ER stress response (*GRP78, eIF2a, ATF4, IRE1, Xbp1, ATF-6, GRP94* and *CHOP*) were evaluated by qPCR, whereas protein levels of eIF2a, p-eIF2a and CHOP were evaluated by Western blot. Our results demonstrated that the five-week empagliflozin treatment resulted in significantly lower mRNA expression of *GRP94, eIF2α, GRP78, IRE1, Xbp1, CHOP* and *ATF6* compared to control ($p = 0.03$, $p = 0.03$, $p = 0.03$, $p = 0.015$, $p = 0.02$, $p = 0.02$ and $p = 0.02$, respectively) (Figure 4).

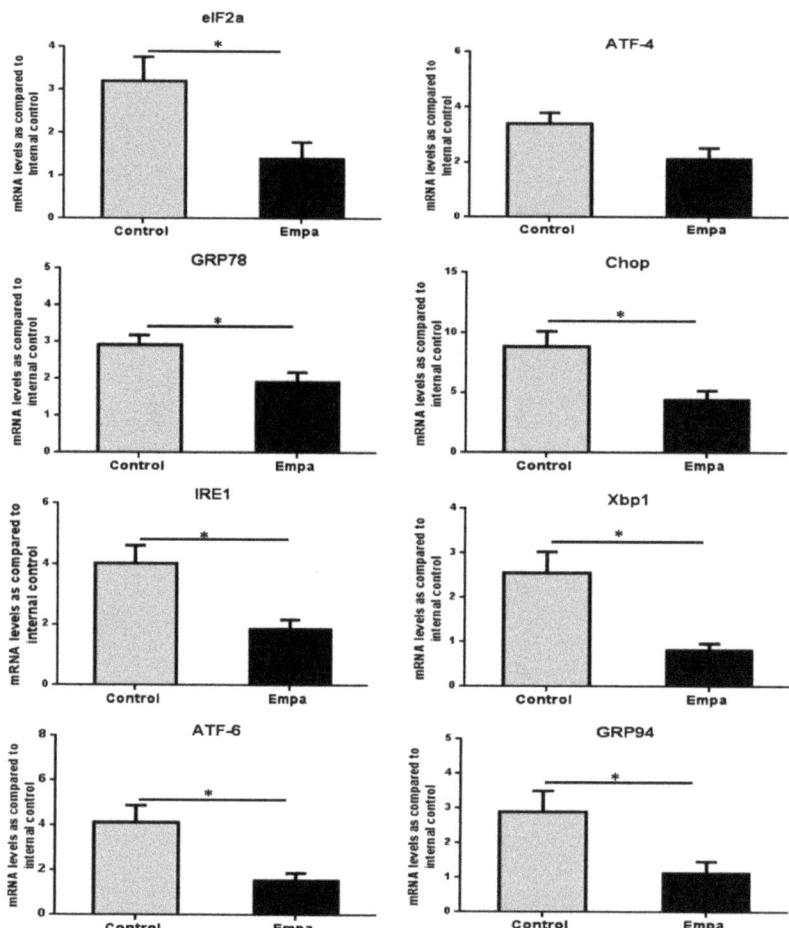

Figure 4. Changes of ER stress core genes mRNA levels after five weeks of empagliflozin/vehicle oral administration in the liver of ApoE$^{(-/-)}$ mice. The mRNA levels of *elf2α*, *ATF-4*, *GRP78*, *CHOP*, *IRE1*, *XbP1*, *ATF-6* and *GRP94* were significantly reduced after five weeks of empagliflozin treatment. Data are shown as the mean ± SEM (*: $p < 0.05$).

Moreover, marginally significant lower *ATF4* mRNA levels were also observed in the Empa group ($p = 0.05$) (Figure 4).

Western blot analysis revealed that CHOP protein levels, as well as the p-eIF2a/eIF2a protein levels ratio, were significantly lower in empagliflozin-treated mice compared to the control group ($p = 0.004$ and $p = 0.04$, respectively) (Figure 5A,B).

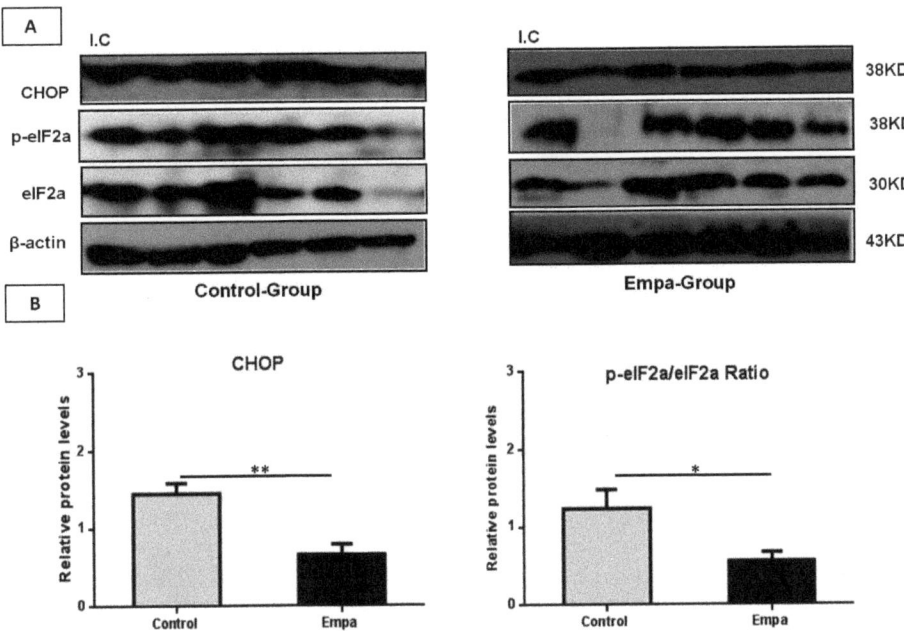

Figure 5. Empagliflozin administration for five weeks reduces protein levels of ER stress markers. (**A**). Western blot analysis of CHOP, total elf-2α and phospho elf-2α in liver tissues. (**B**) Quantitative analyses showed that empagliflozin reduces the protein levels of CHOP, p-elf-2α/elf-2α ratio. Data are expressed as the mean ± SEM (*: $p < 0.05$; **: $p < 0.01$; I.C: Internal control).

2.5. Empagliflozin Administration for Five Weeks Activates the Hepatic Autophagic Flux

Both mRNA and protein levels of autophagy (macro-autophagy) markers were also assessed. Results of the qRT-PCR analysis demonstrated that, compared to the control group, the five-week empagliflozin treatment resulted in significantly lower *mTOR* mRNA levels ($p = 0.03$), while *LC3B* mRNA levels were higher in the Empa group almost reaching statistical significance ($p = 0.06$) (Figure 6A). No differences were observed in *Beclin-1, p62, AMPKa1* and *AMPKa2* mRNA levels between the two groups ($p = 0.2$, $p = 0.5$, $p = 0.12$ and $p = 0.17$, respectively) at the end of the five-week treatment period (data not shown).

However, compared to the control group, p62 protein levels were significantly lower in the Empa group ($p = 0.04$) at the end of this five-week intervention, while Beclin-1 and the ratio of phospho-AMPK/AMPK protein levels were significantly higher ($p = 0.046$ and $p = 0.005$, respectively) (Figure 6B,C).

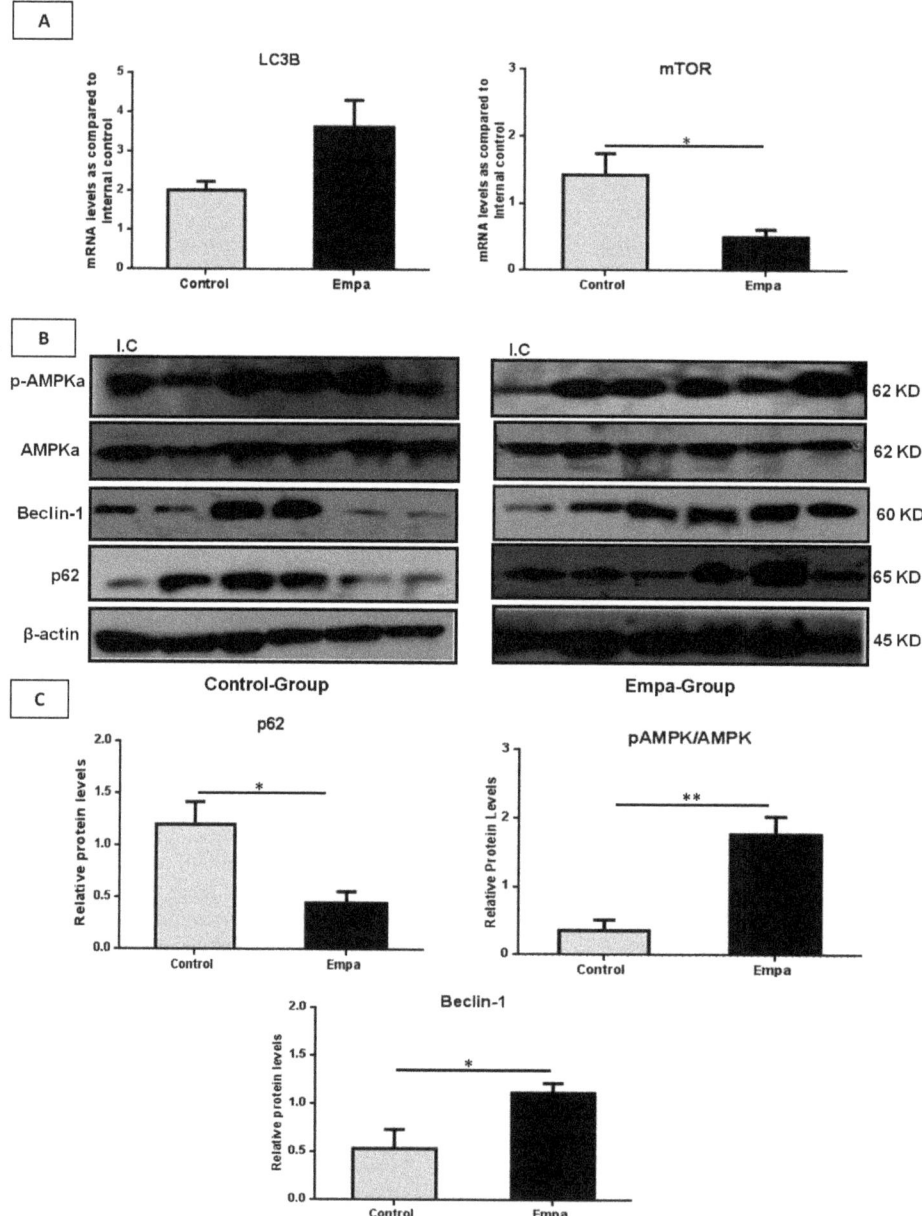

Figure 6. The mRNA and protein expression profiles of the autophagy-related genes. (**A**) Relative mRNA levels of *LC3B* was increased while the *mTOR* mRNA expression was reduced after five weeks of empagliflozin administration. (**B**) Western blot analysis of p62, Beclin-1, total AMPKa and phospho-AMPKa in liver tissues. (**C**) Quantitative analyses showed that empagliflozin reduces p62, while it increases the p-AMPKa/AMPKa ratio and Beclin-1 protein levels. Data are shown as the mean ± SEM (*: $p < 0.05$; **: $p < 0.01$; I.C: Internal control).

2.6. Empagliflozin Administration for Five Weeks Attenuates Hepatic Apoptosis

The *Bcl-2/Bax* ratio is a known indicator of cell susceptibility to apoptosis, thus, we quantified both *Bcl-2* and *Bax* mRNA levels. Our results show that the *Bcl-2/Bax* ratio was significantly higher in the Empa group ($p = 0.02$) compared to the control group at the end of the five-week treatment (Figure 7A). In addition, at this time point, the protein expression of cleaved caspase-8 was found to be significantly lower in the Empa group compared to the control group ($p = 0.006$) (Figure 7B).

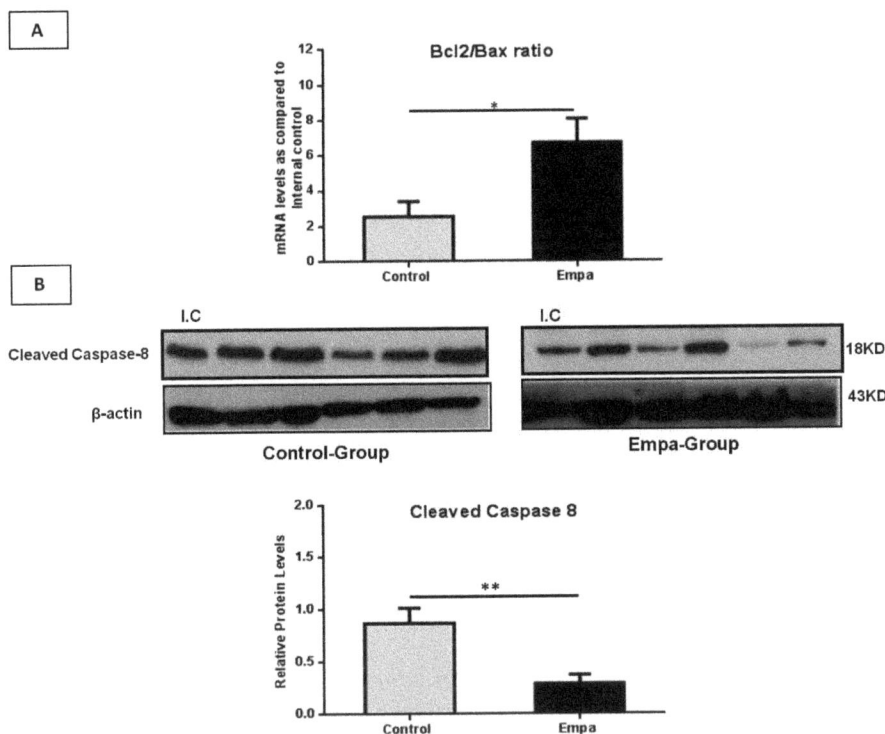

Figure 7. The mRNA and protein levels of apoptosis related molecules. (**A**) Empagliflozin treatment for five weeks significantly increased the mRNA *Bcl2/Bax* ratio. (**B**) Western blot analysis of cleaved caspase-8 with quantitative analyses showing that empagliflozin reduces the protein levels of cleaved caspase-8. Data are shown as the mean ± SEM (*: $p < 0.05$; **: $p < 0.01$; I.C: Internal control).

3. Discussion

The therapeutic potential of SGLT-2i on NAFLD has been previously reported in animal and in human studies [21,23–28]. To shed light on the underlying molecular mechanisms, we present here novel data showing that empagliflozin treatment for five weeks in HFD-fed ApoE$^{(-/-)}$ mice not only decreases fasting glucose, total cholesterol and triglycerides serum levels, but also improves the underlying NAFLD histological features by activating autophagy, alleviating ER stress, and attenuating apoptosis. In the context of this study, HFD-fed ApoE$^{(-/-)}$ mice were used as a NAFLD model since a high-fat, cholesterol-rich diet has been shown to accelerate development of NASH with fibrosis in this animal model [29,30].

Of note, in contrast to human studies [31], in the present study empagliflozin did not reduce the body weight in the treated mice compared to control. Indeed, both ApoE$^{(-/-)}$ mice groups consumed similar amounts of food and gained weight without significant differences between them during the five-week treatment period of our study. This is in accord with previous studies from our group which also showed that canagliflozin and empagliflozin administration for 5 and 10 weeks, respectively, did not promote weight loss in ApoE deficient mice under HFD conditions [9,10]. Interestingly, conflicting results exist in the relevant literature with respect to SGLT-2i effects on body weight in animal models. As such, previous studies have showed that empagliflozin did not affect significantly the body weight of Zucker diabetic fatty (ZDF) rats (a type 2 diabetes animal model) at doses of 10 and 30 mg/kg/day, whereas it can decrease the body weight in ApoE$^{(-/-)}$ mice at a dose of 1–3 mg/kg/day for eight weeks [32,33]. Recently, Petito da Silva et al. reported that empagliflozin administration at a dose of 10 mg/kg/day for five weeks results in decreased body weight in HFD-fed male C57Bl/6 mice [21]. The divergent results in existing animal studies regarding the effects of SGLT-2i on body weight could be attributed, at least in part, to differences in the used animal models, doses and durations of treatment, and underlying diets.

In addition to lowering fasting blood glucose levels, our data further show that in HFD-fed ApoE$^{(-/-)}$ mice empagliflozin can also reduce total cholesterol and triglyceride serum levels over a five-week treatment period. This is in agreement with previous studies from our group and others conducted in various animal models (e.g., ob/ob or wild type mice) and with varying treatment regimens, which showed similar empagliflozin-induced effects on fasting lipid profiles [9,34]. Moreover, in line with our findings, recent studies demonstrated that administration of empagliflozin for 5 and 10 weeks at a dose of 10 mg/jg and 1.5 mg/jg/day, results in significantly reduced serum SGPT levels of HFD-fed male C57BL/6 and ob/ob$^{(-/-)}$ mice, respectively [21,34].

It must be highlighted that, histological findings in the context of the present study showed a marked reduction of liver steatosis, lobular inflammation, ballooning and hepatocellular degeneration in the empagliflozin-treated group, resulting in significantly improved NAS compared to the control group. Similar improvements in hepatic steatosis and steatohepatitis have also been reported in other animal studies with administration of different SGLT-2i, including luseogliflozin, empagliflozin, remogliflozin, ipragliflozin and NGI001 [21,23–27]. Based on these studies, key mechanisms which appear to mediate these effects involve mainly the regulation of insulin resistance/glucose tolerance and changes in the expression of enzymes implicated in beta-oxidation and hepatic de novo lipogenesis [21,23–27]. In line with most of these studies, we found a reduction in the expression of six key-enzymes of lipogenesis which was more pronounced for Screbp-1c, Fasn and pck-1. Of note, Petito da Silva et al. recently reported reduced liver mRNA expression of *Srebp1c*, *Ppar-γ*, *Acc1*, *Scd-1* and *Fasn* in male C57Bl/6 mice treated with empagliflozin for five weeks [21].

The reduction of lipogenesis enzymes following empagliflozin administration could explain—at least in part—the decreased steatosis and fatty droplets area observed within hepatocytes. Accordingly, we found a decreased expression of inflammatory markers, such as *Mcp-1* and *F4/80*, and to a lesser extent *TNF-α* and *IL-6*, with empagliflozin treatment. The decrease in the expression of the aforementioned inflammatory indices has been shown to reduce macrophage infiltration and lobar inflammation in liver leading to alleviation of hepatic steatosis and inflammation [21,23,24,26].

Notably, the present study further expanded on the mechanisms underlying such empagliflozin-induced beneficial effects on NAFLD/NASH, focusing on the gene and protein hepatic expression of factors involved in ER stress, autophagy and apoptosis which are crucial processes implicated in NAFLD development and progression [35–39]. Indeed, it is now well-established that under normal (unstressed) conditions, IRE1, PERK and ATF6 are inactivated upon binding to GRP78/BiP, whereas under stress conditions GRP-78/BiP dissociates from the ER stress sensors, thus activating the three arms of the UPR [37]. Here, we found reduced expression of GRP78/BiP in the liver of the empagliflozin-treated ApoE$^{(-/-)}$ mice compared to control. Overall, existing data regarding GRP78/BiP expression in NAFLD are conflicting [35,36]. Of note, Jo et al. [40] showed that tunicamycin, which can induce liver steatosis, increases GRP78/BiP expression. Moreover, dietary-induced obese mice have been shown to express higher hepatic GRP78/BiP levels compared to lean counterparts [41]. It might be expected here that, since GRP78 is a chaperone responsive to glucose, empagliflozin should decrease its expression through reducing glucose levels. However, using liver tissue from obese mice and cultured rat liver cells, Ozcan et al. found that hyperglycemia did not induce GRP78 expression, suggesting that its regulation is not likely related, at least exclusively, to glycemia [41].

Moreover, we showed here that the three branches of the UPR adaptive pathway, i.e., *PERK, IRE1a* and *ATF6*, were attenuated in the liver tissues of the empagliflozin-treated group compared to control. Specifically, we noted suppression of the PERK-elf2a-ATF4 arm in the liver, as indicated by the decreased phosphorylation of the elf protein and decreased mRNA expression of the transcription factor ATF4. Notably, this pathway is known to regulate lipogenesis and steatosis with ATF4-deficient mice exhibiting decreased synthesis of fatty acids and lower triglyceride serum levels [14].

Furthermore, our results revealed suppression of the IRE1a pathway in the empagliflozin-treated group, as indicated by the decreased mRNA expression of both *IRE1a*, and *Xbp1* which is the transcription factor activated by IRE1a. The IRE1a pathway is also an important regulator of hepatic lipogenesis. Indeed, Xbp1 ablation has been reported to ameliorate liver steatosis and injury, as well as hyperlipidemia in ApoE$^{(-/-)}$ mice [42]. Lee et al. showed that selective deletion of Xbp1 in the liver led to decreased hepatic production of lipids through down regulation of critical lipogenic genes, such as Scd-1, diacyl glycerol acetyltransferase 2 (Dgat2) and acetyl coA carboxylase 2 (Acc2), and subsequently to marked hypocholesterolemia and hypotriglyceridemia [43]. Recently, it has been shown that activation of UPR-IRE-Xbp-1 can trigger activation of the Srebp-1c signalling pathway, leading to increased liver steatosis [44]. Therefore, the decreased activation of both PERK-elf2a-ATF4 and IRE1a-Xbp1 pathways could substantially contribute to the lower total cholesterol and triglyceride serum levels noted with empagliflozin treatment. Similarly, our findings further show that ATF6 expression is also reduced in the liver of the empagliflozin-treated ApoE$^{(-/-)}$ mice compared to control. A recent study by Chen et al. also showed that down-regulation of the ATF6 signalling pathway alleviates the progression of NAFLD by inhibiting ER stress-induced inflammation and apoptosis of liver cells [45].

Interestingly, ATF4, Xbp1 and ATF6 pathways are known to activate UPR target genes implicated in autophagy and apoptosis through regulating CHOP [14]. In our study, the applied five-week empagliflozin treatment resulted in lower mRNA and protein CHOP levels compared to controls. Currently, there are only a few studies exhibiting beneficial effects of SGLT-2i (dapagliflozin and ipragliflozin) on ER stress markers, mostly relating to renal tubular cell inflammation injury in diabetic mice [19,20]. Empagliflozin has also been found to induce a protective effect against diabetic cardiomyopathy by inhibiting IRE1a-Xbp1 and ATF4-CHOP pathways [46], whilst it can also improve β-cell mass in streptozotocin-treated mice through down-regulation of Xbp1, BiP and ATF4 [18]. To the best of our knowledge, there is only one previous study investigating the effects of empagliflozin on ER stress in a diet-induced NAFLD mice model [21]. Indeed, in accord with our findings, Petito da Silva et al. have shown that empagliflozin can mitigate NAFLD development by reducing the expression of genes involved in the elf2α-ATF4-CHOP-GADD45 pathway of UPR activation [21].

As ER stress is a well-established regulator of autophagy via mainly ATF4 and Xbp-1 [17] it is also important to explore autophagic processes in the context of NAFLD. Autophagy breaks down, among others, the intracellular lipids in hepatocytes through a degradation pathway known as lipophagy [20]. Moreover, impaired autophagic flux in the liver is closely related to the development of hepatic steatosis [47]. Overall, the process of autophagosome formation involves three major steps, namely initiation which is mediated by AMPK activation; nucleation with the Beclin-1/class III PI3K complex; and elongation of the isolation membrane with the help of LC3 lipidation [47]. As such, we investigated the effect of empagliflozin on these autophagic processes. Although we noted no significant increase in the mRNA expression of both isoforms of the catalytic subunit of AMPK (AMPKa1 and AMPKa2), our findings demonstrate increased phosphorylation at the N-terminus of the a subunit (Thr172) of AMPK in the liver of empagliflozin-treated ApoE$^{(-/-)}$ mice. The latter is required for full activation of AMPK. In line with our findings, a recent study by Xu et al. reported that administration of empagliflozin for 16 weeks in HFD-induced obese mice increased the phosphorylation of AMPK [48].

It is known that activated AMPK promotes autophagy through various mechanisms, including negative regulation of mTORC1 [49]. Interestingly, we found decreased *mTOR* mRNA expression with empagliflozin treatment, and increased Beclin-1 protein levels which promote the step of nucleation. Furthermore, out data indicate that empagliflozin upregulates the expression of LC3B (both at mRNA and protein level) which is also necessary for the autophagosome formation. In addition, we assessed liver P62/SQSTM1 protein levels which is a selective substrate of autophagy, usually used as an index of impaired autophagic flux [50]. P62/SQSTM1 protein levels were lower in the empagliflozin-treated mice of our study, indicating activation of autophagic flux by this SGLT-2i. It could be argued that the effects of empagliflozin can be attributed primarily to the decrease in glucose levels which could activate the energy-sensor AMPK, causing, in turn, the mTOR-mediated inhibition of autophagy. However, the noted glucose level decrease was not to a degree that can trigger this AMPK-induced mechanism, which is mainly activated under starvation conditions [51].

Taken together, these findings suggest that empagliflozin can activate all these steps of the autophagy process in the liver of HFD-fed ApoE$^{(-/-)}$ mice.

Of note, these findings appear to partly contradict the existing knowledge that decreased ER stress leads to a diminished autophagy [52]. However, it should be noted that SGLT-2i has been found to primarily induce autophagy by a mechanism which has not been fully clarified. Indeed, in the myocardium and immune cells SGLT-2i appear to promote a state that resembles nutrient and oxygen deprivation [53,54]. This state can trigger -among other pathways- AMPK activation which is a main regulator of autophagy [55]. Similarly, compared to control, higher AMPK phosphorylation in the liver of empagliflozin-treated ApoE$^{(-/-)}$ mice was also noted in our study. Additional studies are still required to fully clarify the SGLT-2i-induced effects on autophagy in the liver and other tissues.

Considering that both ER stress and autophagy can eventually regulate apoptosis, here we also investigated the effect of empagliflozin in hepatic apoptosis processes, showing that empagliflozin treatment leads to higher *Bcl-2/Bax* ratio and inactivated caspase-8 in the liver of HFD-fed ApoE$^{(-/-)}$ mice. The former is a well-known apoptosis switch, with a progressive reduction of the *Bcl-2/Bax* ratio having been reported during the progression of NAFLD to NASH which correlates to the apoptosis percentage of hepatocytes [56]. Of interest, CHOP, which according to our results was lower with empagliflozin treatment, has been shown to inhibit Bcl-2 and up-regulate Bax, thus triggering the intrinsic apoptotic pathway [57].

Similarly, the lower hepatic caspase-8 cleavage levels we noted in empagliflozin-treated mice compared to control have also important implications for apoptotic pathways, since activated caspase-8 is required for extrinsic apoptosis and plays a crucial role in Free fatty acid (FFA)-mediated apoptosis in hepatocytes [58]. Interestingly, hepatocyte-specific caspase-8 knockout mice fed a methionine choline-deficient diet (a frequently-used nutritional NASH model) have been shown to exhibit decreased apoptosis and inflammatory processes [59].

Autophagy could also inhibit apoptosis via elimination of p62/SQSTM1, which was found to be lower in the empagliflozin-treated mice of the present study. Of note, SQSTM1/p62 is not only an autophagy-specific substrate, but, when is abnormally accumulated, it can also stimulate the production of reactive oxygen species (ROS) and activate the DNA damage response [60]. As such, our results suggest that activation of autophagy by empagliflozin could directly inhibit hepatic apoptosis by both decreasing caspase-8 activation and eliminating SQSTM1/p62. However, the diminished ER stress (in particular the attenuation of PERK-elfa-ATF-4-CHOP pathway) could also mediate the decreased activation of caspase-8 [61]. The relative contribution of each of these pathways remains unclear and requires further study.

In addition, the reduced ER stress via CHOP could also directly inhibit apoptosis through increasing the Bcl-2/Bax ratio. Thus, it can be hypothesized that a potent autophagic flux due to empagliflozin treatment may attenuate the adaptive HFD-induced ER stress of hepatocytes, in a negative feedback loop. As such, both increased autophagy and reduced ER stress could eliminate hepatic apoptosis and alleviate NAFLD progression. Indeed, it has been demonstrated that autophagy can reduce ER stress, and so it can act protectively by inhibiting apoptosis through caspase inactivation [62]. Of further interest, a study by Zhou et al. in HFD-fed mice showed that inhibition of Scd-1 (a key enzyme in lipid metabolism) enhanced AMPK activity and autophagy (lipophagy), leading to decreased hepatic steatosis [63]. Emphasizing the role of AMPK in hepatic lipogenesis, another recent study documented that AMPK-dependent phosphorylation of insulin-induced gene (Insig) can prevent the activation of Srebp-1c and, consequently, its lipogenic enzymes which regulate triglyceride and fatty acid synthesis, including ATP citrate lyase (ACLY), glycerol-3-phosphate acyltransferase (GPAT), ACC1 and DGAT2 [64]. It becomes evident that, whether empagliflozin can act directly on AMPK which can initiate autophagy and regulate de novo lipogenesis, or on other molecules upstream of AMPK (e.g., Scd-1) remains to be further explored.

Finally, in support of our hypothesis that empagliflozin-triggered increased autophagy can decrease ER stress-induced NAFLD progression, Carloni et al. have demonstrated that rapamycin-induced autophagy inhibits ischemia-induced ER stress, thus protecting against brain injury [65,66]. In this context, administration of 3-methyadenine (an autophagy inhibitor) reversed this beneficial effect and accelerated the ER stress-induced neuronal death [65,66].

Whether the effects of empagliflozin on autophagy, ER stress and apoptosis are mediated directly through SGLT-2 inhibition in the liver tissue is a matter of great scientific interest. According to our data, SGLT-2 was low-expressed in half of the liver samples, without differences in the expression between the control group and Empa group. Interestingly, Obara et al. demonstrated the protein expression of SGLT-2 in human hepatocytes and hepatoma cell lines [67]. More interestingly, SGLT-1 was expressed in the total of the liver tissues (both control and intervention group) suggesting its possible role in the attenuation of NAFLD in our model. Of note, empagliflozin can also bind to SGLT-1, albeit with a lower affinity than SGLT-2; strengthening the suggestion that empagliflozin could act, among others, through SGLT-1, dual SGLT-1/SGLT-2 inhibitor phlorizin recently found to ameliorate NAFLD in Type 2 diabetic mice [68]. Nevertheless, the existence of other, unknown yet, protein(s) which could be a direct target of empagliflozin in hepatocytes cannot be excluded.

Expanding on our previous data [9], we also demonstrated that empagliflozin results in the reduction of pro-atherogenesis markers in aorta, including inflammatory markers (*Il-6*, *Tnf-α*), adhesion molecules (*Vcam-1*) and gelatinolytic activity (*Timp-1/Mmp-2* ratio), although no significant effect on atheroma plaque formation is present at the end of this five-week treatment period (Supplementary Data S1). This is in line with results which we have previously shown, where empagliflozin administered for 10 weeks in ApoE$^{(-/-)}$ mice attenuates the progression of atherosclerotic plaque [9]. Notably, the strong bidirectional relationship between NAFLD and CVD is well established. Indeed, Kim et al. recently showed that NAFLD has prognostic value for identifying individuals who are at higher risk for CVD [69].

A limitation of our study is the lack of body composition assessments of the studied mice. However, the noted changes in total body weight during the five-week study intervention did not differ significantly between the empagliflozin-treated and control groups. Another study limitation is the lack of insulin sensitivity assessments before and after the empagliflozin treatment. Based on the study by Petito da Silva et al., empagliflozin has been shown to increase insulin sensitivity when given for five weeks in diet-induced NAFLD in C57Bl/6 mice [21].

4. Materials and Methods

4.1. Animals

Male C57BL/6J apolipoprotein E (ApoE) knockout mice (ApoE$^{(-/-)}$) were originally purchased from "The Jackson Laboratory" and were bred in the animal facility of the National and Kapodistrian University of Athens. All animals were kept at a specific pathogen free (SPF) controlled environment (22–26 °C temperature, 40–60% humidity and 12 h light/dark cycle), with free access to water and regular chow diet until the age of five weeks. All animal experiments were approved by the local Animal Care and Use Committee (366495-09/07/2019).

4.2. Experimental Protocol

Male ApoE$^{(-/-)}$ mice (n = 16) were used for the study experiments. At five weeks of age, all mice were switched to a high-fat diet (HFD: 20–23% by weight; 40–45% kcal from fat), containing cholesterol (0.2% total). After five weeks on this HFD, the ApoE$^{(-/-)}$ mice were randomly divided into the following two groups: (1) Empagliflozin group (10 mg/kg/day empagliflozin, n = 8), and (2) control group (same volume of 0.5% hydroxyl ethylcellulose per day, n = 8). Empagliflozin or vehicle was administered orally by gavage daily for a period of five weeks. Empagliflozin was purchased from MCE (Cat.No.HY-15409) and dissolved in 0.5% hydroxyl ethylcellulose. During the five-week study treatment, food intake and body weight were measured once weekly. Blood glucose levels were also measured after 8–10 h fasting via tail puncture at baseline (before empagliflozin/vehicle oral administration), and at the study endpoint. At the end of the five-week study treatment, all mice were sacrificed under isoflurane anaesthesia by transection of the diaphragm and the liver and aorta was rapidly excised.

4.3. Serum Analysis of Biochemical Parameters

Venipuncture was performed once at baseline from the facial vein and once by heart puncturing after culling. Serum glucose, total-cholesterol and triglycerides were determined using appropriate enzymatic kits (Biosis TM, Athens, Greece) in a dedicated autoanalyzer.

4.4. RNA Extraction and Quantitative Real-Time PCR

Total RNA was extracted from fresh frozen liver tissues using NucleoSpin RNA Plus kit (Macherey-Nagel, Düren, Germany). The concentration and quality of extracted mRNA were evaluated by a NanoDrop™ instrument (Thermo Scientific, Waltham, MA, USA). Extracted RNA (1000 ng) was reverse transcribed into cDNA using LunaScript® RTsynthesis kit ((New England Biolabs, Ipswich, MA, USA). Real-time PCR analysis was performed as described previously [10]. Expression of key regulatory molecules involved in lipogenesis such as fatty acid synthase (*Fasn*), sterol regulatory element-binding protein 1 (*Screbp-1*), acetyl CoA carboxylase (*Acaca*), stearoyl-CoA desaturase 1 (*Scd-1*), Peroxisome proliferator-activated receptor gamma (*Ppar-γ*) and phosphoenolpyruvate carboxykinase 1 (*Pck-1*), inflammatory markers such as monocyte chemoattractant protein-1(*Mcp-1*), tumour necrosis factor alpha (*TNF-α*), interleukin 6 (*IL-6*) and EGF-like module-containing mucin-like hormone receptor-like 1(*F4/80*), molecules involved in UPR regulation including activating transcription factor 4 (*ATF4*), binding immunoglobulin protein (*GRP78*), IRE1, eukaryotic initiation factor 2 alpha (*eIF2a*), X-box binding protein 1 (*Xbp1*), glucose-regulated protein 94 (*GRP94*), activating transcription factor 6 (*ATF6*) and C/EBP homologous protein (*CHOP*), as well as molecules involved in the regulation of autophagy, such as microtubule-associated protein 1 light chain 3B (*LC3B*), phosphoenolpyruvate carboxykinase 1 (*p62/SQSTM1*), mechanistic target of rapamycin kinase (*mTOR*), Beclin-1, AMP-activated protein kinasesubunit alpha-1 (*AMPKa1*), AMP-activated protein kinasesubunit alpha-2 (*AMPKa2*) acetyl CoA carboxylase (*Acaca*), apoptosis markers such as

B-cell lymphoma 2 (*Bcl-2*) and BCL2-associated X protein (*Bax*), and the hepatic mRNA levels of *SGLT-1* and *SGLT-2* were measured using Luna® Universal qPCR Master Mix (New England Biolabs, Ipswich, MA, USA) on a CFX96 (Bio-RAD, Hercules, CA, USA). A melting curve analysis was performed to confirm the specificity of quantitative polymerase chain reaction (qPCR) products. Fold-changes were calculated using the $2^{-\Delta\Delta Ct}$ method and all values were normalized against 18 s mRNA expression. Differentially expressed genes were identified through fold change filtering where a minimum of two-fold change was considered significant. All reactions were performed in triplicates and repeated at least three times. The sequences of primers used for RT-PCR analysis in this study are listed in Supplementary Table S1.

4.5. Liver Histological Analysis

Mouse liver tissues were fixed in 10% neutral buffered formalin and embedded in paraffin blocks. The 4 µm-thick sections were stained with hematoxylin–eosin (H&E) (Sigma-Aldrich, St. Louis, MO, USA) and used for histopathological analysis while liver fibrosis was evaluated by Masson's trichrome staining. For NAFLD/NASH diagnosis, percentage of steatosis, quantification of lobular inflammation and presence of hepatocellular degeneration were measured according to the NAFLD activity score (NAS). NAS scoring was performed in a blinded manner by two independent pathologists. On average three (2–4) tissue sections from each animal were used for histopathological evaluation.

4.6. SDS-PAGE and Western-Blot Analysis

Western blot analysis was performed as previously described. Briefly, whole protein was extracted from 60 mg of liver tissue using 2× lysis buffer (Cell Signalling Technology, MA, USA) supplemented with PMSF. Samples containing 30 µg of protein were resolved by electrophoresis gels and transferred to a PVDF membrane. After blocking for 1 h with 5% skim milk in TBST, membranes were incubated overnight at 4 °C with antibodies against β-actin (MAB1501 Millipore), LC3B (L7543 Sigma), Beclin-1 (G-11 Santa Cruz Biotechnology), p62 (D-3 Santa Cruz Biotechnology), AMPK (#5831 Cell Signalling), phospho-AMPK (#2531 Cell Signaling), CHOP/GADD153 (H5- Santa Cruz Biotechnology), eIF2a (#9722 Cell Signaling), phospho-eIF2a (Ser51) (#9721 Cell Signalling) and cleaved caspase-8 (Asp387) (#8592 Cell Signalling). Membranes were then probed with goat anti-mouse IgG-HRP (31430, Thermo Scientific) or with goat anti-rabbit IgG-HRP conjugate (12–348, Millipore) secondary antibodies at room temperature for 1 h. An aliquot of pooled standard sample was loaded in one lane of each gel. The pooled sample served as an internal standard to minimize the inter-assay variation for samples run in different gels. Detection of the immuno-reactive bands was performed using the Clarity Western ECL Substrate (BioRad). β-actin served as a loading control. Densitometric analysis was performed using Image J software (NIH, Bethesda, MD, USA).

4.7. Statistical Analysis

Data are presented as mean values ± standard deviation (SD) and percentages, unless stated otherwise. Student's *t*-test, Welch's test or Mann–Whitney test were used, as appropriate, for comparisons of quantitative variables (body weight and biochemical parameters) between the Empa- and control animal groups. Normality of distribution for these variables was tested with the Shapiro–Wilk test and the equality of variances with the Levene's test. Comparisons between groups for qualitative variables were performed with the Fisher's exact test, as appropriate. Within each group, paired t-tests were used to compare levels of each studied parameter before and after the five-week intervention period. A *p* value < 0.05 was considered statistically significant. All statistical analyses were performed using GraphPad Prism Software (v.7) (Graph Pad software, San Diego, CA, USA).

5. Conclusions

We provide novel evidence that empagliflozin treatment for five weeks in HFD-fed ApoE$^{(-/-)}$ mice can attenuate NAFLD by not only improving metabolism and inflammation progression but also by promoting autophagy, reducing HFD-induced ER stress and inhibiting hepatocyte apoptotic processes. Further research studies with longer duration and various empagliflozin doses are required to expand on our present findings and further delineate possible dose and duration-dependent differential effects of empagliflozin on NAFLD development and progression. Clarifying the precise molecular mechanisms underpinning the empagliflozin-induced increase in autophagic flux in hepatocytes will advance our understanding regarding the role of empagliflozin as a potential therapeutic option for NAFLD/NASH prevention and/or treatment.

Supplementary Materials: The following are available online at https://www.mdpi.com/1422-006 7/22/2/818/s1, Data S1: The effect of empagliflozin on atherosclerotic plaque formation; Figure S1: Atherosclerotic plaque and mRNA expression of molecules implicated in atherogenesis in ApoE$^{(-/-)}$ treated with either 10 mg/kg/day Empagliflozin (Empa-group) or vehicle (control-group) for 5 weeks; Table S1: List of primer sequences used for RT-PCR analysis in this study.

Author Contributions: N.N.-A., C.N. and K.P. performed all the experiments. M.S.R. and K.C. performed part of the qPCR experiments. G.K. (Georgios Kyriakopoulos) evaluated the Immunohistochemistry analysis. N.N.-A. and I.K. and G.K. (Georgios Kyriakopoulos) contributed to the writing of the manuscript. N.N.-A., C.N., K.P. and I.K. evaluated the results and contributed to the data analysis and preparing figures. V.K. contributed to the data evaluation and analysis. K.K. was responsible for animal housing conditions and animal care in the animal facility. A.C. and A.G.P. contributed to the interpretation of the results. C.S.M., G.K. (Gregory Kaltsas) and A.G.P. gave critical review of the study's design. H.S.R. and E.K. conceived the project idea, designed and supervised the experiments, interpreted the results and critically revised the manuscript with contribution of N.N.-A. and I.K. H.S.R. and E.K. gave final approval of the version to be published. All authors have read and agreed to the published version of the manuscript.

Funding: This research received no external funding.

Institutional Review Board Statement: All animal experiments were approved by the Athens University Medical School Ethics Committee and by the Veterinary Directorate of the Ministry of Agriculture in agreement with the EU Directive 2010/63/EU for animal experiments (366495-09/07/2019).

Informed Consent Statement: Not applicable.

Data Availability Statement: Data is contained within the article and its supplementary material.

Conflicts of Interest: The authors declare no conflict of interest.

Abbreviations

ApoE	Apolipoprotein E
ATF4	Activating Transcription Factor 4
ATF6	Activating Transcription Factor 6
ALT	Alanine aminotransferase
AST	Aspartate aminotransferase
ACLY	ATP citrate lyase
Acc2	Acetyl coA carboxylase 2
AMPKa1	AMP-activated protein kinase alpha 1
AMPKa2	AMP-activated protein kinase alpha 2
Bcl-2	B-cell lymphoma 2
Bax	BCL2-associated X protein
CHOP	C/EBP homologous protein
CVD	Cardiovascular disease
Dgat2	Diacyl glycerol acetyltransferase 2
DMT2	Diabetes mellitus type 2

Empa	Empagliflozin
ER	Endoplasmic reticulum
eIF2α	Eukaryotic Initiation Factor 2 alpha
Fasn	Fatty acid synthase
F4/80	EGF-like module-containing mucin-like hormone receptor-like 1
FFA	Free fatty acid
GRP78	Binding immunoglobulin protein
GRP94	Glucose-regulated protein 94
GPAT	Glycerol-3-phosphate acyltransferase
HFD	High-fat diet
HbA1c	Hemoglobin A1c
ICAM-1	Intercellular adhesion molecule-1
Il-6	Interleukin 6
Insig	Insulin-induced gene
IRE1α	Inositol-requiring enzyme 1 α
LC3B	Microtubule-Associated Protein 1 Light Chain 3B
mTOR	Mechanistic Target Of Rapamycin Kinase
Mcp-1	Monocyte chemoattractant protein-1
NAFLD	Non-alcoholic fatty liver disease
NASH	Non-alcoholic steatohepatitis
NAS	NAFLD Activity Score
Ppar-γ	Peroxisome proliferator-activated receptor gamma
Pck-1	Phosphoenolpyruvate carboxykinase 1
p62(Sqstm1)	Sequestosome 1
qPCR	Quantitative polymerase chain reaction
ROS	Reactive oxygen species
SGLT-2i	Sodium-glucose cotransporter-2 inhibitors
Screbp-1	Sterol regulatory element-binding protein 1
Scd-1	Stearoyl-CoA desaturase 1
SGOT	Glutamic oxaloacetic transaminase
SGPT	Glutamic-pyruvic transaminase
TNF-α	Tumor necrosis factor alpha
UPR	Unfolded protein response
VCAM-1	Vascular cell adhesion molecule-1
XBP1	X-box binding protein 1
ZDF	Zucker diabetic fatty
γ-GT	Gamma-glutamyl transferase

References

1. Mantovani, A.; Scorletti, E.; Mosca, A.; Alisi, A.; Byrne, C.D.; Targher, G. Complications, morbidity and mortality of nonalcoholic fatty liver disease. *Metabolism* **2020**, *11*, 154170. [CrossRef] [PubMed]
2. Younossi, Z.; Anstee, Q.M.; Marietti, M.; Hardy, T.; Henry, L.; Eslam, M.; George, J.; Bugianesi, E. Global burden of NAFLD and NASH: Trends, predictions, risk factors and prevention. *Nat. Rev. Gastroenterol. Hepatol.* **2018**, *15*, 11–20. [CrossRef] [PubMed]
3. Hazlehurst, J.M.; Tomlinson, J.W. Non-alcoholic fatty liver disease in common endocrine disorders. *Eur. J. Endocrinol.* **2013**, *169*, R27–R37. [CrossRef] [PubMed]
4. Watt, M.J.; Miotto, P.M.; De Nardo, W.; Montgomery, M.K. The Liver as an Endocrine Organ-Linking NAFLD and Insulin Resistance. *Endocr. Rev.* **2019**, *40*, 1367–1393. [CrossRef]
5. Katsiki, N.; Perakakis, N.; Mantzoros, C. Effects of sodium-glucose co-transporter-2 (SGLT2) inhibitors on non-alcoholic fatty liver disease/non-alcoholic steatohepatitis: Ex quo et quo vadimus? *Metabolism* **2019**, *98*, iii–ix. [CrossRef]
6. Ranjbar, G.; Mikhailidis, D.P.; Sahebkar, A. Effects of newer antidiabetic drugs on nonalcoholic fatty liver and steatohepatitis: Think out of the box! *Metabolism* **2019**, *101*, 154001. [CrossRef]
7. Upadhyay, J.; Polyzos, S.A.; Perakakis, N.; Thakkar, B.; Paschou, S.A.; Katsiki, N.; Underwood, P.; Park, K.H.; Seufert, J.; Kang, E.S.; et al. Pharmacotherapy of type 2 diabetes: An update. *Metabolism* **2018**, *78*, 13–42. [CrossRef]
8. Anastasilakis, A.D.; Sternthal, E.; Mantzoros, C.S. Beyond glycemic control: New guidance on cardio-renal protection. *Metabolism* **2019**, *99*, 113–115. [CrossRef]
9. Dimitriadis, G.K.; Nasiri-Ansari, N.; Agrogiannis, G.; Kostakis, I.D.; Randeva, M.S.; Nikiteas, N.; Patel, V.H.; Kaltsas, G.; Papavassiliou, A.G.; Randeva, H.S.; et al. Empagliflozin improves primary haemodynamic parameters and attenuates the development of atherosclerosis in high fat diet fed APOE knockout mice. *Mol. Cell. Endocrinol.* **2019**, *494*, 110487. [CrossRef]

10. Nasiri-Ansari, N.; Dimitriadis, G.K.; Agrogiannis, G.; Perrea, D.; Kostakis, I.D.; Kaltsas, G.; Papavassiliou, A.G.; Randeva, H.S.; Kassi, E. Canagliflozin attenuates the progression of atherosclerosis and inflammation process in APOE knockout mice. *Cardiovasc. Diabetol.* 2018, *17*, 106. [CrossRef]
11. Kahl, S.; Gancheva, S.; Strassburger, K.; Herder, C.; Machann, J.; Katsuyama, H.; Kabisch, S.; Henkel, E.; Kopf, S.; Lagerpusch, M.; et al. Empagliflozin Effectively Lowers Liver Fat Content in Well-Controlled Type 2 Diabetes: A Randomized, Double-Blind, Phase 4, Placebo-Controlled Trial. *Diabetes Care* 2020, *43*, 298–305. [CrossRef]
12. Sattar, N.; Fitchett, D.; Hantel, S.; George, J.T.; Zinman, B. Empagliflozin is associated with improvements in liver enzymes potentially consistent with reductions in liver fat: Results from randomised trials including the EMPA-REG OUTCOME(R) trial. *Diabetologia* 2018, *61*, 2155–2163. [CrossRef]
13. Kim, K.S.; Lee, B.W. Beneficial effect of anti-diabetic drugs for nonalcoholic fatty liver disease. *Clin. Mol. Hepatol.* 2020, *26*, 430–443. [CrossRef]
14. Lebeaupin, C.; Vallee, D.; Hazari, Y.; Hetz, C.; Chevet, E.; Bailly-Maitre, B. Endoplasmic reticulum stress signalling and the pathogenesis of non-alcoholic fatty liver disease. *J. Hepatol.* 2018, *69*, 927–947. [CrossRef]
15. Wu, W.K.K.; Zhang, L.; Chan, M.T.V. Autophagy, NAFLD and NAFLD-Related HCC. *Adv. Exp. Med. Biol.* 2018, *1061*, 127–138.
16. Mota, M.; Banini, B.A.; Cazanave, S.C.; Sanyal, A.J. Molecular mechanisms of lipotoxicity and glucotoxicity in nonalcoholic fatty liver disease. *Metabolism* 2016, *65*, 1049–1061. [CrossRef]
17. Guo, B.; Li, Z. Endoplasmic reticulum stress in hepatic steatosis and inflammatory bowel diseases. *Front. Genet.* 2014, *5*, 242. [CrossRef]
18. Daems, C.; Welsch, S.; Boughaleb, H.; Vanderroost, J.; Robert, A.; Sokol, E.; Lysy, P.A. Early Treatment with Empagliflozin and GABA Improves beta-Cell Mass and Glucose Tolerance in Streptozotocin-Treated Mice. *J. Diabetes Res.* 2019, *2019*, 2813489. [CrossRef]
19. Hosokawa, K.; Takata, T.; Sugihara, T.; Matono, T.; Koda, M.; Kanda, T.; Taniguchi, S.; Ida, A.; Mae, Y.; Yamamoto, M.; et al. Ipragliflozin Ameliorates Endoplasmic Reticulum Stress and Apoptosis through Preventing Ectopic Lipid Deposition in Renal Tubules. *Int. J. Mol. Sci.* 2020, *21*, 190. [CrossRef]
20. Shibusawa, R.; Yamada, E.; Okada, S.; Nakajima, Y.; Bastie, C.C.; Maeshima, A.; Kaira, K.; Yamada, M. Dapagliflozin rescues endoplasmic reticulum stress-mediated cell death. *Sci. Rep.* 2019, *9*, 9887. [CrossRef]
21. Petito-da-Silva, T.I.; Souza-Mello, V.; Barbosa-da-Silva, S. Empaglifozin mitigates NAFLD in high-fat-fed mice by alleviating insulin resistance, lipogenesis and ER stress. *Mol. Cell. Endocrinol.* 2019, *498*, 110539. [CrossRef] [PubMed]
22. Salazar, M.R.; Carbajal, H.A.; Espeche, W.G.; Leiva Sisnieguez, C.E.; Balbin, E.; Dulbecco, C.A.; Aizpurua, M.; Marillet, A.G.; Reaven, G.M. Relation among the plasma triglyceride/high-density lipoprotein cholesterol concentration ratio, insulin resistance, and associated cardio-metabolic risk factors in men and women. *Am. J. Cardiol.* 2012, *109*, 1749–1753. [CrossRef] [PubMed]
23. Nakano, S.; Katsuno, K.; Isaji, M.; Nagasawa, T.; Buehrer, B.; Walker, S.; Wilkison, W.O.; Cheatham, B. Remogliflozin Etabonate Improves Fatty Liver Disease in Diet-Induced Obese Male Mice. *J. Clin. Exp. Hepatol.* 2015, *5*, 190–198. [CrossRef] [PubMed]
24. Qiang, S.; Nakatsu, Y.; Seno, Y.; Fujishiro, M.; Sakoda, H.; Kushiyama, A.; Mori, K.; Matsunaga, Y.; Yamamotoya, T.; Kamata, H.; et al. Treatment with the SGLT2 inhibitor luseogliflozin improves nonalcoholic steatohepatitis in a rodent model with diabetes mellitus. *Diabetol. Metab. Syndr.* 2015, *7*, 104. [CrossRef] [PubMed]
25. Honda, Y.; Imajo, K.; Kato, T.; Kessoku, T.; Ogawa, Y.; Tomeno, W.; Kato, S.; Mawatari, H.; Fujita, K.; Yoneda, M.; et al. The Selective SGLT2 Inhibitor Ipragliflozin Has a Therapeutic Effect on Nonalcoholic Steatohepatitis in Mice. *PLoS ONE* 2016, *11*, e0146337. [CrossRef]
26. Jojima, T.; Tomotsune, T.; Iijima, T.; Akimoto, K.; Suzuki, K.; Aso, Y. Empagliflozin (an SGLT2 inhibitor), alone or in combination with linagliptin (a DPP-4 inhibitor), prevents steatohepatitis in a novel mouse model of non-alcoholic steatohepatitis and diabetes. *Diabetol. Metab. Syndr.* 2016, *8*, 45. [CrossRef]
27. Chiang, H.; Lee, J.C.; Huang, H.C.; Huang, H.; Liu, H.K.; Huang, C. Delayed intervention with a novel SGLT2 inhibitor NGI001 suppresses diet-induced metabolic dysfunction and non-alcoholic fatty liver disease in mice. *Br. J. Pharmacol.* 2020, *177*, 239–253. [CrossRef]
28. Dougherty, J.A.; Guirguis, E.; Thornby, K.A. A Systematic Review of Newer Antidiabetic Agents in the Treatment of Nonalcoholic Fatty Liver Disease. *Ann. Pharmacother.* 2020, *55*, 65–79. [CrossRef]
29. Shibata, M.-A.; Shibata, E.; Fujioka, S.; Harada-Shiba, M. Apolipoprotein E-knockout Mice as a Lifestyle-related Disease Model of Atherosclerosis and Non-alcoholic Fatty Liver Disease. *Int. J. Lab. Med. Res.* 2015, *1*, 107. [CrossRef]
30. Schierwagen, R.; Maybuchen, L.; Zimmer, S.; Hittatiya, K.; Back, C.; Klein, S.; Uschner, F.E.; Reul, W.; Boor, P.; Nickenig, G.; et al. Seven weeks of Western diet in apolipoprotein-E-deficient mice induce metabolic syndrome and non-alcoholic steatohepatitis with liver fibrosis. *Sci. Rep.* 2015, *5*, 12931. [CrossRef]
31. Lee, P.C.; Ganguly, S.; Goh, S.Y. Weight loss associated with sodium-glucose cotransporter-2 inhibition: A review of evidence and underlying mechanisms. *Obes. Rev.* 2018, *19*, 1630–1641. [CrossRef] [PubMed]
32. Steven, S.; Oelze, M.; Hanf, A.; Kroller-Schon, S.; Kashani, F.; Roohani, S.; Welschof, P.; Kopp, M.; Godtel-Armbrust, U.; Xia, N.; et al. The SGLT2 inhibitor empagliflozin improves the primary diabetic complications in ZDF rats. *Redox Biol.* 2017, *13*, 370–385. [CrossRef]

33. Han, J.H.; Oh, T.J.; Lee, G.; Maeng, H.J.; Lee, D.H.; Kim, K.M.; Choi, S.H.; Jang, H.C.; Lee, H.S.; Park, K.S.; et al. The beneficial effects of empagliflozin, an SGLT2 inhibitor, on atherosclerosis in ApoE$^{(-/-)}$ mice fed a western diet. *Diabetologia* **2017**, *60*, 364–376. [CrossRef] [PubMed]
34. Adingupu, D.D.; Gopel, S.O.; Gronros, J.; Behrendt, M.; Sotak, M.; Miliotis, T.; Dahlqvist, U.; Gan, L.M.; Jonsson-Rylander, A.C. SGLT2 inhibition with empagliflozin improves coronary microvascular function and cardiac contractility in prediabetic ob/ob(-/-) mice. *Cardiovasc. Diabetol.* **2019**, *18*, 16. [CrossRef]
35. Gonzalez-Rodriguez, A.; Mayoral, R.; Agra, N.; Valdecantos, M.P.; Pardo, V.; Miquilena-Colina, M.E.; Vargas-Castrillon, J.; Lo Iacono, O.; Corazzari, M.; Fimia, G.M.; et al. Impaired autophagic flux is associated with increased endoplasmic reticulum stress during the development of NAFLD. *Cell Death Dis.* **2014**, *5*, e1179. [CrossRef]
36. Lee, S.; Kim, S.; Hwang, S.; Cherrington, N.J.; Ryu, D.Y. Dysregulated expression of proteins associated with ER stress, autophagy and apoptosis in tissues from nonalcoholic fatty liver disease. *Oncotarget* **2017**, *8*, 63370–63381. [CrossRef]
37. Wang, L.; Chen, J.; Ning, C.; Lei, D.; Ren, J. Endoplasmic Reticulum Stress Related Molecular Mechanisms in Nonalcoholic Fatty Liver Disease (NAFLD). *Curr. Drug Targets* **2018**, *19*, 1087–1094. [CrossRef]
38. Habeos, I.G.; Ziros, P.G.; Chartoumpekis, D.; Psyrogiannis, A.; Kyriazopoulou, V.; Papavassiliou, A.G. Simvastatin activates Keap1/Nrf2 signaling in rat liver. *J. Mol. Med. (Berlin)* **2008**, *86*, 1279–1285. [CrossRef]
39. Rodrigues, G.; Moreira, A.J.; Bona, S.; Schemitt, E.; Marroni, C.A.; Di Naso, F.C.; Dias, A.S.; Pires, T.R.; Picada, J.N.; Marroni, N.P. Simvastatin Reduces Hepatic Oxidative Stress and Endoplasmic Reticulum Stress in Nonalcoholic Steatohepatitis Experimental Model. *Oxid. Med. Cell. Longev.* **2019**, *2019*, 3201873. [CrossRef]
40. Jo, H.; Choe, S.S.; Shin, K.C.; Jang, H.; Lee, J.H.; Seong, J.K.; Back, S.H.; Kim, J.B. Endoplasmic reticulum stress induces hepatic steatosis via increased expression of the hepatic very low-density lipoprotein receptor. *Hepatology* **2013**, *57*, 1366–1377. [CrossRef]
41. Ozcan, U.; Cao, Q.; Yilmaz, E.; Lee, A.H.; Iwakoshi, N.N.; Ozdelen, E.; Tuncman, G.; Gorgun, C.; Glimcher, L.H.; Hotamisligil, G.S. Endoplasmic reticulum stress links obesity, insulin action, and type 2 diabetes. *Science* **2004**, *306*, 457–461. [CrossRef]
42. So, J.S.; Hur, K.Y.; Tarrio, M.; Ruda, V.; Frank-Kamenetsky, M.; Fitzgerald, K.; Koteliansky, V.; Lichtman, A.H.; Iwawaki, T.; Glimcher, L.H.; et al. Silencing of lipid metabolism genes through IRE1alpha-mediated mRNA decay lowers plasma lipids in mice. *Cell Metab.* **2012**, *16*, 487–499. [CrossRef] [PubMed]
43. Lee, A.H.; Scapa, E.F.; Cohen, D.E.; Glimcher, L.H. Regulation of hepatic lipogenesis by the transcription factor XBP1. *Science* **2008**, *320*, 1492–1496. [CrossRef] [PubMed]
44. Dewidar, B.; Kahl, S.; Pafili, K.; Roden, M. Metabolic liver disease in diabetes—From mechanisms to clinical trials. *Metabolism* **2020**, *111*, 154299. [CrossRef]
45. Chen, Z.Y.; Liu, Y.L.; Yang, L.; Liu, P.; Zhang, Y.; Wang, X.Y. MiR-149 attenuates endoplasmic reticulum stress-induced inflammation and apoptosis in nonalcoholic fatty liver disease by negatively targeting ATF6 pathway. *Immunol. Lett.* **2020**, *222*, 40–48. [CrossRef]
46. Zhou, Y.; Wu, W. The Sodium-Glucose Co-Transporter 2 Inhibitor, Empagliflozin, Protects against Diabetic Cardiomyopathy by Inhibition of the Endoplasmic Reticulum Stress Pathway. *Cell. Physiol. Biochem.* **2017**, *41*, 2503–2512. [CrossRef]
47. Mao, Y.; Yu, F.; Wang, J.; Guo, C.; Fan, X. Autophagy: A new target for nonalcoholic fatty liver disease therapy. *Hepat. Med.* **2016**, *8*, 27–37. [CrossRef]
48. Xu, L.; Nagata, N.; Nagashimada, M.; Zhuge, F.; Ni, Y.; Chen, G.; Mayoux, E.; Kaneko, S.; Ota, T. SGLT2 Inhibition by Empagliflozin Promotes Fat Utilization and Browning and Attenuates Inflammation and Insulin Resistance by Polarizing M2 Macrophages in Diet-induced Obese Mice. *EBioMedicine* **2017**, *20*, 137–149. [CrossRef]
49. Holczer, M.; Hajdu, B.; Lorincz, T.; Szarka, A.; Banhegyi, G.; Kapuy, O. A Double Negative Feedback Loop between mTORC1 and AMPK Kinases Guarantees Precise Autophagy Induction upon Cellular Stress. *Int. J. Mol. Sci.* **2019**, *20*, 5543. [CrossRef]
50. Kliosnky, D. Guidelines for the Use and Interpretation of Assays for Monitoring Autophagy (3rd edition) (vol 12, pg 1, 2015). *Autophagy* **2016**, *12*, 443.
51. Kassi, E.; Papavassiliou, A.G. Could glucose be a proaging factor ? *J. Cell. Mol. Med.* **2008**, *12*, 1194–1198. [CrossRef] [PubMed]
52. Song, S.; Tan, J.; Miao, Y.; Zhang, Q. Crosstalk of ER stress-mediated autophagy and ER-phagy: Involvement of UPR and the core autophagy machinery. *J. Cell. Physiol.* **2018**, *233*, 3867–3874. [CrossRef]
53. Xu, C.; Wang, W.; Zhong, J.; Lei, F.; Xu, N.; Zhang, Y.; Xie, W. Canagliflozin exerts anti-inflammatory effects by inhibiting intracellular glucose metabolism and promoting autophagy in immune cells. *Biochem. Pharmacol.* **2018**, *152*, 45–59. [CrossRef]
54. Aragon-Herrera, A.; Feijoo-Bandin, S.; Santiago, M.O.; Barral, L.; Campos-Toimil, M.; Gil-Longo, J.; Pereira, T.M.C.; Garcia-Caballero, T.; Rodriguez-Segade, S.; Rodriguez, J.; et al. Empagliflozin reduces the levels of CD36 and cardiotoxic lipids while improving autophagy in the hearts of Zucker diabetic fatty rats. *Biochem. Pharmacol.* **2019**, *170*, 113677. [CrossRef] [PubMed]
55. Packer, M. Autophagy stimulation and intracellular sodium reduction as mediators of the cardioprotective effect of sodium-glucose cotransporter 2 inhibitors. *Eur. J. Heart Fail.* **2020**, *22*, 618–628. [CrossRef] [PubMed]
56. Li, C.P.; Li, J.H.; He, S.Y.; Li, P.; Zhong, X.L. Roles of Fas/Fasl, Bcl-2/Bax, and Caspase-8 in rat nonalcoholic fatty liver disease pathogenesis. *Genet. Mol. Res.* **2014**, *13*, 3991–3999. [CrossRef] [PubMed]
57. Hu, H.; Tian, M.; Ding, C.; Yu, S. The C/EBP Homologous Protein (CHOP) Transcription Factor Functions in Endoplasmic Reticulum Stress-Induced Apoptosis and Microbial Infection. *Front. Immunol.* **2018**, *9*, 3083. [CrossRef]
58. Akazawa, Y.; Nakao, K. To die or not to die: Death signaling in nonalcoholic fatty liver disease. *J. Gastroenterol.* **2018**, *53*, 893–906. [CrossRef]

59. Hatting, M.; Zhao, G.; Schumacher, F.; Sellge, G.; Al Masaoudi, M.; Gassler, N.; Boekschoten, M.; Muller, M.; Liedtke, C.; Cubero, F.J.; et al. Hepatocyte caspase-8 is an essential modulator of steatohepatitis in rodents. *Hepatology* **2013**, *57*, 2189–2201. [CrossRef]
60. Mathew, R.; Karp, C.M.; Beaudoin, B.; Vuong, N.; Chen, G.H.; Chen, H.Y.; Bray, K.; Reddy, A.; Bhanot, G.; Gelinas, C.; et al. Autophagy Suppresses Tumorigenesis through Elimination of p62. *Cell* **2009**, *137*, 1062–1075. [CrossRef]
61. Iurlaro, R.; Munoz-Pinedo, C. Cell death induced by endoplasmic reticulum stress. *FEBS J.* **2016**, *283*, 2640–2652. [CrossRef]
62. Song, S.; Tan, J.; Miao, Y.; Li, M.; Zhang, Q. Crosstalk of autophagy and apoptosis: Involvement of the dual role of autophagy under ER stress. *J. Cell. Physiol.* **2017**, *232*, 2977–2984. [CrossRef] [PubMed]
63. Zhou, Y.; Zhong, L.; Yu, S.; Shen, W.; Cai, C.; Yu, H. Inhibition of stearoyl-coenzyme A desaturase 1 ameliorates hepatic steatosis by inducing AMPK-mediated lipophagy. *Aging* **2020**, *12*, 7350–7362. [CrossRef] [PubMed]
64. Han, Y.; Hu, Z.; Cui, A.; Liu, Z.; Ma, F.; Xue, Y.; Liu, Y.; Zhang, F.; Zhao, Z.; Yu, Y.; et al. Post-translational regulation of lipogenesis via AMPK-dependent phosphorylation of insulin-induced gene. *Nat. Commun.* **2019**, *10*, 623. [CrossRef] [PubMed]
65. Carloni, S.; Girelli, S.; Scopa, C.; Buonocore, G.; Longini, M.; Balduini, W. Activation of autophagy and Akt/CREB signaling play an equivalent role in the neuroprotective effect of rapamycin in neonatal hypoxia-ischemia. *Autophagy* **2010**, *6*, 366–377. [CrossRef]
66. Carloni, S.; Buonocore, G.; Balduini, W. Protective role of autophagy in neonatal hypoxia-ischemia induced brain injury. *Neurobiol. Dis.* **2008**, *32*, 329–339. [CrossRef] [PubMed]
67. Obara, K.; Shirakami, Y.; Maruta, A.; Ideta, T.; Miyazaki, T.; Kochi, T.; Sakai, H.; Tanaka, T.; Seishima, M.; Shimizu, M. Preventive effects of the sodium glucose cotransporter 2 inhibitor tofogliflozin on diethylnitrosamine-induced liver tumorigenesis in obese and diabetic mice. *Oncotarget* **2017**, *8*, 58353–58363. [CrossRef]
68. David-Silva, A.; Esteves, J.V.; Morais, M.; Freitas, H.S.; Zorn, T.M.; Correa-Giannella, M.L.; Machado, U.F. Dual SGLT1/SGLT2 Inhibitor Phlorizin Ameliorates Non-Alcoholic Fatty Liver Disease and Hepatic Glucose Production in Type 2 Diabetic Mice. *Diabetes Metab. Syndr. Obes.* **2020**, *13*, 739–751. [CrossRef]
69. Kim, J.H.; Moon, J.S.; Byun, S.J.; Lee, J.H.; Kang, D.R.; Sung, K.C.; Kim, J.Y.; Huh, J.H. Fatty liver index and development of cardiovascular disease in Koreans without pre-existing myocardial infarction and ischemic stroke: A large population-based study. *Cardiovasc. Diabetol.* **2020**, *19*, 51. [CrossRef]

MDPI
St. Alban-Anlage 66
4052 Basel
Switzerland
Tel. +41 61 683 77 34
Fax +41 61 302 89 18
www.mdpi.com

International Journal of Molecular Sciences Editorial Office
E-mail: ijms@mdpi.com
www.mdpi.com/journal/ijms

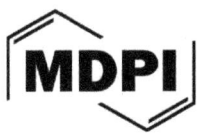

www.ingramcontent.com/pod-product-compliance
Lightning Source LLC
LaVergne TN
LVHW070146100526
838202LV00015B/1903